Churchill Livingstone's

MEDICAL WORD GUIDE

CHURCHILL LIVINGSTONE
NEW YORK, EDINBURGH, LONDON, MELBOURNE, TOKYO

Staff:

Editors Mark Cowell
Ruth Koenigsberg

Computer programming Paulette Lawrence

Production Jeanine Furino

Library of Congress Cataloging-in-Publication Data

Churchill Livingstone's medical word guide.
    p. cm.
  ISBN 0-443-08833-0
  1. Medicine—Terminology. I. Churchill Livingstone (Publisher)
II. Title: Medical word guide.
  [DNLM: 1. Nomenclature. W 15 C563]
R123.C545 1991
610'.14—dc20
DNLM/DLC
for Library of Congress   91-16067
                                                                                                      CIP

© **Churchill Livingstone Inc. 1991**

All rights reserved. No part of this publication may be reproduced, stored in a retrieval system, or transmitted in any form or by any means, electronic, mechanical, photocopying, recording, or otherwise, without prior permission of the publisher (Churchill Livingstone Inc., 1560 Broadway, New York, NY 10036).

Distributed in the United Kingdom by Churchill Livingstone, Robert Stevenson House, 1–3 Baxter's Place, Leith Walk, Edinburgh EH1 3AF, and by associated companies, branches, and representatives throughout the world.

Printed in the United States of America

First published in 1991   7 6 5 4 3 2 1

INTRODUCTION

Churchill Livingstone's Medical Word Guide contains over 40,000 words used in medicine, showing the correct spelling, end-of-line word division, and the stress pattern used in the spoken word. In addition, there are many useful features such as British spellings, alternative word divisions, initial combining forms, grammatical inflections of irregular forms, and glosses to distinguish words that might be confused with one another. Latin words that are part of the multi-word terms that make up anatomical and other medical nomenclature are found in their own alphabetical places.

Names found in eponymous medical terms are divided and pronounced in a separate section beginning on page 309.

In order to use the Word Guide to best advantage, it is suggested that the reader consult the explanatory material in the following sections of this introduction.

Stress and Word Division

The Word Guide uses two stress marks, a bold one (′) placed after the syllable that has the primary stress, and a lighter one (′) placed after syllables spoken with a secondary stress.

A centered dot (·) indicates places where a word may be broken at the end of a line. A permitted word break does not always correspond to an uttered syllable; for example, *isotonic* does not break on the page after the *i*, because by convention one does not break after a single letter that begins a word or before a single letter that ends one. Sometimes a word break is discouraged for other reasons in a sequence where two syllables are pronounced; for example, to prevent a line from ending with two vowels commonly perceived as forming a single syllable (as *ie* in *parietal*, where we do not permit a break between *e* and *t*).

In the system designed for *Churchill Livingstone's Medical Word Guide*, a stress mark alone does not indicate a permitted break; if it

Introduction

coincides with a permitted break, it is followed by a centered dot. Thus the entries

per'i·vas'·cu·lar
cy'·to·plas'm

show that in these words no break is permitted before the *i* or the *m*.

Separate syllables that are not stressed and do not permit breaks are left unmarked. In most cases this causes no problem; the English-speaking reader seeing the entries

elec'·tron
pa·ri'·etal

knows that *electron* must have three syllables and *parietal* must have four. The number may not be readily apparent, however, when two vowels come together, especially in Latin endings. Although speakers of English have become familiar with many of these, such as *nuclei* (plural of *nucleus*) and *radii* (plural of *radius*), the pattern may not be recognized in a word like *cranii* (genitive singular of *cranium*, as in *ossa cranii*). Thus, it should be noted that whereas the sequence *-ae* at the end of Latin words forms a single syllable, as in *fi'·brae* (two syllables), in other two-vowel combinations each vowel represents a separate syllable: *nu'·clei* (three syllables), *cra'·nii* (three), *for·ma'·tio* (four), *dip'·loe* (three).

In spoken language, certain aspects of stress are context-dependent. In particular, a primary stress in an isolated word such as *ami'·no* or *Can'·di·da* may become a secondary stress when these words are part of a multiword unit: *ami'·no ac'·id, Can'·di·da al'·bi·cans*. On the supposition that the reader will be familiar with certain features of word structure, such as the pronunciation of particular word endings or the stress patterns of English words in general, the editors have usually not found it necessary to mark the secondary stress on a final syllable. Given the entries *i'so·tope* and *co·rym'·bi·form*, the reader will quite naturally utter these as *i'so·tope'* and *co·rym'·bi·form'*.

Alternative Word Divisions

In many cases where different pronunciations imply different division points, alternatives are given in square brackets:

cer'·e·brum [ce·re'·brum]

Ideally, one should try to avoid breaking at a point that favors either of the alternative pronunciations, but it is not always possible to do so.

In certain short sequences, however, we suppress the division point altogether while still showing both pronunciations:

    ov′u·late [o′vu·]

In some cases alternatives reflect a divergence in practice between those who prefer to divide between the meaningful elements of a word wherever possible and those who favor a stricter adherence to syllable structure and pronunciation:

    band′·age [ban′·dage]
    ame′·bi·cid′·al [·ci′·dal]

Preferred Division Points

Not all division points are equally good. For instance, when it is necessary to divide a word like *par′a-aor′·tic*, which already contains a fixed hyphen, it should be divided at that hyphen if possible and not elsewhere in the word: *para-/ aortic* rather than *para-aor-/ tic*. In general, it is better to break a compound word between its constituent parts than to interrupt one of those parts; for example, *met′a·car′·po·pha·lan′·ge·al* is preferably broken *metacarpo-/ phalangeal* rather than *metacar-/ pophalangeal* or *metacarpopha-/ langeal*. And the "linking *o*" that joins the parts of a word like *path′·o·gen′·ic* usually goes better with the preceding part (*patho-/ genic*) than with the following part (*path-/ ogenic*).

However, if all the less-than-perfect breaking points were ruled out, the division system would be too rigid for most typesetting programs, forcing many word-space irregularities that are no less disconcerting than bad end-of-line breaks. This Word Guide steers a middle course between the overly stringent division systems used in some dictionaries and spellers and the anything-goes syllabification found in others.

Information in Smaller Print

Various kinds of grammatical and usage information are given in smaller print after an entry word. Except for part-of-speech labels, which are separated from other small-print matter by a wide space, sequences of the same category of information are separated by a comma; sequences in different categories are separated by a semicolon. Thus the entry

    lat′·us   *side; pl.* lat′·era, *gen. sg.* lat′·er·is

Introduction

carries two independent kinds of information: a gloss, *side* (to distinguish it from the word divided *la'·tus*, which means "broad"), and two inflected forms, plural and genitive singular, which are separated by commas. In the entry

    lat'·er·a'·le   *neut. of* lateralis; *pl.* ·lia

the small print matter tells us two things about the word *laterale*: (1) that it is the neuter form of the word *lateralis*, and (2) that it has the plural form *lateralia* (whereas *lateralis* has the plural form *laterales*).

Parts of Speech

If a word has different stresses or divisions for different parts of speech, there are separate entries, with part-of-speech labels added:

    ar'·se·nic   *n.*
    ar·sen'·ic   *adj.*

If a word has more than one medically significant part of speech and there is no difference in stress or division, there is only one entry. Sometimes part-of-speech labels are added if there is an inflection given, just to show that the inflected part of speech is not the only one considered medically significant.

    i'so·late   *n. & v.*   ·lat'·ed, ·lat'·ing
    ma·ture'   *adj. & v.*   ·tured', ·tur'·ing

Glosses

Glosses are synonyms or short defining phrases used to distinguish words that can be confused with one another, such as *afferent* and *efferent*. Glossed entries have the form:

    af'·fer·ent   *conveying toward the center: Cf.* efferent
    ef'·fer·ent   *conveying away from the center: Cf.* afferent

Glosses are also used if a word has more than one meaning and the stress or division pattern differs for each meaning:

    pa'·tent   *unobstructed*
    pat'·ent   *proprietary*

Inflections

Verbs are inflected only when the past or present participle forms are irregular or require a modification in the stem before adding *-ed* or *-ing*.

This occurs most commonly when a final -e is dropped before -ing, or when a final consonant is doubled. The inflected forms are usually truncated to the last syllable or last two syllables; i.e., at the point where they differ from the entry:

    mag'·ni·fy   ·fied, ·fy'·ing
    ra'·di·ate   ·at'·ed, ·at'·ing
    tag   tagged, tag'·ging

Adjective inflections take the form:

    health'y   health'·i·er, health'·i·est

Plurals are not routinely given for nouns that end in -y in the singular and -ies in the plural. Likewise, we have not attempted to give all instances of Latin or Greek plurals when these are formed in a regular manner, although many of them are, in fact, included. The most regular Latin and Greek plural patterns used in medical terms are these:

Singular Ending	Plural Ending	Examples
-sis	-ses	diagnosis: *pl.* diagnoses
-itis	-itides	meningitis: *pl.* meningitides
-um	-a	flagellum: *pl.* flagella
-oma	-omata	angioma: *pl.* angiomata (*or* angiomas)

In the case of *-oma*, the regular English *-s* plural can always be used instead of *-omata*, except when the word is part of a Latin phrase, e.g., *condyloma latum*: pl. *condylomata lata*.

The following plural patterns are very common but less predictable than those shown above:

Singular Ending	Plural Ending	Examples
-a	-ae	vertebra: *pl.* vertebrae (*but compare* trauma: *pl.* traumata *or* traumas)
-us	-i	gyrus: *pl.* gyri (*but compare* plexus: Latin *pl.* plexus, English *pl.* plexuses)
-on	-a	ganglion: *pl.* ganglia (*but compare* neuron: *pl.* neurons)

Introduction

As the foregoing table shows, some words are both English and Latin, and are treated differently depending on the language under consideration. Thus the noun *sinus* forms a regular plural *sinuses* in English but has the plural form *sinus* in Latin; the word *anterior* as an English adjective remains unaltered in all contexts, whereas as a Latin adjective it takes plural, genitive, and other grammatical forms. For nouns, a plural used only in Latin is given thus:

    lens   *L. pl.* len'·tes

and it is understood that the English plural (in this case *lenses*) is formed in the usual way.

If a plural or other inflected form is identical to the entry word, it is shown but not divided:

    spe'·cies   *pl.* species

Spelling and Other Variants

There are two kinds of variant in the Word Guide:

1. Morphemic variants, such as *physiologic* and *physiological*, or *dermoplasty* and *dermatoplasty*.

2. Spelling variants, such as *disk* and *disc*, *intern* and *interne*; also, British spellings, such as *anaesthesia* for *anesthesia*, and spacing or hyphenation variants, such as *gallbladder* and *gall bladder*.

With regard to British spellings, it should be noted that the regular but optional spelling of the suffix *-ize* as *-ise* (*-ization* as *-isation*, etc.) is not shown for the entries in this book. It is to be understood, however, that all terms with the suffix *-ize* (*-iz-*) may also appear with *-ise* (*-is-*), for example, *immunize / immunise*, *ionization / ionisation*. (On the other hand, British readers should remember that not all words ending in *-ise* can be spelled with *-ize*; *incise* and *compromise*, for example, have no variants with *z*.)

Variants are entered in their own places if they are more than five entries away from the more common form:

    ar'·te·fact   *var. of* artifact

The variant word is not routinely given at the principle entry word, although it may be shown when both are common or important. The

British spellings of basic words such as *oesophagus* appear both at the American spelling and at their own alphabetical places:

 esoph′·a·gus *Brit.* oe·soph′·
 oe·soph′·a·gus *Brit. spel. of* esophagus

Derivative words, however, such as *oesophagitis*, appear in their own places only.

If the variant would be within five entries, it is not entered separately but the variation is shown at the principal entry:

 cu·rette′ *also* ·ret′
 phys′·i·o·log′·ic *also* ·i·cal

Single Word Policy

The Word Guide is organized to help find the one word in a multiword medical term that the user needs to divide or spell correctly. There are countless chemical or pharmaceutical compounds ending in the words *acid* or *hydrochloride*, enzymes ending in *kinase*, etc., but there is no point to taking up space in the book by repeating these words hundreds of times. The reader need only look up *acid, hydrochloride*, and *kinase* in their own alphabetical places. The same is true for many Latin words that form the second or a further element in a medical term; e.g., *simplex, neonatorum, congenita*. However, since the form of a Latin noun or adjective depends on its relationship to the word it modifies, we have given most of the inflections one is likely to encounter in the medical literature. Thus, the occurrence of such terms as *nevus pigmentosus, retinitis pigmentosa,* and *xeroderma pigmentosum* is reflected in a single entry:

 pig′·men·to′·sus *fem.* ·sa, *neut.* ·sum

To make the text more readable, we have adopted the convention that when the masculine singular form (traditionally used as the basic form in Latin) must show inflections both for case and number and for gender, the feminine and/or neuter forms are entered separately:

 ac′·ces·so′·ria *fem. of* accessorius; *pl. & gen. sg.* ·ri·ae
 ac′·ces·so′·ri·us *pl. & gen. sg.* ·rii

Latin anatomical entries show the inflections that occur in Nomina Anatomica terminology.

There are two kinds of exceptions to the single-word policy:

1. Certain foreign phrases are best kept together for various reasons, for example, because their constituent words have no medical significance (*déjà vu, in vitro*), or because it is useful to contrast a two-word adverbial phrase with its adjectival counterpart:

    post′ par′·tum   *adv.*
    post·par′·tum   *adj.*

2. Species names are kept under the genus name. As most specific epithets are limited to one or two genera, the reader should find that listing species in this manner is efficient and convenient. (Some specific epithets, such as *coli* or *intestinalis*, are, in fact, found as non-italicized entry words or inflected forms.)

Combining Forms

In dictionaries, prefixes and initial combining forms end in a hyphen, (e.g., *anti-, cardio-, hemato-*). In the Word Guide, divided combining forms end in a centered dot, to show that there is no hyphen in the combined word. (A hyphen is commonly used, however, when the combination results in adjacent identical letters: *anti-infectious, post-traumatic*, although there are many exceptions, such as *microorganism*.) Including the combining form enables the reader to spell and divide many more terms than a book of this kind has room for. Since these forms are not used in isolation, they are given the division and stress pattern (usually secondary only) they will have when combined with any independent word.

When variant spellings or alternative stress and/or word divisions are given at a combining form, for example

    cer′·e·bro·   [ce·re′·bro·]
    he′·ma·to·   *Brit.* hae′·ma·to·

and these apply to all subsequent words beginning with that combining form, the variants or alternatives are not repeated at each word but are understood as applying.

However, in cases where the alternative division or variant spelling does not always apply, or where there are two combining forms with similar spellings, the alternatives are repeated at those words to which they apply:

ped′o·　　　　　　foot
pe′·do·　　　　　　child; also pae′·do·
pe′·do·don′·tist　　also pae′·
pe·dom′·e·ter
pe′·do·mor′·phic　also pae′·

Footnotes

Footnotes are used for usage and other information that does not fit into the column format of this book. They are signaled by a superscript number to the right of the entry word.

Some footnotes describe notation conventions tied to the word in question, (e.g., enzyme numbering at *enzyme*), but we have made no attempt to be comprehensive. Most notation systems used in the biomedical sciences, as for genetics or immunology, are far too complex to be given here. However, in many cases where such information does fit into a footnote, the editors have considered its inclusion to be in keeping with the purpose of the Word Guide.

Abbreviations Used in This Book

adj.	adjective
adv.	adverb *or* adverbial phrase
Brit.	British
Cf.	compare (*Latin* confer)
fem.	feminine
gen.	genitive
L.	Latin
masc.	masculine
n.	noun
neut.	neuter
pl.	plural
sg.	singular
spel.	spelling
v.	verb
var.	variant

WORD GUIDE

A

a′bac·te′·ri·al
aban′·don·ment
ab·ap′·i·cal
abar′·og·no′·sia
ab′·ar·thro′sis pl. ·ses
ab′·ar·tic′·u·lar
ab′·ar·tic′·u·la′·tion
aba′·sia
abate′ abat′·ed, abat′·ing
abate′·ment
ab·ax′·i·al
ab′·do·men [ab·do′·men] gen. ab·do′·mi·nis
ab·dom′·i·nal
ab·dom′·i·nal′·gia
ab·dom′·i·na′·lis neut. ·le
ab·dom′·i·no·
ab·dom′·i·no·an·te′·ri·or
ab·dom′·i·no·car′·di·ac
ab·dom′·i·no·cen·te′·sis pl. ·ses
ab·dom′·i·no·jug′·u·lar
ab·dom′·i·no·lum′·bar
ab·dom′·i·no·per′·i·ne′·al
ab·dom′·i·no·plas′·ty
ab·dom′·i·no·pos·te′·ri·or
ab·dom′·i·no·tho·rac′·ic
ab·dom′·i·no·vag′·i·nal
ab·dom′·i·no·ves′·i·cal

ab·du′·cens pl. ab′·du·cen′·tes, gen. sg.
ab′·du·cen′·tis
ab·du′·cent
ab·duct′
ab·duc′·tion movement from median axis: Cf. adduction
ab·duc′·tor L. pl. ab′·duc·to′·res
ab′·em·bry·on′·ic
ab′·en·ter′·ic
ab′·e·quose
ab·er′·rans pl. ab′·er·ran′·tes
ab·er′·rant
ab′·er·ra′·tion
a′be′·ta·lip′o·pro′·tein·e′·mia [·li′po·] Brit. ·ae′·mia
abey′·ance
ab′·i·ent
a′bi′o·gen′·e·sis
a′bi′o·ge·net′·ic
a′bi′·o·log′·ic
a·bi·o′·sis
a′bi·ot′·ic
a′bi′·o·tro′·phic [·troph′·ic]
a′bi·ot′·ro·phy
ab·ir′·ri·tant
ab′·lac·ta′·tion
a′blas·te′·mic
ab·late′ ·lat′·ed, ·lat′·ing
ab·la′·tio
ab·la′·tion
ableph′·a·rous

ableph′·a·ry
ab′·lu·ent
ab·lu′·tion
ab·mor′·tal moving from damaged tissue: Cf. admortal
ab·neu′·ral
ab·nor′·mal
ab′·nor·mal′·i·ty
ab′·oma·si′·tis
ab′·oma′·sum
ab·o′rad
ab·o′ral
abort′
abort′·er
abor′tient
abor′·ti·fa′·cient
abor′·ti·gen′·ic
abor′·tin
abor′·tion
abor′·tive
abor′·tus L. pl. & gen. sg. abortus
a′bouche·ment′
abou′·lia var. of abulia
abra′·chia
abra′·chio·ceph′·a·lus
abra′·chio·ceph′·a·ly
abra′·chi·us
abrad′·ant
abrade′ abrad′·ed, abrad′·ing
abra′·sio pl. abra′·si·o′·nes
abra′·sion
abra′·sive
abra′·sor
ab′·re·ac′·tion

a′brin
a′brism
ab′·ro·ta′·num
ab·rup′·tio
ab·rup′·tion
a′brus
A′brus prec′·a·to′·ri·us
ab·sce′·dens
ab′·scess
ab·sces′·sus pl.
  abscessus
ab·scis′sion
ab·scon′·sio
ab·sco′·pal
ab′·sence
ab·sen′·tia
Ab·sid′·ia
ab′·sinthe also ·sinth
ab·sin′·thin
ab′·sin·this′m [·sinth·is′m]
ab·sin′thi·um
ab′·sin·thol
ab′·so·lute′
ab·sorb′·a·ble
ab·sor′·bance [·sorb′·ance]
ab·sor′·be·fa′·cient
ab·sor′·ben·cy also ·ban·cy
ab·sor′·bent [·sorb′·ent]
ab·sorb′·er
ab·sorp′·ti·om′·e·ter
ab·sorp′·ti·om′·e·try
ab·sorp′·tion a taking into: Cf. adsorption
ab·sorp′·tive
ab·ster′·gent
ab′·sti·nence
ab·strac′·tion
ab·tor′·sion
abu′·lia
abu′·lic
abuse′ n. & v.
  abused′, abus′·ing
abut′·ment
aca′·cia

acal′·ci·co′·sis
a′cal·cu′·lia
acamp′·sia
Acan′·tha·moe′·ba
  [Acanth′·amoe′·ba]
  A. cul′·bert·so′·ni
acan′·tha·moe·bi′·a·sis
  [acanth′·amoe·]
acanth′·es·the′·sia
  [acan′·thes·] Brit.
  ·aes·the′·
acan′·thi·on
acan′·tho·
acan′·tho·am′·e·lo·blas·to′·ma
Acan′·tho·ceph′·a·la
acan′·tho·ceph′·a·lan
acan′·tho·ceph′·a·li′·a·sis
acan′·tho·ceph′·a·lous
Acan′·tho·ceph′·a·lus
Acan′·tho·chei′·lo·ne′·ma
acan′·tho·cyte
acan′·tho·cy·to′·sis
acan′·thoid
ac′·an·thol′·y·sis
acan′·tho·lyt′·ic
ac′·an·tho′·ma pl.
  ·mas or ·ma·ta
Ac′·an·tho′·phis
acan′·thor·rhex′·is
ac′·an·tho′·sis
ac′·an·thot′·ic
a cap′·i·te ad cal′·cem
acap′·nia
acap′·nic also ·ni·al
acap′·su·lar
acap′·su·la′·tum
acar′·bia
acar′·dia
acar′·di·ac
a′car·di′·a·cus
acar′·d·ius
ac′·a·ri′·a·sis
acar′·i·cide
ac′·a·rid
Acar′·i·dae

ac′·a·ri·di′·a·sis [acar′·i·]
ac′·a·rine
ac′·a·ri·no′·sis
acar′·i·o′·sis
ac′·a·ro·
ac′·a·ro·der·ma·ti′·tis
ac′·a·roid
ac′·a·rol′·o·gy
ac′·a·ro·pho′·bia
ac′·a·ro·tox′·ic
Ac′·a·rus
acar′y·ote var. of
  akaryote
acat′·a·las·e′·mia
  Brit. ·ae′·mia
acat′·a·la′·sia
acat′·a·lep′·sia
acat′·a·lep′·sy
acat′·a·lep′·tic
acat′·a·pha′·sia
ac′·a·thec′·tic [a′ca·]
ac′·a·thex′·is [a′ca·]
ac′·a·this′·ia [a′ca·]
  var. of akathisia
acau′·dal
acau′·date
ac·cel′·er·ans
ac·cel′·er·ant
ac·cel′·er·at′·ed
ac·cel′·er·a′·tion
ac·cel′·er·a′·tor
ac·cel′·er·a·to′·ry
ac·cel′·er·in
ac·cel′·er·om′·e·ter
ac·cen′·tu·a′·tion
ac·cen′·tu·a′·tor
ac·cep′·tor
ac′·cess
ac·ces′·si·bil′·i·ty
ac·ces′·si·ble
ac′·ces·so′·ria fem. of accessorius; pl. & gen. sg. ·ri·ae
ac′·ces·so′·ri·us pl. & gen. sg. ·rii
ac·ces′·so·ry
ac′·ci·dent

ac'·ci·den'·tal
ac'·ci·den'tal·is'm
ac·cip'·i·ter
ac·cli'·ma·ta'·tion
ac'·cli·ma'·tion
ac·cli'·ma·ti·za'·tion
ac·cli'ma·tize ·tized,
 ·tiz'·ing
ac·com'·mo·da'·tion
ac·com'·mo·da'·tive
ac·com'·mo·dom'·e·ter
ac·couche·ment' [ac·
 couche'·ment]
ac·cou·cheur'
ac·cou·cheuse'
ac·cred'·i·ta'·tion
ac'·cre·men·ti'·tion
ac·cre'·tio
ac·cre'·tion
ac·cre'·tion·ar'y
ac'·cro·chage'
ac·cul'·tur·a'·tion
ac·cu'·mu·la'·tor
ac'·cu·ra·cy
ace'·cli·dine
ac'·e·dap'·sone
acel'·lu·lar
ace'·lo·mate var. of
 acoelomate
ace'·nes·the'·sia
ace'·no·cou'·ma·rol
acen'·tric
a'ce·pha'·lia
a'ce·phal'·ic
aceph'a·lo·bra'·chia
aceph'·a·lo·car'·dia
aceph'·a·lo·chei'·ria
 also ·chi'·ria
aceph'·a·lo·cyst
aceph'·a·lo·gas·te'·ria
 also ·gas'·tria
aceph'·a·lo·po'·dia
aceph'·a·lor·rha'·chia
aceph'·a·lo·sto'·mia
aceph'·a·lo·tho·ra'·cia
aceph'·a·lous
aceph'·a·lus
aceph'·a·ly

ac'·er·ate
acer'bo·pho'·bia
acer'·e·bral [a'ce·re'·]
ac'·er·o'·la
ac'·ero·pho'·bia
ace'·ro·tous
acer'·vate
acer'·vu·line
acer'·vu·lo'·ma
acer'·vu·lus pl. ·li
aces'·o·dyne
ac'·e·tab'·u·lar
Ac'·e·tab·'u·lar'·ia
ac'·e·tab'·u·la'·ris
ac'e·tab'·u·lec'·to·my
ac'·e·tab'·u·lo·plas'·ty
ac'·e·tab'·u·lum pl.
 ·la, gen. sg. ·li
ac'·e·tal'
ac'·et·al'·de·hyde
acet'·a·mide [ac'et·
 am'·ide]
ac'·et·am'·i·dine
ac'et·amin'·o·phen
 [acet'·]
ac'·et·an'·i·lide also
 ·lid
ac'·et·an·i'si·dine
ac'·e·tan'·nin
ac'·et·ar'·sol
ac'·et·ar'·sone
ac'·e·tate
ac'et·azol'·a·mide
ace'·tic
ac'·e·tim'·e·ter
ac'·e·tin
ac'e·to· [ace'·to·]
ace'·to·ac'·e·tate
 [ac'e.to·]
ac'e·to·ace'·tic
Ace'·to·bac'·ter
ac'e·to·car'·mine
ace'·to·form
ac'e·to·hex'·amide
acet'·o·in [ac'e·to'·in]
ac'e·to·ki'·nase
ac'·e·tol
ac'e·to·lac'tic

ac'e·tol'y·sis
ac'e·tom'·e·ter
ac'e·to·mor'·phine
ac'·e·to·na'·tion
ac'·e·tone
ac'·e·ton·e'·mia [·to·
 ne'·] Brit. ·ae'·mia
ac'·e·ton·e'·mic [·to·
 ne'·] Brit. ·ae'·mic
ac'·e·ton·gly'cos·u'·ria
 [·co·su'·]
ac'e·to·ni'·trile
ac'·e·ton·u'·ria [·to·
 nu'·]
ac'e·to-or'·ce·in
ac'e·to·phen'·a·zine
ac'e·to·phe·net'·i·din
ac'e·to·py'·rine
ac'e·to·sul'·fone
 Brit. ·phone
ac'et·phen·ar'·sine
ac'et·phe·net'·i·din
ac'et·py'·ro·gall
ac'e·tri·zo'·ate
ace'·tum gen. ·ti
ace'·tyl [ac'e·tyl]
ace'·tyl·ami'·no·ben'·
 zine
ace'·tyl·ami'·no·flu'o·
 rene
ace'·tyl·an'·i·line
acet'·y·lase
acet'·y·la'·tion
ace'·tyl·car·bro'·mal
ace'·tyl·cho'·line
 [acet'·yl·]
ace'·tyl·cho·lin·es'·ter·
 ase [acet'·yl·]
ace'·tyl·co·en'·zyme
ace'·tyl·cys'·te·ine
 [acet'·yl·]
ace'·tyl·dig'·i·tox'·in
acet'·y·lene
ace'·tyl·ga·lac·tos'·
 amine
ace'·tyl·glu·cos'·amine
acet'·y·lide
ace'·tyl·meth'·a·dol

ace'·tyl·mu·ram'·ic
ace'·tyl·neur·amin'·ic
ace'·tyl·phen'·yl·hy'·dra·zine
ace'·tyl·pro'·ma·zine
ace'·tyl·sal'·i·cyl'·a·mide
ace'·tyl·sa·lic'·y·late
ace'·tyl·sal'·i·cyl'·ic
ace'·tyl·ser'·ine
ace'·tyl·stro·phan'·thi·din
ace'·tyl·tan'·nin
ace'·tyl·trans'·fer·ase
ach'a·la'·sia
Ach'·a·ti'·na fu·li'·ca
ache *n. & v.* ached, ach'·ing
achei'·lia
achei'·lous
achei'·ria
achei'·ro·po'·dia
achei'·rous
achieve'·ment
achi'·lia *var. of* acheilia
Achil'·les *gen.* Achil'·lis
achil'·lo·bur·si'·tis
achil'·lo·dyn'·ia
achil'·lo·gram
ach'il·lor'·rha·phy
achil'·lo·te·not'·o·my
ach'il·lot'·o·my
achi'·lous *var. of* acheilous
achi'·ria *var. of* acheiria
achi'·ro·po'·dia *var. of* acheiropodia
achi'·rous *var. of* acheirous
a'chlor·hy'·dria
a'chlor·hy'·dric
achlo'·ric
a'chlo·rop'·sia
a'cho·lan'·gic
acho'·lic

a'·cho·lu'·ric
achon'·dro·gen'·e·sis
achon'·dro·pla'·sia
achon'·dro·plas'·tic
achon'·dro·plas'·ty
achor'·dal
achor'·date
a'cho·re'·sis
achro'·a·cy·to'·sis
achroi'a
achro'·ma
a'chro·ma'·sia [ach'ro·]
ach'ro·mat
ach'ro·mate
ach'ro·mat'ic [a'chro·]
achro'·ma·tin
achro'·ma·tin'·ic
achro'·ma·tis'm
a'chro·mat'o·cy·to'·sis [achro'·ma·to·]
a'chro·mat'·o·phil [achro'·ma·to·]
achro'·ma·to·phil'·ia [a'chro·mat'·o·]
achro'·ma·to'·pia
achro'·ma·to'·pic
achro'·ma·top'·sia
achro'·ma·to'·sis
achro'·ma·tu'·ria
achro'·mia
achro'·mo·der'·ma
achro'·mo·phil
achro'·mo·trich'·ia
achy'·lia
acic'·u·lar
acic'·u·late
ac'·id
ac'·i·de'·mia *Brit.* ·dae'·
ac'·id-fast'
acid'·ic
acid'·i·fi·ca'·tion
acid'·i·fy fied, ·fy'·ing
ac'·i·dim'·e·ter
acid'·i·met'·ric
ac'·i·dim'·e·try
acid'·i·ty

acid'·o·gen'·ic [ac'·i·do·]
acid'·o·phil *also* ·phile
acid'·o·phil'·ia [ac'·i·do·]
acid'·o·phil'·ic [ac'·i·do·]
ac'·i·doph'·i·lus
ac'·i·do'·sis
ac'·i·dot'·ic
ac'·i·du'·ria
ac'·i·du'·ric
ac'·i·nar *also* acin'·ic
Ac'·i·ne'·to·bac'·ter
acin'·i·form
ac'·i·no·tu'·bu·lar
ac'·i·nous
ac'·i·nus *pl.* ·ni
ack'·ee [ackee']
ac'·me
ac'·ne
ac'·ne·gen'·ic
ac'·ne·i·form [ac·ne'·i·] *also* ac'·ne·form
ac·ne'·i·for'·mis
ac·ni'·tis
Ac'·o·can'·thera
ac'·o·can'·ther·in
acoe'·lo·mate
acoe'·naes·the'·sia *Brit. spel. of* acenesthesia
acol'·lis
acom'·ple·men·te'·mia *Brit.* ·tae'·
acon'·i·tase
ac'·o·nite
ac'·o·nit'·ic
acon'·i·tine
Ac'·o·ni'·tum
a'co·re'a
acor'·mus
acous'·ma
acous'·tic *also* ·ti·cal
acous'·ti·co·fa'·cial
acous'·ti·co·mo'·tor
acous'·ti·co·spi'·nal

acous'·tics[1]
acous'·to·gram   *also*
·ti·
ac·quired'
ac'·qui·si'tion
ac'·qui·si'·tus   *fem.*
·ta, *neut.* ·tum
ac'·ral
acra'·nia
acra'·ni·al
Ac'·re·mo'·ni·el'·la
ac'·rid
ac'·ri·dine
ac'·ri·sor'·cin
a'crit'·i·cal
ac'·ro·
ac'·ro·ag·no'·sia
ac'·ro·an'·es·the'·sia
  Brit. ·an'·aes·
ac'·ro·ar·thri'·tis
ac'·ro·blast
ac'·ro·blas'·tic
ac'·ro·brach'y·ceph'·a·ly
ac'·ro·cen'·tric
ac'·ro·ce·phal'·ic
ac'·ro·ceph'·a·lo·pol'y·syn·dac'·ty·ly
ac'·ro·ceph'·a·lo·syn·dac'·ty·ly
ac'·ro·ceph'·a·ly
ac'·ro·cy'·a·no'·sis
ac'·ro·der'·ma·ti'·tis
ac'·ro·der'·ma·to'·sis
  pl. ·ses
ac'·ro·dol'·i·cho·me'·lia
ac'·ro·dyn'·ia
ac'·ro·dys·pla'·sia
ac'·ro·dys·tro'·phic
  [·troph'·ic]
ac'·ro·dys'·tro·phy
ac'·ro·fa'·cial
ac'·ro·ge'·ria [·ger'·ia]
ac'·rog·no'·sia

ac'·rog·no'·sis
ac'·ro·hy'·per·hi·dro'·sis
ac'·ro·hy'·po·ther'·my
ac'·ro·ker'·a·to·elas'·toi·do'·sis
ac'·ro·ker·at·os'·is
  pl. ·ses
ac'ro·ki·ne'·sia   *also*
  ·sis
acro'·le·in
ac'·ro·mac'·ria
ac'·ro·mas·ti'·tis
ac'·ro·me·gal'·ic
ac'·ro·meg'·a·loid
ac'·ro·meg'·a·loid·is'm
ac'·ro·meg'·a·ly   *also*
  ·me·ga'·lia
ac'·ro·mel·al'·gia
ac'·ro·me'·lia
ac'·ro·mel'·ic [·me'·lic]
ac'·ro·met'a·gen'·e·sis
acro'·mi·al
acro'·mi·a'·lis   *neut.*
  ·le
ac'·ro·mi'·cria
acro'·mio·cla·vic'·u·lar
acro'·mio·cla·vic'·u·la'·ris   *neut.* ·re
acro'·mio·cor'·a·coid
acro'·mio·hu'·mer·al
acro'·mi·on
acro'·mi·on·ec'·to·my
acro'·mio·scap'·u·lar
acro'·mio·tho·rac'·ic
acrom'·pha·lus
ac'·ro·neu·rop'·a·thy
ac'·ro·nine
ac'·ro·nyx
ac'·ro-os'·te·ol'·y·sis
ac'·ro·pach'y
ac'·ro·pa·ral'·y·sis
ac'·ro·par'·es·the'·sia
  Brit. ·aes·the'·

acrop'·a·thy
ac'·ro·pho'·bia
ac'·ro·pig·men·ta'·tion
ac'·ro·pur'·pu·ra
ac'·ro·scle'·ro·der'·ma
ac'·ro·scle·ro'·sis
ac'·ro·som'·al [·so'·mal]
ac'·ro·some
ac'·ro·sphe'·no·syn·dac·tyl'·ia
ac'·ro·spi·ro'·ma
acros'·te·al'·gia
ac'·ro·ter'·ic
acrot'·ic
ac'·ro·tis'm
ac'·ro·tro'·pho·neu·ro'·sis
ac'·ry·late
acryl'·ic
ac'·ry·lo·ni'·trile
ac'·tin
ac·tin'·ic
ac'·ti·nide
ac·tin'·i·form
ac'·ti·nin
ac·tin'·i·um
ac'·ti·no· [ac·tin'o·]
ac'·ti·no·bac'·il·lo'·sis
Ac'·ti·no·ba·cil'·lus
ac'·ti·no·der'·ma·ti'·tis
ac'·ti·nom'·e·ter
ac'·ti·nom'·e·try
Ac'·ti·no·my'·ces
  A. bo'·vis
  A. is'·ra·el'·ii
  A. naes·lun'·dii
ac'·ti·no·my'·cete
  [·my·cete']
ac'·ti·no·my·ce'·tin
ac'·ti·no·my·ce'·tous
ac'·ti·no·my'·cin
ac'·ti·no·my·co'·ma
  pl. ·mas *or* ·ma·ta

---

[1] When denoting the science, *acoustics* is treated as a singular noun; when describing sound quality, it is treated as plural.

actinomycosis / adenolipoma 6

ac'·ti·no·my·co'·sis
   pl. ·ses
ac'·ti·no·my·cot'·ic
ac'·ti·no·my·co'·tin
ac'·ti·non
ac'·ti·no·rho'·dine
ac'·ti·no·spec'·ta·cin
ac·tin'o·spore [ac'·ti·no·]
ac'·ti·no·ther'·a·peu'·tics
ac'·ti·no·ther'·a·py
ac'·tion
ac'·ti·vate ·vat'·ed, ·vat'·ing
ac'·ti·va'·tion
ac'·ti·va'·tor
ac'·tive
ac·tiv'·i·ty
ac'·to·my'·o·sin
ac'·tu·ar'·i·an
ac'·tu·ar'y
ac'u·clo'·sure
ac'u·fi'·lo·pres'·sure
acu'·i·ty
acu'·mi·na'·ta neut.
   pl. & fem. sg. of
   acuminatus; pl. ·tae
acu'·mi·nate
acu'·mi·na'·tum neut.
   of acuminatus; pl. ·ta
acu'·mi·na'·tus
ac''u·pres'·sure
ac''u·punc'·ture
ac''u·sec'·tion
ac''u·sec'·tor
acu'·sis
acu'·sti·ca fem. of
   acusticus; pl. & gen.
   sg. ·cae
acu'·sti·cum neut. of
   acusticus
acu'·sti·cus pl. & gen.
   sg. ·ci
acute'
ac'u·tor'·sion
acu'·tus fem. ·ta
a'cy'·a·not'·ic

acy'·clic
acy'·clo·vir
a'cy·e'·sis
ac'·yl
ac'·yl·ase
ac'·yl·a'·tion
acyl'·o·in
ac'·yl·trans'·fer·ase
acys'·tia
acys'·tic
adac'·tyl·is'm
adac'·ty·ly also a'dac·tyl'·ia
ad'·a·man'·tine
ad'·a·man'·ti·no·car'·ci·no'·ma pl. ·mas or ·ma·ta
ad'·a·man'·ti·no'·ma
   pl. ·mas or ·ma·ta
ad'·a·man'·ti·num
ad'·a·man'·to·blast
ad'·a·man'·to·blas·to'·ma pl. ·mas or ·ma·ta
ad'·ams·ite
ad'·an·so'·ni·an
adapt'·a·bil'·i·ty
adapt'·a·ble
ad'·ap·ta'·tion
adapt'·er also adap'·tor
adap'·tive
ad'·ap·tom'·e·ter
ad·ax'·i·al
ad'·der
ad'·dict n.
ad·dict' v.
ad·dic'·tion
ad·dic'·tive
ad'·di·so'·ni·an
ad'·di·son·is'm
ad'·di·tive
ad·du'·cent
ad·duct'
ad·duc'·ta fem. of
   adductus
ad·duc'·tion
   movement toward

   median axis: Cf.
   abduction
ad·duc'·tor gen. ad'·duc·to'·ris
ad'·duc·to'·ri·us neut.
   ·ri·um
ad·duc'·to·va'·rus
ad·duc'·tus fem. ·ta
ad'·e·nal'·gia
ad'·e·nase
a'den·drit'·ic
ad'·e·nec'·to·my
ade'·nic
aden'·i·form [ade'·ni·]
ad'·e·nine
ad'·e·ni'·tis
ad'·e·no·
ad'·e·no·ac'·an·tho'·ma
   pl. ·mas or ·ma·ta
ad'·e·no·am'·e·lo·blas·to'·ma pl. ·mas or ·ma·ta
ad'·e·no·car'·ci·no'·ma
   pl. ·mas or ·ma·ta
ad'·e·no·cele
ad'·e·no·cys'·tic
ad'·e·no·cys·to'·ma
   pl. ·mas or ·ma·ta
ad'·e·no·fi·bro'·ma
   pl. ·mas or ·ma·ta
ad'·e·no·hy'·po·phys'·e·al [·hy·poph'·y·se'·al] var. of adenohypophysial
ad'·e·no·hy·poph'·y·sec'·to·my
ad'·e·no·hy'·po·phys'·i·al
ad'·e·no·hy·poph'·y·sis
   gen. ·hy·po·phys'·e·os
ad'·e·noid
ad'·e·noi'·dal
ad'·e·noid·ec'·to·my
ad'·e·noid·is'm
ad'·e·noid·i'·tis
ad'·e·no·li·po'·ma pl.
   ·mas or ·ma·ta

ad'·e·no·li·po'·ma·to'·sis
ad'·e·no·lym'·pho·cele
ad'·e·no·lym·pho'·ma *pl.* ·mas *or* ·ma·ta
ad'·e·no'·ma *pl.* ·mas *or* ·ma·ta
ad'·e·no'ma·toid [·nom'a·]
ad'·e·no'·ma·to'·sis
ad'·e·no'·ma·to'·sum
ad'·e·nom'a·tous [·no'ma·]
ad'·e·no·my·o'·ma *pl.* ·mas *or* ·ma·ta
ad'·e·no·my'·o·ma·to'·sis
ad'·e·no·my·om'a·tous [·o'ma·]
ad'·e·no·my·o'·sis
ad'·e·nop'·a·thy
ad'·e·no·sal'·pin·gi'·tis
ad'·e·no·sar·co'·ma *pl.* ·mas *or* ·ma·ta
aden'·o·sine
ad'·e·no'·sis
aden'·o·syl·ho'·mo·cys'·te·ine
aden'·o·syl·me·thi'·o·nine
aden'·o·syl·trans'·fer·ase
ad'·e·no·tome
ad'·e·not'·o·my
ad'·e·no·ton'·sil·lec'·to·my
ad'·e·no·var'·ix *pl.* ·var'·i·ces
ad'·e·no·vi'·rus
ad'·e·nyl
aden'·y·late
ad'·e·nyl'·ic
ad'·e·nyl'o·suc'·ci·nate
ad'·e·nyl'·yl
ad'·eps
ader'·mo·gen'·e·sis
ad·hae'·rens *pl.* ad'·hae·ren'·tes; *var. of* adherens

ad·here' ·hered', ·her'·ing
ad·her'·ence
ad·he'·rens *pl.* ad'·he·ren'·tes
ad·her'·ent
ad·he'·si·ec'to·my
ad·he'·sin
ad·he'·sio *pl.* ad·he'·si·o'·nes
ad·he'·sion
ad·he'·si·ot'·o·my
ad·he'·sive
adi'·ac·tin'·ic
adi'·a·do'·cho·ki·ne'·sia *also* ·do'·ko·, ·sis
adi'·a·pho·re'·sis
adi'·a·pho·ret'·ic
adi'a·spi'·ro·my·co'·sis
adi'a·spi·ro'·sis
adi'·a·ther'·mance *also* ·man.cy
ad'·i·ent
ad'·i·pec'·to·my
ad'·i·phen'·ine
adip'·ic
ad'·i·po·
ad'·i·po·cele
ad'·i·po·cel'·lu·lar
ad'·i·po·cere
ad'·i·po·cyte
ad'·i·po·gen'·ic *also* ad'·i·pog'·e·nous
ad'·i·po·ki·ne'·sis
ad'·i·po·ki·net'·ic
ad'·i·po·ne·cro'·sis
ad'·i·po·pec'·tic *also* ·pex'·ic
ad'·i·po·pex'·is *also* ·pex'·ia
ad'·i·po'·sa *fem. of* adiposus; *pl.* ·sae
ad'·i·pose
ad'·i·po'·sis
ad'·i·po'·si·tas
ad'·i·pos'·i·ty
ad'·i·po'·so·gen'·i·ta'·lis

ad'·i·po'·sus *fem.* ·sa, *neut.* ·sum
adip'·sia
ad'·i·tus *pl.* aditus
ad'·junct
ad·junc'·tive
ad'·ju·vant
ad'·ju·van·tic'·i·ty
ad·max'·il·lar'y
ad'·mi·nic'·u·lum *pl.* ·la
ad·mix'·ture
ad·mor'·tal *moving toward damaged tissue:* Cf. abmortal
ad·na'·sal
ad'·nate
ad nau'·se·am
ad·neu'·ral
ad·nex'a
ad·nex'·al
ad'·nex·i'·tis
ad'·oc·cip'·i·tal
ad'·o·les'·cence
ad'·o·les'·cent
ad·o'ral
adre'·nal
adre'·nal·ec'·to·mize ·mized, ·miz'·ing
adre'·nal·ec'·to·my
adren'·a·line
ad'·ren·ar'·che [ad'·ren·ar'·che]
ad'·re·ner'·gic
adre'·no·
adre'·no·cep'·tive
adre'·no·cep'·tor
adre'·no·chrome
adre'·no·cor'·ti·cal
adre'·no·cor'·ti·coid
adre'·no·cor'·ti·co·mi·met'·ic
adre'·no·cor'·ti·co·ste'·roid
adre'·no·cor'·ti·co·tro'·pic [·trop'·ic]
adre'·no·cor'·ti·co·tro'·pin

adre'·no·dox'·in
adre'·no·gen'·i·tal
adre'·no·glo·mer'·u·lo·tro'·pin
adre'·no·leu'·ko·dys'·tro·phy
adren'·o·lyt'·ic
adre'·no·med'·ul·lar'y
adre'·no·re·cep'·tor *var. of* adrenoceptor
adre'·no·stat'·ic
adre'·no·sym'·pa·thet'·ic
adre'·no·tro'·phic [·troph'·ic]
adre'·no·tro'·pic [·trop'·ic]
adre'·no·tro'·pin *also* ·phin
ad·sorb'
ad·sor'·bent [·sorb'·ent]
ad·sorp'·tion
  adherence of fluid to a surface: *Cf.* absorption
ad·ster'·nal
ad·tor'·sion
adult' [ad'·ult]
adul'·ter·ant
adul'·ter·ate ·at'·ed, ·at'·ing
adul'·ter·a'·tion
ad·vance'·ment
ad'·ve·hens *pl.* ad'·ve·hen'·tes
ad'·ve·hent
ad'·ven·ti'·tia
ad'·ven·ti'·tial
ad'·ven·ti'·tious
ad·ver'·sive
a'dy·nam'·ia [·na'·mia]
a'dy·nam'·ic
ae-*See also words beginning* e-

Ae'·des[2]
A. ae·gyp'·ti
A. al'·bo·pic'·tus
A. leu'·co·ce·lae'·nus
A. tae'·nio·rhyn'·chus
A. tri'·ser·i·a'·tus
ae·lu'·ro·pho'·bia *var. of* ailurophobia
ae·qua'·tor *var. of* equator
ae·quo'·rin
aer'·ate [a'er·ate] ·at·ed, ·at·ing
aer·a'·tion
aer·e'·mia *Brit.* ·ae'·mia
aer·if'·er·ous
aer'·i·fi·ca'·tion
aer'o· [a'ero·]
Aer'·o·bac'·ter
aer'·obe [a'er·]
aer·o'·bic
aer'o·bi·ol'·o·gy
aer'o·bi·o'·sis
aer'o·bi·ot'·ic
aer'·o·cele
Aer'o·coc'·cus
aer'·o·col'·pos
aer'·odon·tal'·gia
aer'·o·don'·tia
aer'·o·don'·tics
aer'o·em'·bo·lis'm
aer'o·em·phy·se'·ma
aer'·o·gen
aer'·o·gen'·e·sis
aer'·o·gen'·ic
aer·og'·e·nous
aer'o·med'·i·cine
aer·om'·e·ter
aer'·o·mo'·nad
Aer'·o·mo'·nas

aer'o·neu·ro'·sis
aer'o·odon·tal'·gia *var. of* aerodontalgia
aer'o·oti'·tis *var. of* aerotitis
aer'o·per·i·to·ne'·um
aer'·o·pha'·gia
aer'·o·phag'·ic
aer·oph'·a·gy
aer'·o·phil
aer'·o·phil'·ic
aer·oph'·i·lous
aer'o·pho'·bia
aer'·o·phore
aer'o·ple·thys'·mo·graph
aer'·o·scope
aer·os'·co·py
aer'o·si·nus·i'·tis
aer·o'·sis
aer'·o·sol
aer'·o·sol'·i·za'·tion
aer·o·tax'·is
aer'o·ther·a·peu'·tics
aer'o·ther'·a·py
aer·oti'·tis
aer'o·tol'er·ant
aer'o·to·nom'e·ter
aer'o·to·nom'e·try
aer'o·tro'·pism
aes·the'·sia *var. of* esthesia
aes·the'·sio· *var. of* esthesio-
aes·thet'·ic *var. of* esthetic
aes·thet'·ics *var. of* esthetics
aes'·ti·val *Brit. spel. of* estival
aes'·ti·va'·lis *neut.* ·le
aes'·ti·va'·tion *Brit. spel. of* estivation

---

2 This is sometimes spelled *Aëdes* to show that the *A* and the *e* do not form a diphthong but are pronounced separately: *A-e'-des*. However, diacritical marks are not used in the official taxonomic nomenclature.

ae′·ther[3] *a Brit. spel.
of* ether
ae′·ti·o· *Brit. spel. of*
etio-
ae′·ti·ol′·o·gy *Brit.
spel. of* etiology
afe′·brile [afeb′·rile]
afe′·tal
af′·fect *n.*
af·fec′·tive
af′·fec·tiv′·i·ty
af·fec′·to·mo′·tor
af′·fer·ens *neut. pl.*
af′·fer·en′·tia
af′·fer·ent *conveying toward the center: Cf.* efferent
af′·fer·en·ta′·tion
af·fil′·i·a′·tion
af·fi′·nal
af·fin′·i·ty
af′·flux
af·flux′·ion
a′fi·brin′·o·gen·e′·mia *Brit.* ·ae′·mia
af′·la·tox′·in
afron′·tal
af′·ter·birth
af′·ter·brain
af′·ter·care
af′·ter·con·trac′·tion
af′·ter·cur′·rent
af′·ter·damp
af′·ter·ef·fect′
af′·ter·glow
af′·ter·im′·age
af′·ter·load
af′·ter·po·ten′·tial
af′·ter·sen·sa′·tion
af′·ter·stain
af′·ter·treat′·ment
af′·ter·vi′·sion
afunc′·tion·al

aga·lac′·tia
aga·lac′·tic
a′ga·lac·to′·sis
agal′·or·rhe′a *Brit.*
·rhoe′a
agam′·ete [ag′a·mete]
a′ga·met′·ic
agam′·ic
a′gam′·ma·glob′·u·lin·e′·mia *Brit.* ·ae′·mia
ag′a·mo·cy·tog′·e·ny
*Ag′a·mo·fi·lar′·ia
[Agam′o·]*
ag′a·mo·gen′e·sis
[agam′o·]
ag′a·mo·ge·net′·ic
[agam′o·]
ag′·a·mont [agam′·ont]
ag′·a·mous
a′gan′·gli·on′·ic
a′gar [ag′ar]
a′gar-a′gar [ag′ar-ag′ar]
ag′·a·ric [agar′·ic]
agar′·i·cin
Agar′·i·cus
ag′·a·rose
agas′·tria
agas′·tric
age *n. & v.* aged, ag′·ing *or* age′·ing
agen′e·sis
agen′·i·tal·is′m
a′gent
ageu′·sia
ageu′·sic
ag′ger *pl.* ·ger·es, *gen. sg.* ·ger·is
ag·glu′·ti·na·ble
ag·glu′·ti·nant
ag·glu′·ti·nate
ag·glu′·ti·na′·tion
ag·glu′·ti·na·tive
ag·glu′·ti·nin

ag·glu′·ti·no·gen
ag·glu′·ti·no·gen′·ic
ag·glu′·ti·no·phil′·ic
ag′·glu·tom′·e·ter
ag′·gre·gate *n. & v.*
·gat′·ed, ·gat′·ing
ag′·gre·ga′·ti
ag′·gre·ga′·tion
ag′·gre·gom′·e·ter
ag′·i·tans
ag′·i·ta′·tor *L. pl.* ag′·i·ta·to′·res
ag′·i·to·pha′·sia
Ag·kis′·tro·don
aglan′du·lar
a′glo·mer′·u·lar
agly′·cone
ag′·mi·nat′·ed
ag′·mi·na′·tion
ag·na′·thia
ag·na′·thous
ag′·no·gen′·ic
ag·no′·sia
ag·no′·sic *also* ag·nos′·tic
a′go·nad′·al
ag′·o·nal *also* agon′·ic
ag′·o·nist
ag′·o·nis′·tic
ag′·o·ny
ag′·o·ra·pho′·bia
ag′·o·ra·pho′·bic
agram′·ma·tis′m
agran′·u·lar
agran′·u·lo·cyt′·ic
agran′·u·lo·cy·to′·sis
agran′·u·lo′·sis
agraph′·ia
agraph′·ic
agryp′·nia
a′gryp·not′·ic [ag′rip·]
a′gue
agy′·ria

---

[3] *Aether* and *ether* are alternative British spellings for the hypothetical medium of electromagnetic waves, and formerly also for highly volatile substances including those used in anesthesia. In the modern chemical sense, however, only *ether* is used.

agy′·ric
aich′·mo·pho′·bia
aid *help:* Cf. aide
aide *helper:* Cf. aid
AIDS
ail′·ment
ai·lu′·ro·pho′·bia
ai·nhum′
air′-borne[4]
air′·way
Ajel′·lo·my′·ces
akar″y·o·cyte
akar″y·ote
aka·ta′·ma
ak′·a·this′·ia
akee′ [ak′ee] *var. of*
   ackee
a′ki·ne′·sia [ak′i·]
a′ki·ne′·sic [ak′i·]
a′ki·net′·ic
a′la *pl. & gen. sg.*
   a′lae
a′lac·ta′·sia
ala′·lia
al′·a·nine
a′lar
ala′·re *neut. of* alaris;
   pl. ·ria
ala′·ris *pl.* ·res
a′la·ryn′·ge·al
alas′·trim
a′late
ala′·tus
al′·ba *fem. sg. & neut.*
   pl. of albus
al·be′·do
al′·bi·cans *pl.* al′·bi·
   can′·tes, *gen.* al′·bi·
   can′·tia
al′·bi·dus
al·bin′·ic
al′·bi·nis′m
al′·bi·nis′·mus

al·bi′·no
al·bi′·no·is′m
al′·bi·not′·ic
al′·bi·punc·ta′·tus
al′·bu·gin′·ea
al′·bu·gin′·e·ot″·o·my
al′·bu·gin′·e·ous
al·bu′·gi·ni′·tis
al·bu′·go *pl.* al·bu′·gi·
   nes
al′·bum *neut. of* albus
al·bu′·men
al′·bu·mim′·e·try
al·bu′·min
al·bu′·mi·nim′·e·try
al·bu′·min·oid [·mi·
   noid]
al·bu′·mi·nose
al·bu′·mi·nous
al·bu′·min·u′·ria [·mi·
   nu′·ria]
al′·bus *fem.* ·ba, *neut.*
   ·bum
Al″·ca·lig′·e·nes
   A. fae·ca′·lis
al·cap′·ton *var. of*
   alkapton
al·cap′·ton·u′·ria [·to·
   nu′·] *var. of* alkap-
   tonuria
al·cap′·ton·u′·ric [·to·
   nu′·] *var of* alkapto-
   nuric
al′·co·hol
al′·co·hol·e′·mia *Brit.*
   ·ae′·mia
al′·co·hol′·ic
al′·co·hol·is′m
al′·co·hol·i·za′·tion
al′·co·hol·om′·e·ter
al′·co·hol·u′·ria
al·co·hol′·y·sis
al′·co·ho·lyt′·ic

al′·de·hyde
al′·di·mine [ald″·i·]
al′·do·bi″·uron′·ic
al′·do·hex″·ose
al′·dol
al′·do·lase
al·don′·ic
al′·do·pen′·tose
al′·dose
al·dos′·ter·one [al′·do·
   ster′·]
al·dos′·ter·on·is′m [al′·
   do·ster′·]
al·dos′·ter·on·o′·ma
al·dos′·ter·on·u′·ria [·o·
   nu′·ria]
al′·do·tet′·rose
al·dox′·ime
al′·drin
alec′·i·thal
alem′·mal
a′leu·ke′·mic *Brit.*
   ·kae′·
aleu′·kia *also* ·cia
aleu″·ko·cy·the′·mic
   Brit. ·co·cy·thae′·
aleu″·ko·cy·to′·sis
al′·eu·rone
alex′·ia
alex′·ic
alex″·i·phar′·mac
aley′dig·is′m
al′·gae
al′·gal
al·gan′·es·the′·sia [alg′·
   an·] *Brit.* ·aes·the′·
al′·ge·don′·ic
al·ge′·sia
al·ge′·sic
al′·ge·sim′·e·ter
al′·ge·sim′·e·try
al·ge″·si·o·gen′·ic
al′·ges·the′·sia *Brit.*
   ·gaes·; *also* ·the′·sis

---

4 This term is ordinarily spelled *airborne* (no hyphen) in reference to aircraft or military personnel, but preferably *air-borne* (on the pattern of *water-borne, arthropod-borne*) in describing microorganisms, pollutants, etc.

al·get′·ic
al′·gi·cide
al′·gid
al′·gin
al·gi·nate
al·gin′·ic
al′·gio·
al′·go·
al′·go·cep′·tor
al′·go·gen′·e·sis
al′·go·gen′·ic
al′·go·lag′·nia
al·gom′·e·ter
al·gom′·e·try
al′·go·pho′·bia
al′·gor
al′·go·rith′m
al′i·cy′·clic
a′lien·a′·tion
a′lien·ist
al′i·form [a′li·]
align′
align′·ment
al′·i·ment
al′·i·men·ta′·ri·us
al′·i·men′ta·ry
al′·i·men·ta′·tion
al′i·na′·sal [a′li·]
alinement *misspelling of* alignment
al′·i·phat′·ic
al′·i·quot
al′i·sphe′·noid [a′li·]
aliz′·a·rin
al′·ka·le′·mia *Brit.*
 ·lae′·mia
al′·ka·les′·cens-dis′·par
al′·ka·li *pl.* ·lis *or* ·lies
al′·ka·lim′·e·ter
al′·ka·line
al′·ka·lin′·i·ty
al′·ka·li·nu′·ria
al′·ka·loid
al′·ka·lo′·sis *pl.* ·ses
al′·ka·lot′·ic
al′·kane
al·kan′·nin
al·kap′·ton

al·kap′·ton·u′·ria [·to·nu′·ria]
al·kap′·ton·u′·ric [·to·nu′·ric]
al′·kene
alk·ox′·ide
alk·ox′y
al′·kyl
al′·kyl·at′·ing
al′·kyl·a′·tion
al′·kyne
al′·la·ches·the′·sia
  Brit. ·chaes·
al′·lan·ti′·a·sis
al·lan′·to·
al·lan′·to·cho′·ri·on′·ic
al·lan′·to·en·ter′·ic
al′·lan·to′·ic
al·lan′·toid
al′·lan·toi′·do·an′·gi·op′·a·gous
al·lan′·to·in
al·lan′·to·is *pl.* al′·lan·to′·i·des
al·lele′
al·le′·lic
al·lel′·ism
al·le′·lo·
al·le′·lo·morph
al′·ler·gen
al′·ler·gen′·ic
al·ler′·gic
al·ler′·gid
al′·ler·gist
al′·ler·gol′·o·gy
al′·ler·gy
Al′·les·che′·ria
al′·les·che·ri′·a·sis
al′·les·the′·sia *Brit.*
  ·laes·
al·le′·vi·ant
al·le′·vi·ate ·at′·ed, ·at′·ing
al′·li·cin
al′·lied [al·lied′]
al′·li·ga′·tion
al′·li·in
Al′·li·*um*

al′·lo·
al′·lo·an′·ti·bod′y
al′·lo·an′·ti·gen
al′·lo·bar′·bi·tal
al′·lo·chei′·ria
al′·lo·ches·the′·sia
  Brit. ·chaes·; *var. of* allachesthesia
al′·lo·cor′·tex
Al′·lo·der′·ma·nys′·sus
al′·lo·dip′·loid
al′·lo·erot′·i·cis′m
  also ·er′·o·tis′m
al′·lo·es·the′·sia *Brit.*
  ·aes·; *var. of* allesthesia
al·log′·a·my
al′·lo·ge·ne′·ic *also*
  ·gen′·ic
al′·lo·graft
al′·lo·ki·ne′·sis
al′·lo·ki·net′·ic
al′·lo·met·ric
al·lom′·e·try
al′·lo·morph
al′·lo·mor′·phic
al′·lo·mor′·phism
al′·lo·path
al′·lo·path′·ic
al·lop′·a·thy
al′·lo·phene
al′·lo·phen′·ic
al′·lo·plas′·tic
al′·lo·plas′·ty
al′·lo·ploid
al′·lo·ploi′·dy
al′·lo·pol′y·ploid
al′·lo·pol′y·ploi′·dy
al′·lo·pu′·ri·nol
al′·lo·rhyth′·mic
al′·lose
al′·lo·some
al′·lo·ster′·ic [·ste′·ric]
al′·lo·tet′·ra·ploid
al′·lo·tet′·ra·ploi′·dy
al′·lo·to′·pia
al′·lo·top′·ic
al′·lo·trans·plan·ta′·tion
al·lot′·ri·o·

al·lot′·ri·o·geus′·tia
al′·lo·trope
al′·lo·tro′·phic [·troph′·ic]
al′·lo·tro′·pic [·trop′·ic]
al·lot′·ro·py
al′·lo·type
al′·lo·typ′·ic
al′·lo·ty′·py
al·lox′·an
al·lox′·a·zine
al′·lox′·ure′·mia
al′·lox·u′·ria
al′·lox·u′·ric
al′·loy [al·loy′]
al′·lo·zyme
al′·lyl
al′·lyl·mer·cap′·tan
al′·ly·sine
al′·oe
al′·o·et′·ic
alo′·gia
al′·o·in *also* alo′·e·tin
al′·o·pe′·cia
al′·o·pe′·cic
al′·pha
al′·pha·lyt′·ic
al′·pha·mi·met′·ic
al′·pha·nu·mer′·ic
al′·pha·pro′·dine
al′·pha·vi′·rus
al·pren′·o·lol
al′·ser·ox′·y·lon
al′·sto·nine
al′·te·plase
al′·ter
al′·ter·ant
al′·ter·a·tive
al′ter·nans
Al′·ter·nar′·ia
al·ter·nar′·ia·tox·i·co′·sis
al′·ter·nate *adj. & v.*
  ·nat′·ed, ·nat′·ing
al′·ter·na′·tion

al′·ter·no·bar′·ic
al′·ti·tude
al′·ti·tu′·di·nal
al·tri′·cial
al′·tri·gen′·der·is′m
  also ·gen′·drism
al′·trose
al′·um
alu′·mi·na
al′·u·min′·i·um⁵ *var.*
  of aluminum
alu′·mi·no′·sis
alu′·mi·nous
alu′·mi·num
al′·ve·at′·ed
al′·vei *pl. & gen. sg.*
  of alveus
al′·veo·bron′·chi·o·li′·tis
al′·veo·den′·tal *var.*
  of alveolodental
al′·ve·o·gen′·i·ca
al·ve′·o·lar
al′·ve·o·la′·re *neut. of* alveolaris
al′·ve·o·la′·ris *pl.* ·res
al·ve′·o·late
al·ve′·o·lat′·ed [al′·ve·]
al′·ve·o·lec′·to·my [al·ve′·]
al·ve′·o·li *pl. & gen.*
  sg. of alveolus
al′·veo·lin′·gual
al′·ve·o·li′·tis
al·ve′·o·lo·
al·ve′·o·lo·ba′·sal
al·ve′·o·lo·cap′·il·lar′y
al·ve′·o·lo·den′·tal
al·ve′·o·lo·plas′·ty
al′·ve·o·lot′·o·my [al·ve′·]
al·ve′·o·lus *pl.* ·li
al′·ve·o·plas′·ty
al′·ve·us *pl.* ·vei
al′·vine

al′·vus *pl. & gen. sg.*
  ·vi
alym′·pho·pla′·sia
a′maas
am′·a·crine
amal′·gam
amal′·gam·a′·tor [·ga·ma′·]
Am′·a·ni′·ta
  A. *mus·car′·ia*
  A. *phal·loi′·des*
  A. *vi·ro′·sa*
am′a·ni′·tin
aman′·ta·dine
am′·as·then′·ic
amas′·tia
amas′ti·gote
am′·au·ro′·sis
am′·au·rot′·ic
amax′o·pho′·bia
am′·be·no′·ni·um
am′·ber
am′·ber·gris
am′·bi·
am′·bi·dex·ter′·i·ty
  also ·dex·tral′·i·ty
am′·bi·dex′·trous
am′·bi·ent
am·big′·uo·spi′·no·tha·lam′·ic
am·big′·u·ous
am·big′·u·us
am′·bi·lat′·er·al
am′·bi·sex′·u·al
am′·bi·sex·u·al′·i·ty
am′·bi·ten′·den·cy
am·biv′·a·lence
am·biv′·a·lent
am′·bly·a′·phia
am′·bly·chro·mat′·ic
Am′·bly·om′·ma
  A. *amer′·i·ca′·num*
  A. *ca′·jen·nen′·se*
am′·bly·ope
am′·bly·o′·pia

---

5 The form *aluminium* is widely used outside the United States.

am'·bly·o'·pic
am'·bly·o·scope
am'·bo   var. of ambon;
   pl. am·bo'·nes
am'·bo·   var. of ambi-
am'·bo·cep'·tor
am'·bo·my'·cin
am'·bon
Am·bro'·sia
am'·bu·lance
am'·bu·lance·man'
am'·bu·lans
am'·bu·lant
am'·bu·la·to'·ry
am'·bu·phyl'·line
ame'·ba   also amoe'·
   ba; pl. ·bas or ·bae
ame'·ba·cid'·al [·ci'·
   dal]   var. of amebi-
   cidal
ame'·ba·cide   var. of
   amebicide
am'·e·bi'·a·sis
ame'·bi·c
ame'·bi·cid'·al [·ci'·dal]
ame'·bi·cide
ame'·bi·form
ame'·bi·o'·sis   var. of
   amebiasis
ame'·bo·cyte
ame'·boid
am'·e·bo'·ma
am'·e·bo'·sis   var. of
   amebiasis
ame'·bu·la   pl. ·las or
   ·lae
a'mel·a·not'·ic
ame'·lia
am'·e·lo·
ame'·e·lo·blast
am'·e·lo·blas'·tic
am'·e·lo·blas·to'·ma
am'·e·lo·gen'·e·sis
am'·e·lus [ame'·lus]

amen'·or·rhe'a   Brit.
   ·rhoe'a
amen'·or·rhe'·ic   Brit.
   ·rhoe'·ic
amen'·stru·al
a'ment
amen'·tia
am'·er·is'·tic
a'me·tab'·o·lous
am'·e·thop'·ter·in
am'·e·trom'·e·ter
am'·e·tro'·pia
am'·e·tro'·pic [·trop'·
   ic]
am'·i·an·ta'·cea
am'·i·dase
am'·ide
am'·i·din
am'·i·dine
am'·i·di'·no
am'·i·di'·no·trans'·fer·
   ase
am'·i·do· [ami'·do·]
am'·i·do·py'·rine
amim'·ia
am'·ine [amine']
ami'·no[6]
ami'·no·ac'·e·tate
ami'·no·ace'·tic
ami'·no·ac'·id·e'·mia
   Brit. ·ae'·mia
ami'·no·ac'·id·op'·a·thy
ami'·no·ac'·id·u'·ria
ami'·no·ac'·yl
ami'·no·ben'·zo·ate
ami'·no·ben·zo'·ic
ami'·no·bu·tyr'·ic
ami'·no·ca·pro'·ic
ami'·no·cy'·cli·tol
ami'·no·glu·tar'·ic
ami'·no·gly'·co·side
ami'·no·hip'·pur·ate
ami'·no·hip·pu'·ric
ami'·no·i'so·bu'·ta·nol

ami'·no·i'so·bu·tyr'·ic·
   acid·u'·ria
ami'·no·pep'·ti·dase
ami'·no·phyl'·line
am'·i·nop'·ter·in
ami'·no·py'·rine
ami'·no·quin'·o·line
ami'·no·sa·lic'·y·late
ami'·no·sal'·i·cyl'·ic
ami'·no·sug'·ar
ami'·no·trans'·fer·ase
a'mi·to'·sis
a'mi·tot'·ic
am'·me·ter
am·mo'·nia
am·mo'·ni·ac
am'·mo·ni'·a·cal
am·mo'·nia-ly'·ase
am·mo'·ni·a'·tum
am·mo'·ni·fi·ca'·tion
am·mo'·ni·um
am'·mo·ther'·a·py
am·ne'·sia
am·ne'·si·ac
am·ne'·sic
am·nes'·tic
am'·nio·
am'·ni·on'·ic
am'·ni·o·cele
am'·nio·cen·te'·sis
   pl. ·ses
am'·nio·cho'·ri·on'·ic
am'·ni·o·clep'·sis
am'·nio·em'bry·on'·ic
am'·nio·gen'·e·sis
am'·ni·og'·ra·phy
am'·ni·on
am'·ni·on·i'·tis
am'·ni·o·scope
am'·ni·os'·co·py
Am'·ni·o'·ta
am'·ni·ote
am'·ni·ot'·ic
am'·ni·o·tome

---

6 Symbols for amino acids consist of three letters, the first of which is capitalized: Arg (arginine), Cys (cysteine), etc.

am'·ni·ot'·o·my
am'o·bar'·bi·tal
am'o·di'·a·quin
Amoe'·ba
amoe'·ba pl. ·bae or
  ·bas; var. of ameba
am'·oe·bi'·a·sis var.
  of amebiasis
amoe'·bic var. of
  amebic
amoe'·bi·cid'·al var.
  of amebicidal
amoe'·bi·cide var. of
  amebicide
amoe'·bi·form var. of
  amebiform
amoe'·bo·cyte var. of
  amebocyte
amoe'·boid var. of
  ameboid
am'·oe·bo'·ma var. of
  ameboma
Amoe'·bo·tae'·nia
amoe'·bu·la var. of
  amebula; pl. ·lae or ·las
amor'·phic
amor'phin·is'm
amor'phog·no'·sia
  also ·sis
amor'·phous
amor'·phus pl. ·phi
am'·o·site
amox'·i·cil'·lin
am'·per·age
am'·pere
am·phet'·a·mine
am'·phi·
am'·phi·ar·thro'·di·al
am'·phi·ar·thro'·sis
  pl. ·ses
am'·phi·as'·ter
am'·phi·bol'·ic
am·phib'·o·lous
am'·phi·cen'·tric
am'·phi·cra'·nia
am'·phi·cyte
am'·phi·di'·ar·thro'·di·
  al

am'·phi·di'·ar·thro'·sis
  pl. ·ses
am·phig'·o·ny
am'·phi·mic'·tic
am'·phi·mix'·is
am'·phi·stome
am'·phi·tene
am·phit'·ri·chous
  also ·chate
am'·pho·
am'·pho·lyte
am'·pho·my'·cin
am'·pho·phil
am'·pho·phile
am'·pho·phil'·ic
am·phor'·ic
am'·pho·ter'·ic
am'·pho·ter'·i·cin
am'·pi·cil'·lin
am'·pli·fi·ca'·tion
am'·pli·tude
am·pul'·la pl. & gen.
  sg. ·lae
am·pul'·lar
am'·pul·la'·re neut. of
  ampullaris; pl. ·ria
am'·pul·la'·ris
am·pul'·la·ry [am'·pul·
  lar'y]
am'·pule also ·poule
am'·pul·li'·tis
am·pul'·lu·la pl. ·lae
am'·pu·tate tat'·ed,
  ·tat'·ing
am'·pu·ta'·tion
am'·pu·tee'
amu'·sia
amyc'·tic
am'y·dri'·a·sis
amyd'·ri·caine
a'my·e'·lia [am'y·]
a'my·el'·ic
ảmy'·e·lin·at'·ed
amy'·e·lin·a'·tion
a'my·e·lin'·ic
a'my·e·lon'·ic
amy'·e·lous
amyg'·da·la pl. ·lae

amyg'·da·lec'·to·my
amyg'·da·lin
amyg'·da·line
amyg'·da·lo·
amyg'·da·loid
amyg'·da·loid·ec'·to·
  my
amyg'·da·loi'·de·um
amyg'·da·lot'·o·my
am'·yl
am'·y·la'·cea
am'·y·la'·ceous
am'·y·lase
am'·y·las·u'·ria
am'·y·lo·
am'·y·lo·bar'·bi·tone
am'·y·lo·dex'·trin
am'·y·lo·dys·pep'sia
am'·y·loid
am'·y·loid·e'·mia [·loi·
  de'·mia] Brit. ·ae'·
  mia
am'·y·loi'·do·gen'·ic
am'·y·loi·do'·sis [·loid·
  o'·]
am'·y·lo·pec'·tin
am'·y·lo·pec'·ti·no'·sis
  [·tin·o'·]
am'·y·lo·pha'·gia
am'·y·lose
am'·y·los·u'·ria
am'·yl·pen'·i·cil'·lin
am'·y·lum
amy'·o·pla'·sia
amy'·os·the'·nia
amy'·os·then'·ic
amy'·o·to'·nia
amy'·o·tro'·phia
amy'·o·tro'·phic
  [·troph'·ic]
a'my·ot'·ro·phy [am'y·]
amyx'·or·rhe'a Brit.
  ·rhoe'a
an'a
anab'·a·sis
an'·a·bat'·ic
an'a·bi·ot'·ic
an'·a·bol'·ic

anab′·o·lis′m
anab′·o·lite
an′·a·cho′·lia
an′·a·cho·ret′·ic
an′·acid′·i·ty
anac′·la·sis
anac′·li·sis
an·a·clit′·ic
an′·a·crot′·ic
anac′·ro·tis′m
an′·a·cu′·sis *also*
·cou′·sia
an′a·di·crot′·ic
an′a·di′·cro·tis′m
anae′·mia *Brit. spel.
of* anemia
an′·aer·obe [an·aer′·obe]
an′·aer·o′·bic
an′·aero·bi·o′·sis [an·aer′o·]
an′·aer·o·gen′·ic [an·aer′·]
an′·aer·o′·sis
an′·aes·the′·sia *Brit.
spel. of* anesthesia
an′·aes·the′·si·ol′·o·gy
Brit. spel. of anesthesiology
an′·aes·thet′·ic *Brit.
spel. of* anesthetic
anaes′·the·tist *Brit.
spel. of* anesthetist
anaes′·the·tize *also*
·tise; ·tized *or* ·tised,
·tiz′·ing *or* ·tis′·ing;
Brit. spel. of
anesthetize
an′·a·gen
an′·a·go·cyt′·ic
an′·a·go·tox′·ic
an′·a·ku′·sis *var. of*
anacusis
a′nal
an′·a·lep′·tic

ana′·les *pl. of* analis
an′·al·ge′·sia
an′·al·ge′·sic
an′·al·get′·ic
an·al′·gia
an·al′·gic
ana′·lis *pl.* ·les
anal′·i·ty
an′·al·ler′·gic
anal′o·gous
an′·a·logue[7] *also* ·log
anal′·o·gy
an′·al′·pha·lip′o·pro′·tein·e′·mia [·li′po·]
Brit. ·ae′·mia
anal′·y·sand
an′·a·lyse ·lysed,
·lys′·ing; *Brit. spel. of*
analyze
an′·a·lys′·er *Brit.
spel. of* analyzer
anal′·y·sis *pl.* ·ses
an′·a·lyst
an′·a·lyte
an′·a·lyt′·ic *also* ·i·cal
an′·a·lyze ·lyzed,
·lyz′·ing; *Brit.* ·lyse,
·lysed, ·lys′·ing
an′·a·lyz′er
an′·am·ne′·sis *pl.* ·ses
an′·am·nes′·tic
an′·am·ni·ot′·ic
an′·an·kas′·tic *also*
·cas′·
an′a·phase
an′a·pho·ret′·ic
[anaph′·o·]
an′a·pho′·ria
an′·aph′·ro·dis′·i·ac
an′a·phy·lac′·tic
an′a·phy·lac′·tin
an′a·phy·lac′·to·gen
an′a·phy·lac′·to·gen′·ic
an′a·phy·lac′·toid
an′a·phy·lac′·to·tox′·in

an′a·phyl′a·tox′·in
also ·phyl′o·
an′a·phy·lax′·is
an′·a·pla′·sia
an′·a·plas·mo′·sis
an′·a·plas′·tic
an′·a·ple·rot′·ic
an·ap′·no·graph
an·ap′·tic
an·ar′·thria
an·ar′·thric
an′·a·sar′·ca
an′a·schis′·tic
an·as′·tig·mat′·ic
anas′·to·mose
·mosed, ·mos′·ing
anas′·to·mo′·sis *pl.*
·ses
anas′·to·mot′·ic
anas′·to·mot′·i·cus
fem. ·ca, *neut.* ·cum
an′·a·tom′·ic *also* ·i·cal
an′·a·tom′·i·co·path′·o·log′·ic *also* ·i·cal
an′·a·tom′·i·cus *fem.*
·ca, *neut. sg.* ·cum
anat′·o·mist
anat′·o·mo·pa·thol′·o·gy
anat′·o·my
an′a·tox′·ic
an′a·tox′·in
an′a·tox′i·re·ac′·tion
an′a·tri·crot′·ic
an′a·tro′·pia
an′a·tro′·pic [·trop′·ic]
an·az′·o·lene
an′·chor·age
an′·chy·lo· *var. of*
ankylo-
an′·cil′·lar′y [an·cil′·la·ry]
an′·co·nad
an′·co·nal [an·co′·]

---

[7] The spelling *analog* is preferred when contrasted with *digital*.

an·co′·ne·al
an·co′·ne·us *pl. &
   gen. sg.* ·nei
an′·co·ni′·tis
an′·cy·lo· *var. of*
   ankylo-
An′·cy·los′to·ma
A. bra·zil′·i·en′·se
A. ca·ni′·num
A. du·o′·de·na′·le
an·cyl′·o·stome
an′·cy·lo·sto·mi′·a·sis
[·los′·to·]
an′·dri·at′·rics
an·dri′·a·try
an′·dro·
an′·dro·blas·to′·ma
   pl. ·mas *or* ·ma·ta
an′·dr·ogen
an′·dro·gen′·e·sis
an′·dro·ge·net′·ic
an′·dro·gen′·ic
an′·dro·ge·nic′·i·ty
an·drog′·e·nize
   ·nized, ·niz′·ing
an·drog′·e·nous
an′·dro·gyne
an′·dro·gyn′·ic [·gy′·nic]
an·drog′·y·nous
an·drog′·y·ny
an′·droid
an·drol′·o·gy
an·drom′·e·do·tox′·in
an′·dro·mi·met′·ic
an′·dro·phil′·ic
an′·dro·stane
an′·dro·stane′·di·ol
an′·dro·stane′·di·one
an′·dro·stene′·di·ol
an′·dro·stene′·di·one
an·dros′·ter·one
an′·ec·dot′·al [·do′·tal]
an′·echo′·ic
an′·elec·tro·ton′·ic
an′·elec·trot′·o·nus
ane′·mia *Brit.* anae′·mia

ane′·mic *Brit.* anae′·mic
an·em′o· [an′·emo·]
anem′·o·nin
an′·en·ce·phal′·ic
an′·en·ceph′·a·lous
an′·en·ceph′·a·ly *also*
   ·ce·pha′·lia
an·en′·ter·ous
aneph′·ric
an·ep′·i·plo′·ic
an′·er·gas′·tic
an·er′·gia
an·er′·gic
an′·er·gize ·gized, ·giz′·ing
an′·er·gy
an′·er·oid
an′·er·y·throp′·sia
an·es′·the·ki·ne′·sia *also* ·ci·ne′·sia
an′·es·the′·sia *Brit.* ·aes·the′·; *pl.* ·si·ae *or* ·si·as
an′·es·the·sim′·e·ter
an′·es·the′·si·ol′·o·gist
an′·es·the′·si·ol′·o·gy
an′·es·thet′·ic
anes′·the·tist
anes′·the·ti·za′·tion
anes′·the·tize ·tized, ·tiz′·ing
an·es′·trous
an·es′·trus *also* ·trum
an′·e·to·der′·ma
an·eu′·ga·my
an′·eu·ploid
an′·eu·ploi′·dy
aneu′·ria
aneu′·ri·lem′·mic
aneu′·rin
aneurism *misspelling of*
   aneurysm
a′neu·ro·gen′·ic [aneu′·]
an′·eu·rys′m
an′·eu·rys′·mal
an′·eu·rys·mec′·to·my

an′·eu·rys·mog′·ra·phy
an′·eu·rys′·moid
an′·eu·rys′·mo·plas′·ty
an′·eu·rys·mor′·rha·phy
an·gei′·al
an·gel′·i·ca
an′·gi·ec·ta′·sia *also*
   ·ec′·ta·sis
an′·gi·ec·tat′·ic
an′·gi·ec′·to·my
an′·gi·i′tis
an·gi′·na [an′·gi·]
an′·gi·nal [an·gi′·]
an′·gi·noid
an′·gi·nose
an′·gi·no′·sus
an′·gi·nous
an′·gio·
an′·gio·ac′·cess
an′·gi·o·blast
an′·gio·blas·to′·ma
   pl. ·mas *or* ·ma·ta
an′·gio·car′·di·o·gram
an′·gio·car′·di·o·graph
an′·gio·car·di·og′·ra·phy
an′·gio·car′·dio·ki·net′·ic
an′·gio·car·di′·tis
an′·gio·cin·e·ma·tog′·ra·phy
an′·gio·cyst
an′·gio·der′·ma·ti′·tis
an′·gio·dys′·ge·net′·ic
an′·gio·dys·pla′·sia
an′·gio·dys′·tro·phy
   also ·dys·tro′·phia
an′·gio·ec·tat′·ic
an′·gio·ede′·ma
an′·gio·en′·do·the·li·o′·ma *pl.* ·mas *or* ·ma·ta
an′·gio·en′·do·the·li·o′·ma·to′·sis
an′·gio·fi′·bro·li·po′·ma
an′·gio·fi·bro′·ma *pl.* ·mas *or* ·ma·ta

an'·gio·fi·bro'·sis
an'·gio·fol·lic'·u·lar
an'·gio·gen'·e·sis
an'·gi·o·gen'·ic
an'·gi·o·gram
an'·gi·o·graph
an'·gi·o·graph'·ic
an'·gi·og'·ra·phy
an'·gi·o·gen'·ic
an'·gi·o·gram
an'·gi·o·graph
an'·gi·og'·ra·phy
an'·gio·hy·per·to'·nia
an'·gio·hy'·per·tro'·phic [·troph'·ic]
an'·gio·hy'·po·to'·nia
an'·gi·oid
an'·gio·ker'·a·to'·ma
  pl. ·mas or ·ma·ta
an'·gio·ker'·a·to'·sis
  pl. ·ses
an'·gio·lip'o·fi·bro'·ma [·li'po·]
an'·gio·lip'o·lei'o·my·o'·ma [·li'po·]
an'·gio·li·po'·ma pl. ·mas or ·ma·ta
an'·gi·o·lith'·ic
an'·gi·o·lo'·gia
an'·gi·o·log'·ic
an'·gi·ol'·o·gy
an'·gio·lym·phan'·gi·o'·ma
an'·gio·lym·pho'·ma
  pl. ·mas or ·ma·ta
an'·gi·ol'·y·sis
an'·gi·o'·ma pl. ·mas or ·ma·ta
an'·gi·o'·ma·to'·sa
an'·gi·o'·ma·to'·sis
an'·gi·om'a·tous [·o'ma·]
an'·gio·my'o·fi·bro'·ma
an'·gio·my'o·li·po'·ma
an'·gio·my'o·o'·ma pl. ·mas or ·ma·ta
an'·gio·my'o·neu·ro'·ma

an'·gio·my'o·sar·co'·ma
an'·gio·neu·rec'·to·my
an'·gio·neu'·ro·ede'·ma
  Brit. ·neu'·ro·oe·de'·
an'·gio·neu·ro'·ma
  pl. ·mas or ·ma·ta
an'·gio·neu·rop'·a·thy
an'·gio·neu·rot'·ic
an'·gio·oe·de'·ma
  Brit. spel. of angioedema
an'·gi·o·path'·ic
an'·gio·pa·thol'·o·gy
an'·gi·op'·a·thy
an'·gio·pha·ko'·ma·to'·sis also ·pha·co'·
an'·gi·o·plas'·tic
an'·gi·o·plas'·ty
an'·gio·poi·e'·sis
an'·gio·poi·et'·ic
an'·gio·pres'·sure
an'·gio·ret'·i·nog'·ra·phy
an'·gi·or'·rha·phy
an'·gio·sar·co'·ma pl. ·mas or ·ma·ta
an'·gi·os'·co·py
an'·gio·sco·to'·ma pl. ·mas or ·ma·ta
an'·gio·spas'm
an'·gio·spas'·tic
an'·gi·os'·to·my
an'·gio·stron'·gy·li'·a·sis
An'·gio·stron'·gy·lus
  A. can'·to·nen'·sis
an'·gi·o·ten'·sin
an'·gi·o·ten'·sin·ase
an'·gi·o·ten·sin'·o·gen
an'·gi·o·tome
an'·gio·to·mog'·ra·phy
an'·gi·ot'·o·my
an'·gio·ton'·ic
an'·gi·o·to'·nin
an·gi'·tis var. of angiitis
an'·gor

ang'·strom
an'·gu·la'·ris
an'·gu·la'·tion
an'·gu·lus pl. & gen. sg. ·li
an·hap'·to·glo'·bin·e'·mia Brit. ·ae'·mia
an'·he·do'·nia
an'·he·don'·ic
an·he'·mo·poi·e'·sis Brit. ·hae'·mo·
an·hep'·a·tog'·e·nous
an'·hi·dro'·sis
an'·hi·drot'·ic
an·hy'·drase
an'·hy·dra'·tion
an'·hy·dre'·mia Brit. ·drae'·mia
an·hy'·dride
an'·hy'·drite
an·hy'·dro·
an'·hy·drot'·ic
an·hy'·drous
a'ni gen. of anus
an'·ic·ter'·ic
anid'·e·us
an'·il·er'·i·dine
an'·i·lide
an'·i·line
a'ni·lin'·gus also ·linc'·tus
an'·i·lin·is'm
an'·i·lis'm also ·lin·is'm
an'·i·ma
an'·i·mal
an'·i·mal'·cule
an'·i·mus
an'·i'on
an'·ion'·ic
an'·irid'·ia
an'·i·sa·ki'·a·sis
An'·i·sa'·kis
an'·is·chu'·ria [·isch·u'·]
an·i'sei·ko'·nia
an·i'sei·kon'·ic
an·i'so·

anisochromatic / anorganic

an·i′so·chro·mat′·ic
an·i′so·chro′·mia
an·i′so·co′·ria
an·i′so·cy·to′·sis
an′·isog′·a·mous
an′·isog′·a·my
an·i′so·ico′·nia *var.
of* aniseikonia
an·i′so·mas′·tia
an·i′so·me′·lia
an·i′so·mel′·ic [·me′·lic]
an·i′so·met′·ric
an·i′so·me·tro′·pia
an·i′so·me·tro′·pic [·trop′·ic]
an·i′so·pho′·ria
an·i′so·poi′·ki·lo·cy·to′·sis
an·i′so·sthen′·ic [·i′sos·then′·]
an·i′so·ton′·ic
an·i′so·tro′·pic [·trop′·ic]
an′·isot′·ro·py
an′·kle
an′·ky·lo·
an′·ky·lo·bleph′·a·ron
an′·ky·lo·glos′·sia
an′·ky·lose ·losed, ·los′·ing
an′·ky·lo′·sis[8] *pl.* ·ses
an′·ky·lo·sto·mi′·a·sis *var. of* ancylostomiasis
an′·ky·lot′·ic
an′·ky·lot′·o·my
an′·ky·roid
an′·la·ge *pl.* an′·la·gen
an·neal′·ing
an·nec′·tens *pl.* an′·nec·ten′·tes
an′·ne·lid

An·nel′·i·da
an′·nu·lar
an′·nu·la′·re *neut. of* annularis
an′·nu·la′·ris *pl.* ·res
an′·nu·let
an′·nu·li *pl. & gen. sg. of* annulus
an′·nu·lo·plas′·ty
an′·nu·lor′·rha·phy
an′·nu·lot′·o·my
an′·nu·lus[9] *pl. & gen. sg.* ·li
a′no *ablative of* anus
a′no·
an′o·chro·ma′·sia [a′no·]
ano′·ci·as·so′·ci·a′·tion
a′no·coc·cyg′·e·al
a′no·coc·cyg′·e·um *neut. of* anococcygeus
a′no·coc·cyg′·e·us *pl.* ·ei
an·od′·al [·o′·dal]
an′·ode
an·od′·ic [·o′·dic]
an′·odon′·tia
an′·o·dyne
an′·o·e′·sis
an·oes′·trous *Brit. spel. of* anestrous
an·oes′·trus *Brit. spel. of* anestrus
an′·o·et′·ic
a′no·gen′·i·tal
anom′·a·lad
anom′·a·lo·scope
anom′·a·lous
anom′·a·ly
an′·o·mer
ano′·mia
anom′·ic [ano′·mic]

an′·o·mie
an·onych′·ia
anon′·y·ma
anon′·y·mous
a′no·pel′·vic
Anoph′·e·les
A. al′·bi·man′·us
A. di′·rus
A. fu·nes′·tus
A. gam′·bi·ae
A. la·bran′·chi·ae
A. mac′·u·li·pen′·nis
A. quad′·ri·mac′·u·la′·tus
anoph′·e·li·cide
anoph′·e·line
anoph′·e·lis′m
an′o·pho′·ria *var. of* anaphoria
an′·oph·thal′·mia
an′·oph·thal′·mic
an·o′·pia
a′no·plas′·ty
An′·o·plu′·ra
an·op′·sia
an·or′·chid
an′·or·chid′·ic
an·or′·chism *also* ·chi·dis′m
a′no·rec′·tal *involving anus and rectum: Cf.* anorectic
an′·orec′·tic *involving lack of appetite: Cf.* anorectal
an′·oret′·ic *var. of* anorectic
an′·orex′·ia
an′·orex′·i·ant
an′·orex′·ic
an·orex′·i·gen′·ic
an′·or·gan′·ic

---

[8] In contrast to the plural form of the noun, the 3rd person singular of the verb *ankylose* is divided *an′·ky·los′·es*.

[9] The spelling *anulus* is the correct Latin form and is preferred in the Nomina Anatomica, but the double *n* is common in both clinical and anatomical usage and is reinforced by related terms such as *annular* and *annuloplasty*.

an'·or·tho'·pia
a'no·scro'·tal
an·os'·mia
an·os'·mic
ano'·sog·no'·sia
ano'·sog·no'·sic
an'·os·phre'·sia   also
   ·phra'·sia
a'no·spi'·nal
an'·os·to'·sis
an·o'·tia
an'o·tro'·pia   var. of
   anatropia
a'no·vag'·i·nal [·va·gi'·nal]
an·ov'u·lar [·o'vu·]
an·ov'u·la'·tion [·o'vu·]
an·ov'u·la·to'·ry [·o'vu·]
an'·ox·e'·mia   Brit.
   ·ae'·mia
an'·ox·e'·mic   Brit.
   ·ae'·mic
an·ox'·ia
an·ox'·ic
an'·sa   pl. & gen. sg.
   an'·sae
an'·sate
an'·ser·i'·nus   fem. ·na
an'·si·form
an·sot'·o·my
ant·ac'·id
an·tag'·o·nis'm
an·tag'·o·nist
an·tag'·o·nis'·tic
an·tal'·gic
ant'·an·al·ge'·sia
ant'·ar·thrit'·ic
ant'·asth·mat'·ic
an·taz'·o·line
an'·te
an'·te·
an'·te·bra'·chi·al
an'·te·bra'·chi·a'·lis
an'·te·bra'·chi·um   pl.
   ·bra'·chia, gen. sg.
   ·bra'·chii
an'·te·car'·di·um

an'·te ci'·bum [cib'·um]
an'·te·co'·lic
an'·te·cu'·bi·tal
an'·te·flex'·ion
an'·te·grade
ant'·emet'·ic
an'·te mor'·tem   adv.
an'·te·mor'·tem   adj.
an'·te·na'·tal
an·ten'·na   pl. ·nae
an'·te·par'·tal
an'·te·par'·tum
an'·te pran'·di·um
ant'·ereth'·ic
an·te'·ri·ad
an·te'·ri·or   pl. ·ri·o'·res, gen. sg. ·ri·o'·ris, gen. pl. ·ri·o'·rum
an·te'·ri·us   neut. of anterior; pl. ·ri·o'·ra
an'·tero·
an'·tero·clu'·sion
an'·ter·o·grade
an'·tero·in·fe'·ri·or
an'·tero·lat'·er·al
an'·tero·lat'·er·a'·lis
an'·tero·me'·di·al
an'·tero·me'·di·an
an'·tero·pos·te'·ri·or
an'·tero·pul'·sion
an'·tero·sep'·tal
an'·tero·su·pe'·ri·or
an'·te·ver'·sion
ant·he'·lix   pl. ·hel'·i·ces, gen. sg. ·hel'·i·cis
an'·thel·min'·tic [ant'·hel·]   also ·min'·thic
ant·hem'·or·rhag'·ic Brit. ·haem'·; var. of antihemorrhagic
ant'·her·pet'·ic   var. of antiherpetic
an'·thi·o'·li·mine
an'·thra·cene
an·thrac'·ic
an'·thra·co·
an'·thra·coid

an'·thra·co'·ma
an'·thra·co·ne·cro'·sis
an'·thra·co·sil'·i·co'·sis
an'·thra·co'·sis
an'·thra·cot'·ic
an'·thra·lin
an'·thra·my'·cin
an·thran'·i·late
an'·thra·nil'·ic
an'·thrax
an'·throne
an'·thro·po·
an'·thro·po·bi·ol'·o·gy
an'·thro·po·cen'·tric
an'·thro·po·cen'·trism
an'·thro·po·gen'·ic
an'·thro·poid
An'·thro·poi'·dea
an'·thro·po·log'·ic
   also ·i·cal
an'·thro·pol'·o·gist
an'·thro·pol'·o·gy
an'·thro·pom'·e·ter
an'·thro·po·met'·ric
an'·thro·pom'·e·try
an'·thro·po·mor'·phic
an'·thro·po·mor'·phism
an'·thro·po·no'·sis
an'·thro·po·not'·ic
an'·thro·po·phil'·ic
   also ·poph'·i·lous
an'·thro·po·zo'·o·no'·sis
an'·thro·po·zo'·o·phil'·ic
an'·ti·
an'·ti·abor'·ti·fa'·cient
an'·ti·ad'·re·ner'·gic
an'·ti·al·ler'·gic
an'·ti·ame'·bic   also ·amoe'·
an'·ti·ane'·mia   Brit. ·anae'·
an'·ti·ane'·mic   Brit. ·anae'·
an'·ti·an'·gi·nal [·an·gi'·nal]
an'·ti·an'·ti·bod'y

an'·ti·ar·rhyth'·mic
an'·ti·ar·thrit'·ic
an'·ti·ath'·er·o·gen'·ic
an'·ti·bac·te'·ri·al
an'·ti·bi·o'·sis
an'·ti·bi·ot'·ic
an'·ti·bod'y
an'·ti·bra'·chi·al var.
  of antebrachial
an'·ti·bra'·chi·um
  var. of antebrachium
an'·ti·bro'·mic
an'·ti·ca·chec'·tic
an'·ti·car·cin'·o·gen
  [·car'·ci·no·]
an'·ti·car'·ci·no·gen'·ic
an'·ti·car'·di·um var.
  of antecardium
an'·ti·ca·thex'·is
an'·ti·ceph'·a·lal'·gic
an'·ti·car'·i·ous
an'·ti·chlo·rot'·ic
an'·ti·cho'·lin·er'·gic
an·tic'·i·pate   ·pat'·ed,
  ·pat'·ing
an·tic'·i·pa'·tion
an'·ti·cli'·nal
an'·ti·cne'·mi·on
an'·ti·co·ag'·u·lant
an'·ti·co·ag'·u·la·tive
an'·ti·co'·don
an'·ti·com'·ple·men'·ta·ry
an'·ti·con·vul'·sant
  [·vuls'·ant]
an'·ti·con·vul'·sive
an·ti'·cus
an'·ti·de·pres'·sant
an'·ti·di'·a·bet'·ic
an'·ti·di'·ar·rhe'·al
  also ·rhe'·ic; Brit.
  ·rhoe'·
an'·ti·di'·u·re'·sis
an'·ti·di'·u·ret'·ic
an'·ti·dot'·al [·do'·tal]
an'·ti·dote
an'·ti·drom'·ic [·dro'·mic]

an'·ti·dys'·en·ter'·ic
an'·ti·edem'·a·tous
an'·ti·emet'·ic
an'·ti·en'·zyme
an'·ti·ep'·i·lep'·tic
an'·ti·ep'·i·the'·li·al
an'·ti·fe'·brile [·feb'·rile]
an'·ti·fer·til'·i·ty
an'·ti·fi'·bril·la·to'·ry
an'·ti·fi'·bri·no·ly'·sin
an'·ti·fi'·bri·no·lyt'·ic
an'·ti·fi·lar'·i·al
an'·ti·flat'·u·lent
an'·ti·fun'·gal
an'·ti·gen
an'·ti·gen·e'·mia Brit.
  ·ae'·mia
an'·ti·gen'·ic
an'·ti·ge·nic'·i·ty
an'·ti·glob'·u·lin
an'·ti·go·nad'·o·tro'·pic
  [·gon'·a·do·, ·trop'·ic]
an'·ti·go·nad'·o·tro'·pin
  [·gon'·a·do·]
an'·ti·grav'·i·ty
an'·ti·growth'
an'·ti·he'·lix var. of
  anthelix
an'·ti·hel·min'·tic
  var. of anthelmintic
an'·ti·he'·mo·lyt'·ic
an'·ti·hem'·or·rhag'·ic
  Brit. ·haem'·
an'·ti·hi·drot'·ic
an'·ti·his'ta·mine
an'·ti·his'·ta·min'·ic
an'·ti·hy·drop'·ic
an'·ti·hy'·per·cho·les'·ter·ol·e'·mic Brit.
  ·ae'·mic
an'·ti·hy'·per·gly·ce'·mic Brit. ·cae'·mic
an'·ti·hy'·per·ten'·sive
an'·ti·im·mune'
an'·ti·in·fec'·tive also
  ·tious

an'·ti·in·flam'·ma·to'·ry
an'·ti·ke'·to·gen'·ic
an'·ti·lar'·val
an'·ti·leish·man'·i·al
an'·ti·le·prot'·ic
an'·ti·leu·ke'·mic
  Brit. ·kae'·mic
an'·ti·lew'·is·ite
an'·ti·li·pe'·mic Brit.
  ·pae'·mic
an'·ti·lith'·ic
an'·ti·lu·et'·ic
an'·ti·lym'·pho·cyte
an'·ti·lym'·pho·cyt'·ic
an'·ti·ly'·sin
an'·ti·ly'·sis
an'·ti·ma·lar'·i·al
an'·ti·me·nin'·go·coc'·cal also ·coc'·cic
an'·ti·men'·or·rhag'·ic
an'·ti·me·tab'·o·lite
an'·ti·mi·cro'·bi·al
  also ·cro'·bic
an'·ti·mi·tot'·ic
an'·ti·mo'·ni·al
an'·ti·mo'·ny
an·tim'·o·nyl·tar'·trate
an'·ti·morph
an'·ti·mor'·phic
an'·ti·mus'·ca·rin'·ic
an'·ti·mu'·ta·gen
an'·ti·mu'·ta·gen'·ic
an'·ti·mu'·ta·tor
an'·ti·my'·as·then'·ic
an'·ti·my·cot'·ic
an'·ti·nar·cot'·ic
an'·ti·na'·tal·is'm
an'·ti·nau'·se·ant
an'·ti·ne'·o·plas'·tic
an'·ti·neu·rit'·ic
an'·ti·no'·ci·cep'·tive
an'·ti·nu'·cle·ar
an'·ti·oe·dem'·a·tous
  Brit. spel. of anti-
  edematous
an'·ti·ov'u·la·to'·ry
  [·o'vu·]
an'·ti·ox'·i·dant

an'·ti·par'·a·lyt'·ic
an'·ti·par'·kin·son
an'·ti·par'·kin·so'·ni·an
an'·ti·pa·thet'·ic
an'·ti·pe·dic'·u·lar
an'·ti·pe·dic'·u·lot'·ic
an'·ti·pe'·ri·od'·ic
an'·ti·per'·i·stal'·sis
an'·ti·per'·i·stal'·tic
an'·ti·per'·spi·rant
an'·ti·phag'·o·cyt'·ic
an'·ti·phlo·gis'·tic
an'·ti·phthi'·ri·ac[10]
an'·ti·plas'·min
an'·ti·plas·mo'·di·al
an'·ti·plas'·tic
an'·ti·plate'·let
an'·ti·pneu'·mo·coc'·cal *also* ·coc'·cic
an·tip'·o·dal
an'·ti·port
an'·ti·pro·throm'·bin
an'·ti·pru·rit'·ic
an'·ti·pso'·ri·at'·ic
an'·ti·psy·chot'·ic
an'·ti·pthi'·ri·ac[11]
an'·ti·py'·o·gen'·ic
an'·ti·py·re'·sis
an'·ti·py·ret'·ic
an'·ti·ra'·bic
an'·ti·ra'·bies
an'·ti·ra·chit'·ic
an'·ti·re·tic'·u·lar
an'·ti·rheu·mat'·ic
an'·ti·rick·ett'·si·al
an'·ti·sca'·bi·et'·ic
an'·ti·schis'·to·so'·mal
an'·ti·scor·bu'·tic
an'·ti·seb'·or·rhe'·ic *Brit.* ·rhoe'·ic
an'·ti·se·cre'·to·ry
an'·ti·self'
an'·ti·sense

an'·ti·sep'·sis
an'·ti·sep'·tic
an'·ti·sep'·ti·cize ·cized, ·ciz'·ing
an'·ti·se'·rum *pl.* ·se'·ra *or* ·se'·rums
an'·ti·si·al'·a·gog'·ic [·si'·a·la·]
an'·ti·si·al'·a·gogue [·si'·a·la·]
an'·ti·si·al'·ic
an'·ti·spas·mod'·ic
an'·ti·spas'·tic
an'·ti·staph'·y·lo·coc'·cal *also* ·coc'·cic
an'·ti·ste·ril'·i·ty
an'·ti·strep'·to·coc'·cal *also* ·coc'·cic
an'·ti·strep'·to·ly'·sin
an'·ti·su'·do·rif'·ic
an'·ti·syph'·i·lit'·ic
an'·ti·te·tan'·ic
an'·ti·the'·nar [an·tith'·e·nar]
an'·ti·throm'·bin
an'·ti·throm'·bo·plas'·tin
an'·ti·throm·bot'·ic
an'·ti·thy'·ro·glob'·u·lin
an'·ti·thy'·roid
an'·ti·thy'·ro·tox'·ic
an'·ti·tox'·ic
an'·ti·tox'·in
an'·ti·tox·in'·o·gen
an'·ti·trag'·i·cus *pl.* ·ci
an'·ti·tra'·go·hel'·i·cine
an'·ti·tra'·go·hel'·i·ci'·na
an'·ti·tra'·gus *pl.* ·gi
an'·ti·trep'·o·ne'·mal
an'·ti·try·pan'·o·so'·mal

an'·ti·tryp'·sin
an'·ti·tryp'·tic
an'·ti·tu·ber'·cu·lot'·ic
an'·ti·tu·ber'·cu·lous
an'·ti·tu'·mor *Brit.* ·mour
an'·ti·tu'·mor·i·gen'·ic
an'·ti·tus'·sive
an'·ti·urat'·ic
an'·ti·ven'·in
an'·ti·vi'·ral
an'·ti·xer'·oph·thal'·mic
an'·tra *pl. of* antrum
an'·tral
an·trec'·to·my
an·tri'·tis
an'·tro·
an'·tro·du·o·de·nec'·to·my
an'·tro·my·co'·sis
an'·tro·na'·sal
an·trorse' [an'·trorse]
an'·tro·scope
an'·tro·stome
an·tros'·to·my
an·trot'·o·my
an'·tro·tym·pan'·ic
an'·trum *pl.* an'·tra, *gen. sg.* an'·tri
anu'·cle·ar
anu'·cle·ate
an'·u·lus[12] *pl. & gen. sg.* ·li
anu'·ran
an'·ure'·sis
an'·uret'·ic
an·u'·ria
a'nus *gen.* a'ni, *ablative* a'no, *accusative* a'num
anx·i'·ety
anx'·i·o·lyt'·ic

---

10 See footnote at *Pthirus*.
11 See footnote at *Pthirus*.
12 See footnote at *annulus*.

aor′·ta *gen.* aor′·tae
aor′·tic
aor′·ti·ca *fem. sg. &
neut. pl. of* aorticus
aor′·ti·co·pul′·mo·nar′y
aor′·ti·co·re′·nal
aor′·ti·co·re·na′·le *pl.*
·lia
aor′·ti·cus *pl. & gen.
sg.* ·ci
a′or·ti′·tis
aor′·to·ca′·val
aor′·to·gram
aor′·to·graph′·ic
a′or·tog′·ra·phy
aor′·to·pul′·mo·nar′y
aor′·to·sub·cla′·vi·an
a′or·tot′·o·my
apal′·les·the′·sia *Brit.*
·laes·
a′pa·min
a′par·a·lyt′·ic
a′para·thy′·roid·is′m
ap′·ar·thro′·sis
ap′·a·thet′·ic
ap′·a·thy
ap′·a·tite
ap′·a·zone
a′pep·sin′·ia
ape′·ri·ent
a′pe·ri·od′·ic
aper′·i·tive
aper′·ta
ap′·er·tu′·ra *pl. &
gen. sg.* ·rae
ap′·er·ture
a′pex *pl.* ap′i·ces, *gen.
sg.* ap′i·cis
a′pex·car′·di·o·gram
a′pex·car′·di·og′·ra·phy
apha′·gia
aph′·ake
apha′·kia
apha′·kic
a′pha·lan′·gia
apha′·sia
apha′·si·ac
apha′·sic

apha′·si·ol′·o·gist
apha′·si·ol′·o·gy
aph′er·e′·sis [apher′·e·
sis]
apho′·nia
aphon′·ic [apho′·nic]
aphose′
aphos′·pho·ro′·sis
aphra′·sia
aph′·ro·dis′·i·ac
aph′·thae *sg.* aph′·tha
aph·tho′·sa
aph·tho′·sis
aph′·thous
ap′i·cal [a′pi·cal]
ap′·i·ca′·le *neut. of*
apicalis
ap′·i·ca′·lis *pl.* ·les
a′pi·cec′·to·my [ap′·i·]
var. of apicoectomy
ap′i·ces [a′pi·] *pl. of*
apex
ap′i·cis *gen. of* apex
ap′i·co· [a′pi·co·]
ap′i·co·ec′·to·my
ap′i·col′·y·sis
Ap′i·com·plex′a
ap′i·co·pos·te′·ri·or
gen. ·ri·o′·ris
ap′i·cos′·to·my
ap′i·ec′·to·my [a′pi·]
var. of apicoectomy
a′pio·ther′·a·py
a′pi·sin
a′pi·tu′·i·tar·is′m
a′pla·cen′·tal
ap′·la·nat′·ic
aplan′o·gam′·ete [·ga·
mete′]
apla′·sia
aplas′·tic
apleu′·ria
ap′·nea [ap·ne′a]
Brit. ·noea
ap·ne′·ic *Brit.* ·noe′·ic
ap·neu′·sis
ap′o·at′·ro·pine
ap′o·can′·no·side

ap′·o·chro′·mat
ap′o·chro·mat′·ic
ap′·o·cop′·tic
ap′·o·crine
apoc′·y·nin
Apoc′·y·num
ap′·o·dal
apo′·dia *also* ap′·o·dy
ap′·o·dous
ap′o·en′·zyme
ap′·o·gee
apo′·lar
ap′o·lip′o·pro′·tein
[·li′po·]
ap′·o·mix′·is
ap′o·mor′·phine
ap′·o·neu·rec′·to·my
ap′·o·neu·ror′·rha·phy
ap′·o·neu·ro′·sis *pl.*
·ses
ap′·o·neu·ro·si′·tis
ap′·o·neu·rot′·ic
ap′·o·neu·rot′·i·ca
ap′·o·neu′·ro·tome
ap′·o·neu·rot′·o·my
apoph′·y·sate
ap′·o·phys′·e·al
[apoph′·y·se′·al]
var. of apophysial
ap′·o·phys′·i·al
ap′·o·phys′·i·ar′y
apoph′·y·sis *pl.* ·ses
apoph′·y·si′·tis
ap′·o·plas·mat′·ic
ap′·o·plec′·tic
ap′·o·plec′·ti·form
ap′·o·plec′·toid
ap′·o·plex′y
ap′o·pro′·tein
ap′o·re·pres′·sor
ap′·o·some
apos′·ta·sis
apos′·thia
ap′·o·tha·na′·sia
apoth′·e·car′y
ap′·o·them *also*
·theme
ap′·ox·em′·e·na

apox′·e·sis
ap′·o·zem *also* ·zeme
  or apoz′·e·ma
ap′·pa·ra′·to·ther′·a·py
  [·rat′o·]
ap·pa·ra′·tus
ap·pend′·age
ap′·pen·dec′·to·my
ap·pen′·di·cal
ap·pen′·di·ce′·al
  [ap′pen·di′·ceal] *also*
  ap·pen′·di·cal *or* ap′·
  pen·di′·cial
ap·pen′·di·ces *pl. of*
  appendix
ap·pen′·di·cis *gen. of*
  appendix
ap·pen′·di·ci′·tis
ap·pen′·di·co·
ap·pen′·di·col′·y·sis
  [·co·ly′·sis]
ap·pen′·di·cos′·to·my
ap′·pen·dic′·u·lar
ap′·pen·dic′·u·la′·ris
ap·pen′·dix *pl.* ·dix·es
  or ·di·ces, *gen.* ·di·cis
ap′·per·cep′·tion
ap′·pe·stat
ap′·pe·tite
ap′·pe·ti′·tive [ap·pet′·
  i·tive]
ap′·pla·nate
ap′·pla·na′·tion
ap′·pla·nom′·e·ter
ap·pli′·ance
ap′·pli·ca′·tion
ap′·pli·ca′·tor
ap·plied′
ap·pose′ ·posed′,
  ·pos′·ing
ap′·po·site
ap′·po·si′·tion
ap·prais′·al
ap′·pre·hen′·sion
ap′·pre·hen′·sive·ness
ap·prox′·i·mal
ap·prox′·i·mate
ap·prox′·i·ma′·tor

aprac′·tic
aprac′·tog·no′·sia
aprax′·ia
aprax′·ic
ap′·ro·bar′·bi·tal
aproc′·tia
ap′·ro·sex′·ia
ap′ro·so′·pia [a′pro·]
apro′·tic
ap′·ti·tude
ap·ty′·a·lis′m [apty′·]
ap′·ud·o′·ma
ap′·u·lo′·sis *pl.* ·ses
ap′·u·lot′·ic
a′pus
apyk′·no·mor′·phous
ap′·y·rase
a′py·ret′·ic
a′py·rex′·ia
a′py·rex′·i·al
aq′ua *pl.* aq′·uae
aq′·uae·duc′·tus *var.*
  of aqueductus
aq′·ue·duct
aq′·ue·duc′·tus *pl. &*
  gen. sg. aqueductus
a′que·ous [aq′·ue·ous]
aquo′·sus
ar′·a·bic
arab′·i·nose
ar′·a·bin′·o·side [arab′·
  i·no·]
arab′·i·tol
arach′·i·don′·ic
arach′·nid
Arach′·ni·da
arach′·nid·is′m
ar′·ach·ni′·tis
arach′·no·
arach′·no·dac′·ty·ly
arach′·noid
ar′·ach·noi′·dal
ar′·ach·noi′·dea *fem.*
  of arachnoideus
ar′·ach·noi′·de·a′·lis
  pl. ·les
ar′·ach·noi′·de·us
arach′·noid·i′·tis

ar′·ach·nol′·y·sin
  [arach′·no·ly′·sin]
ara′·ne·o′·sus
ara′·ne·us
ar′·bor
ar′·bo·res′·cent
ar′·bo·ri·za′·tion
ar′·bo·vi′·rus *also* ar′·
  bor·
ar·bu′·tin
arc
ar·cade′
arch
Ar′·chae·bac·te′·ria
ar·cha′·ic
arch′·en·ceph′·a·lon
arch·en′·ter·on
ar′·che·typ′·al
ar′·che·type
ar′·chi·cor′·tex
ar′·chi·gon′·o·cyte
ar′chil
ar′·chi·pal′·li·um
ar′·chi·tec·ton′·ics
ar′·cho·cele
ar′·ci·form
arc·ta′·tion
ar′·cu·a′·ta *fem. of*
  arcuatus; *pl.* ·tae
ar′·cu·ate
ar′·cu·a′·tion
ar′·cu·a′·tus *fem.* ·ta,
  neut. ·tum
ar′·cus *pl. & gen. sg.*
  arcus
a′rea *L. pl. & gen. sg.*
  a′re·ae
a′re·a′·tus *fem.* ·ta,
  neut. ·tum
a′re·flex′·ia
a′re·flex′·ic
ar′·e·na′·ceous
are′·na·vi′·rus
are′·o·la *pl.* ·lae
are′·o·lar
ar′·e·o·la′·ris *pl.* ·res
ar′·e·o·la′·ta
are′·o·late

areolitis / arthroclasia 24

ar′·e·o·li′·tis
ar′·e·om′·e·ter
ar′·e·o·met′·ric
Ar′·gas
ar·gas′·id
Ar·gas′·i·dae
ar·gen′·taf·fin
ar·gen′·taf·fin·o′·ma [·fi·no′·]
ar′·gen·ta′·tion
ar·gen′·to·
ar·gen′·to·phil′·ic
ar′·gi·nase
ar′·gi·nine
ar′·gi·nin·e′·mia [·ni·ne′·] Brit. ·ae′·mia
ar′·gi·ni′·no·suc′·ci·nate
ar′·gi·ni′·no·suc·cin′·ic
ar·gi·ni′·no·suc·cin′·ic·ac′·id·u′·ria
ar′·gon
ar·gyr′·ia also ar′·gy·ris′m
ar′·gy·ri′·a·sis
ar′·gy·ro·phil
ar′·gy·ro′·sis
arhin′·en·ceph′·a·ly [arhi′·nen·] var. of arrhinencephaly
arhi′·nia var. of arrhinia
ari′·bo·fla′·vin·o′·sis
ar′·i·do·sil′·i·qua′·ta
arith′·mo·ma′·nia
ar′·ma·men·tar′·i·um pl. ·ia
Ar·mig′·e·res
arm′·pit
ar′·o·mat′·ic
aro′·ma·ti·za′·tion
arous′·al
ar′·o·yl
ar·rache·ment′
ar·ray′
ar·rec′·tor pl. ar′·rec·to′·res
ar·rest′

ar·rha′·phia
ar·rhe′·no· [ar′·rhe·no·]
ar·rhe′·no·blas·to′·ma pl. ·mas or ·ma·ta
ar′·rhe·no′·ma pl. ·mas or ·ma·ta
ar′·rhe·not′·o·ky
ar·rhin′·en·ceph′·a·ly
ar·rhi′·nia
ar·rhi′·no·ceph′·a·ly
ar·rhyth′·mia
ar·rhyth′·mic
ar′·row·root′
ar′·sa·nil′·ic
ar′·se·nate
ar′·se·nic n.
ar·sen′·ic adj.
ar·sen′·i·cal
ar·sen′·i·cal·is′m
ar′·se·nide
ar·se′·ni·ous
ar′·se·nite
ar′·se·no·ben·zene′
ar′·se·no·cep′·tor [ar·sen′·o·]
ar′·se·nol′·y·sis
ar′·se·no·re·sis′·tant
ar′·se·no·ther′·a·py
ar′·se·nous var. of arsenious
ar′·sen·ox′·ide
ar′·sine
ars·phen′·a·mine
ar′·te·fact var. of artifact
ar′·te·fac′·ta
ar′·te·fac·ti′·tious var. of artifactitious
ar′·te·re′·nol
ar·te′·ria pl. & gen. sg. ·ri·ae, gen. pl. ·ri·a′·rum
ar·te′·ri·al
ar·te′·ri·al·i·za′·tion
ar·te′·rio·
ar·te′·rio·cap′·il·lar′y
ar·te′·rio·di·lat′·ing
ar·te′·rio·gen′·e·sis

ar·te′·ri·o·gram
ar·te′·ri·o·graph
ar·te′·ri·og′·ra·phy
ar·te′·ri·o′·la pl. ·lae
ar·te′·ri·o′·lar
ar·te′·ri·ole
ar·te′·ri·o·lith
ar·te′·ri·o·li′·tis
ar·te′·ri·o′·lo·ne·cro′·sis
ar·te′·ri·o′·lo·scle·ro′·sis
ar·te′·ri·o′·lo·scle·rot′·ic
ar·te′·ri·o′·lo·ve′·nous
ar·te′·ri·o′·lo·ven′·u·lar
ar·te′·rio·mo′·tor
ar·te′·rio·neph′·ro·scle·ro′·sis
ar·te′·ri·op′·a·thy
ar·te′·ri·or′·rha·phy
ar·te′·ri·or·rhex′·is
ar·te′·rio·scle·ro′·sis
ar·te′·rio·scle·rot′·ic
ar·te′·ri·o′·si pl. of arteriosus
ar·te′·ri·os′·i·ty
ar·te′·rio·spas′m
ar·te′·rio·spas′·tic
ar·te′·rio·ste·no′·sis
ar·te′·ri·o′·sum neut. of arteriosus
ar·te′·ri·o′·sus pl. ·si
ar·te′·ri·ot′·o·my
ar·te′·rio·ve′·nous
ar′·ter·i′·tis
ar′·tery
ar·thral′·gia
ar·thral′·gic
ar·threc′·to·my
ar·thrit′·ic
ar·thrit′·i·cum
ar·thri′·tis pl. ar·thrit′·i·des
ar′·thro·
ar·throc′·a·ce
ar′·thro·cen·te′·sis
ar′·thro·cla′·sia

ar'·thro·cli'·sis
Ar'·thro·der'·ma
ar·throd'·e·sis [ar'·
  thro·de'·sis]
ar·thro'·dia
ar·thro'·di·al
ar'·thro·dys·pla'·sia
ar'·thro·erei'·sis
ar·throg'·e·nous
ar'·thro·gram
ar'·thro·graph
ar'·thro·graph'·ic
ar·throg'·ra·phy
ar'·thro·gry·po'·sis
ar'·thro·hy'·al
ar'·thro·klei'·sis   var.
  of arthroclisis
ar'·thro·lith
ar'·thro·li·thi'·a·sis
ar'·thro·lo'·gia
ar·throl'·o·gy
ar·throl'·y·sis
ar·throm'·e·ter
ar·throm'·e·try
ar'·thro-oph'·thal·
  mop'·a·thy
ar'·thro-os'·teo-on'·y·
  cho·dys·pla'·sia
ar·throp'·a·thy
ar'·thro·pho·nom'·e·try
ar'·thro·phyte
ar'·thro·plas'·ty
ar'·thro·pneu'·mo·
  roent'·gen·og'·ra·phy
ar'·thro·pod
Ar·throp'·o·da
ar'·thro·scope
ar'·thro·scop'·ic
ar·thros'·co·py
ar·thro'·sis
ar'·thro·spore
ar'·thro·tome
ar'·thro·to·mog'·ra·phy
ar·throt'·o·my
ar'·thro·tro'·pic [·trop'·
  ic]
ar·throx'·e·sis
ar·tic'·u·lar

ar·tic'·u·la'·re   neut.
  of articularis; pl. ·ria
ar·tic'·u·la'·ris   pl. ·res
ar·tic'·u·late
ar·tic'·u·la'·tio   pl. ·ti·
  o'·nes, gen. sg. ·ti·o'·
  nis, gen. pl. ·ti·o'·num
ar·tic'·u·la'·tion
ar·tic'·u·la'·tor
ar·tic'·u·la·to'·ry
ar·tic'·u·lus   pl. & gen.
  sg. ·li, ablative ·lo
ar'·ti·fact
ar'·ti·fac'·tu·al
ar'·y·ep·i·glot'·tic
ar'·y·ep·i·glot'·ti·cus
  fem. ·ca
ar'·yl
ar'·yl·es'ter·ase
ar'·y·te'·no·ep·i·glot'·
  tic
ar'·y·te'·noid
ar'·y·te·noi'·dea   fem.
  of arytenoideus; pl. &
  gen. sg. ·de·ae
ar'·y·te·noi'·de·us
ar'·y·te'·noid·ec'·to·my
ar'·y·te·noi'·de·us
ar'·y·te'·noid·i'·tis
ar'·y·te·noi'·do·pex'y
ar'y·vo·ca'·lis
as'·a·fet'·i·da   also
  foet'·
as'·a·rum
as·bes'·tos
as'·bes·to'·sis
as·bol'·i·cum
as'·ca·ri'·a·sis
as·car'·i·cide
as'·ca·rid
As·car'·i·dae
as·car'·i·di'·a·sis [as'·
  ca·ri·] var. of
  ascariasis
As'·ca·rid'·i·dae
as·car'·i·do'·sis [as'·ca·
  ri·]   var. of ascariasis
As'·ca·ris

A. lum'·bri·coi'·des
As'·ca·rops
as·cen'·dens   pl. as'·
  cen·den'·tes, gen. sg.
  as'·cen·den'·tis
as·cen'·sus
Asc'·hel·min'·thes
  [As'·chel·]
as'·ci   pl. of ascus
as·ci'·tes
as·cit'·ic
as'·ci·tog'·e·nous
as·cog'·e·nous
as'·co·my'·cete [·my·
  cete']
As'·co·my·ce'·tes
as'·co·my·ce'·tous
ascor'·bate
ascor'·bic
as'·co·sin
as'·cus   pl. ·ci
a'se·cre'·to·ry
ase'·mia
asep'·sis
asep'·tate
asep'·tic
asep'·ti·cis'm
ase'·quence
asex'·u·al
a'sex·u·al'·i·ty
asex'·u·al·i·za'·tion
a'si·a'·lia
asi'·a·lor·rhe'a   Brit.
  ·rhoe'a
asid'·er·o'·sis
aso'·cial
aso'·ma   pl. aso'·ma·ta
aso'·ma·tog·no'·sia
aso'·mus
aso'·nia
Aso'pia
as·par'·a·gi·nase
as·par'·a·gine
as·par'·tame [as'·par·]
as·par'·tase [as'·par·]
as·par'·tate [as'·par·]
as·par'·tic
as·par'·to·cin

as·par′·to·ki′·nase
as·par′·tyl·gly′·cos·ami·
nu′·ria [·amin·u′·]
aspas′·tic
as′·pect
as′·per
as′per·gil′·li   pl. of
aspergillus
as′·per·gil′·lic
as′·per·gil′·lin
as′·per·gil·lo′·ma   pl.
·mas or ·ma·ta
as′·per·gil′·lo·my·co′·
sis
as′·per·gil·lo′·sis
As′·per·gil′·lus
A. fla′·vus
A. fu′·mi·ga′·tus
A. par′·a·sit′·i·cus
as′·per·gil′·lus   pl. ·li
asper′·ma·tis′m
a′sper′·ma·to·gen′·e·sis
[a′sper·mat′o·]
asper′·mia
as′·per·ous
aspher′·ic   also ·i·cal
as·phyx′·ia
as·phyx′·i·al
as·phyx′·i·ant
as·phyx′·i·ate   ·at′·ed,
·at′·ing
as·phyx′·i·a′·tion
as·pid′·i·um
as′·pi·do·sper′·ma
as′·pi·do·sper′·mine
as′·pi·rate   ·rat′·ed,
·rat′·ing
as′·pi·ra′·tion
as′·pi·ra′·tor
as′·pi·rin
asple′·nia
asplen′·ic
as′·po·ro·gen′·ic
[a′spo·]
as′·po·rog′·e·nous
[a′spo·]
aspor′·u·late
as·sault′
as·saul′·tive
as′·say [as·say′]
as·sess′·ment
as′·si·dent
as·sign′·ment
as·sim′·i·la·ble
as·sim′·i·la′·tion
as·sis′·tant [·sist′·ant]
as·so′·ci·ate   ·at′·ed,
·at′·ing
as·so′·ci·a′·tion
as·so′·ci·a·tive
as·so′·ci·us
as′·so·nance
as·sort′·ment
asta′·sia
asta′·sia-aba′·sia
astat′·ic
as′·ta·tine
as′·ter
aste′·reo·cog′·no·sy
aste′·re·og·no′·sis
as·te′·ric
as·te′·ri·on   pl. ·ria
as′·ter·ix′·is
aster′·nal
aster′·nia
as′·ter·oid
as·the′·nia
as·then′·ic
as′·the·no·co′·ria [as·
the′·no·]
as′·the·nom′·e·ter
as′·the·no′·pia
as′·the·no′·pic
as′·the·no·sper′·mia
asth′·ma
asth·mat′·ic
asth·mat′·i·cus
asth′·mo·gen′·ic
as′·tig·mat′·ic
astig′·ma·tis′m
astig′·ma·tom′·e·ter
   var. of astigmometer
as′·tig·mom′·e·ter
as′·tig·mom′·e·try
astig′·mo·scope
asto′·ma·tous
asto′·mia
as·trag′·a·lar
as·trag′·a·lec′·to·my
as·trag′·a·lus   pl. &
gen. sg. ·li
as′·tral
as·trin′·gent
as′·tro·
as′·tro·blast
as′·tro·blas·to′·ma   pl.
·mas or ·ma·ta
as′·tro·cyte
as′·tro·cy·to′·ma   pl.
·mas or ·ma·ta
as′·tro·cy·to′·ma·to′·sis
as′·tro·cy·to′·sis
as·trog′·lia [as′·tro·
gli′a]
as′·tro·gli·o′·ma
as′·tro·sphere
a′syl·la′·bia
asy′·lum
a′sym·bo′·lia
a′sym·met′·ri·cal
[as′ym·]   also ·met′·
ric
asym′·me·tros
asym′·me·try
a′symp·to·mat′·ic
a′syn·ap′·sis   pl. ·ses
asyn′·chro·nous
asyn′·chro·ny
asyn′·cli·tis′m
a′syn·er′·gia
a′syn·er′·gic
asyn′·er·gy
a′syn·tax′·ia
asys′·to·le
a′sys·tol′·ic
atac′·tic
at′·a·rac′·tic   also
·rax′·ic
atav′·i·cus
at′·a·vis′m
at′·a·vis′tic
atax′·ia
atax′·ia·gram
atax′·ia·graph

atax′·i·am′·e·ter
atax′·ic var. of atactic
at′·e·lec′·ta·sis
at′·e·lec·tat′·ic
ate′·li·o′·sis also ·lei·o′·
ate′·li·ot′·ic also ·lei·ot′·
at′·e·lo·
at′·e·lo·car′·dia
at′·e·lo·chei′·ria also ·chi′·ria
at′·e·lo·my·e′·lia
at′·e·lo·po′·dia
ath′·er·ec′·to·my
ather′·man·cy
ather′·ma·nous
ath′·ero·
ath′·ero·em′·bo·lis′m
ath′·ero·gen′·e·sis
ath′·er·o·gen′·ic
ath′·er·o′·ma pl. ·mas or ·ma·ta
ath′·er·o′·ma·to′·sis
ath′·er·o′·ma·tous [·om′a·]
ath′·ero·scle·ro′·sis pl. ·ses
ath′·ero·scle·rot′·ic
ath′·e·toid
ath′·e·to′·sis pl. ·ses
ath′·e·tot′·ic also ·to′·sic
ath·let′·i·cum
athrep′·sia
ath′·ro·cy·to′·sis
athy′·re·o′·sis
athy′·re·ot′·ic
at·lan′·tad
at·lan′·tal
at·lan′·tis gen. of atlas
at·lan′·to·
at·lan′·to·ax′·i·al
at·lan′·to·ax′·i·a′·lis
at·lan′·to·did′·y·mus
at·lan′·to·ep·i·stro′·phic
at·lan′·toid

at·lan′·to·mas′·toid
at·lan′·to-oc·cip′·i·tal
at·lan′·to-oc·cip′·i·ta′·lis neut. ·le
at·lan′·to·odon′·toid
at′·las gen. at·lan′·tis
at·mol′·y·sis
at·mom′·e·ter
at′·mo·sphere
at′·mo·spher′·ic
at′·om
atom′·ic
at′·om·is′m
at′·om·ize ·ized, ·iz′·ing
at′·om·iz′·er
ato′·nia
ato′·nia-asta′·sia
aton′·ic
at′o·nic′·i·ty [a′to·]
at′·o·ny
at′·o·pen
atop′·ic [ato′·pic]
atop′·og·no′·sia also ·no′·sis
at′·o·py
atox′·ic
atox′·i·gen′·ic
at′·rac·tyl′·ic
atrac′·ty·lo·side
a′trans·fer′·rin·e′·mia Brit. ·ae′·mia
a′trau·mat′·ic
A′trax
atre′·sia
atret′·ic also atre′·sic
atret′·i·cum
atre′·to· [at′·re·to·]
atre′·to·ce·pha′·lia
atre′·to·gas′·tria
at′·re·top′·sia [a′tre·]
a′tria pl. of atrium
a′tri·al
a′tri·a′·lis
a′tri·al·ized
atrich′·ia
at′·ri·chous [atrich′·ous]

a′trii gen. of atrium
a′trio·
a′trio·sep′·to·plas′·ty
a′tri·ot′·o·my
a′trio·ven·tric′·u·lar
a′trio·ven·tric′·u·la′·ris neut. ·re
a′tri·um pl. a′tria, gen. sg. a′trii
atro′·phia
atroph′·ic [atro′·phic]
atro′·phi·ca pl. ·cae
atro′·phi·cans
at′·ro·pho·der′·ma
at′·ro·phy n. & v. ·phied, ·phy·ing
at′·ro·pine
at′·ro·pin·is′m
at′·ro·pin·i·za′·tion
at·tack′
at′·tar
at·ten′·tion
at·ten′·u·ant
at·ten′·u·ate ·at′·ed, ·at′·ing
at·ten′·u·a′·tion
at·ten′·u·a′·tor
at·ten′·u·a′·tus
at′·tic
at′·ti·co·an′·tral
at′·ti·co·an·trot′·o·my
at′·ti·co·mas′·toid
at′·ti·cot′·o·my
at·tol′·lens
at·trac′·tant [at·tract′·ant]
at·trac′·tion
at′·tra·hens
at′·tri·bute
at·tri′·tion
atyp′·ia
atyp′·i·cal
au′·dio·
au′·dio·an·al·ge′·sia
au′·di·o·gen′·ic
au′·di·o·gram
au′·di·ol′·o·gist
au′·di·ol′·o·gy

au′·di·om′·e·ter
au′·di·o·met′·ric
au′·di·o·me·tri′·cian
au·di·om′e·try
au′·dio·vis′·u·al
au·di′·tion
au·di·ti′·va *pl. & gen. sg.* ·vae
au′·di·to·psy′·chic
au′·di·to′·ri·us
au′·di·to′·ry
au′·di·to·sen′·so·ry
au·di′·tus *gen.* auditus
aug·men′·tor
au′·la
au′·ra
au′·ral
au′·ra·mine
au′·ran·ti′·a·sis
au′·rem *accusative of* auris
Au′·reo·ba·sid′·i·um
au′·res *pl. of* auris
au′·ric
au′·ri·cle
au·ric′·u·la *pl. & gen. sg.* ·lae
au·ric′·u·lar
au·ric′·u·la′·re *neut. of* auricularis; *pl.* ·ria
au·ric′·u·la′·ris *pl.* ·res
au·ric′·u·lo·tem′·po·ral
au·ric′·u·lo·tem′·po·ra′·lis *ablative* ·li
au·ric′·u·lo·ven·tric′·u·lar
au′·rin
au′·ri·nar′·i·um *pl.* ·ia *or* ·iums
au′·ris *pl.* ·res, *gen. sg.* ·ris, *gen. pl.* ·ri·um
au′·ri·scope
au′·ri·sec′·tor
au′·rist
au′·ro·
au′·ro·chro′·mo·der′·ma

au′·ro·ther′·a·py
au′·ro·thi′o·glu′·cose
au′·ro·thi′o·gly′·ca·nide
au′·ro·thi′o·gly′·col·an′·i·lide
au′·ro·thi′o·ma′·late
au′·ro·thi′o·sul′·fate *Brit.* ·phate
au′·rous
aus·cult′
aus′·cul·tate   ·tat′·ed, ·tat′·ing
aus′·cul·ta′·tion
aus·cul′·ta·to′·ry
Aus·tra′·lo·pith′·e·ci′·nae [Aus′·tra·]
aus·tra′·lo·pith′·e·cine [aus′·tra·]
Aus·tra′·lo·pith′·e·cus [Aus′·tra·, ·pi·the′·cus]
Aus′·tro·bil·har′·zia
au′·ta·coid
au·te′·cious *also* au·toe′·
au′·tism
au·tis′·tic
au′·to·
au′·to·ag·glu′·ti·na′·tion
au′·to·ag·glu′·ti·nin
au′·to·al·ler′·gic
au′·to·al′·ler·gi·za′·tion
au′·to·al′·ler·gy
au′·to·anal′·y·sis *pl.* ·ses
au′·to·an′·a·lyz′·er
au′·to·an′·ti·bod′y
au′·to·an′·ti·gen
au′·to·ca·tal′·y·sis
au′·to·cat′·a·lyt′·ic
au′·to·cath′·e·ter·is′m
au′·to·cho′·le·cys·tec′·to·my
au′·to·cho′·le·cys′·to·du′·o·de·nos′·to·my
au·toch′·tho·nous
au′·to·clave

au′·to·cy·tol′′·y·sis
au′·to·cy′·to·lyt′·ic
au′·to·der′·mic
au′·to·di·ges′·tion
au′·to·dip′·loid
au′·to·ech′o·la′·lia
au′·to·ech′o·prax′·ia
au′·toe′·cious *var. of* autecious
au′·to·ec·ze′ma·ti·za′·tion [·zem′a·]
au′·to·ep′·i·la′·tion
au′·to·erot′·ic
au′·to·erot′·i·cis′m
au′·to·er′·o·tis′m *var. of* autoeroticism
au′·to·eryth′·ro·cyte
au′·to·flu′o·ro·scope
au·tog′·a·mous
au·tog′·a·my
au·tog′·e·nous *also* au′·to·gen′·ic
au·tog′·e·ny
au′·to·graft
au′·to·hem′·ag·glu′·ti·nin *Brit.* ·haem′·
au′·to·he′·mo·ly′·sin *Brit.* ·hae′·
au′·to·he·mol′′·y·sis *Brit.* ·hae·
au′·to·he′·mo·ther′·a·py *Brit.* ·hae′·
au′·to·hyp·no′·sis
au′·to·im·mune′
au′·to·im·mu′·ni·ty
au′·to·im′·mu·ni·za′·tion
au′·to·in·fec′·tion
au′·to·in·oc′·u·la′·tion
au′·to·in·tox′·i·ca′·tion
au′·to·ki·ne′·sis
au′·to·ki·net′·ic
au·tol′·o·gous
au·tol′·y·sate
au·tol′·y·sin
au·tol′·y·sis *pl.* ·ses
au′·to·lyt′·ic

au′·to·lyze ·lyzed,
·lyz′·ing; *Brit.* ·lyse,
·lysed, ·lys′·ing
au′·to·mat′·ic
au·tom′·a·tis′m
au·tom′·a·ton *pl.* ·ta
au′to·mix′·is *pl.*
·mix′·es
au′·to·nom′·ic
au′·to·nom′·i·cum
gen. sg. ·ci, *gen. pl.*
·nom′·i·co′·rum
au·ton′·o·mous
au′·to-ox′·i·da′·tion
au′to·pha′·gia *also*
au·toph′·a·gy
au′·to·pha′·gic [·phag′·ic]
au′·to·phag′·o·some
au′·to·phene
aut′·oph·thal′·mo·scope
au′·to·plast
au′·to·plas′·tic
au′·to·plas′·ty
au′·to·ploid
au′·to·ploi′·dy
au′·to·po′·di·um *pl.*
·dia
au′·to·pol′y·mer
au′·to·pol′y·ploid
au′·to·pol′y·ploi′·dy
au′·to·pro·throm′·bin
au′·top·sy
au′·to·ra′·di·o·gram
au′·to·ra′·di·o·graph
au′·to·ra·di·og′·ra·phy
au′·to·reg·u·la′·tion
au′·to·scop′·ic
au·tos′·co·py
au′·to·sen′·si·ti·za′·tion
au′·to·sen′·si·tize
·tized, ·tiz′·ing
au′·to·sex′·ing
au′·to·site
au′·to·sit′·ic
au′·to·som′·al [·so′·mal]

au′·to·so′·ma·tog·no′·sis
au′·to·some
au′·to·sple·nec′·to·my
au′·to·sug·gest′·i·bil′·i·ty
au′·to·sug·ges′·tion
au′·to·sym′·pa·thec′·to·my
au′·to·tech′·ni·con
au′·to·to′·mo·graph′·ic
au′·to·to·mog′·ra·phy
au′·to·top′·ag·no′·sia
au′·to·tox′·ic
au′·to·tox′·i·cus
au′·to·tox′·in
au′·to·trans·fu′·sion
au′·to·trans′·plant
au′·to·trans·plan·ta′·tion
au′·to·troph
au′·to·tro′·phic
[·troph′·ic]
au′·to·vac·ci·na′·tion
au′·to·vac·cine′
au·tox′·i·da′·tion [aut·ox′·] *var. of* auto-oxidation
au′·to·zy′·gous
aux′·a·no· [aux·an′o·]
aux′·a·no·dif′·fer·en′·ti·a′·tion
aux·an′·o·gram
aux′·a·no·graph′·ic
aux′·a·nog′·ra·phy
aux·e′·sis
aux·et′·ic
aux·il′·ia·ry
aux·il′·io·mo′·tor
aux′·in
aux′o·
aux′·o·car′·dia
aux′·o·cyte
aux′·o·drome
aux·ol′·o·gy
aux′o·ton′·ic
aux′·o·troph

aux′·o·tro′·phic
[·troph′·ic]
avail′·a·bil′·i·ty
av′·a·lanche
aval′vu·lar
avas′·cu·lar
avas′·cu·lar·i·za′·tion
av′·er·age *n., adj. & v.*
·aged, ·ag·ing
a′ver·mec′·tin
aver′·sion
aver′·sive
a′vi·ad′·e·no·vi′·rus
a′vi·an
av′·i·din
avid′·i·ty
a′vil·lo′·sum
avir′·u·lent
avi′·ta·min·o′·sis
avi′·ta·min·ot′·ic
avoid′·ance
av′·oir·du·pois′
avulse′ avulsed′,
avuls′·ing
avul′·sion
a′xen′·ic
ax′·es *pl. of* axis
ax′·i·al
ax′·i·a′·tion
ax·if′·u·gal
ax′·i·lem′·ma *var. of*
axolemma
ax·il′·la *pl. & gen. sg.*
·lae
ax′·il·la′·ris *pl.* ·res
ax′·il·lar′y [ax·il′·la·ry]
ax′·il·lo·fem′·o·ral
ax′·io·ap′·pen·dic′·u·lar
ax·ip′·e·tal
ax′·is *pl.* ax′·es, *gen.*
sg. axis
ax′o·
ax′o-ax′·o·nal
ax′o-ax·on′·ic
ax′o·den′·drite
ax′o·den·drit′·ic
ax′o·den′·dro·so·mat′·ic

ax·of′·u·gal   var. of
    axifugal
ax′o·lem′·ma
ax·ol′·y·sis
ax·om′·e·ter
ax′·on   also ·one
ax′·o·nal
ax′·o·neme
ax′·o·nom′·e·ter
ax′·o·not·me′·sis
ax·op′·e·tal   var. of
    axipetal
ax′·o·plas′m
ax′·o·plas′·mic
ax′·o·po′·di·um   pl.
    ·dia
ax′o·so·mat′·ic
ax′·o·style
az′a·gua′·nine
az′a·me·tho′·ni·um
az′a·pro′·pa·zone
    [a′za·]
az′a·ri′·bine
az′a·ser′·ine [·se′·rine]
az′a·thi′·o·prine
az′a·u′ri·dine
aze′·o·trope [a′ze·]
aze′·o·tro′·pic [a′ze·,
    ·trop′·ic]
az′e·pin′·a·mide [a′ze·]
az′·ide [a′zide]
az′·i·do·thy′·mi·dine
az′o·   [a′zo·]
az′o·bil′·i·ru′·bin
az′o·car′·mine
azo′·ic
az′·ole
az′o·lit′·min
az′o·my′·cin
azo′·o·sper′·ma·tis′m
azo′·o·sper′·mia
az′o·ru′·bin
az′o·te′·mia   Brit.
    ·tae′·
az′o·te′·mic   Brit.
    ·tae′·
Azo′·to·bac′·ter

az′o·tor·rhe′a [azo′·]
    Brit. ·rhoe′a
az′o·tu′·ria
az′o·tu′·ric
az·tre′·o·nam
az′·ure
az′u·res′·in
az′u·ro·phil [azu′·]
az′u·ro·phil′·ic [azu′·]
az′y·go·gram
az′·y·gog′·ra·phy
az′·y·gos   gen. az′·y·
    gou
azy′·go·spore
az′y·gous [azy′·]
azym′·ic [azy′·mic]

B

Ba·be′·sia
    B. mi·cro′·ti
bab′·e·si′·a·sis
Ba·be′·si·el′·la
ba·be′·si·o′·sis
bac′·cate
bac′·ci·form
bac′·il·lar′y [ba·cil′·la·
    ry]
bac′·il·le′·mia   Brit.
    ·lae′·
ba·cil′·li   pl. of bacillus
ba·cil′·li·form
ba·cil′·lin
bac′·il·lo′·sis
bac′·il·lu′·ria
Ba·cil′·lus
    B. an′·thra·cis
    B. meg′·a·te′·ri·um
    B. sub′·ti·lis
ba·cil′·lus   pl. ·li
bac′·i·tra′·cin
back′·bone
back′·cross
back′·flow
back′·light′·ing
back′·scat′·ter
back′·up

bac′·lo·fen
bac′·ter·e′·mia   Brit.
    ·ae′·mia
bac′·ter·e′·mic   Brit.
    ·ae′·mic
bac·te′·ria   pl. of
    bacterium
bac·te′·ri·al
bac·te′·ri·cid′·al [·ci′·
    dal]
bac·te′·ri·cide
bac·te′·ri·cid′·in [·ci′·
    din]
bac′·ter·id   also ·ide
bac·te′·ri·e′mia   var.
    of bacteremia
bac′·ter·in
bac′·ter·in′·ia
bac·te′·rio·
bac·te′·ri·o·cid′·in [·ci′·
    din]   var. of bacteri-
    cidin
bac·te′·ri·o·cin
bac·te′·ri·ol′·o·gist
bac·te′·ri·ol′·o·gy
bac·te′·rio·ly′·sin
bac·te′·ri·ol′·y·sis
bac·te′·ri·o·lyt′·ic
bac·te′·ri·o·phage′
bac·te′·ri·o·phag′·ic
bac·te′·ri·o·pha·gol′·o·
    gy
bac·te′·ri·o·phy·to′·ma
bac·te′·rio·rho·dop′·sin
bac·te′·ri·o′·sis
bac·te′·rio·sta′·sis
bac·te′·ri·o·stat′
bac·te′·rio·stat′·ic
bac·te′·rio·ther′·a·py
bac·te′·ri·o·tro′·pic
    [·trop′·ic]
bac·te′·ri·o·tro′·pin
Bac·te′·ri·um
bac·te′·ri·um   pl. ·ria
bac·te′·ri·u′·ria
bac′·ter·oid
Bac′·ter·oi·da′·ce·ae
Bac′·ter·oi′·des

B. biv′·i·us
B. cor·ro′·dens
B. dis′·i·ens
B. frag′·i·lis
B. mel′·a·ni′·no·gen′·i·cus
bac′·ter·oi′·des
bac′·ter·oi·do′·sis
bac′·ter·u′·ria var. of bacteriuria
bac′·to·pren′·ol
badge
ba·gasse′
bag′·as·so′·sis
bal′·ance n. & v.
 ·anced, ·anc·ing
ba·lan′·ic
bal′·a·ni′·tis
bal′·a·no·
bal′·a·no·cele
bal′·a·no·plas′·ty
bal′·a·no·pos·thi′·tis
bal′·a·no·pre·pu′·tial
bal′·a·nor·rha′·gia
bal′·an·tid′·i·al
bal′·an·ti·di′·a·sis [ba·lan′·]
bal′·an·tid′·i·o′·sis var. of balantidiasis
Bal′·an·tid′·i·um
ba·lan′·ti·do′·sis var. of balantidiasis
Bal′·bi·a′·nia
bal·bu′·ti·es
ball′·ing
bal′·lism
bal·lis′·mus
bal·lis′·tic
bal·lis′·tics
bal·lis′·to·car′·di·o·gram
bal·lis′·to·car′·di·o·graph
bal·lis′·to·car′·di·og′·ra·phy
bal·loon′
bal·loon′·ing
bal·lot′·ta·ble

bal·lotte′·ment′ [bal·lotte′·ment]
balm
bal′·ne·ol′·o·gy
bal′·neo·ther′·a·peu′·tics
bal′·neo·ther′·a·py
bal′·ne·um
bal′·sam
bal·sam′·ic
bal′·te·um
ban′·crof·ti′·a·sis also ·to′·sis
band′·age [ban′·dage]
ban′·da·let′·ta
band′·ing
band′·width
bap′·ti·sin
bar′·ag·no′·sis
 inability to sense weight: Cf. barognosis; also ·sia
bar′·an·es·the′·sia
 Brit. ·aes·
bar′·ba gen. ·bae
barb·al′·o·in
bar·bei′·ro
bar′·bi·tal
bar′·bi·tone var. of barbital
bar·bi′·tu·rate
bar′·bi·tu′·ric
bar·bi′·tur·is′m [bar′·bi·] also ·tu·is′m
bar′bo·tage′
bar′·es·the′·sia Brit. ·aes·the′·
bar′·hyp·es·the′·sia
 Brit. ·aes·the′·
bar′·ia·tri′·cian
bar′·iat′·rics
bar′·ic
bar′·i·to′·sis
bar′·i·um
bar′o·
bar′o·ag·no′·sis var. of baragnosis

bar′·o·cep′·tor var. of baroreceptor
bar′·odon·tal′·gia
bar′·og·no′·sis ability to sense weight: Cf. baragnosis
ba·rom′·e·ter
bar′·o·met′·ric
bar′o·oti′·tis var. of barotitis
bar′o·re·cep′·tor
bar′o·si′·nus·i′·tis
bar′·o·stat
bar′·otal′·gia
bar′·oti′·tis
bar′o·trau′·ma
bar′o·trau·mat′·ic
bar′·ri·er
bar′·tho·lin′·i·an
bar′·tho·lin·i′·tis
Bar′·ton·el′·la
 B. ba·cil′·li·for′·mis
bar′·ton·el·lo′·sis also ·li′·a·sis
bar′y·
bar′·ye
bar′y·es·the′·sia Brit. ·aes·the′·; var. of baresthesia
bar′y·la′·lia
ba·ry′·ta
bar′·y·to′·sis var. of baritosis
ba′·sad
ba′·sal
ba·sa′·le neut. of basalis; pl. ·lia
ba·sa′·lis pl. ·les
ba′·sa·loid
base
base′·line
base′·ment
base′·plate
ba′·ses pl. of basis
bas′·es pl. of base
bas-fond′
ba′·si·
ba′·si·al

ba'·si·al·ve"·o·lar
ba'·si·bran'·chi·al
ba·sic'·i·ty
ba'·si·cra'·ni·al
ba·sid'·ia *pl. of*
  basidium
ba·sid'·io·
*Ba·sid'i·ob"·o·lus
B. ra·na"·rum*
ba·sid'·io·my"·cete
  pl. ·my"·cetes
*Ba·*sid'·io·my·ce"·tes
ba·sid'·io·spore
ba·sid'·i·um *pl.* ba·sid'·ia
ba'·si·fa"·cial
ba'·si·hy"·al *also* ·hy"·oid
bas'·i·lad
bas'·i·lar
bas'·i·la"·ris
ba'·si·lat'·er·al
ba·sil'·ic
ba·sil'·i·ca
bas'·i·lo·pha·ryn'·ge·al
ba'·sio· *var. of* basi-
ba'·sio·breg·mat'·ic
ba'·si·oc·cip'·i·tal
ba"·si·on
ba'·si·o"tic
ba·sip'·e·tal
ba'·si·pha·ryn'·ge·al
ba'·si·pha·ryn'·ge·us
ba'·si·pre·sphe"·noid
ba'·si·rhi'·nal
ba'·sis *pl.* ·ses, *gen. pl.* ·si·um
ba'·si·sphe"·noid
ba'·si·squa"·mous
ba'·si·tem"·po·ral
ba'·si·ver'·te·bral
ba'·si·ver'·te·bra"·lis
  pl. ·les
ba'·so·
ba"·so·cer'·vi·cal
ba"·so·cyte
ba"·so·cy'·to·pe"·nia
ba"·so·cy·to"·sis

ba'·so·graph
ba"·so·lat'·er·al
ba"·so·phil *also* ·phile
ba"·so·phil'·ia
ba"·so·phil'·ic
ba·soph'·i·lis'm
ba·soph'·i·lous
ba'·so·plas'm
ba'·so·squa"·mous
bas'·si·net'
bas'·so·rin
bath'·es·the"·sia *Brit.*
  ·aes·; *var. of* bathyes-
  thesia
bath'·mo·tro"·pic
  [·trop'·ic]
bath'·mo·tro"·pism
bath'o·
bath'·o·chro"·mic
bath'·o·mor'·phic
bath'o·phe·nan"·thro·line [·phen·an'·]
bath'y·
bath'y·an'·es·the"·sia
  Brit. ·aes·
bath'y·car'·dia
bath'y·es·the"·sia
  Brit. ·aes·
bath'y·hy"·per·es·the"·sia *Brit.* ·aes·
bath'y·hy"·po·es·the"·sia *also* ·hyp'·es·;
  Brit. ·aes·
bat'·ra·cho·tox"·in [ba·trach'o·]
bat'·ta·ris'm
bat'·ta·ris"·mus
bat'·ter·ing
bat'·tery
bat'·yl
baud
bayes'·i·an
bay'·o·net' [bay"·o·net]
Bdel'·lo·vib"·rio
bea'·ker [beak"·er]
bear'·ber'·ry
beard
be·bee'·rine

be·can'·thone
bech'·ic
bec'·lo·meth"·a·sone
bec'·que·rel'
be·dew'·ing
bed'·fast
bed'·rid'·den
Bed·so"·nia
bed'·sore
bed'·wet'·ting
bees'·wax
bee'·tle
Beg'·gi·a·to'a
beg'·ma
be·hav'·ior *Brit.* ·iour
be·hav'·ior·al *Brit.* ·iour·
be·hav'·ior·is'm *Brit.* ·iour·
be·hav'·ior·ist *Brit.* ·iour·
be·hav'·ior·is"·tic *Brit.* ·iour·
be·hen'·ic
bej'·el
Bel·as"·ca·ris
belch
be·lem'·noid [bel"·em·]
bel'·la·don'·na
bel'·lows
bel'·ly
bel'·ly·ache
bel'·ly·but'·ton
bel'·o·noid
bel'·o·no·ski·as"·co·py
bem'·e·gride
ben·ac'·ty·zine
Be·na"·cus
ben'·da·zac
ben'·dro·flu"·a·zide
ben'·dro·flu"·me·thi"·a·zide
ben'·e·fi"·ci·ary
ben·eth"·a·mine
ben·gal'
be·nign'
be·nig'·nant
be·nig'·num

be·nor′·ter·one
ben·ox′·i·nate
ben′·ton·ite
benz·al′·de·hyde
benz′·al·ko′·ni·um
benz′·a·mine
ben′·za·thine
ben′·zene [ben·zene′]
ben′·ze·noid
ben·zeth′·a·mine
benz′·e·tho′·ni·um
benz·hy′·dra·mine
ben′·zi·dine
benz′·im·id·az′·ole
ben′·zo·ate
ben′·zo·caine
ben·zoc′·ta·mine
ben·zo·dep′a
ben′·zo·di·az′·e·pine
ben′·zo·di·ox′·an
ben·zo′·ic
ben′·zo·in
ben′·zol
ben′·zol·is′m
ben′·zo·pur′·pu·rine
ben′·zo·py′·rene
ben′·zo·qui·none′ [·quin′·one]
ben′·zo·qui·no′·ni·um
ben′·zo·sul′·fi·mide
ben′·zo·yl
ben′·zo·yl·meth′·yl·ec′·go·nine
ben′·zo·yl·pas
benz·phet′·a·mine
benz·py′·rene
benz′·py·rin′·i·um
benz·thi′·a·zide
benz·tro′·pine
ben·zyd′·a·mine
ben′·zyl
ben·zyl′·ic
ben′·zyl·ox′y·car′·bon·yl

ben′·zyl·pen′·i·cil′·lin
be·phe′·ni·um [·phen′·i·]
ber′·ber·ine
ber′i·ber′i
berke′·li·um[13]
ber′·ry
be·ryl′·li·o′·sis
be·ryl′·li·um
be·ryth′·ro·my′·cin
bes′·ti·al′·i·ty
be′·ta
be′·ta·cis′m
be′·ta·ine
be′·ta·meth′·a·sone
be′·ta·tron
be′·ta·zole
be′·tel
be·than′·e·chol [·tha′·ne·]
be·than′·i·dine
bet′·u·la
be·tween′-brain *also* betweenbrain
bex
be′·zoar
bi′·al·am′·i·col
bi′·ar·tic′·u·lar
bi′·ar·tic′·u·late
bi′·as
bi′·au·ric′·u·lar
bi·ax′·i·al
bi·bal′·lism
bib′·lio·
bib′·li·o·clast
bib′·lio·ma′·nia
bib′·lio·ther′·a·py
bib′·u·lous
bi·cam′·er·al
bi·cam′·er·a′·tus
bi·cap′·su·lar
bi·car′·bon·ate
bi·car′·bon·a·te′·mia *Brit.* ·tae′·

bi·cel′·lu·lar
bi·ceph′·a·lus
bi′·ceps[14] *L. pl.* bi·cip′·i·tes, *gen. sg.* bi·cip′·i·tis
bi·cil′·i·ate
bi·cip′·i·tal
bi·cip′·i·ta′·lis
bi·cip′·i·to·ra′·di·al
bi·cip′·i·to·ra′·di·a′·lis
bi·clon′·al [·clo′·nal]
bi·col′·lis
bi′·con·cave′ [·con′·cave]
bi·con′·dy·lar
bi·con′·dy·la′·ris
bi′·con·vex′ [·con′·vex]
bi·cor′·nate
bi·cor′·nis
bi·cor′·nous
bi·cor′·nu·ate *also* ·cor′·nate *or* ·cor′·nute
bi·cou′·date
bi·cuc′·ul·line
bi·cus′·pal
bi·cus′·pid
bi·cus′·pi·dal
bi·cus′·pid·i·za′·tion
bi·dac′·ty·ly
bi·den′·tate
bi′·di·rec′·tion·al
bi′·dis·coi′·dal
bi·du′o·ter′·tian
bid′·u·ous
bi·en′·ni·al
bi·fa′·cial
bi′·fas·cic′·u·lar
bi·fer′·i·ous *var. of* bisferious
bi′·fid [bif′·id]
Bif′·i·do·bac·te′·ri·um

---

[13] This is sometimes pronounced *ber-kē′-li-um*, but more properly *berk′-li-um*, as in Berkeley, California, where the element was first produced and identified.

[14] The proper English plural is *bi′·ceps·es*. Popularly, however, *biceps* is used in English for both singular and plural.

bi′·fi·dus [bif′·i·dus]
  fem. ·da, *neut.* ·dum
bi·fix′·ate
bi·fo′·cal
bi·fo′·rate [bi′·fo·]
bi′·fo·ris
bi·fur′·cate [bi′·fur·]
  also ·cat′·ed
bi′·fur·ca′·tio *pl.* ·ca′·
  ti·o′·nes
bi′·fur·ca′·tion
bi′·fur·ca′·tum
bi·gem′·i·nal
bi·gem′·i·num *neut.*
  of bigeminus; *pl.* ·na
bi·gem′·i·nus *pl.* ·ni
bi·gem′·i·ny
bi·ger′·mi·nal
bi·go′·ni·al
bi·is′·chi·al [-isch′·i·al]
bi′·la·mel′·lar
bi·lam′·el·late [bi′·la·
  mel′·late] *also* ·lat·
  ed
bi·lam′·i·nar
bi·lat′·er·al
bi·lat′·er·a′·lis
bi·lat′·er·al·is′m
bi′·lay′·er
Bil·har′·zia
bil·har′·zi·al
bil′·har·zi′·a·sis
bil·har′·zi·o′·ma
bil·har′·zi·o′·sis
bil′i [bi′·li·]
bil′·i·a′·ris
bil′·i·ar′y
bil′i·di·ges′·tive
bil′·i·fac′·tion
bi′·li·fer *pl.* bi·lif′·eri
bi·lif′·er·ous
bil′·i·fi·ca′·tion
bil′·i·fus′·cin
bil′i·gen′·e·sis
bil′i·ge·net′·ic
bil′·i·gen′·ic
bi·lig′·u·late
bi′·lin

bil′·i·o′·sa *pl.* ·sae
bil′·ious
bil′·ious·ness
bil′·i·ra′·chia
bil′·i·ru′·bin
bil′·i·ru′·bin·e′·mia
  [·bi·ne′·mia] *Brit.*
  ·ae′·mia
bil′·i·ru′·bin·u′·ria [·bi·
  nu′·ria]
bil′·i·u′·ria
bil′·i·ver′·din
bi·lo′·bate
bi′·lobed
bi·lob′·u·lar
bi·lob′·u·late
bi·loc′·u·lar
bi·loc′·u·la′·ris *neut.*
  ·re
bi·loc′·u·late
bi·loc′·u·la′·tion
bi·ma′·lar
bi′·mal·le′·o·lar
bi·man′·u·al
bi·mas′·toid
bi·max′·il·lar′y
bi·mod′·al [·mo′·dal]
bin′·an′·gle
bi′·na·ry
bi·na′·sal
bin·au′·ral
bin·au·ric′·u·lar
bind bound, bind′·ing
bind′·er
bin·oc′·u·lar
bin·o′·tic
bin·ov′u·lar [·o′vu·]
bi·nu′·cle·ar
bi·nu′·cle·ate
bi′·nu·cle′·o·late
bi′o·
bi′o·ac·cu′·mu·la′·tion
bi′o·acous′·tic
bi′o·ac′·tive
bi′o·ac·tiv′·i·ty
bi′o·as·say′ [·as′·say]
bi′o·au·tog′·ra·phy
bi′o·avail′·a·bil′·i·ty

bi′·o·blast
bi′·o·ce·no′·sis *also*
  ·coe·no′·
bi′o·chem′·i·cal
bi′o·chem′·is·try
bi′·o·cid′·al [·ci′·dal]
bi′·o·cide
bi′·o·coe·no′·sis *var.*
  of biocenosis
bi′o·com·pat′·i·bil′·i·ty
bi′o·con·cen·tra′·tion
bi·oc′·u·lar
bi′·o·cy′·tin
bi′o·de·grad′·a·ble
bi′o·deg′·ra·da′·tion
bi′o·di·al′·y·sis *pl.*
  ·ses
bi′o·dy·nam′·ics
bi′o·elec′·tric
bi′o·elec·tric′·i·ty
bi′o·elec·tron′·ic
bi′o·en′·er·get′·ic
bi′o·eth′·i·cal
bi′o·eth′·ics
bi′o·feed′·back
bi′o·fla′·vo·noid
bi′o·gen′·e·sis
bi′o·ge·net′·ic
bi′·o·gen·ic
bi′o·glass
bi′o·haz′·ard
bi′o·hy·drau′·lic
bi′o·ki·net′·ics
bi′·o·log′·ic
bi′·o·log′·i·cal *n. &*
  adj.
bi·ol′·o·gy
bi′o·lu′·mi·nes′·cence
bi·ol′·y·sis
bi′·o·lyt′·ic
bi′o·mag·net′·ic
bi′o·mag′·ne·tom′·e·ter
bi′o·mass
bi′·ome
bi′o·me·chan′·i·cal
bi′o·me·chan′·ics
bi′o·med′·i·cal
bi′o·med′·i·cine

biometer / bladevent

bi·om′·e·ter
bi′·o·met′·ric
bi′·o·me·tri′·cian
bi′·o·met′·rics
bi·om′·e·try
bi′·o·mi′·cro·scope
bi′·o·mi·cros′·co·py
Bi·om′·pha·lar′·ia
  B. al′·ex·an·dri′·na
  B. gla·bra′·ta
bi′·o·ne·cro′·sis
bi·on′·ic
bi′·o·nom′·ics
bi′·o·phage
bi′·oph′·a·gous
bi·oph′·a·gy
bi′·o·phar′·ma·ceu′·ti·cal
bi′·o·phar′·ma·ceu′·tics
bi′·o·phore
bi′·o·pho·tom′·e·ter
bi′·o·phy·lac′·tic
bi′·o·phy·lax′is
bi′·o·phys′·i·cal
bi′·o·phys′·ics
bi′·o·phys′·i·og′·ra·phy
bi′·o·plas′m
bi′·o·plas′·mic
bi′·o·plast
bi′·o·pol′y·mer
bi′·op·sy
bi·op′·ter·in
bi·op′·tic
bi·or′·bit·al
bi′·o·rhe·ol′·o·gy
bi′·o·rhyth′m
bi′·o·sen′·sor
bi·o′·sis
bi′·o·sphere
bi′·o·sta·tis′·tics
bi′·o·syn′·the·sis *pl.*
 ·ses
bi′·o·syn·thet′·ic
bi·o′·ta
bi′·o·tax′·is
bi′·o·tax′y
bi′·o·tech·nol′·o·gy
bi′·o·te·lem′·e·try

bi·ot′·ic
bi′·o·tin
bi′·o·tin′·yl
bi′·o·tox′·i·col′·o·gy
bi′·o·tox′·in
bi′·o·trans′·for·ma′·tion
bi′·o·type
bi·ov′u·lar [·o′vu·]
bi′·pa·ren′·tal
bi′·pa·ri′·etal
bip′·a·rous
bi·par′·tite
bi′·ped
bi·ped′·al
bi·ped′·i·cle
bi·pen′·nate
bi′·pen·na′·tus
bi·pen′·ni·form
bi·per′·i·den
bi·pha′·sic
bi·phen′·a·mine
bi·phe′·nyl [·phen′·yl]
bi·phet′·a·mine
bi·po′·lar
bi′·po·lar′·i·ty
bi′·po·ten′·ti·al′·i·ty
bi·ra′·mous
bird′·pox
bi·re·frac′·tive
bi′·re·frin′·gence
bi′·re·frin′·gent
bi·rhi′·nia
birth′·ing
birth′·mark
birth′·rate
birth′·weight *var. of*
  birth weight
bis·ac′o·dyl [bis′·aco′·dyl]
bis′·acro′·mi·al
bis′·al·bu′·min·e′·mia
  Brit. ·ae′·mia
bis·ax′·il·lar′y
bis′·cuit
bi·sect′
bi·sec′·tion
bi·sep′·tate
bi·sex′·u·al

bi′·sex′·u·al′·i·ty
bis·fer′·i·ous
bis·il′·i·ac
bis′·muth
bis′·muth·is′m
bis′·muth·o′·sis
bis′·o·brin
bis·ox′·a·tin
bis·phos′·phate
bi·spi′·nous
bi′·sta′·ble
bi·stra′·tal
bis′·tri·min
bi·sul′·fate *Brit.*
 ·phate
bi·sul′·fite *Brit.* ·phite
bi·tar′·trate
bi·tem′·po·ral
bite′·wing
bi·ther′·mal
bi·thi′·o·nol
bi·thi′·o·no·late
Bi·thyn′·ia
bit′·ing
Bi′·tis
bi·tro′·chan·ter′·ic
bi·tro′·pic [·trop′·ic]
bit′·ters
bi·tu′·ber·al
bi·tu′·men
bi·tu′·mi·no′·sis
bi·un′·du·lant
bi′·u·ret [bi′·u·ret′]
bi·va′·lent
bi·ven′·ter [bi′·ven·]
bi·ven′·tral
bi′·ven·tric′·u·lar
bi′·vi·tel′line
bix′·in
bi′·zy′·go·mat′·ic
black′·bod′y *pl.*
 ·bod′·ies
black′·fly
black′·head
black′·out
blad′·der
blad′·der·worm
blade′·vent

blastema / borrelidin

blas·te′·ma *pl.* ·mas *or* ·ma·ta
blas·te′·mal
blas·te′·mic [·tem′·ic]
blas′·tid *also* ·tide
blas′·tin
blas′·to·
blas′·to·coele *also* ·cele *or* ·coel
blas′·to·coe′·lic *also* ·ce′·lic
blas′·to·cyst
blas′·to·cyte
blas′·to·cy·to′·ma *pl.* ·mas *or* ·ma·ta
blas′·to·derm
blas′·to·disk *also* ·disc
blas′·to·gen′·e·sis
blas′·to·gen′·ic
blas·tog′·e·ny
blas·tol′·y·sis
blas·to′·ma *pl.* ·mas *or* ·ma·ta
blas′·to·mere
blas′·to·mer·ot′·o·my
Blas′·to·my′·ces
B. der′·ma·tit′·i·dis
blas′·to·my·cete′ [·my′·cete]
blas′·to·my′·cin
blas′·to·my·co′·sis
blas′·to·my·cot′·ic
blas′·to·my·cot′·i·ca
blas′·to·neu′·ro·pore
blas′·to·phore
blas′·toph·tho′·ria
blas′·to·phyl′·lum
blas′·to·pore
blas′·to·sphere
blas′·to·stro′·ma
blas·tot′·o·my
blas′·tu·la *pl.* ·las *or* ·lae
blas′·tu·la′·tion
Blat′·ta
Blat·tel′·la
B. ger·man′·i·ca
blat′·tic

Blat′·ti·dae
bleach′·ing
bleb
bleed bled, bleed′·ing
bleed′·er
blem′·ish
blen′·no·
blen′·noid
blen′·nor·rha′·gia
blen′·nor·rhag′·ic
blen′·nor·rhe′a *Brit.* ·rhoe′a
blen′·nor·rhe′·al *Brit.* ·rhoe′·al
blen·nu′·ria
ble′o·my′·cin
bleph′·ar·ad′·e·ni′·tis
bleph′·a·ral
bleph′·a·rec′·to·my
bleph′·a·ris′m
bleph′·a·rit′·ic
bleph′·a·ri′·tis
bleph′·a·ro·
bleph′·a·ro·ad′·e·no′·ma
bleph′·a·ro·ath′·er·o′·ma
bleph′·a·ro·chal′·a·sis
bleph′·a·ro·con·junc′·ti·vi′·tis
bleph′·a·ro·der′·ma·chal′·a·sis
bleph′·a·ro·plast
bleph′·a·ro·plas′·tic
bleph′·a·ro·plas′·ty
bleph′·a·rop·to′·sis [·ro·pto′·sis]
bleph′·a·ro·spas′m
bleph′·a·ro·sphinc′·ter·ec′·to·my
bleph′·a·ro·stat
bleph′·a·rot′·o·my
blind′·ness
blis′·ter
bloat
block·ade′
block′·age
block′·er

blood′·let·ting
blood′·shot
blood′·stream *also* blood stream
blood′y blood′·i·er, blood′·i·est
blow′·fly
bo′·den·plat′·te
Bo′·do
B. cau·da′·tus
B. sal′·tans
B. u′ri·na′·ri·us
bod′y *pl.* bod′·ies
bod′y-rock′·ing
boil
bol′·e·nol
bo·lom′·e·ter
bo′·lus
bom·be′·sin
bone′·let
bone′-salt
bone′·set·ter
bon′y bon′·i·er, bon′·i·est
boom′·slang
Bo·oph′·i·lus
boost′·er
bo·rac′·ic
bo′·rate
bo′·rax
bor′·bo·ryg′·mus *pl.* ·mi
Bor′·de·tel′·la
B. par′a·per·tus′·sis
B. per·tus′·sis
bo′·ric
bo′·ride
bo′·rism
bor′·ne·ol
bor′·nyl
bo′·ro·caine
bo′·ron
bo′·ro·sal′·i·cyl′·ic
Bor·rel′·ia
B. burg·dor′·feri
B. dut·to′·nii
B. re′·cur·ren′·tis
bor·rel′·i·din

bor·rel′·i·o′·sis
bo′·son
boss
bos′·se·lat′·ed
bos′·se·la′·tion
boss′·ing
bot
bo·tan′·ic *also* ·i·cal
bot′·a·ny
bot′·fly
both·rid′·i·um *pl.* ·ia
both′·rio·ceph·a·li′·a·
  sis
Both′·rio·ceph′·a·lus
both′·ri·um *pl.* ·ria
Bo′·throps
  B. at′·rox
bot′·o·gen′·in
bot′·ry·oid
bot′·ry·o·my′·ces
bot′·ry·o·my·co′·ma
bot′·ry·o·my·co′·sis
bot′·ry·o·my·cot′·ic
bot′·tle
bot′·tro·my′·cin
bot′·u·li·form
bot′·u·lin
bot′·u·li′·nus[15] *neut.*
  ·num
bot′·u·lis′m
bouf·fée′
bou·gie′
bou′·gie·nage′ *also*
  ·gi·nage′
bouil′·lon
bou·lim′·ia *var. of*
  bulimia
bound′·ary
bou·quet′
bout
bou·ton′
bou′·ton·neuse′
bou′·ton·nière′

Bo·vic′·o·la
bo′·vine
bo·vi′·nus *fem.* ·na,
  neut. ·num
bow′·el
bow′·en·oid
bow′·leg
bow′·leg′·ged [·legged]
box′·i·dine
brace′·let
bra′·chi·
bra′·chia *pl. of*
  brachium
bra′·chi·al
bra′·chi·al′·gia
bra·chi·a′·lis *pl.* ·les
bra′·chii *gen. of*
  brachium
bra′·chio·
bra′·chio·bra′·chi·al
bra′·chio·ce·phal′·ic
bra′·chio·ce·phal′·i·ca
  fem. of brachiocepha-
  licus; *pl.* ·cae
bra′·chio·ce·phal′·i·cus
bra′·chio·cru′·ral
bra′·chio·cu′·bi·tal
bra′·chio·fa′·cial
bra′·chio·ra′·di·al
bra′·chio·ra′·di·a′·lis
bra′·chi·um *pl.* ·chia,
  gen. sg. ·chii
brach′·y·
brach′·y·ba′·sia
brach′·y·car′·dia
brach′·y·ce·pha′·lia
brach′·y·ce·phal′·ic
brach′·y·ceph′·a·lis′m
brach′·y·ceph′·a·lous
brach′·y·ceph′·a·ly
  also ·ce·pha′·lia
brach′·y·chei′·lia *also*
  ·chi′·lia

brach′·y·cne′·mia
brach′·y·cne′·mic
brach′·y·dac·tyl′·ic
brach′·y·dac′·ty·ly
  also ·dac·tyl′·ia
brach′·y·don′·tia
brach′·y·esoph′·a·gus
  also ·oe·soph′·
brach′·y·fa′·cial
brach′·y·glos′·sal
brach′·y·gna′·thia
brach′·y·gna′·thous
  [bra·chyg′·na·thous]
brach′·y·met′a·car′·pal·
  is′m
brach′·y·met′a·car′·pia
brach′·y·me·tap′·o·dy
brach′·y·met′a·tar′·sia
brach′·y·me·tro′·pia
brach′·y·me·tro′·pic
  [·trop′·ic]
brach′·y·mor′·phic
brach′·y·odont
brach′·y·odon′·tia *var.*
  of brachydontia
brach′·y·pel′·lic
brach′·y·pha·lan′·gia
bra·chyp′·o·dous
brach′·y·pro·so′·pic
brach′·y·rhi′·nia
brach′·y·ther′·a·py
brach′·y·typ′·i·cal
brack′·et
brad′·y·
brad′·y·ar·rhyth′·mia
brad′·y·ar′·thria
brad′·y·car′·dia
brad′·y·car′·di·ac
brad′·y·crot·ic
brad′·y·ki·ne′·sia
brad′·y·ki·ne′·sis
brad′·y·ki·net′·ic
brad′·y·ki′·nin

---

[15] In reference to the toxin, the neuter form comes from the species name *Clostridium botulinum*, while the masculine form is based on the organism's earlier name, *Bacillus botulinus*.

brad'y·la'·lia
brad'y·lex'·ia
brad'y·pep'·tic
brad'y·pha'·sia
brad'y·phre'·nia
brad'y·pne'a *Brit.*
·pnoe'a
brad'y·pra'·gia
brad'y·rhyth'·mia
brad'y·tach'y·car'·dia
brad'y·zo'·ite
braille
brain
brain'·case
brain'-dam·aged
brain'-dead
brain'·stem *also* brain stem
branch'·er
bran'·chia *pl.* ·chi·ae
bran'·chi·al
bran'·chi·o·gen'·ic
bran'·chi·og'·e·nous
bran'·chi·o'·ma *pl.* ·mas *or* ·ma·ta
bran'·chi·o·mere
brawn'y brawn'·i·er, brawn'·i·est
bra·ye'·ra
breast
breath
breathe breathed, breath'·ing
breath'-hold·ing
breech
breg'·ma *pl.* ·ma·ta
breg·mat'·ic
breg'·ma·to·dym'·ia
breg'·mo·car'·di·ac
brems'·strahl'·lung
breph'·o·plas'·tic
breph'·o·plas'·ty
bre·tyl'·i·um
brev'e *neut. of* brevis; *pl.* brev'·ia
brev'i·
brev'i·col'·lis
brev'i·flex'·or

brev'i·lin'·e·al
brev'i·ra'·di·ate
brev'·is *pl.* ·es
bridge
bridge'·work
brise·ment'
brit'·tle
broach
broad'-spec'·trum
bro'·ken
bro'·mate
bro'·ma·to·
bro'·ma·to·ther'·a·py
bro'·ma·to·tox'·in
bro·maz'·e·pam
brom·chlo'·re·none
brom·cre'·sol
bro'·me·lain *also* ·lin
brom·hex'·ine
brom'·hi·dro'·sis
bro'·mic
bro'·mide
bro'·mid·is'm
bro'·mi·dro'·sis *var. of* bromhidrosis
bro'·mi·nate ·nat'·ed, ·nat'·ing
bro'·min·di'·one
bro'·mine
bro'·mism *also* ·min·is'm
bro'·mite
bro'·mi·za'·tion
bro'·mo·
bro'·mo·ac'·e·tate
bro'·mo·crip'·tine
bro'·mo·de·ox'y·u'ri·dine
bro'·mo·der'·ma
bro'·mo·di'·phen·hy'·dra·mine
bro'·mo·i'o·dis'm
bro'·mo·ma'·nia
bro'·mo·men'·or·rhe'a *Brit.* ·rhoe'a
bro'·mo·meth'·ane
bro'·mo·phe'·nol *also* brom·phe'·nol

bro'·mo·thy'·mol *also* brom·thy'·mol
bro'·mo·u'ra·cil
brom'·phen·ir'·a·mine
brom·phe'·nol
brom·thy'·mol
bronch'·ad'·e·ni'·tis
bron'·chi *pl. & gen. sg. of* bronchus
bron'·chi· *var. of* broncho-
bron'·chia *pl. of* bronchium
bron'·chi·al
bron'·chi·a'·lis *pl.* ·les
bron'·chic
bron'·chi·ec·ta'·sia
bron'·chi·ec·ta'·sic
bron'·chi·ec'·ta·sis
bron'·chi·ec·tat'·ic
bron·chil'·o·quy
bron'·chi·o·cele *var. of* bronchocele
bron'·chi·o·gen'·ic
bron·chi'·o·lar [bron'·chi·o'·lar]
bron'·chi·ole
bron'·chi·o·lec'·ta·sis [·ol·ec'·]
bron'·chi·o·li'·tis
bron·chi'·o·lo· [bron'·chi·o'·lo·]
bron·chi'·o·lo·al·ve'·o·lar
bron·chi'·o·lus *pl.* ·li
bron'·chio·spas'm *var. of* bronchospasm
bron'·chio·ste·no'·sis *var. of* bronchostenosis
bron·chit'·ic
bron·chi'·tis
bron'·chi·um *pl.* ·chia
bron'·cho·
bron'·cho·ad'·e·ni'·tis
bron'·cho·ae·goph'·o·ny *Brit. var. of* bronchoegophony
bron'·cho·al·ve'·o·lar

bron'·cho·al'·ve·o·li'·
tis
bron'·cho·as'·per·gil·
lo'·sis
bron'·cho·bil'·i·ar'y
bron'·cho·cav'·ern·ous
bron'·cho·cele
bron'·cho·con·stric'·
tion
bron'·cho·con·stric'·tor
bron'·cho·dil'·a·ta'·tion
also ·di·la'·tion
bron'·cho·di·la'·tor
[·di'·la·]
bron'·cho·egoph'·o·ny
bron'·cho·esoph'·a·ge'·
al
bron'·cho·esoph'·a·ge'·
us
bron'·cho·esoph'·a·
gos'·co·py
bron'·cho·fi'·ber·scope
Brit. ·fi'·bre·
bron'·cho·gen'·ic
bron·chog'·e·nous
bron'·cho·gram
bron·chog'·ra·phy
bron'·cho·lith
bron'·cho·li·thi'·a·sis
bron'·cho·ma·la'·cia
bron'·cho·me'·di·as·ti'·
nal
bron'·cho·me'·di·as'·ti·
na'·lis
bron'·cho·mon'i·li'·a·
sis [·mo'ni·]
bron'·cho·mo'·tor
bron'·cho·my·co'·sis
bron'·cho-oe·soph'·a·
ge'·al Brit. var. of
bronchoesophageal
bron'·cho-oe·soph'·a·
ge'·us var. of
bronchoesophageus
bron'·cho-oe·soph'·a·
gos'·co·py Brit.
var. of bronchoesopha-
goscopy

bron·chop'·a·thy
bron'·cho·phon'·ic
[·pho'·nic]
bron·choph'·o·ny
bron'·cho·plas'·ty
bron'·cho·pleu'·ral
bron'·cho·pneu·mo'·nia
bron'·cho·pneu·mon'·ic
bron'·cho·pul'·mo·na'·
lis pl. ·les
bron'·cho·pul'·mo·
nar'y
bron'·chor·rha'·gia
bron'·chor·rhe'a Brit.
·rhoe'a
bron'·cho·scope
bron'·cho·scop'·ic
bron·chos'·co·py
bron'·cho·spas'm
bron'·cho·spi·rom'·e·
ter
bron'·cho·spi·rom'·e·
try
bron'·cho·ste·no'·sis
bron·chos'·to·my
bron·chot'·o·my
bron'·cho·tra'·che·al
bron'·cho·ve·sic'·u·lar
bron'·chus pl. & gen.
sg. ·chi
broth
Bru·cel'·la
B. abor'·tus
B. mel'·i·ten'·sis
B. su'·is
bru·cel'·la pl. ·lae or
·las
bru·cel'·lar
bru·cel'·lin
bru'·cel·lo'·sis
bru'·cine
Bru'·gia
B. ma·lay'i
bruis'·a·bil'·i·ty
bruise
bruisse·ment'
bruit
bru·nes'·cens

bru·nes'·cent
brush'·ing
brux'·ism
brux'o·ma'·nia
bry·o'·nia
bu'·ba
bu'·bo pl. ·boes
bu·bon'·ic
bu·bon'·i·ca
bu·bon'·o·cele
buc'·ca pl. & gen. sg.
·cae
buc'·cal
buc·ca'·lis pl. ·les
buc'·ci·na'·tor
buc'·ci·na·to'·ri·us
pl. ·ria
buc'·co-
buc'·co·cer'·vi·cal
buc'·co·fa'·cial
buc'·co·gin'·gi·val
[·gin·gi'·]
buc'·co·la'·bi·al
buc'·co·lin'·gual
buc'·co·pha·ryn'·gea
buc'·co·pha·ryn'·ge·al
buc'·co·pha·ryn'·ge·a'·
lis
buc'·co·ver'·sion
bu'·cli·zine
bud bud'·ded, bud'·
ding
bu'·fa·gin
buff'·er
bu'·fo·
bu·for'·min
bu'·fo·tox'·in
bul'·bar
bul'·bi gen. of bulbus
bul·bi'·tis
bul'·bo·
bul'·bo·cap'·nine
bul'·bo·cav'·er·no'·sus
bul'·bo·cav'·ern·ous
bul'·bo·gas'·trone
bul·boi'·dea
bul'·bo·mem'·bra·nous
bul'·bo·mim'·ic

bul′·bo·nu′·cle·ar
bul′·bo·pon′·tine
bul′·bo·spi′·nal
bul′·bo·spi′·ral
bul′·bo·spon′·gi·o′·sus
bul′·bo·ure′·thral
bul′·bo·u′re·thra′·lis
bul′·bous
bul′·bo·ven·tric′·u·lar
bul′·bus *pl. & gen. sg.*
·bi
bu·lim′·ia
bu·lim′·ic
Bu·li′·mus
B. *af′·ri·ca′·nus*
B. *fuch′·si·a′·nus*
B. *leach′·ii*
B. *trun·ca′·tus*
Bu·li′·nus
bul′·la *pl.* ·lae
bul·lec′·to·my
bul·lo′·sus *fem.* ·sa,
 neut. ·sum
bul′·lous
bu·nam′·i·dine [·na′·
 mi·]
bun′·dle
bun′·ga·ro·tox′·in
Bun′·ga·rus
bu·ni′·o·dyl
bun′·ion
bun′·ion·ec′·to·my
bun′·ya·vi′·ral
Bun′·ya·vi′·ri·dae
bun′·ya·vi′·rus
buph·thal′·mia *var. of*
 buphthalmos
buph·thal′·mos
bu·piv′·a·caine
bur[16] *also* burr
bu′·ra·mate
bu·ret′ *also* ·rette′
bur′·nish·er
bur′·sa *pl. & gen. sg.*
 ·sae

bur′·sal
bur·sa′·ta
bur′·sate
bur·sec′·to·my
bur·si′·tis
bur′·so·lith
bur·sot′·o·my
bu′·ser·el′·in
bu·sul′·fan
bu′·ta·bar′·bi·tal
bu′·ta·caine
bu′·ta·di·az′·a·mide
bu·tal′·bi·tal
bu·tam′·ben
bu′·tane
bu′·tane·di′·ol
bu′·ta·nol
bu′·ta·per′·a·zine
bu′·ta·pro′·benz
but·eth′·a·mine
bu·thi′·a·zide
but·ox′·a·mine
but′·ter·fly
but′·tock
bu′·tyl
bu′·tyl·ac′·e·tate
bu′·tyl·ene
bu′·tyl·par′·a·ben
bu′·ty·ra′·ceous
bu·tyr′·ic
bu′·ty·ro·
bu′·ty·roid
bu′·ty·ro·phe′·none
bu′·tyr·yl
by′·pass
bys′·si·no′·sis

C

cac′·es·the′·sia *Brit.*
 ·aes·the′·
ca·chec′·tic
ca·chec′·tin
ca·chet′

ca·chex′·ia *also*
 ·chex′y
cach′·in·na′·tion
cac′·o·
cac′·o·don′·tia
cac′·o·dyl
cac′·o·dyl′·ic
cac′·o·gen′·ic
cac′·o·geu′·sia
cac′·o·la′·lia
ca·cos′·mia
ca·cu′·men *pl.* ·mi·na
ca·cu′·mi·nal
ca·dav′·er·
ca·dav′·er·ic
ca·dav′·er·ine
ca·dav′·er·ous
cad′·mi·um
ca·du′·ca
ca·du′·ce·us
cae- *See also words*
 beginning ce-
cae·ca′·lis *pl.* ·les
cae′·cum *var. of*
 cecum; *pl.* ·ca
cae′·cus
cae′·no·
cae′·no·gen′·e·sis
cae·sar′·e·an *also* ·i·
 an; *var. of* cesarean
caf·fe′·ic
caf·feine′ [caf′·feine]
caf′·fein·is′m
ca·hin′·cic
caj′·e·put *also* caj′·u·
 put
caj′·e·put·ol *also* caj′·
 u·put·ol
ca·lac′·tin
cal′·a·mine
cal′·a·mus
cal·ca′·nea *fem. of*
 calcaneus
cal·ca′·ne·al *also* ·ne·
 an

---

16 The spelling *bur* is preferred for the dental drill bit; the spelling *burr* is preferred for
 the tool used in cutting bone.

cal·ca′·nei gen. of
  calcaneus
cal·ca′·ne·i′tis
cal·ca′·neo·ca′·vus
cal·ca′·neo·cu′·boid
cal·ca′·neo·cu·boi′·de·
  us fem. ·dea, neut.
  ·de·um
cal·ca′·ne·o·dyn′·ia
cal·ca′·neo·fib′·u·lar
cal·ca′·neo·na·vic′·u·
  lar
cal·ca′·neo·tib′·i·al
cal·ca′·neo·val′·go·ca′·
  vus
cal·ca′·neo·val′·gus
cal·ca′·neo·va′·rus
cal·ca′·ne·um pl.
  ·nea; var. of calcaneus
cal·ca′·ne·us pl. &
  gen. sg. ·nei
cal′·car pl. cal·car′·ia
cal·ca′·rea
cal·car′·e·ous
cal′·ca·rine
cal′·ca·ri′·nus fem.
  ·na
cal′·ci·
cal′·ci·co′·sis
cal·cif′·er·ol
cal·cif′·er·ous
cal·cif′·ic
cal·cif′·i·cans
cal′·ci·fi·ca′·tion
cal′·ci·fy ·fied, ·fy′·ing
cal·cig′·er·ous
cal·cim′·e·ter
cal′·ci·na′·tion
cal′·ci·no′·sis pl. ·ses
cal′·cio·
cal′·cio·ki·ne′·sis
cal′·cio·ki·net′·ic
cal′·ci·or·rha′·chia
cal′·ci·pec′·tic
cal′·ci·pe′·nia

cal′·ci·pe′·nic
cal′·ci·pex′·ic
cal′·ci·pex′·is
cal′·ci·pex′y
cal′·ci·phy·lax′·is
cal′·ci·phy·lac′·tic
cal′·ci·priv′·ia
cal′·ci·priv′·ic
cal′·cis gen. of calx
cal′·cite
cal′·ci·to′·nin
cal′·ci·tri′·ol
cal′ci·um
cal′·ci·u′·ria
cal′·co·
cal′·co·dyn′·ia
cal′·co·sphe′·rite
  [·spher′·ite]
cal′·cu·lif′·ra·gous
cal′·cu·lo·gen′·e·sis
cal′·cu·lo′·sis
cal′·cu·lous
cal′·cu·lus pl. ·li
cal′·e·fa′·cient
cal′·e·fac′·tion
calf pl. calves
cal′·i·ber also ·bre
cal′·i·brate ·brat′·ed,
  ·brat′·ing
cal′·i·bra′·tion
cal′·i·bra′·tor
cal′·i·ce′·al [ca′·li·]
cal′·i·cec′·ta·sis [ca′·li·]
  pl. ·ses
cal′·i·cec′·to·my [ca′·
  li·]
ca′·li·ces [cal′·i·ces]
  pl. of calix
ca′·li·cine
ca·lic′·u·lus pl. ·li
cal′·i·ec′·ta·sis [ca′·li·]
cal′·i·ec′·to·my [ca′·li·]
cal′·i·for′·ni·um
cal′·i·per

cal′·is·then′·ics [·i·
  sthen′·] Brit. cal′·
  lis·
ca′·lix[17] pl. ·li·ces
cal′·li·cre′·in var. of
  kallikrein
Cal·liph′·o·ra
Cal′·li·phor′·i·dae
Cal′·li·tro′·ga
cal·lo′·sal
cal·los′·i·ty
cal·lo′·so·mar′·gin·al
cal·lo′·sum neut. of
  callosus; gen. ·si
cal·lo′·sus
cal′·lous adj.
cal′·lus n.
calm′·a·tive [cal′·ma·
  tive]
cal·mod′·u·lin
cal′·o·mel
Cal′·o·mys
cal′·or
ca·lo′·ri·
ca·lo′·ric
Cal′·o·rie 1000
  calories
cal′·o·rie
cal′·o·ri·fa′·cient [ca·
  lo′·ri·]
cal′·o·rif′·ic
cal′·o·ri·gen′·ic [ca·lo′·
  ri·]
cal′·o·rim′·e·ter
cal′·o·ri·met′·ric [ca·
  lo′·ri·]
cal′·o·rim′·e·try
cal′·o·ry var. of
  calorie
cal′·o·tro′·pin
ca·lotte′
cal′·pain
cal′·pa·stat′·in
cal·var′·ia pl. ·i·ae
cal·var′·i·al

---

17 See note at *calyx*.

calvarium / canthectomy

cal·var′·i·um   *incorrect var. of* calvaria
cal·vi′·ti·es
calx   *pl.* cal″·ces, *gen. sg.* cal″·cis
cal′·y·ce′·al [ca′·ly·]   *var. of* caliceal
cal′·y·cec′·ta·sis [ca′·ly·]   *var. of* calicectasis
cal′·y·cec′·to·my [ca′·li·]   *var. of* calicectomy
ca·lyc′·i·form
ca′·ly·cine   *var. of* calicine
ca·lyc″·u·lus   *var. of* caliculus
Ca·lym′·ma·to·bac·te′·ri·um gran′·u·lo′·ma·tis
ca″·lyx[18]   *pl.* ·li·ces; *var. of* calix
cam′·bi·um
cam·bo′·gia
cam′·e·ra   *L. pl. & gen. sg.* ·rae
cam′·i·sole
cam′·o·mile   *var. of* chamomile
cam′·phene
cam′·phor   *also* cam·pho″·ra
cam′·pho·ra″·ceous
cam′·phor·at′·ed
cam·pho′·ric
cam′·phor·is′m
cam′·phyl
cam·pim′·e·ter
cam·pim′·e·try
cam′·po·spas′m
camp′·to·
camp′·to·cor′·mia

camp′·to·dac·tyl′·ia   *var. of* camptodactyly
camp′·to·dac·tyl′·ic
camp′·to·dac′·ty·ly   *also* ·tyl·is′m
camp′·to·mel′·ic [·me′·lic]
camp″·to·spas′m
camp′·to·the″·cin
cam′·pus
Cam′·py·lo·bac′·ter
   C. fe′·tus
   C. je·ju′·ni
   C. py·lo′·ri
cam′·py·lo·bac·te″·ri·o″·sis
cam′·py·lo·gna′·thia
cam′·sy·late
ca·nal′
can′·a·lic″·u·lar
can′·a·lic″·u·li′·tis
can′·a·lic″·u·lus   *pl.* ·li
ca·nal′·i·for′·mis
ca·na′·lis   *pl.* ·les, *gen. sg.* ·lis
ca·nal″·i·za′·tion [can′·a·li·]
can′·a·lized
can′·a·van′·in
can·av′·a·nine
can′·cel·lous
can·cel′·lus   *pl.* ·li
can′·cer
can′·cer·i·cid′·al [·ci′·dal]   *also* can′·cer·o·
can′·cer·i·za′·tion
can′·cer·ol″·o·gy
can′·cero·pho″·bia
can′·cero·stat″·ic
can′·cer·ous
can′·cri·form
can′·croid
can′·crum

can·de′·la [·del′a]
can′·di·ci′·din
Can′·di·da
   C. al″·bi·cans
   C. trop′·i·ca″·lis
can′·di·dal
can′·di·di″·a·sis   *pl.* ·ses
can′·di·did   *also* can′·di·dide
can′·di·do″·sis   *var. of* candidiasis
can·di·ru′
ca·nes′·cent
ca′·nine
ca·ni′·ni·form
ca·ni′·nus   *pl. & gen. sg.* ca·ni′·ni
ca·ni″·ti·es
can′·ker
can·nab′·i·nol
can′·na·bis
can′·na·bis′m
can′·nu·la   *pl.* ·lae *or* ·las
can′·nu·late   ·lat′·ed, ·lat′·ing
can′·nu·la″·tion   *also* ·li·za″·tion
can′·thal
can′·tha·ri″·a·sis
can·thar′·i·dal
can·thar″·i·des   *pl. of* cantharis
can′·tha·rid′·i·al   *var. of* cantharidal
can·thar″·i·din
can·thar″·i·dis′m
Can′·tha·ris
   C. ves′·i·ca·to″·ria
can′·tha·ris   *pl.* can·thar″·i·des
can·thec′·to·my

---

18 *Calix* is the correct Latin spelling for a cuplike structure such as a subdivision of the renal pelvis, while *calyx* properly refers to the outer covering of a flower bud or the sepals of the mature flower. The two words have long been confused, however, and many anatomists continue to use *calyx* in the sense of *calix*.

can'·thi *pl. & gen. sg.*
  of canthus
can·thi'·tis
can'·tho·
can·thor'·rha·phy
can·thot'·o·my
can'·thus *pl. & gen.*
  sg. ·thi
can'·u·la *var. of*
  cannula
ca·pac'·i·tance
ca·pac'·i·ta'·tion
ca·pac'·i·tor
ca·pac'·i·ty
cap'·il·la'·re *pl.* ·la'·
  ria
Cap'·il·lar'·ia
  C. phil'·ip·pi·nen'·sis
cap'·il·la·ri'·a·sis
cap'·il·lar'·i·os'·co·py
cap'·il·la·ri'·tis
cap'·il·lar'·i·ty
cap'·il·la·rop'·a·thy
cap'·il·la·ros'·co·py
  var. of capillarioscopy
cap'·il·lar'y
ca·pil'·li *sg.* ca·pil'·lus
cap'·il·lo·ve'·nous
cap'·is·tra'·tion
cap'·i·ta *pl. of* caput
cap'·i·tal
cap'·i·tate
cap'·i·ta'·tum
cap'·i·tel'·lum
cap'·i·tis *gen. of* caput
ca·pit'·u·lar
ca·pit'·u·lum *pl.* ·la,
  gen. sg. ·li
cap'·no·
cap·nog'·ra·phy
cap·nom'·e·try
cap'·no·phil'·ic
cap'·o·ben'·ic
cap'·re·o·my'·cin
cap'·ric
ca·pril'·o·quis'm
cap'·ri·pox'·vi'·rus
cap'·ro·ate

ca·pro'·ic
cap'·ry·late
ca·pryl'·ic
cap·sa'·i·cin
cap'·si·cin
cap'·si·cum
cap'·sid
cap'·so·mere *also*
  ·mer
cap·sot'·o·my *var. of*
  capsulotomy
cap'·su·la *pl. & gen.*
  sg. ·lae
cap'·su·lar
cap'·su·la'·re
cap'·su·la'·tion
cap'·sule
cap'·su·lec'·to·my
cap'·su·li'·tis
cap'·su·lo·
cap'·su·lo·gan'·gli·on'·
  ic
cap'·su·lo·len·tic'·u·lar
cap'·su·lo·plas'·ty
cap'·su·lo·pu'·pil·la'·ris
cap'·su·lor'·rha·phy
cap'·su·lo·tha·lam'·ic
cap'·su·lo·tome
cap'·su·lot'·o·my
cap'·to·di'·a·mine
cap'·to·pril
cap'·ut *pl.* cap'·i·ta,
  gen. sg. cap'·i·tis
car'a·a'·te *var. of*
  carate
ca·ram'·i·phen
ca·ra'·te
car'·ba·chol
car'·ba·mate
car'·ba·maz'·e·pine
car'·ba·mide
carb'·a·mi'·no
carb'·a·mi'·no·he'·mo·
  glo'·bin *Brit.* ·hae'·
  mo·glo'·
car·bam'·o·yl
car·bam'·o·yl·a'·tion

car·bam'·o·yl·trans'·
  fer·ase
car'·ba·myl *var. of*
  carbamoyl
carb·an'·i'on
car'·ba·zide
car'·bene
car·ben'·i·cil'·lin
car'·ben·ox'·o·lone
car·be'·ta·pen'·tane
carb·he'·mo·glo'·bin
  Brit. ·hae'·mo·glo'·
car'·bide
car'·bi·do'·pa
car·bi'·ma·zole
car'·bi·nox'·a·mine
car'·bo·benz·ox'y
car'·bo·cat'·i'on
car'·bo·cho'·line
car'·bo·clo'·ral *also*
  ·chlo'·ral
car'·bo·cy'·clic
car'·bo·di·im'·ide
car'·bo·hy'·drase
car'·bo·hy'·drate
car'·bol·fuch'·sin
car·bol'·ic
car'·bo·li'·gase
car'·bo·lis'm
car'·bo·my'·cin
car'·bon
car'·bon·ate
car·bon'·ic
car'·bon·u'·ria [·bo·
  nu'·ria]
car'·bo·nyl
car·box'y·bi'·o·tin
car·box'y·he'·mo·glo'·
  bin *Brit.* ·hae'·mo·
  glo'·
car·box'y·ki'·nase
car·box'·yl
car·box'·yl·ase
car·box'·yl·a'·tion
car·box'·yl·es'·ter·ase
car'·box·yl'·ic
car·box'·yl·trans'·fer·
  ase

car·box′y-ly′·ase
car·box′y·meth′·yl
car·box′y·meth′·yl·cel′·
 lu·lose
car·box′y·pep′·ti·dase
car·bro′·mal
car′·bun·cle
car·bun′·cu·lar
car·bun′·cu·lo′·sis
car·bun′·cu·lus *pl.* ·li
car·bu′·ta·mide
car·byl′·a·mine
car′·ci·nec′·to·my
car′·ci·no·
car′·ci·no·em′·bry·on′·
 ic
car·cin′′·o·gen [car′·ci·
 no·gen′]
car′·ci·no·gen′·e·sis
car′·ci·no·gen′·ic
car′·ci·no·ge·nic′·i·ty
car′·ci·noid
car′·ci·no·ly′·sin
car′·ci·nol′·y·sis
car′·ci·no·lyt′·ic
car′·ci·no′·ma *pl.*
 ·mas *or* ·ma·ta
car′·ci·no′·ma·toid
 [·nom′a·]
car′·ci·no′·ma·toi′·des
car′·ci·no′·ma·to′·sis
car′·ci·nom′a·tous
 [·no′ma·]
car′·ci·no′·mel·co′·sis
 [·nom′·el·]
car′·ci·no·sar·co′·ma
 pl. ·mas *or* ·ma·ta
car′·ci·no′·sis
car′·ci·no·stat′·ic
car′·ci·nous
car′·del·my′·cin
car·de′·no·lide
car′·dia
car′·di·ac *of the heart
 or the gastric cardia:
 Cf.* cardial
car·di′·a·ca *pl. of*
 cardiacum; *fem. of*

cardiacus; *pl. & gen.
 sg.* ·cae
car·di′·a·cum *neut. of*
 cardiacus; *pl.* ·ca
car·di′·a·cus *pl. &
 gen. sg.* ·ci
car′·di·al *of the
 gastric cardia only: Cf.*
 cardiac
car′·di·al′·gia
car′·di·ant
car′·di·ec′·ta·sis
car′·di·ec′·to·my
car′·di·o·
car′·di·o·ac·cel′·er·a·tor
car′·di·o·ac′·tive
car′·di·o·an′·gi·og′·ra·
 phy
car′·di·o·an′·gi·ol′·o·gy
car′·di·o·asth′·ma
car′·di·o·au′·di·to′·ry
car′·di·o·cen·te′·sis
car′·di·o·cha·la′·sia
car′·di·o·cir·rho′·sis
car′·di·o·dy·nam′·ic
car′·di·o·esoph′·a·ge′·al
 Brit. -oe·soph′·
car′·di·o·fa′·cial
car′·di·o·gen′·e·sis
car′·di·o·gen′·ic
car′·di·o·gram
car′·di·o·graph
car′·di·o·graph′·ic
car′·di·og′·ra·phy
car′·di·o·in·hib′·i·tor
car′·di·o·in·hib′·i·to′·ry
car′·di·o·ki·net′·ic
car′·di·o·ky·mog′·ra·
 phy
car′·di·o·lip′·in
car′·di·o·lith
car′·di·ol′·o·gist
car′·di·ol′·o·gy
car·di·ol′·y·sis
car′·di·o·ma·la′·cia
car′·di·o·meg′·a·ly
car′·di·om′·e·ter
car′·di·o·met′·ric

car′·di·om′·e·try
car′·di·o·my′·o·li·po′·sis
car′·di·o·my′·o·path′·ic
car′·di·o·my·op′·a·thy
car′·di·o·my′·o·plas′·ty
car′·di·o·my·ot′·o·my
car′·di·o·nec′·tor
car′·di·o·neph′·ric
car′·dio-oe·soph′·a·ge′·
 al *Brit. spel. of* cardio-
 esophageal
car′·di·o·pal′·u·dis′m
car′·di·o·path′·ic
car′·di·o·pa·thol′·o·gy
car′·di·op′·a·thy
car′·di·o·per′·i·car′·di·o·
 pex′y
car′·di·o·per′·i·car·di′·
 tis
car′·di·o·plas′·ty
car′·di·o·ple′·gia
car′·di·o·ple′·gic
car′·di·o·pneu·mat′·ic
car′·di·o·pneu′·mo·
 graph
car′·di·o·pneu′·mo·no·
 pex′y
car′·di·o·pul′·mo·nar′y
car′·di·o·re′·nal
car′·di·or′·rha·phy
car′·di·o·scle·ro′·sis
car′·di·o·scope
car′·di·o·spas′m
car′·di·o·ta·chom′·e·ter
car′·di·o·ta·chom′·e·try
car′·di·o·ther′·a·py
car′·di·o·tho·rac′·ic
car′·di·ot′·o·my
car′·di·o·ton′·ic
car′·di·o·tox′·ic
car′·di·o·vas′·cu·lar
car′·di·o·ver′·sion
car′·di·o·vert′
car′·di·o·vert′·er
car′·di·o·vi′·rus
car·di′·tis
car′·ies *pl.* caries

ca·ri′·na *pl.* ·nae *or* ·nas
car′·i·nate
car′·io·
car′·io·gen′·e·sis
car′·i·o·gen′·ic
car′·i·os′·i·ty
car′·io·stat′·ic
car′·i·ous
ca·ri′·so·pro′·dol
car·mal′·um
car·min′·a·tive [car′·mi·na·]
car′·mine
car·min′·ic
car·nas′·si·al
car′·nea *pl.* ·ne·ae
car′·ne·ous
car′·ni·tine
Car·niv′·o·ra
car′·ni·vore
car·niv′·o·rous
car′·no·sine
car′·no·sin·e′·mia [·si·ne′·mia] *Brit.* ·ae′·mia
car′·o·tene
car′·o·ten·e′·mia [·te·ne′·mia] *Brit.* ·ae′·mia
ca·rot′·e·noid *also* ·i·noid
car′·o·te·no′·sis
ca·rot′·i·ca *fem. of* caroticus
ca·rot′·i·ci *pl. & gen. sg. of* caroticus
ca·rot′·i·co·cli′·noid
ca·rot′·i·co·tym·pan′·i·ca *fem. of* caroticotympanicus; *pl.* ·cae
ca·rot′·i·co·tym·pan′·i·cus *pl.* ·ci
ca·rot′·i·co·tym·pan′·ic
ca·rot′·i·cum *neut. of* caroticus
ca·rot′·i·cus *pl. & gen. sg.* ·ci

ca·rot′·id
ca·ro′·ti·dis *gen. of* carotis
ca·rot′·i·do·sym′·pa·tho·a′tri·al
ca·rot′·i·do·va′·go·a′tri·al
ca·rot′·i·do·ven·tric′·u·lar
car′·o·ti·ne′·mia *var. of* carotenemia
car′·o·ti·no′·sis
ca·ro′·tis *pl.* ·ti·des, *gen. sg.* ·ti·dis
car′·pal
car·pa′·le *neut. of* carpalis; *pl.* ·lia
car·pa′·lis *pl.* ·les
car·pec′·to·my
car·phol′·o·gy *also* car′·pho·lo′·gia
car′·pi *pl. & gen. sg. of* carpus
car·pi′·tis
car′·po·
car′·po·car′·pal
car′·po·met′a·car′·pal
car′·po·met′a·car·pa′·le *neut. of* carpometacarpalis; *pl.* ·lia
car′·po·met′a·car·pa′·lis *pl.* ·les
car′·po·ped′·al
car′·po·pha·lan′·ge·al
car′·pop·to′·sis
car′·pus *pl. & gen. sg.* ·pi
car′·ra·geen *also* ·gheen
car′·ra·geen′·an *also* ·gheen′·in
car′·ri·er
car′·ti·lage
car′·ti·lag′·i·nes *pl. of* cartilago
car′·ti·la·gin′·e·us *fem.* ·gin′·ea
car′·ti·la·gin′·i·form

car′·ti·lag′·i·noid
car′·ti·lag′·i·nous
car′·ti·la′·go *pl.* ·lag′·i·nes, *gen. sg.* ·lag′·i·nis
car′·un·cle
ca·run′·cu·la *pl.* ·lae
ca·run′·cu·lar
car′yo· *var. of* karyo·
cas·cade′
cas·car′a
ca′·se·a′·tion
ca′·sein [ca·sein′]
ca′·se·ous
ca′·se·um
cas′·trate ·trat′·ed, ·trat′·ing
cas·tra′·tion
cas′·troid
cas′·u·al·ty
cas′·u·is′·tic
cas′·u·is·try
cat′a·
ca·tab′·a·sis
cat′·a·bat′·ic
cat′a·bi·o′·sis
cat′a·bi·ot′·ic
cat′·a·bol′·ic
ca·tab′·o·lin
ca·tab′·o·lis′m
ca·tab′·o·lite
ca·tab′·o·lize ·lized, ·liz′·ing
cat′·a·crot′·ic
cat′a·di·crot′·ic
cat′a·did′·y·mus
cat′a·di·op′·tric
cat′·a·gen
cat′·a·lase
cat′·a·lat′·ic
cat′·a·lep′·sy
cat′·a·lep′·tic
cat′·a·lo′·gia
ca·tal′·y·sis *pl.* ·ses
cat′·a·lyst
cat′·a·lyt′·ic
cat′·a·lyze ·lyzed, ·lyz′·ing; *Brit.* ·lyse, ·lysed, ·lys′·ing

catamenia / cecoplication   **46**

cat'·a·me'·nia
cat'·a·me'·ni·al
cat'·a·mite
cat'·a·pha'·sia
cat'a·pho·re'·sis
cat'a·pho'·ria
cat'·a·phre'·nia
cat'a·phy·lax'·is
cat'·a·pla'·sia
cat'·a·plas'm
cat'·a·plec'·tic
cat'·a·plex'y
cat'·a·poph'·y·sis
cat'·a·ract
cat'·a·rac'·to·gen'·ic
cat'·a·rac'·tous
ca·tarrh'
ca·tar'·rhal
Cat'·ar·rhi'·na
cat'·ar·rhine
ca·tas'·tro·phe
cat'·a·stroph'·ic
ca·tat'·a·sis
cat'·a·thy'·mia
cat'·a·to'·nia
cat'·a·ton'·ic
ca·tat'·o·noid
cat'a·tri·crot'·ic
cat'a·tro'·pia
cat'·e·chol
cat'·e·chol'·a·mine
cat'·e·chu
cat'·elec'·tro·ton'·ic
cat'·elec·trot'·o·nus
cat'·e·nat'·ed
cat'·e·noid
ca·ten'·u·late
cat'·er·pil'·lar
cat'·gut
cath'·a·rom'·e·ter
ca·thar'·sis   *pl.* ·ses
ca·thar'·tic
ca·thect'
ca·thep'·sin
cath'·e·ter
cath'·e·ter·i·za'·tion
cath'·e·ter·ize   ·ized,
  ·iz'·ing

cath'·e·ter·o·stat'
cath'·e·tom'·e·ter
ca·thex'·is   *pl.* ·thex'·
  es
cath'·i·so·pho'·bia
cath·od'·al [·o'·dal]
cath'·ode
ca·thod'·ic
ca·thol'·i·con
cat'·i'on
cat'·ion·ic
cat·op'·tric
cat·op'·tro·scope
cat'o·tro'·pia   *var. of*
  catatropia
cau'·ca·soid   *also*
  Caucasoid
cau'·da   *pl. & gen. sg.*
  ·dae
cau'·dad
cau'·dal
cau·da'·lis   *neut.* ·le
cau'·dal·ward
cau'·date
cau·da'·to·len·tic'·u·lar
cau·da'·tus   *gen.* ·ti
cau'·do·ceph'·a·lad
caul
caus'·al
cau·sal'·gia
cau·sa'·tion
caus'·a·tive
cause
caus'·tic
cau'·ter
cau'·ter·ant
cau'·ter·i·za'·tion
cau'·tery
ca'·va   *pl. of* cavum,
  fem. of cavus; *pl. &*
  gen. sg. ·vae, *gen. pl.*
  ·ca·va'·rum
ca'·val
ca'·va·scope
cav'·e·o'·la [ca·ve'·o·
  la]
cav'·ern
ca·ver'·na   *pl.* ·nae

cav'·er·ni'·tis
cav'·er·no'·ma   *pl.*
  ·mas *or* ·ma·ta
cav'·er·no'·sa   *pl. of*
  cavernosum, *fem. of*
  cavernosus
cav'·er·no·si'·tis
cav'·er·nos'·to·my
cav'·er·no'·sum   *neut.*
  of cavernosus; *pl.* ·sa,
  gen. sg. ·si
cav'·er·no'·sus   *pl. &*
  gen. sg. ·si
cav'·ern·ous
Ca'·via
cav'·i·tar'y
cav'·i·tas   *pl.* cav'·i·
  ta'·tes, *gen. sg.* ·ta'·tis
cav'·i·ta'·tion
ca·vi'·tis
cav'·i·ty
ca'·vo·gram
ca·vog'·ra·phy
ca'·vo·mes'·en·ter'·ic
ca'·vo·sur'·face
ca'·vo·val'·gus
ca'·vum   *adj. & n.*
  neut. of cavus; *pl.* ·va
ca'·vus   *pl. & gen. sg.* ·vi
ce·as'·mic
ce'·cal   *Brit.* cae'·
ce·ca'·lis   *var. of*
  caecalis
ce·cec'·to·my   *Brit.*
  cae'·
ce·ci'·tis   *Brit.* cae'·
ce'·co   *Words*
  beginning thus have
  the British spelling
  caeco-
ce'·co·ap'·pen·dic'·u·
  lar
ce'·co·co'·lo·pex'y
ce'·co·co·los'·to·my
ce'·co·cys'·to·plas'·ty
ce'·co·il'·e·os'·to·my
ce'·co·pex'y
ce'·co·pli·ca'·tion

ce'·co·sig'·moid·os'·to·my
ce·cos'·to·my
ce·cot'·o·my
ce'·cum *also* cae'·cum
cef'·a·clor
cef'·a·drox'·il
cef'·a·man'·dole
cef'·a·tri'·zine
cef·az'·o·lin
cef·met'·a·zole
ce·fon'·i·cid
cef'·o·per'·a·zone
ce·fo'·ra·nide
cef'·o·tax'·ime
cef'·o·ti'·am
ce·fox'·i·tin
cef·sul'·o·din
cef'·ti·zox'·ime
cef'·tri·ax'·one
cef'·ur·ox'·ime
ce·la'·tion
ce'·li·ac *also* coe'·li·ac
ce·li'·a·cus *var. of*
  coeliacus; *fem.* ·ca
ce'·li·ec'·to·my *also*
  coe'·
ce'·lio· *also* coe'·lio·
ce'·lio·cen·te'·sis
ce'·lio·col·pot'·o·my
ce'·lio·my'·o·mec'·to·my
ce'·lio·my'·o·si'·tis
ce'·lio·py·o'·sis
ce'·li·or'·rha·phy
ce'·li·os'·co·py
ce'·li·ot'·o·my
ce'·li·pro'·lol
cell
cel'·la *pl. & gen. sg.*
  ·lae
cel·lif'·u·gal *var. of*
  cellulifugal
cel·lip'·e·tal *var. of*
  cellulipetal
cel'·lo·bi'·ose
cel·loi'·des
cel·loi'·din

cel'·lu·la *pl. & gen.*
  sg. ·lae
cel'·lu·lar
cel'·lu·lar'·i·ty
cel'·lu·lase
cel'·lule
cel'·lu·lif'·u·gal
cel'·lu·lip'·e·tal
cel'·lu·lit'·ic
cel'·lu·li'·tis
cel'·lu·lo·
cel'·lu·lo·cu·ta'·ne·ous
cel'·lu·lo·fi'·brous
cel'·lu·lo·neu·ri'·tis
cel'·lu·lo·ra·dic'·u·lo·
  neu·ri'·tis
cel'·lu·lo'·sa
cel'·lu·lose
cel'·lu·los'·i·ty
cel'·lu·lo·tox'·ic
ce'·lo· *hernia*
ce'·lo· *cavity; var. of*
  coelo-
ce'·lom *var. of* coelom
ce·lom'·ic *var. of*
  coelomic
ce'·lo·phle·bi'·tis
ce·los'·chi·sis
ce'·lo·scope
ce'·lo·so'·mia
ce'·lo·vi'·rus *also*
  CELO virus
ce'·lo·zo'·ic *var. of*
  coelozoic
Cel'·si·us
ce·ment'
ce·men'·tal
ce'·men·ta'·tion
ce·men'·ti·cle
ce·men'·ti·fi·ca'·tion
ce·men'·ti·fy'·ing
ce·men'·to·
ce·men'·to·blast
ce·men'·to·blas·to'·ma
ce·men'·to·cla'·sia
ce·men'·to·cyte
ce·men'·to·den'·tin·al
ce·men'·to·enam'·el

ce·men'·to·gen'·e·sis
ce·ment'·oid [·men'·
  toid]
ce'·men·to'·ma *pl.*
  ·mas *or* ·ma·ta
ce'·men·to'·sis
ce·men'·tum
cen'·es·the'·sia *Brit.*
  coen'·aes·
cen'·es·thet'·ic *Brit.*
  coen'·aes·
cen·es'·tho·path'·ic
  Brit. coen·aes'·
ce'·no· *var. of* coeno-
  & caeno-
ce·no'·bi·um *var. of*
  coenobium
ce'·no·cyte *var. of*
  coenocyte
ce'·no·gen'·e·sis *var.*
  of caenogenesis
ce'·no·site *var. of*
  coenosite
cen·tal'·gia
cen'·ter *also* ·tre
cen·te'·sis
cen'·ti·
cen'·ti·grade
cen'·ti·gram
cen'·ti·li'·ter *Brit.* ·tre
cen'·ti·me'·ter *Brit.* ·tre
cen'·ti·mor'·gan
cen'·ti·nor'·mal
cen'·ti·pede
cen'·ti·poise
cen'·ti·stoke
cen'·tra *pl. of* centrum
cen'·trad
cen'·tral
cen·tra'·le *neut. of*
  centralis
cen·tra'·lis *pl.* ·les
cen'·trax·o'·ni·al
cen'·tre *var. of* center
cen'·tren'·ce·phal'·ic
cen'·tri·
cen'·tri·ac'·i·nar

cen'·tric
cen'·tri·cip'·i·tal
cen·tric'·i·put
cen·trif'·u·gal
cen·trif'·u·ga'·tion
cen'·tri·fuge
cen·trif'·u·gum
cen'·tri·lob'·u·lar
cen'·tri·ole
cen·trip'·e·tal
cen'·tro·
cen'·tro·ac'·i·nar
cen'·tro·blast
cen'·tro·blas'·tic
Cen'·tro·ces'tus
cen'·tro·cyte
cen'·tro·cyt'·ic
cen'·tro·des'·mus
   also ·mose
cen'·tro·lec'·i·thal
cen'·tro·lob'·u·lar
cen'·tro·me'·di·an
cen'·tro·mere
cen'·tro·mer'·ic
cen'·tro·nu'·cle·ar
cen'·tro·pos·te'·ri·or
cen'·tro·some
cen'·tro·sphere
cen'·trum   *pl.* ·tra
Cen'·tru·roi'·des
ceph'·a·ce·trile'
ce·pha'·eline
ceph'·a·lad
ceph'·a·lal'·gia   *also*
   ce·phal'·gia
ceph'·al·ede'·ma   Brit.
  ·oe·de'·
ceph'·a·le'·ma·to·cele'
  [·le·mat'o·] *var. of*
  cephalohematocele
ceph'·a·le'·ma·to'·ma
  var. of cephalohe-
  matoma
ceph'·a·lex'·in
ceph'·al·he'·ma·to·cele'
  [·he·mat'o·] *var. of*
  cephalohematocele

ceph'·al·he'·ma·to'·ma
  var. of cephalohe-
  matoma
ceph'·al·hy'·dro·cele
ce·phal'·ic
ce·phal'·i·ca
ceph'·a·lin
ceph'·a·li·za'·tion
ceph'·a·lo·
ceph'·a·lo·cau'·dad
ceph'·a·lo·cau'·dal
ceph'·a·lo·cen·te'·sis
ceph'·a·lo·cer'·cal
ceph'·a·lo·did'·y·mus
ceph'·a·lo·dym'·ia
ceph'·a·lod'·y·mus
ceph'·a·lo·dyn'·ia
ceph'·al·oe·de'·ma
  Brit. spel. of
  cephaledema
ceph'·a·lo·gas'·ter
ceph'·a·lo·gly'·cin
ceph'·a·lo·gram
ceph'·a·lo·gy'·ric
ceph'·a·lo·he'·ma·to·
  cele' [·he·mat'o·]
  Brit. ·hae'·
ceph'·a·lo·he'·ma·to'·
  ma Brit. ·hae'·
ceph'·a·lom'·e·lus
ceph'·a·lom'·e·ter
ceph'·a·lo·met'·ric
ceph'·a·lom'·e·try
ceph'·a·lo'·nia
ceph'·a·lop'·a·gus
ceph'·a·lo·pal'·pe·bral
ceph'·a·lop'·a·thy
ceph'·a·lo·pel'·vic
ceph'·a·lo·pel·vim'·e·
  try
ceph'·a·lo·ple'·gia
ceph'·a·lo·ra·chid'·i·an
  also ·rha
ceph'·a·lor'·i·dine
ceph'·a·lo·spo'·rin
  also ·rine
ceph'·a·lo·spo'·rin·ase
Ceph'·a·lo·spo'·ri·um

ceph'·a·lo·stat
ceph'·a·lo·style
ceph'·a·lo·thin
ceph'·a·lo·tho'·ra·co·ili·
  op'·a·gus
ceph'·a·lo·tho'·ra·cop'·
  a·gus
ceph'·a·lo·tho'·rax
ceph'·a·lo·tri·gem'·i·nal
ceph'·a·lo·tro'·pic
  [·trop'·ic]
ceph'·a·my'·cin
ceph'·a·pi'·rin
ce·ra'·ceous
cer'·a·mide
cer'·a·sine
Ce·ras'·tes
ce'·rate
cer'·a·to·   *var. of*
  kerato-
cer'·a·to·cri'·coid
cer'·a·to·cri·coi'·de·us
  neut. ·de·um
cer'·a·to·glos'·sus
cer'·a·to·hy'·al
cer'·a·to·pha·ryn'·ge·al
cer'·a·to·pha·ryn'·ge·us
  fem. ·gea
Cer'·a·to·phyl'·li·dae
Cer'·a·to·phyl'·lus
Cer'·a·to·po·gon'·i·dae
cer·car'·ia *pl.* ·i·ae
cer·car'·i·al
cer·car'·i·cid'·al [·ci'·
  dal]
cer'·ci *pl. of* cercus
cer·clage'
cer'·co·cyst
cer'·co·mer
Cer'·co·mo'·nas
Cer'·co·pith'·e·coi'·dea
cer'·cus *pl.* ·ci
ce'·re·al
cer'·e·bel'·lar
cer'·e·bel·la'·ris *gen.*
  pl. ·ri·um
cer'·e·bel'·li *gen. of*
  cerebellum

cer′·e·bel·lif′·u·gal
  also ·lof′·u·gal
cer′·e·bel·lip′·e·tal
cer′·e·bel·li′·tis
cer′·e·bel′·lo·
cer′·e·bel′·lo·med′·ul·lar′y
cer′·e·bel′·lo·med′·ul·la′·ris
cer′·e·bel′·lo·ol′·i·var′y
cer′·e·bel′·lo·pa·ren′·chy·mal
cer′·e·bel′·lo·pon′·tine
  also ·tile
cer′·e·bel′·lo·pon′·tis
cer′·e·bel′·lo·ru′·bral
cer′·e·bel′·lo·ru·bra′·lis
cer′·e·bel′·lo·ru′·bro·spi′·nal
cer′·e·bel′·lo·spi′·nal
cer′·e·bel′·lo·tha·lam′·ic
cer′·e·bel′·lo·tha·lam′·i·cus
cer′·e·bel′·lo·ves·tib′·u·lar
cer′·e·bel′·lum gen. ·li
cer′·e·bral [ce·re′·]
cer′·e·bra′·lis neut. ·bra′·le
cer′·e·bri gen. of cerebrum
ce·re′·bri·form
cer′·e·brif′·u·gal
cer′·e·brip′·e·tal
cer′·e·bro· [ce·re′·bro·]
cer′·e·bro·car′·di·ac
cer′·e·bro·cer′·e·bel′·lar
cer′·e·bro·hep′·a·to·re′·nal
cer′·e·broid
cer′·e·bro·mac′·u·lar
cer′·e·bro·oc′·u·lar
cer′·e·brop′·a·thy
cer′·e·bro·pon′·tine
cer′·e·bro·pu′·pil·lar′y
cer′·e·bro·ret′·i·nal
cer′·e·bro·side
cer′·e·bro·si·do′·sis
cer′·e·bro·spi′·nal
cer′·e·bro·spi′·nant
cer′·e·bros′·to·my
cer′·e·bro·ten′·di·nous
cer′·e·bro·to′·nia
cer′·e·bro·ty′·phus
cer′·e·bro·vas′·cu·lar
cer′·e·brum [ce·re′·brum] gen. ·bri
cere′·cloth
ce·re′·o·lus pl. ·li
ce′·ri·um
cer′o·
ce′·roid
ce′·roid-lip′o·fus′·cin·o′·sis [-li′po·]
ce·rot′·ic
cer′·ti·fi′·a·ble
cer′·ti·fi·ca′·tion
ce·ru′·le·us fem. ·lea
ce·ru′·lo·plas′·min
ce·ru′·men
ce·ru′·mi·no′·sa pl. ·sae
ce·ru′·mi·no′·sis
ce·ru′·mi·nous also ·nal
cer′·vi·cal
cer′·vi·ca′·le neut. of cervicalis
cer′·vi·ca′·lis pl. ·les, gen. pl. ·li·um
cer′·vi·cec′·to·my
cer′·vi·cis gen. of cervix
cer′·vi·ci′·tis
cer′·vi·co·
cer′·vi·co·ax′·il·lar′y
cer′·vi·co·bra′·chi·al
cer′·vi·co·col·pi′·tis
cer′·vi·co·fa′·cial
cer′·vi·co·med′·ul·lar′y
cer′·vi·co·scap′·u·lar
cer′·vi·co·tho·rac′·ic
cer′·vi·co·tho·rac′·i·cum
cer′·vi·co·u′·ter·ine
cer′·vi·co·vag′·i·nal
cer′·vi·co·vag′·i·na′·lis pl. ·les
cer′·vi·co·vag′·i·ni′·tis
cer′·vi·co·ves′·i·cal
cer′·vix pl. ·vi·ces, gen. sg. ·vi·cis
ce·sar′·e·an also cae·, ·i·an
ce′·si·um
Ces·to′·da
ces′·tode
ces′·to·di′·a·sis
ces′·toid
Ces·toi′·dea
ce·ta′·ce·um
ce′·tri·mide
ce′·tyl
ce′·tyl·py′·ri·din′·i·um
cev′·a·dine
Cha·ber′·tia
chafe chafed, chaf′·ing
cha·go′·ma
cha·la′·sia
cha·las′·to·der′·mia
  also chal′·a·zo·
cha·la′·za pl. ·zae or ·zas
cha·la′·zi·on pl. ·zia
chal·ci′·tis
chal′·co·my′·cin
chal·co′·sis copper deposition: Cf. chalicosis
chal′·i·co′·sis stone dust pneumoconiosis: Cf. chalcosis
chal·ki′·tis var. of chalcitis
chal′·lenge
chal′·one
cha·lu′·ni
cham′·ber
cham′·o·mile
chance′·bone

chan′·cre
chan′·cri·form
chan′·croid
chan·croi′·dal
chan′·crous
chan′·nel
cha′·o·tro′·pic [·trop′·ic]
chap   chapped, chap′·ping
char′·ac·ter
char′·ac·ter·is′·tic
char·bon′
char′·coal
char′·la·tan
char′·la·tan·is′m
char′·ley·horse′
char′·ring
char′·ta   pl. ·tae
char·treu′·sin
char′·tu·la   pl. ·lae
chas′·ma
chaude′-pisse′
chaul·moo′·gra
chaul·moo′·gric
check′·bite
check′·up
cheek′·bone
chei·lec′·to·my
cheil′·ec·tro′·pi·on
chei·li′·tis
chei′·lo·
chei′·lo·plas′·ty
chei·lor′·rha·phy
chei·los′·chi·sis
chei·lo′·sis
chei′·lo·sto′·ma·to·plas′·ty
chei·lot′·o·my
Chei′·ra·can′·thi·um   var. of Chiracanthium
chei′·ro   also chi′·ro·
chei′·ro·kin′·es·the′·sia   Brit. ·aes·the′·
chei′·ro·kin′·es·thet′·ic   Brit. ·aes·thet′·
chei′·ro·lin
chei′·ro·meg′·a·ly

chei′·ro·plas′·ty
chei′·ro·pom′·pho·lyx
chei′·ro·spas′m
che′·late   n. & v. ·lat′·ed, ·lat′·ing
che·la′·tion
che·lic′·era   pl. ·er·ae
chel′·i·don
che′·loid   var. of keloid
che′·loi·do′·sis
chem′·abra′·sion
chem′·i·cal
chem′·i·co·
chem′i·lu′·mi·nes′·cence [che′·mi·]
chem′·ist
chem′·is·try
che′·mo·
che′·mo·au′·to·troph
che′·mo·au′·to·tro′·phic [·troph′·ic]
che′·mo·cau′·tery
che′·mo·cep′·tor   var. of chemoreceptor
che′·mo·co·ag′·u·la′·tion
che′·mo·dec·to′·ma   pl. ·mas or ·ma·ta
che′·mo·dif′·fer·en′·ti·a′·tion
che′·mo·em′·bo·li·za′·tion
che′·mo·ki·ne′·sis
che′·mo·ki·net′·ic
che′·mo·lith′·o·troph
che′·mo·lith′·o·tro′·phic [·troph′·ic]
che′·mo·nu′·cle·ol′·y·sis
che′·mo·or·gan′·o·troph
che′·mo·pal′·li·dec′·to·my
che′·mo·pal′·li·do·thal′·a·mec′·to·my
che′·mo·pro′·phy·lax′·is   pl. ·es
che′·mo·re·cep′·tor

che′·mo·re′·flex
che′·mo·re·sis′·tant
che′·mo·sen′·si·tive
che′·mo·sen′·so·ry
che′·mo·se′·ro·ther′·a·py
che·mo′·sis
che′·mo·stat [chem′·o·]
che′·mo·ster′·i·lant
che′·mo·sup·pres′·sion
che′·mo·sur′·gery
che′·mo·sur′·gi·cal
che′·mo·syn′·the·sis   pl. ·ses
che′·mo·tac′·tic
che′·mo·tax′·is
che′·mo·thal′·a·mec′·to·my
che′·mo·thal′·a·mot′·o·my
che′·mo·ther′·a·peu′·tic
che′·mo·ther′·a·py
che·mot′·ic
che′·mo·trans′·mit·ter
che′·mo·troph
che′·mo·tro′·phic [·troph′·ic]
che′·mo·tro′·pic [·trop′·ic]
che′·mo·tro′·pism
che′·no·de·ox′y·cho′·lic
che′·no·po′·di·um
cher′·ub·is′m
Chey′·le·ti·el′·la
chi′·asm   var. of chiasma
chi·as′·ma   pl. ·ma·ta, gen. sg. ·ma·tis
chi′·as·mat′·ic   also chi·as′·mic
chi′·as·mom′·e·ter
chick′en·pox   also chicken pox
chig′·ger
chig′·oe   also chig′o
chik′·un·gun′·ya
chil′·blain

child′·bed
child′·bear·ing
child′·birth
child′·proof
chi·li′·tis *var. of* cheilitis
chi′·lo· *var. of* cheilo-
chi′·lo·mas′·ti·gi′·a·sis
Chi′·lo·mas′·tix
  C. *mes·nil′i*
Chi·lop′·o·da
chi·los′·chi·sis *var. of* cheiloschisis
chi·me′·ra *also* chi·mae′·ra
chi·me′·ric
chi·me′·rism
chin′·cap *also* chin cap
chinch
chi·ni′·o·fon
chi·no′·i·dine
chi′·on·ablep′·sia
Chi′·ra·can′·thi·um
chi′·ral
chi·ral′·i·ty
chi′·ro· *var. of* cheiro-
chi′·ro·meg′·a·ly *var. of* cheiromegaly
chi′·ro·po′·di·cal
chi·rop′·o·dist
chi·rop′·o·dy
chi′·ro·prac′·tic
chi′·ro·prac′·tor
Chi·rop′·tera
chi′·ro·spas′m *var. of* cheirospasm
chi·rur′·geon
chi·rur′·gery
chi·rur′·gic
chi·rur′·gi·cus *fem.*
  ·ca, *neut.* ·cum
chis′·el
chi′-square
chi′·tin
chi′·tin·ous
chlam′·y·de′·mia
  Brit. ·dae′·mia

Chla·myd′·ia
  C. *psit′·ta·ci*
  C. *tra·cho′·ma·tis*
chla·myd′·ia *pl.* ·i·ae
  or ·i·as
Chla·myd′·i·a′·ce·ae
chla·myd′·i·al
chla·myd′·i·o′·sis
chla·myd′·o·spore
chlo·as′·ma
chlor·ac′·e·tate
chlor′·ace′·tic
chlor·ac′·ne
chlo′·ral
chlo′·ral·is′m
chlo′·ral·ize
chlo·ram′·bu·cil
chlo′·ra·mine
chlor′·am·phen′·i·col
chlor′·anil′·ic
chlo′·rate
chlor·bu′·tol [chlor′·bu·]
chlor·cy′·cli·zine
chlor′·de·cone
chlor′·di·az′·ep·ox′·ide
chlo·rel′·lin
chlo·re′·mia *Brit.* ·rae′·
chlo·ret′·ic
chlor·hex′·i·dine
chlor·hy′·dria
chlor·hy′·drin
chlo′·ric
chlo′·ride
chlo′·ri·du′·ria [·rid·u′·ria] *var. of* chloruria
chlo′·ri·nat′·ed
chlo′·ri·na′·tion
chlo′·ri·na′·tor
chlo′·rine
chlor′·i·son′·da·mine
chlo′·rite
chlor·mer′·o·drin
chlor·mez′·a·none
chlo′·ro·
chlo′·ro·ace′·tic
chlo′·ro·bu′·ta·nol

chlo′·ro·cru′·o·rin
chlo′·ro·di·ni′·tro·ben′·zene [·ben·zene′]
chlo′·ro·flu′o·ro·car′·bon
chlo′·ro·form
chlo′·ro·gen′·ic
chlo′·ro·gua′·nide
chlo′·ro·leu·ke′·mia
  Brit. ·kae′·
chlo·ro′·ma *pl.* ·mas *or* ·ma·ta
chlo′·ro·meth′·ane
chlo·rom′·e·try
chlo′·ro·pe′·nia
chlo′·ro·per′·cha
chlo′·ro·pex′·ia
chlo′·ro·phane
chlo′·ro·phyll
chlo′·ro·pic′·rin
Chlo·rop′·i·dae
chlo′·ro·plast *also* chlo′·ro·plas′·tid
chlo′·ro·pro′·caine
chlo·rop′·sia *also* ·ro′·pia
chlo′·ro·pyr′·i·lene
chlo′·ro·quine
chlo·ro′·sis
chlo′·ro·sul·fon′·ic
chlo′·ro·then
chlo′·ro·thi′·a·zide
chlo·rot′·ic
chlo′·rous
chlo·rox′·ine
chlor′·phen·ir′·a·mine
chlor′·phen·ox′·a·mine
chlor·pro′·ma·zine
chlor·pro′·pa·mide
chlor′·pro·thix′·ene
chlor′·quin·al′·dol
chlor′·tet′·ra·cy′·cline
chlor·thal′·i·done
chlor′·ure′·sis
chlor′·uret′·ic
chlor·u′ria
chlo′·ryl
chlor·zox′·a·zone

cho′·a·na *pl.* ·nae
cho′·a·nal
cho′·a·nate
cho′·a·noid
Cho′·a·no·tae′·nia
choke   choked, chok′·ing
cho′·la·gog′·ic
cho′·la·gogue
cho′·lane
cho·lan′·ge·i′tis *var.*
 of cholangitis
cho·lan′·gi·ec′·ta·sis
 also ·ec·ta′·sia
cho·lan′·gio·
cho·lan′·gio·ad′·e·no′·ma
cho·lan′·gio·car′·ci·no′·ma
cho·lan′·gio·en′·ter·os′·to·my
cho·lan′·gio·gas·tros′·to·my
cho·lan′·gi·o·gram
cho·lan′·gi·og′·ra·phy
cho·lan′·gio·hep′·a·ti′·tis
cho·lan′·gio·hep′·a·to′·ma
cho·lan′·gio·je′·ju·nos′·to·my
cho·lan′·gi·ole
cho·lan′·gi·o·lit′·ic
cho·lan′·gi·o·li′·tis
cho·lan′·gi·o′·ma
cho·lan′·gi·os′·to·my
cho·lan′·gi·ot′·o·my
cho′·lan·git′·ic
cho′·lan·gi′·tis
cho·lan′·ic
cho′·la·no·poi·e′·sis
 [cho·lan′o·]
cho′·la·no·poi·et′·ic
 [cho·lan′o·]
cho′·le·
cho′·le·cal·cif′·er·ol
cho′·le·cys′·tec·ta′·sia
cho′·le·cys·tec′·to·my

cho′·le·cyst·elec′·tro·co·ag′·u·lec′·to·my
cho′·le·cyst′·en·ter′·ic
cho′·le·cyst·en′·tero·anas′·to·mo′·sis
cho′·le·cyst·en′·ter·or′·rha·phy
cho′·le·cyst·en′·ter·os′·to·my
cho′·le·cyst·gas·tros′·to·my
cho′·le·cys′·tic
cho′·le·cys′·tis
cho′·le·cys·ti′·tis
cho′·le·cyst·ne·phros′·to·my
cho′·le·cys′·to·
cho′·le·cys′·to·cele
cho′·le·cys′·to·cho·lan′·gi·o·gram
cho′·le·cys′·to·co·lon′·ic
cho′·le·cys′·to·co·los′·to·my
cho′·le·cys′·to·co·lot′·o·my
cho′·le·cys′·to·du′·o·de′·nal
cho′·le·cys′·to·du′·o·de′·no·co′·lic
cho′·le·cys′·to·du′·o·de·nos′·to·my
cho′·le·cys′·to·elec′·tro·co·ag′·u·lec′·to·my
cho′·le·cys′·to·en′·tero·anas′·to·mo′·sis
 var. of cholecystentero-anastomosis
cho′·le·cys′·to·en′·ter·os′·to·my *var. of* cholecystenterostomy
cho′·le·cys′·to·gas·tros′·to·my *var. of* cholecystgastrostomy
cho′·le·cys′·to·gram
cho′·le·cys·tog′·ra·phy

cho′·le·cys′·to·il′e·os′·to·my
cho′·le·cys′·to·in·tes′·ti·nal
cho′·le·cys′·to·je′·ju·nos′·to·my
cho′·le·cys′·to·ki′·nin
cho′·le·cys′·to·ne·phros′·to·my
cho′·le·cys′·to·pex′y
cho′·le·cys′·to·py′·e·los′·to·my
cho′·le·cys·tor′·rha·phy
cho′·le·cys·tos′·to·my
cho′·le·cys·tot′·o·my
cho′·le·doch′·al [cho·led′·o·chal]
cho′·le·do·chec′·to·my [cho·led′·o·]
cho′·le·do·chi′·tis [cho·led′·o·]
cho·led′·o·cho·
cho·led′·o·cho·cho·led′·o·chos′·to·my
cho·led′·o·cho·cys·tos′·to·my
cho·led′·o·cho·du′·o·de′·nal
cho·led′·o·cho·du′·o·de·nos′·to·my
cho·led′·o·cho·en′·ter·os′·to·my
cho·led′·o·chog′·ra·phy
cho·led′·o·cho·il′·e·os′·to·my
cho·led′·o·cho·je′·ju·nos′·to·my
cho·led′·o·cho·li·thi′·a·sis
cho·led′·o·cho·li·thot′·o·my
cho·led′·o·chor′·rha·phy
cho·led′·o·cho·scope
cho·led′·o·chos′·to·my
cho·led′·o·chot′·o·my
cho·led′·o·chous

cho·led′·o·chus gen.
·chi
cho′·le·glo′·bin
cho′·le·lith
cho′·le·li·thi′·a·sis
cho·le′·mia Brit. ·lae′·
cho·le′·mic Brit. ·lae′·
cho′·le·poi·e′·sis
cho′·le·poi·et′·ic
chol′·era
chol′·e·ra′·ic
cho′·le·re′·sis
cho′·le·ret′·ic
chol′·er·i·form
chol′·er·i·for′·mis
cho·les′·tane
cho′·le·sta′·sis
cho′·le·stat′·ic
cho·les′·te·a·to′·ma
  pl. ·mas or ·ma·ta
cho·les′·te·a·tom′·a·tous
cho·les′·ter·e′·mia
  Brit. ·ae′·mia
cho·les′·ter·in·o′·sis [·i·no′·sis]
cho·les′·ter·in·u′·ria [·i·nu′·] var. of cholesteroluria
cho·les′·ter·ol
cho·les′·ter·ol·e′·mia
  Brit. ·ae′·mia
cho·les′·ter·ol·o′·sis
cho·les′·ter·ol·u′·ria
cho·les′·ter·o′·sis
cho′·le·styr′·a·mine
cho′·lic
cho′·line
cho′·lin·er′·gic
cho′·lin·es′·ter·ase
cho′·li·no·cep′·tive
cho′·li·no·lyt′·ic
cho′·li·no·mi·met′·ic
cho′·li·no·re·cep′·tor
cho′·lo· var. of chole-
cho′·lo·tho′·rax
cho·lu′·ria
chon′·dral

chon·drec′·to·my
chon′·dri·fi·ca′·tion
chon′·dri·fy ·fied, ·fy′·ing
chon′·drio·
chon·dri′·tis
chon′·dro·
chon′·dro·blast
chon′·dro·blas·to′·ma
  pl. ·mas or ·ma·ta
chon′·dro·cal′·ci·no′·sis
chon′·dro·cla′·sis
chon′·dro·clast
chon′·dro·cos′·tal
chon′·dro·cra′·ni·um
chon′·dro·cu·ta′·ne·ous
chon′·dro·cyte
chon′·dro·der′·ma·ti′·tis
chon′·dro·dys·pla′·sia
chon′·dro·dys·tro′·phic [·troph′·ic]
chon′·dro·dys′·tro·phy
  also ·dys·tro′·phia
chon′·dro·ep′·i·phys′·e·al [·epiph′·y·se′·al]
chon′·dro·epiph′·y·si′·tis
chon′·dro·gen′·e·sis
chon′·dro·gen′·ic
chon′·dro·glos′·sus
chon′·droid
chon·dro′·i·tin
chon′·dro·li·po′·ma
  pl. ·mas or ·ma·ta
chon·drol′·o·gy
chon·drol′·y·sis
chon·dro′·ma pl. ·mas or ·ma·ta
chon′·dro·ma·la′·cia
chon′·dro·ma·to′·sis
chon·dro′·ma·tous [·drom′·a·]
chon′·dro·mere
chon′·dro·met′·a·pla′·sia
chon′·dro·mu′·cin

chon′·dro·mu′·coid
chon′·dro·my·o′·ma
chon′·dro·myx′·oid
chon′·dro·ne·cro′·sis
chon′·dro-os′·teo·dys′·tro·phy
chon′·dro-os′·te·o′·ma
chon·drop′·a·thy
chon′·dro·pha·ryn′·gea
chon′·dro·pha·ryn′·ge·al
chon′·dro·phyte
chon′·dro·pla′·sia
chon′·dro·plast
chon′·dro·plas′·tic
chon′·dro·plas′·ty
chon·dro′·sa·mine
chon′·dro·sar·co′·ma
chon·dro′·sis
chon′·dro·ster′·nal
chon′·dro·ster′·no·plas′·ty
chon·drot′·o·my
chon′·dro·tro′·phic [·troph′·ic]
chon′·dro·xiph′·oid
chor·an′·gi·o′·ma var. of chorioangioma
chor′·da pl. & gen. sg. ·dae
chor′·dal [chord′·al]
chor′·da·mes′o·derm
Chor·da′·ta
chor′·date having a notochord: Cf. cordate
chor·dee′ [chor′·dee]
chor·di′·tis inflammation of vocal cord: Cf. corditis
chor′·do·
chor·do′·ma pl. ·mas or ·ma·ta
chor′·do·pex′y var. of cordopexy
chor·dot′·o·my
cho·re′a
cho·re′·al
cho·re′·ic

cho·re′·iform
cho′·reo·ath′·e·to′·sis
cho′·re·oid
cho′·reo·ma′·nia
cho′·ri·al
cho′·rio·
cho′·rio·ad′·e·no′·ma
cho′·rio·al′·lan·to′·ic
cho′·rio·al·lan′·to·is
cho′·rio·am′·ni·on′·ic
cho′·rio·am′·ni·on·i′·tis
cho′·rio·an′·gio·fi·bro′·ma
cho′·rio·an′·gi·o′·ma
cho′·rio·cap′·il·la′·ris
cho′·rio·cap′·il·lar′y
cho′·rio·car′·ci·no′·ma
cho′·rio·ep′·i·the′·li·o′·ma
cho′·ri·oid *var. of* choroid
cho′·ri·oi′·dea *var. of* choroidea
cho′·ri·o′·ma *pl.* ·mas *or* ·ma·ta
cho′·rio·men′·in·gi′·tis
cho′·ri·on
cho′·ri·on′·ic
cho′·rio·pla·cen′·tal
cho′·rio·plaque
Cho′·ri·op′·tes
cho′·ri·op′·tic
cho′·rio·ret′·i·nal
cho′·rio·ret′·i·ni′·tis
cho′·rio·ret′·i·nop′·a·thy
cho·ris′·ta
cho′·ris·to′·ma *pl.* ·mas *or* ·ma·ta
cho′·roid
cho·roi′·dal
cho·roi′·dea *fem. of* choroideus; *pl. & gen. sg.* ·de·ae
cho′·roid·ec′·to·my
cho′·roi·de·re′·mia [·roid·ere′·]

cho·roi′·de·um *neut. of* choroideus
cho·roi′·de·us
cho′·roid·i′·tis
cho·roi′·do·
cho·roi′·do·iri′·tis
cho′·roid·op′·a·thy
cho·roi′·do·ret′·i·ni′·tis *var. of* chorioretinitis
chro′·maf·fin
chrom′·af·fin′·i·ty
chro′·maf·fin·o′·ma [·fi·no′·ma]
chro′·maf·fi·nop′·a·thy
chro′·man
chro′·ma·phil *var. of* chromophil
chrom′·ar·gen′·taf·fin
chro′·mate
chro·mat′·ic
chro′·ma·tid
chro′·ma·tin
chro′·ma·tis′m
chro′·ma·to· [chro·mat′o·]
chro·mat′·o·cyte [chro′·ma·to·]
chro·mat′·o·gram
chro·mat′·o·graph
chro·mat′·o·graph′·ic [chro′·ma·to·]
chro′·ma·tog′·ra·phy
chro′·ma·tol′·y·sis
chro′·ma·to·lyt′·ic
chro′·ma·tom′·e·ter
chro·mat′o·phil [chro′·ma·to·] *also* ·phile; *var. of* chromophil
chro·mat′o·phil′·ia [chro′·ma·to·]
chro·mat′o·phil′·ic [chro′·ma·to·] *var. of* chromophilic
chro·mat′o·phore [chro′·ma·to·]
chro′·ma·to·pho·ro·tro′·pic [·trop′·ic]

chro′·ma·toph′·o·rous
chro′·ma·to·plas′m [chro·mat′o·]
chro′·ma·to·plast [chro·mat′o·]
chro′·ma·top′·sia
chro′·ma·to′·sis
chro′·ma·to·tax′·is
chro′·ma·tot′·ro·pis′m [·to·tro′·] *var. of* chromotropism
chrome
chrom′·es·the′·sia *Brit.* ·aes·the′·
chrom′·hi·dro′·sis *also* chrom′·i·
chro′·mic
chro·mid′·i·al
chro·mid′·i·um *pl.* ·mid′·ia
chro′·mi·um
chro′·mo·
Chro′·mo·bac·te′·ri·um
chro′·mo·blast
chro′·mo·blas′·to·my·co′·sis
chro′·mo·cen′·ter *Brit.* ·tre
chro′·mo·cyte
chro′·mo·gen
chro′·mo·gen′·ic
chro·mol′·y·sis *var. of* chromatolysis
chro′·mo·mere
chro·mom′·e·ter
chro′·mo·my′·cin
chro′·mo·my·co′·sis
chro′·mo·nar
chro′·mo·ne′·ma *pl.* ·ma·ta; *also* chro′·mo·neme
chro′·mo·phil *also* ·phile
chro′·mo·phil′·ic
chro′·mo·phobe
chro′·mo·pho′·bia
chro′·mo·phore
chro′·mo·phose

chro′·mo·plas′m
chro′·mo·plast *also*
  chro′·mo·plas′·tid
chro′·mo·pro′·tein
chro·mop′·sia *var. of*
  chromatopsia
chro′·mo·scope
chro·mos′·co·py
chro′·mo·som′·al [·so′·mal]
chro′·mo·some
chro′·mo·trich′·i·al
chro′·mo·tro′·pic
  [·trop′·ic]
chro·mot′·ro·pis′m
  [chro′·mo·tro′·pism]
chron′·ax·im′·e·ter
chron·ax′·i·met′·ric
chron′·ax·im′·e·try
chron′·axy *also* ·ax·ie
  or chron·ax′·ia
chron′·ic
chro·nic′·i·ty
chron′·i·cus *fem.* ·ca,
  neut. ·cum
chron′o·
chron′o·bi·ol′·o·gy
chron′·o·graph
chron′·o·log′·ic *also*
  ·i·cal
chro·nom′·e·try
chron′o·my·om′·e·ter
chron′·o·scope
chron′·o·tro′·pic
  [·trop′·ic]
chro·not′·ro·pis′m
chrys′·a·ro′·bin
chry·si′·a·sis
chrys′o·
chrys′·o·der′·ma
Chrys′·o·my′·ia
chrys′·o·phan′·ic
Chrys′·ops
  C. di·mid′·i·a′·ta
  C. dis·ca′·lis
  C. si·la′·cea
chry·so′·sis *var. of*
  chrysiasis

chrys′o·ther′·a·py
chrys′·o·tile
chyl·an′·gi·o′·ma
chyle
chyl′·ec·ta′·sia
chy·le′·mia *Brit.* ·lae′·
chyl′·li *gen. of* chylus
chy′·li· *var. of* chylo-
chy′·li·fa′·cient
chy′·li·fac′·tion
chy·lif′·er·ous
chy′·li·fi·ca′·tion
chy′·li·form
chy′·lo·
chy′·lo·cele
chy′·lo·cyst
chy′·lo·der′·ma
chy′·lo·mi′·cron
chy′·lo·mi′·cro·ne′·mia
  [·cron·e′·mia] *Brit.*
  ·nae′·
chy′·lo·per′·i·car·di′·tis
chy′·lo·per′·i·car′·di·um
chy′·lo·per′·i·to·ne′·um
chy′·lo·poi·e′·sis
chy′·lo·poi·et′·ic
chy′·lor·rhe′a *Brit.*
  ·rhoe′a
chy·lo′·sis
chy′·lo·tho′·rax
chy′·lous
chy·lu′·ria
chy′·lus *gen.* ·li
chyme
chy·mif′·er·ous
chy′·mi·fi·ca′·tion
chy′·mo·pa·pa′·in
chy′·mo·poi·e′·sis
chy′·mo·sin
chy′·mo·tryp′·sin
chy′·mo·tryp·sin′·o·gen
chy′·mo·tryp′·tic
ci′·bus *accusative* ·bum
cic′·a·trec′·to·my
cic′·a·tri′·cial
cic′·a·trix *pl.* cic′·a·tri′·ces

cic′·a·tri′·zant
cic′·a·tri·za′·tion
cic′·a·trize ·trized,
  ·triz′·ing
cic′·u·tis′m
ci′·dal
ci′·gua·ter′a
cil′·ia *pl. of* cilium
cil′·i·a′·re *neut. of*
  ciliaris
cil′·i·a′·ris *pl.* ·res
cil′·i·ar′·i·scope
cil′·i·a·rot′·o·my
cil′·i·ar′y
cil′·i·ate
cil′·i·at′·ed
cil′·io·irid′·i·al
Cil′·i·oph′·o·ra
cil′·io·ret′·i·nal
cil′·io·scle′·ral
cil′·io·spi′·nal
cil′·i·um *pl.* cil′·ia
ci·met′·i·dine
Ci′·mex
  C. he·mip′·ter·us
  C. lec′·tu·lar′·i·us
Ci·mic′·i·dae
cin·cho′·na
cin·chon′·ic
cin·chon′·i·dine [·cho′·ni·]
cin′·cho·nine
cin′·cho·nis′m
cin′·cho·phen
cin′e· *var. of* kine-
cin′e·an′·gio·car′·di·og′·ra·phy
cin′e·an′·gi·o·graph′·ic
cin′·e·an′·gi·og′·ra·phy
cin′e·flu′o·rog′·ra·phy
cin′e·flu′o·ros′·co·py
cin′·e·mat′·ics
cin′·e·mat′·o·graph′·ic
cin′·e·ma·tog′·ra·phy
cin′·e·ole
cin′e·phle·bog′·ra·phy
cin′·e·plas′·ty
cin′e·ra′·di·og′·ra·phy

ci·ne′·re·us *fem.* ·rea,
 neut. ·re·um
cin′e·roent′·gen·og′·ra·
 phy
ci·ne′·sio· *var. of*
 kinesio-
ci·net′o· *var. of*
 kineto-
cin′·gu·late
cin′·gu·lec′·to·my
cin′·gu·lot′·o·my
cin′·gu·lum *pl.* ·la,
 gen. sg. ·li
cin′·na·bar
cin′·na·me′·in
cin·nam′·ic
cin′o· [ci′·no·] *var. of*
 kino-
ci′·o·no·
cir′·ca·di′·an [cir·ca′·
 di·an]
cir′·ci·na′·ta
cir′·ci·nate
cir′·cuit
cir′·cu·la′·re *neut. of*
 circularis
cir′·cu·la′·ris *pl.* ·res
cir′·cu·la′·tion
cir′·cu·la·to′·ry
cir′·cu·lus *pl. & gen.*
 sg. ·li
cir′·cum·
cir′·cum·a′nal
cir′·cum·ax′·il·lar′y
cir′·cum·ca′·val
cir′·cum·cise ·cised,
 ·cis′·ing
cir′·cum·ci′·sion
cir′·cum·cor′·ne·al
cir′·cum·duc′·tion
cir·cum′·fer·ence
cir·cum′·fer·en′·tia
cir·cum′·fer·en′·tial
cir′·cum·flex
cir′·cum·flex′a *fem.*
 of circumflexus; *pl. &*
 gen. sg. ·flex′·ae
cir′cum·flex′·us

cir′·cum·len′·tal
cir′·cum·nu′·cle·ar
cir′·cum·oc′·u·lar
cir′·cum·o′ral
cir′·cum·pen′·nate
cir′·cum·scribed
cir′·cum·scrip′·tus
 fem. ·ta
cir′·cum·stan′·ti·al′·i·ty
cir′·cum·val′·late
cir′·cum·vo·lu′·tio
cir·rho′·sis
cir·rhot′·ic
cir′·rus *pl.* cir′·ri
cir′·so·
cir′·soid
cir·som′·pha·los
cir′·soph·thal′·mia
cis′·tern
cis·ter′·na *pl. & gen.*
 sg. ·nae
cis·ter′·nal
cis′·ter·nog′·ra·phy
cis′·tron
cit′·ral
cit′·rate
cit′·ric
cit′·rin
Cit′·ro·bac′·ter
cit′·ro·nel′·la
cit′·rul·line [ci·trul′·
 line]
cit′·rul·li·ne′·mia [·lin·
 e′·mia] *Brit.* ·nae′·
cit′·rul·li·nu′·ria [·lin·
 u′·ria]
ci·tru′·ria
clad′·i·nose
clad′·i·o′·sis
clad′·o·spo′·ri·o′·sis
Clad′·o·spo′·ri·um
clair·au′·di·ence
clair·voy′·ance
clam·ox′y·quin
cla·pote·ment′
clap′·ping
cla·rif′·i·cant
clar′·i·fi·ca′·tion

clas·mat′·o·cyte
clas′·ma·to′·sis
clas′·sic *also* ·si·cal
clas′·si·fi·ca′·tion
clas′·tic
clas′·to·gen′·ic
clath′·rate
clau′·di·cant
clau′·di·ca′·tion
clau′·di·ca·to′·ry
claus′·tral
claus′·tro·pho′·bia
claus′·trum *pl* ·tra
cla′·va *pl.* ·vae
clav′·a·cin
cla′·val
cla′·vate
cla·va′·tion
Clav′·i·ceps
clav′·i·cle
clav′i·cor′·a·co·ax′·il·
 lar′y
clav′·i·cot′·o·my
cla·vic′·u·la *pl. &*
 gen. sg. ·lae
cla·vic′·u·lar
cla·vic′·u·la′·ris
cla·vic′·u·late
cla·vic′·u·lec′·to·my
clav′·i·for′·min
clav′i·pec′·to·ral
clav′i·pec′·to·ra′·lis
cla′·vus *pl.* ·vi
claw′·hand *also* claw
 hand
clear′·ance
cleav′·age
cleft
clei′·do·
clei′·do·cos′·tal
clei′·do·cra′·ni·al
clei′·do·ep′i·troch′·le·
 ar
clei′·do·hu′·mer·al
clei′·do·hy′·oid
clei′·do·mas′·toid
clei′·do·mas·toi′·de·us
clei′·do·oc·cip′·i·tal

clei'·do·scap'·u·lar
clei'·do·ster'·nal
clei·dot'·o·my
clem'·as·tine
clem'·i·zole
cle'·oid
clep'·to·ma'·nia
cli'·do· *var. of* cleido-
cli'·ent
cli'·mac·ter'·ic [·mac'·ter·]
cli'·mac·ter'·i·um
cli'·mac·tic
cli'·ma·to·ther'·a·peu'·tics
cli'·ma·to·ther'·a·py
cli'·max
clin'·da·my'·cin
clin'·ic
clin'·i·ca
clin'·i·cal
cli·ni'·cian
clin'·i·co·
clin'·i·co·ge·net'·ic
clin'·i·co·path'·o·log'·ic *also* ·i·cal
clin'·i·co·pa·thol'·o·gy
cli'·no·
cli'·no·ce·phal'·ic
cli'·no·ceph'·a·ly
cli'·no·dac'·ty·ly *also* ·tyl·is'·m
cli'·noid
cli·noi'·de·us
clit'·i·on
clit'·o·ral
clit'·o·ri·dec'·to·my
clit'·o·ris *gen.* cli·to'·ri·dis
clit'·o·ri'·tis
clit'·o·ro·meg'·a·ly
cli'·val
cli'·vus
clo·a'·ca *pl. & gen. sg.* ·cae
clo·a'·cal
clo'·a·co·gen'·ic
clo·faz'·i·mine

clo·fi'·brate
clo'·mi·phene
clo·mip'·ra·mine
clon'·al [clo'·nal]
clo·na'·ze·pam
clone *also* clon
clon'·ic
clo·nic'·i·ty
clon'·i·co·ton'·ic
clo'·ni·dine
clon'·ism *also* clo·nis'·mus
clon'·o·graph
clo·nor·chi'·a·sis
Clo·nor'·chis si·nen'·sis
clon'o·spas'm
clo'·nus
clo·pam'·ide
clo·raz'·e·pate
clo'·ra·zep'·ic
clo'·ro·phene
clor·ter'·mine
Clos·trid'·i·um
  C. bot'·u·li'·num
  C. dif·fic'·i·le
  C. his'·to·lyt'·i·cum
  C. per·frin'·gens
  C. tet'·a·ni
clos·trid'·i·um *pl.* ·trid'·ia
clo'·sure
clot clot'·ted, clot'·ting
clo·trim'·a·zole
cloud'y ·i·er, ·i·est
clox'·a·cil'·lin
club'·bing
club'·foot *pl.* ·feet
club'·hand
clu'·ne·al
clu'·nes *sg.* ·nis, *gen. pl.* ·ni·um
clus'·ter
cly'·sis *pl.* ·ses
clys'·ma
clys'·ter
cne'·mi·al

cne'·mis *pl.* ·mi·des, *gen. sg.* ·mi·dis
co·ac'·er·vate
co'·ad·ap·ta'·tion
co'·ag·glu'·ti·na'·tion
co·ag'·u·la *pl. of* coagulum
co·ag'·u·la·bil'·i·ty
co·ag'·u·la·ble
co·ag'·u·lant
co·ag'·u·lase
co·ag'·u·late ·lat'·ed, ·'lat·ing
co·ag'·u·la'·tion
co·ag'·u·la'·tive
co·ag'·u·la'·tor
co·ag'·u·lop'·a·thy
co·ag'·u·lo·vis'·co·sim'·e·ter
co·ag'·u·lum *pl.* ·la
co'·apt
co'·ap·ta'·tion
co·arct' *var. of verb* coarctate
co·arc'·tate *adj. & v.* ·tat'·ed, ·tat'·ing
co'·arc·ta'·tion
co·ax'·i·al
co·bal'·a·min
co'·balt
co'·ban
co'·bra
co'·bra·ly'·sin
co'·ca
co·caine'
co·cain'·ism
co'·cain·i·za'·tion
co'·car·cin'·o·gen [·car'·ci·no·]
co·car'·ci·no·gen'·e·sis
coc'·ci *pl. of* coccus
Coc·cid'·ia
coc·cid'·ia *pl. of* coccidium
coc·cid'·i·al
coc·cid'·i·an
coc·cid'·i·oi'·dal

Coc·cid'·i·oi'·des im·
  mi'·tis
coc·cid'·i·oi'·din
coc·cid'·i·oi·do'·ma
coc·cid'·i·oi'·do·men'·
  in·gi'·tis
coc·cid'·i·oi'·do·my·
  co'·sis also ·cid'·io·
  my·
coc·cid'·i·oi·do'·sis
coc·cid'·i·o'·sis
coc·cid'·i·o·stat
coc·cid'·i·um pl. ·ia
coc'·co·bac'·il·lar'y
  [·ba·cil'·la·ry]
coc'·co·ba·cil'·lus pl.
  ·li
coc'·co·gen'·ic
coc'·coid
coc'·cu·lin
coc'·cu·lus
Coc'·cus
coc'·cus pl. ·ci
coc'·cy·al'·gia
coc'·cy·dyn'·ia
coc'·cyg·al'·gia
coc·cyg'·ea fem. of
  coccygeus
coc·cyg'·e·al
coc'·cy·gec'·to·my
coc·cyg'·eo·pu'·bic
coc·cyg'·e·um neut.
  of goccygeus
coc·cyg'·e·us pl. &
  gen. sg. ·ei
coc'·cy·gis [coc·cy'·
  gis] gen. of coccyx
coc'·cy·go·dyn'·ia
  also coc'·cy·o·
coc'·cy·got'·o·my
coc'·cyx pl. coc'·cy·
  ges, gen. sg. ·cy·gis
coch'·i·neal' [coch'·i·
  neal]
coch'·lea pl. & gen.
  sg. ·le·ae
coch'·le·ar

coch'·le·a'·re neut. of
  cochlearis
coch'·le·a'·ri·for'·mis
coch'·le·a'·ris
coch'·le·ate
coch'·le·og'·ra·phy
coch'·leo·pal'·pe·bral
coch'·leo·sta·pe'·di·al
coch'·le·os'·to·my
coch'·leo·ves·tib'·u·lar
Coch'·li·o·my'·ia
  C. hom'·i·ni·vo'·rax
  C. mac'·el·la'·ria
cock·ade'
cock'·roach
cock'·tail
co'·con'·scious
coc'·tion
co'·de'·hy·drog'·e·nase
co'·deine
co'·dex pl. co'·di·ces
cod'·o·cyte
co·dom'·i·nance
co·dom'·i·nant
co'·don
coe- See also words
  beginning ce-
co'·ef·fi'·cient
Coe·len'·ter·a'·ta
coe·len'·ter·ate
coe'·li·ac var. of
  celiac
coe·li'·a·ca neut. pl.
  & fem. sg. of coe·li'·a·
  cus
coe·li'·a·cus pl. &
  gen. sg. ·ci
coe'·lio· var. of celio-
coe'·li·o·cy·e'·sis
coe'·li·ot'·o·my
coe'·lo·
coe'·lom
coe'·lo·mate
coe·lom'·ic
coe'·lo·my·ar'·i·al
coe'·lo·scope var. of
  celoscope
coe'·lo·so'·my

coe'·lo·zo'·ic
coen'·aes·the'·sia
  Brit. spel. of cenes-
  thesia
coen·aes'·tho·path'·ic
  Brit. spel. of cenestho-
  pathic
coe'·no·
coe·no'·bi·um pl. ·bia
coe'·no·cyte aseptate
  cell mass: Cf. coenosite
coe'·no·cyt'·ic
coe'·no·site free-living
  commensal: Cf.
  coenocyte
coe·nu'·rus pl. ·ri
co·en'·zyme
co'·ex'·ci·ta'·tion
co'·fac'·tor
cog·ni'·tion
cog'·ni·tive
co·her'·ent
co·he'·sion
co·he'·sive
co·ho'·ba
co·hor'·mone
co'·hort
co'·hosh
coil
co'·in'·di·ca'·tion
co'·in·fec'·tion
coi'·no· var. of coeno-
coi'·no·site var. of
  coenosite
co'·in·sur'·ance
co'·i'so·gen'·ic
co'·ital
co·i'tion
co'·itus pl. & gen. sg.
  coitus, accusative ·itum
co·lan'·ic
col'·ce·mide
col'·chi·cine
cold'·blood'·ed
cold'·sen'·si·tive
cold'·sore also cold
  sore
co·lec'·to·my

col′·eo·
col′·eo·cys·ti′·tis
co·les′·ti·pol
co′·li   gen. of colon
co′·li·bac′·il·le′·mia
   Brit. ·lae′·mia
co′·li·bac′·il·lo′·sis
co′·li·bac′·il·lu′·ria
co′·lic   of the colon
col′·ic   abdominal
   disorder
co′·li·ca   fem. of
   colicus
col′·i·cin [co′·li·]
col′·i·cin′·o·gen [co′·
   li·]
col′·i·cin′·o·gen′·ic
   [co′·li·]
col′·icky
co′·li·cus   pl. & gen.
   sg. ·ci
co′·li·cys·ti′·tis
co′·li·cys′·to·py′·e·li′·
   tis
co′·li·form [col′·i·]
co·lin′·e·ar′·i·ty
co′·li·phage [col′·i·]
co′·li·pli·ca′·tion   var.
   of coloplication
co·lis′·tin
co·li′·tis   pl. co·lit′·i·
   des
co′·li·tox·e′·mia   Brit.
   ·ae′·mia
col′·la·gen
col·lag′e·nase [col′·a·
   gen·ase]
col′·la·gen·a′·tion
col′·la·ge·nol′·y·sis
col′·la·gen′·o·lyt′·ic
col′·la·ge·no′·ma   pl.
   ·mas or ·ma·ta
col′·la·ge·no′·sis
col·lag′·e·nous
col·lapse′   ·lapsed′,
   ·laps′·ing
col′·lar

col′·lar·bone   also
   collar bone
col′·lar·ette′
col·lat′·er·al
col·lat′·er·a′·le   neut.
   of collateralis; pl. ·lia
col·lat′·er·a′·lis
col′·li   gen. of collum
col·lic′·u·lec′·to·my
col·lic′·u·li′·tis
col·lic′·u·lus   pl. &
   gen. sg. ·li, gen. pl.
   col·lic′·u·lo′·rum
col′·li·ga′·tive
col′·li·gens
col′·li·ma′·tion
col′·li·ma′·tor
col·lin′·e·ar
col′·li·qua′·tion
col·liq′·ua·tive
col·li′·sion
col·lo′·di·on
col′·loid
col·loi′·dal
col·loi′·do·pex′y
col′·lum   pl. & gen. sg.
   ·li
col′·lu·to′·ri·um   pl.
   ·ria
col·lyr′·i·um   pl. ·lyr′·
   ia
co′·lo·
col′·o·bo′·ma   pl. ·mas
   or ·ma·ta
co′·lo·ce·cos′·to·my
   Brit. ·cae·cos′·
co′·lo·cen·te′·sis   pl.
   ·ses
co·loc′·ly·sis [co′·lo·
   cly′·sis]
co′·lo·co′·lic
co′·lo·co·los′·to·my
co′·lo·cynth   also co′·
   lo·cyn′·this
co′·lo·cyn′·thi·dis′m
co′·lo·fix·a′·tion
co′·lo·hep′·a·to·pex′y
co·lol′·y·sis

co′·lon   gen. co′·li
co·lo′·ni·al
co·lon′·ic
col′·o·ni·za′·tion
col′·o·nize   ·nized,
   ·niz′·ing
co·lon′·o·scope
co′·lo·nos′·co·py
col′·o·ny
co′·lo·pex′y
co·loph′·o·ny
co′·lo·pli·ca′·tion
co′·lo·proc·tec′·to·my
co′·lo·proc·ti′·tis
co′·lo·proc·tos′·to·my
co′·lop·to′·sis
col′·or   Brit. ·our
col′·or·blind′   Brit.
   ·our·; also color blind
col′·or·blind′·ness
   Brit. ·our·; also color
   blindness
co′·lo·rec′·tal
co′·lo·rec·ti′·tis
co′·lo·rec·tos′·to·my
col′·or·im′·e·ter
col′·or·im′·e·try
co′·lo·sig′·moid·os′·to·
   my [·moi·dos′·]
co·los′·to·my
co·los′·trum
co·lot′·o·my
co′·lo·vag′·i·nal
co′·lo·ves′·i·cal
col·pal′·gia
col·pec′·to·my
col′·peu·ryn′·ter
col′·peu′·ry·sis
col·pi′·tis
col′·po·
col′·po·cele
col′·po·ce′·li·ot′·o·my
   Brit. ·coe′·li·
col′·po·clei′·sis   pl.
   ·ses
col′·po·cys·ti′·tis
col′·po·cys′·to·cele
col′·po·cys·tot′·o·my

col′·po·epis′′·i·or′′·rha·
 phy
col′·po·hy′·per·pla′′·sia
col′·po·per′·i·ne·or′·
 rha·phy
col′·po·pex′y
col′·po·plas′·ty
col′·po·poi·e′·sis
col·por′·rha·phy
col′·po·scope
col·pos′·co·py
col′·po·stat
col′·po·ste·no′′·sis
col′·po·ste·not′·o·my
col·pot′·o·my
col′·po·ure′·ter·ot′·o·
 my
col′·po·xe·ro′′·sis
col′·u·brid
Co·lu′·bri·dae
col′·u·mel′·la *pl.* ·lae
col′′·umn
co·lum′·na *pl. & gen.*
 sg. ·nae
co·lum′·nar
co′·ma
co′·ma·tose
com′·e·do *pl.* com′·e·
 do′′·nes
com′·e·do·car′·ci·no′′·
 ma *pl.* ·mas *or* ·ma·
 ta
co′·mes *pl.* com′·i·tes
co·mes′·ti·ble
com′·i·tance
com′·i·tans *pl.* com′·i·
 tan′·tes
com′·i·tant
com′·i·tes *pl. of*
 comes
co·mi′·tial
com·men′·sal
com·men′·sal·is′m
com′·mi·nut′·ed
com′·mi·nu′·tion
com′·mis·su′·ra *pl. &*
 gen. sg. ·rae

com·mis′′·su·ral [com′·
 mi·su′·ral]
com′·mis·sure
com·mis′′·su·ro·spi′′·nal
com′·mis·sur·ot′·o·my
com·mit′·ment
com·mo′·tio
com·mu′·ne *neut. of*
 communis
com·mu′·ni·ca·ble
com·mu′·ni·cans *pl.*
com·mu′·ni·can′′·tes
com·mu′·ni·cat′·ing
com·mu′·nis *pl.* ·nes
com′·pact [com·pact′′]
com·pac′·tion
com·pac′·tus *fem.* ·ta,
 neut. ·tum
com·pa′·ges
com·par′·a·tor
com′·part·men′·tal·i·
 za′′·tion
com·part′·men·ta′·tion
com·pat′·i·bil′′·i·ty
com·pat′·i·ble
com′·pen·sat′·ing
com′·pen·sa′·tion
com′·pen·sa′·tor
com·pen′′·sa·to′·ry
com′·pe·tence
com′·pe·ten·cy
com·pim′·e·ter
com′·ple·ment
com′·ple·men·tar′′·i·ty
com′·ple·men′·ta·ry
com′·ple·men·ta′·tion
com·ple′·ta
com′·plex
com·plex′·ion
com·plex′·us *pl. &*
 gen. sg. complexus
com·pli′·ance
com′·pli·ca′·tion
com·po′·nent
com′·pos men′·tis
com·pos′·i·ta
com·pos′·ite
com′·pound

com′′·press
com·press′′
com·pres′·si·bil′′·i·ty
com·pres′·sion
com·pres′·sive
com·pres′·sor
com·pul′·sion
com·pul′·sive
com·put′·ed
com·put′·er
con′·al·bu′·min
co·nar′·i·um *gen.* co·
 nar′′·ii
co·na′·tion
con′·ca·nav′·a·lin
con·cat′·e·nate
con·cat′·e·na′·tion
con′·cave [con·cave′′]
con·cav′·i·ty
con·ca′′·vo·con′′·cave
 [·con·cave′′]
con·ca′′·vo·con′′·vex
 [·con·vex′′]
con′·cen·trate ·trat′·
 ed, ·trat′·ing
con′·cen·tra′·tion
con·cen′·tric
con′·cept
con·cep′·tion
con·cep′·tive
con·cep′·tus
con′·cha *pl. & gen.*
 sg. chae, *gen. pl.* con·
 cha′·rum
con′·chal
con′·cho·tome
con·chot′·o·my
con·coc′·tion
con·cor′·dance
con·cor′·dant
con′·cre·ment
con·cres′·cence
con·cre′·tio
con·cre′·tion
con·cus′·sion
con′·den·sa′·tion
con·dens′·er
con·di′·tion

con·di′·tioned
con·di′·tion·er
con·di′·tion·ing
con′·dom
con·du′·cens
con·duct′
con·duc′·tance [·duct′·ance]
con·duc′·tion
con·duc′·tive
con′·duc·tiv′·i·ty
con·duc′·to·met′·ric
con′·duc·tom′·e·try
con·duc′·tor
con′·duit
con·du′·pli·cate
con·du′·pli·ca′·to
con′·dy·lar
con′·dy·la′·ris
con′·dyl·ar·thro′·sis
con′·dyle
con′·dyl·ec′·to·my [·dy·lec′·]
con′·dy·li pl. of condylus
con·dyl′·i·cus
con·dyl′·i·on
con′·dy·loid
con′·dy·loi′·de·us pl. & gen. sg. ·dei
con′·dy·lo′·ma pl. ·mas or ·ma·ta
con′·dy·lo′·ma·to′·sis
con′·dy·lo′·ma·tous [·lom′a·]
con′·dy·lo′·sis
con′·dy·lot′·o·my
con′·dy·lus pl. ·li
co·nex′·us var. of connexus
con·fab′·u·la′·tion
con·fec′·tio pl. ·fec′·ti·o′·nes
con·fec′·tion
con′·fer·ence
con′·fi·den′·ti·al′·i·ty
con·fig′·u·ra′·tion
con·fine′·ment

con·fir′·ma·to′·ry
con′·flict
con′·flu·ence
con′·flu·ens
con′·flu·ent
con·fo′·cal
con′·for·ma′·tion
con·form′·er
con·fu′·sion
con·fu′·sion·al
con′·ge·la′·tio gen. ·la·ti·o′·nis
con′·ge·la′·tion
con′·ge·ner
con′·ge·ner′·ic
con·gen′·er·ous
con·gen′·ic
con·gen′·i·tal
con·gen′·i·ta′·lis neut. ·le
con·gen′·i·tus fem. ·ta, neut. ·tum
con·gest′·ed
con·ges′·tin
con·ges′·tion
con·ges′·tive
con·glo′·bate [con′·glo·]
con·glom′·er·ate
con·glu′·ti·na′·tion
con·glu′·ti·nin
con′·gress
con·gres′·sus
co′·ni pl. & gen. sg. of conus
con′·ic also ·i·cal
co·nid′·i·um pl. ·ia
co′·ni·ine
co′·ni·is′m
co′·nio·cor′·tex var. of koniocortex
co′·ni·om′·e·ter var. of koniometer
co′·ni·ot′·o·my
co′·ni·um
con′·i·za′·tion [co′·ni·]
con·joined′
con′·ju·gant

con′·ju·ga′·ta
con′·ju·gate
con′·ju·gat′·ed
con′ju·ga′·tion
con′·junc·ti′·va fem. of conjunctivus; pl. & gen. sg. ·vae
con′·junc·ti′·val
con·junc′·ti·va′·lis pl. ·les
con·junc′·ti·vi′·tis
con′·junc·ti′·vo·dac′·ryo·cys·tos′·to·my
con′·junc·ti′·vo·plas′·ty also ·ti′·vi·
con′·junc·ti′·vo·rhi·nos′·to·my
con′·junc·ti′·vum neut. of conjunctivus; gen. ·vi
con′·junc·ti′·vus pl. & gen. sg. ·vi
con·na′·tal
con′·nate
con·nec′·tion Brit. con·nex′·ion
con·nec′·tive
con·nec′·tor
con·nex′·us
co′·noid
co·noi′·de·um
co′·no·scope
con′·qui·nine
con′·san·guin′·e·ous
con′·san·guin′·i·ty
con′·scious
con·sen′·su·al
con·sent′
con′·ser·va′·tion
con·ser′·va·tive
con·serve′ ·served′, ·serv′·ing
con·sis′·ten·cy
con·sol′·i·dant
con·sol′·i·da′·tion
con′·so·nat′·ing
con′·spe·cif′·ic
con·sper′·gent

con·sper'·sus
con'·stan·cy
con'·stant
con'·stel·la'·tion
con'·sti·pate   ·pat'·ed,
    ·pat'·ing
con'·sti·pa'·tion
con·sti'·tu·ent
con'·sti·tu'·tion
con'·sti·tu'·tion·al
con'·sti·tu'·tive
con·strict'
con·stric'·tion
con·stric'·tive
con·stric'·tor   L. pl.
    con'·stric·to'·res, gen.
    sg. ·ris
con·sult'
con·sul'·tant [·sult'·
    ant]
con'·sul·ta'·tion
con·sum'·er
con·sump'·tion
con·sump'·tive
con'·tact
con·tac'·tant
con·ta'·gion
con·ta'·gi·o'·sus   fem.
    ·sa, neut. ·sum
con·ta'·gious
con·ta'·gi·um   pl. ·gia
con·tam'·i·nant
con·tam'·i·nate
con·tam'·i·na'·tion
con'·ti·gu'·ity
con·tig'·u·ous
con'·ti·nence
con·tor'·tus   pl. ·ti
con'·tra·
con'·tra·cep'·tion
con'·tra·cep'·tive
con·tract'
con·trac'·tile
con'·trac·til'·i·ty
con·trac'·tion
con·trac'·ture
con'·tra·fis'·sure
con'·tra·in'·di·cant

con'·tra·in'·di·cate
    ·cat'·ed, ·cat'·ing
con'·tra·in'·di·ca'·tion
con'·tra·lat'·er·al
con'·tra·stim'·u·lant
con'·tra·ver'·sive
con'·tre·coup'
con'·trec·ta'·tion
con·trol'   ·trolled',
    ·trol'·ling
con·tuse   ·tused', ·tus'·
    ing
con·tu'·sion
con·tu'·sive
Co'·nus
co'·nus   pl. co'·ni
con'·va·lesce'
    ·lesced', ·lesc'·ing
con'·va·les'·cence
con'·va·les'·cent
con·val'·la·tox'·in
con·vec'·tion
con·ver'·gence
con·ver'·gent
con·ver'·sion
con·ver'·tase
con·ver'·tin
con'·vex [con·vex']
con·vex'·i·ty
con·vex'o·con'·cave
    [·con·cave']
con·vex'o·con'·vex
    [·con·vex']
con'·vo·lu'·ta
con'·vo·lut'·ed
con'·vo·lu'·tion
con·vul'·sant
con·vul'·sion
con·vul'·sive
con'·vul·si'·vus
co-os'·si·fy   ·fied, ·fy'·
    ing
co'·pe·pod
Co·pep'·o·da
cop'·ing
cop'·i·o'·pia
co·pol'y·mer
cop'·per

cop'·per·as
cop'·per·head
co'·pre·cip'·i·tat'·ing
co'·pre·cip'·i·ta'·tion
co'·pre·cip'·i·tin
cop·rem'·e·sis
cop'·ro·
cop'·ro·an'·ti·bod'y
cop'·ro·lag'·nia
cop'·ro·la'·lia
cop'·ro·lith
cop·rol'·o·gy
cop'·ro·pha'·gia   also
    cop·roph'·a·gy
cop·roph'·a·gous
cop'·ro·phil   also
    ·phile
cop'·ro·phil'·ia
cop'·ro·por·phyr'·ia
cop'·ro·por'·phy·rin
cop'·ro·zo'a   sg. ·zo'·
    on
cop'·ro·zo'·ic
cop'·u·la   pl. ·lae
cop'·u·la'·tion
co·quille'
cor   gen. cor'·dis
cor'·a·cid'·i·um   pl.
    ·cid'·ia
cor'·a·co·acro'·mi·al
cor'·a·co·acro'·mi·a'·le
cor'·a·co·bra'·chi·al
cor'·a·co·bra'·chi·a'·lis
cor'·a·co·cla·vic'·u·la'·
    re
cor'·a·co·cla·vic'·u·lar
cor'·a·co·hu'·mer·al
cor'·a·co·hu'·mer·a'·le
cor'·a·co·hy'·oid
cor'·a·coid
cor'·a·coi'·de·us
cor'·a·coid·i'·tis
cor'·a·co·ra'·di·a'·lis
cor'·a·co·ul·na'·ris
cord
cord'·al
cor'·date   heart-
    shaped: Cf. chordate

cor·dec′·to·my
cor′·di·form
cor′·di·for′·mis
cor′·dis *gen. of* cor
cord′·ite
cor·di′·tis *inflammation of spermatic cord: Cf.* chorditis
cor′·do·pex′y
cor·dot′·o·my *var. of* chordotomy
Cor′·dy·lo′·bia
cor′·e·cli′·sis
co·rec′·tome
cor′·ec·to′·pia
cor′e·di·al′·y·sis
co·rel′·y·sis [cor′e·ly′·sis]
cor′·en·cli′·sis
cor′·e·om′·e·ter
cor′·e·om′·e·try
cor′·e·pex′y
cor′·e·plas′·ty *also* cor′·e·o·
co′·re·pres′·sor
co·ret′·o·my
co′·ri·a′·ceous
co′·ri·um *gen.* ·rii
cor′·nea *L. pl. & gen. sg.* ·ne·ae
cor′·ne·al
cor′·ne·i′tis
cor′·neo·bleph′·a·ron
cor′·neo·iri′·tis
cor′·neo·man·dib′·u·lar
cor′·neo·scle′·ra
cor′·neo·scle′·ral
cor′·ne·ous
cor′·ne·um
cor·nic′·u·late
cor·nic′·u·la′·tus *fem.* ·ta, *neut.* ·tum
cor·nic′·u·lo·pha·ryn′·ge·al
cor·nic′·u·lum
cor′·ni·fi·ca′·tion
cor′·nu *pl.* ·nua, *gen. sg.* ·nus

cor′·nu·al
cor′·nu·ate
cor′·nu·ra·dic′·u·lar
cor′·o *var. of* core-
cor′·o·cli′·sis *var. of* coreclisis
co·rom′·e·ter
co·ro′·na *pl.* ·nae
cor′·o·nad [co·ro′·nad]
cor′·o·nal [co·ro′·nal]
cor′·o·na′·lis *neut* ·le
cor′·o·na′·ria *fem. of* coronarius; *pl. & gen. sg.* ·ri·ae
cor′·o·na′·ri·um *neut. of* coronarius; *gen.* ·rii
cor′·o·na′·ri·us *pl. & gen. sg.* ·rii
cor′·o·nar′y
co·ro′·na·vi′·rus
cor′·o·ner
co·ro′·ni·on *pl.* ·nia
cor′·o·ni′·tis
cor′·o·noid
cor′·o·noid·ec′·to·my
cor′·o·noi′·de·us *fem.* ·dea
cor′·o·par·el′·cy·sis
cor′·o·plas′·ty *var. of* coreplasty
co·rot′·o·my
cor′·po·ra *pl. of* corpus
cor′·po·ral
cor′·po·ra′·tion
cor·po′·re·al
corps *pl.* corps
corpse
cor′·pus *pl.* cor′·po·ra, *gen. sg.* ·ris, *gen. pl.* ·rum
cor′·pus·cle
cor·pus′·cu·lar
cor·pus′·cu·lum *pl.* ·la
cor·rec′·tion
cor·rec′·tive
cor′·re·la′·tion

cor′·re·spon′·dence [·spond′·ence]
cor′·ri·gent
cor′·ri·noid
cor·ro′·sive
cor′·ru·ga′·tion
cor′·ru·ga′·tor
cor′·set
cor′·tex *pl.* cor′·ti·ces
cor′·ti·cal
cor′·ti·ca′·lis
cor′·ti·cal·i·za′·tion
cor′·ti·cate
cor′·ti·cif′·u·gal
cor′·ti·cip′·e·tal
cor′·ti·co·
cor′·ti·co·adre′·nal
cor′·ti·co·af′·fer·ent
cor′·ti·co·au′·to·nom′·ic
cor′·ti·co·bul′·bar
cor′·ti·co·bul·ba′·ris
cor′·ti·co·cer′·e·bel′·lar
cor′·ti·co·col·lic′·u·lar
cor′·ti·co·ef′·fer·ent
cor′·ti·cof′·u·gal *var. of* corticifugal
cor′·ti·co·ge·nic′·u·late
cor′·ti·co·gram
cor′·ti·co·hy′·po·tha·lam′·ic
cor′·ti·co·hy′·po·tha·lam′·i·cus *pl. & gen. sg.* ·ci
cor′·ti·coid
cor′·ti·co·lib′·er·in
cor′·ti·co·med′·ul·lar′y
cor′·ti·co·ni′·gral
cor′·ti·co·nu′·cle·ar
cor′·ti·co·nu′·cle·a′·ris
cor′·ti·co-oc′·u·lo·ceph′·a·lo·gy′·ric
cor′·ti·co·pal′·li·dal
cor′·ti·co·pe·dun′·cu·lar
cor′·ti·cop′·e·tal *var. of* corticipetal
cor′·ti·co·pon′·tile

cor′·ti·co·pon·ti′·na
  fem. of corticopontinus;
  pl. ·nae
cor′·ti·co·pon′·tine
cor′·ti·co·pon·ti′·nus
cor′·ti·co·pon′·to·cer·e·
  bel′·lar
cor′·ti·co·pu′·pil·lar′y
cor′·ti·co·re·tic′·u·la′·
  ris pl. ·res
cor′·ti·co·ru′·bral
cor′·ti·co·spi′·nal
cor′·ti·co·spi·na′·lis
  pl. ·les
cor′·ti·co·ste′·roid
cor′·ti·cos′·ter·one
  [·co·ste′·rone]
cor′·ti·co·stri′·ate
cor′·ti·co·stri·a′·to·ni′·
  gral
cor′·ti·co·stri·a′·to·spi′·
  nal
cor′·ti·co·tha·lam′·ic
cor′·ti·co·tha·lam′·i·ca
  pl. ·cae
cor′·ti·co·troph
cor′·ti·co·tro′·phic
  [·troph′·ic]
cor′·ti·co·tro′·pic
  [·trop′·ic]
cor′·ti·co·tro′·pin
cor′·tin
cor′·ti·sol
cor′·ti·sone
cor′·us·ca′·tion
co·ryd′·a·lis
co·rym′·bi·form
cor′·ym·bose
cor′·y·ne·bac·te′·ri·o·
  phage
Cor′·y·ne·bac·te′·ri·um
  C. diph·the′·ri·ae
  C. xe·ro′·sis
cor′·y·ne·bac·te′·ri·um
  pl. ·ria
co·ryn′·e·form [co·ry′·
  ne·]
co·ry′·za

cos·met′·ic
cos′·ta pl. & gen. sg.
  ·tae, gen. pl. cos·ta′·
  rum
cos′·tal
cos·ta′·le neut. of
  costalis
cos·tal′·gia
cos·ta′·lis pl. ·les
cos′·tate
cos·tec′·to·my
cos′·ti·
cos′·tive
cos′·to· also cos′·ti·
cos′·to·cen′·tral
cos′·to·cer′·vi·cal
cos′·to·cer′·vi·ca′·lis
cos′·to·chon′·dral
cos′·to·chon·dra′·lis
  pl. ·les
cos′·to·chon·dri′·tis
cos′·to·cla·vic′·u·lar
cos′·to·cla·vic′·u·la′·ris
  neut. ·re
cos′·to·co′·lic
cos′·to·cor′·a·coid
cos′·to·di′·a·phrag·
  mat′·ic
cos′·to·di′·a·phrag·
  mat′·i·cus
cos′·to·me′·di·as′·ti·
  na′·lis
cos′·to·pec′·to·ral
cos′·to·per′·i·car′·di·ac
cos′·to·phren′·ic
cos′·to·pleu′·ral
cos′·to·pneu′·mo·pex′y
cos′·to·scap′·u·lar
cos′·to·scap′·u·la′·ris
cos′·to·ster′·nal
cos′·to·tome
cos′·to·trans′·ver·sa′·
  ri·us fem. ·ria, neut.
  ·ri·um
cos′·to·trans·verse′
cos′·to·trans′·ver·sec′·
  to·my
cos′·to·ver′·te·bral

cos′·to·ver′·te·bra′·lis
  pl. ·les
cos′·to·xiph′·oid [·xi′·
  phoid]
cos′·to·xi·phoi′·dea
co′·syn·tro′·pin
co′·throm′·bo·plas′·tin
co′·trans·duc′·tion
co′·tri·mox′·a·zole
cot′·ton·mouth
co′-twin
cot′·y·le′·don
cot′·y·loid
cough
cou′·lomb
cou′·ma·rin
coun′·sel·ing also ·sel·
  ling
count′·er
coun′·ter·
coun′·ter·act′
coun′·ter·ac′·tion
coun′·ter·ac′·tive
coun′·ter·cur′·rent
coun′·ter·ex·ten′·sion
coun′·ter·im·mu′·no·
  elec′·tro·pho·re′·sis
coun′·ter·in·ci′·sion
coun′·ter·in′·di·cate
  ·cat′·ed, ·cat′·ing; var.
  of contraindicate
coun′·ter·ir′·ri·tant
coun′·ter·ir′·ri·ta′·tion
coun′·ter·o′pen·ing
coun′·ter·pho′·bia
coun′·ter·pho′·bic
coun′·ter·pul·sa′·tion
coun′·ter·punc′·ture
coun′·ter·shock
coun′·ter·stain
coun′·ter·trac′·tion
coun′·ter·trans·fer′·
  ence
coup
cou′·ple ·pled, ·pling
coup′·ler
co·va′·lence also ·len·
  cy

co·va′·lent
co·var′·i·ance
co·var′·i·ate
cov′·er·glass *also*
  cover glass
cov′·er·slip
co′·vert [co·vert′,
  cov′·ert]
cowl
cow′·per·i′·tis
cow′·pox
cox′a *pl.* & *gen. sg.*
  cox′·ae
cox·al′·gia
cox·ar′·thro·lis·thet′·ic
cox′·ar·throp′·a·thy
cox′·ar·thro′·sis
Cox′·i·el′·la bur·net′·ii
cox·it′·ic
cox·i′·tis
cox′o·fem′·o·ral
cox·sack′·ie·vi′·rus
  also Coxsackie virus
cra′·dle
cra′·ni·ad
cra′·ni·al
cra′·ni·a′·le *neut. of*
  cranialis
cra′·ni·a′·lis *pl.* ·les
Cra′·ni·a′·ta
cra′·ni·ec′·to·my
cra′·nii *gen. sg. of*
  cranium
cra′·nio·
cra′·nio·buc′·cal
cra′·ni·o·cele
cra′·ni·oc′·la·sis
cra′·ni·o·clast
cra′·nio·did′·y·mus
cra′·nio·fa′·cial
cra′·nio·fe·nes′·tria
cra′·ni·o·graph
cra′·ni·og′·ra·phy
cra′·nio·hy′·po·phys′·i·al
cra′·nio·la·cu′·nia
cra′·ni·o·log′·ic *also*
  ·i·cal

cra′·ni·ol′·o·gy
cra′·nio·man·dib′·u·lar
cra′·ni·om′·e·ter
cra′·ni·o·met′·ric
cra′·ni·om′·e·try
cra′·ni·op′·a·gus
cra′·nio·pha·ryn′·ge·al
cra′·nio·pha·ryn′·gi·o′·ma
cra′·ni·o·plas′·ty
cra′·nio·ra·chis′·chi·sis
  also cra′·ni·or·rha·
cra′·ni·or·rha·chid′·i·an
cra′·nio·sa′·cral
cra′·ni·os′·chi·sis
cra′·ni·os′·co·py
cra′·nio·si′·nus
cra′·nio·spi′·nal
cra′·nio·ste·no′·sis
cra′·nio·syn′·os·to′·sis
cra′·nio·ta′·bes
cra′·nio·tel′·en·ce·phal′·ic
cra′·ni·o·tome
cra′·ni·ot′·o·my
cra′·nio·to·pog′·ra·phy
cra′·ni·um *pl.* ·nia,
  gen. sg. ·nii
crap′·u·lent
crap′·u·lous
cras′·sum *gen.* ·si
cra′·ter
cra·ter′·i·form
cra′·ter·i·za′·tion
cra·vat′
craw′-craw *var. of*
  kra-kra
cream
crease
cre′·atine
cre′·atin·e′·mia [·ati·ne′·] *Brit.* ·ae′·mia
cre·at′·i·nine
cre′·atin·u′·ria [·ati·nu′·]
cre′·a·tox′·in *var. of*
  kreotoxin
crèche

cre·mas′·ter
cre′·mas·ter′·ic
cre′·mas·ter′·i·ca
cre·ma′·tion
crem′·or
cre′·na *pl.* ·nae
cre′·nate
cre·na′·tion
cre′·no·cyte
cre′·no·cy·to′·sis
cren′·u·la′·tion
cre′·o·lin
cre′·o·sote
cre′o·tox′·in *var. of*
  kreotoxin
crep′·i·tant
crep′·i·ta′·tion
crep′·i·tus *pl.* crepitus
cres·cen′·do
cres′·cent
cres·cen′·tic
cre′·sol
cre·sor′·ci·nol
cres·ox′y·di′·ol
cres·ox′y·pro·pane′·di·ol [·pro′·pane·di′·ol]
crest
cres′·ta
cres′·to·my′·cin
cres′·yl
cre′·ta
cre′·tin
cre′·tin·is′m
cre′·tin·oid
cre′·tin·ous
crev′·ice
cre·vic′·u·lar
crib′·ral
crib′·rate
crib′·ri·form
crib′·ro·eth′·moid
cri·bro′·sus *fem.* ·sa
crib′·rum *pl.* ·ra
crick
cri′·co·ar′·y·te′·noid
cri′·co·ar′·y·te·noi′·de·us *fem.* ·dea, *neut.* ·de·um

cri′·co·esoph′·a·ge′·us
   also -oe·soph′·
cri′·coid
cri·coi′·dea   *pl. & gen.
   sg.* ·de·ae
cri′·coid·ec′·to·my
cri′·co·pha·ryn′·ge·al
cri′·co·pha·ryn′·ge·us
   fem. ·gea, *neut.* ·ge·um
cri′·co·thy′·roid
cri′·co·thy·roi′·dea
   fem. of cri′·co·thy·roi′·
   de·us
cri′·co·thy·roi′·de·um
   neut. of cri′·co·thy·roi′·
   de·us
cri′·co·thy·roi′·de·us
   pl. & gen. sg. ·dei
cri′·co·thy·rot′·o·my
cri·cot′·o·my
cri′·co·tra′·che·al
cri′·co·tra′·che·a′·le
cri′·co·tra′·che·ot′·o·
   my
cri′·co·vo·ca′·lis
cri′ du chat′
crim′·i·nal·is′m
crim′·i·nol′·o·gy
crip′·ple   ·pled, ·pling
cri′·sis   *pl.* ·ses
cris·pa′·tion
cris′·pa·tu′·ra
cris′·ta   *pl. & gen. sg.*
   ·tae
cris′·tal   *of a crest: Cf.*
   crystal
cris′·tate
cri·te′·ri·on   *pl.* ·ria
Cri·thid′·ia
cri·thid′·ia
crit′·i·cal
crit′·i·cal′·i·ty
Cro-Mag′·non
cro′·mo·gly′·cate
cro′·mo·lyn
cross′·bite   *also* cross
   bite

cross′·breed   ·bred,
   ·breed′·ing
cross′-eye
cross′·ing-o′ver
cross′-link′·ing
cross′-match′ing
cross′·o′ver
cross′-re·ac′·tion
cross′-sec′·tion   *also*
   cross section
Cro·tal′·i·dae
Crot·a·li′·nae
Crot′·a·lus
cro·taph′·i·on
cro′·ton
cro·ton′·ic
cro′·ton·is′m
cro′·to·nyl   *also* cro·
   ton′·o·yl
croup
croup′·ous
croup′y
crown
cru′·ci·ate
cru′·ci·a′·tus   *fem.* ·ta,
   neut. ·tum
cru′·ci·ble
cru′·ci·form
cru′·ci·for′·mis   *neut.*
   ·me
cru′·or
cru′·ra   *pl. of* crus
cru′·ral
cru·ra′·lis
cru′·ris   *gen. of* crus
cru′·ro·cru′·ral
cru·rot′·o·my
crus   *pl.* cru′·ra, *gen.
   sg.* cru′·ris
crus′·ta   *pl.* ·tae
Crus·ta′·cea
crus·ta′·cean
crux   *L. pl.* cru′·ces
cry′·al·ge′·sia
cry′·an·es·the′·sia
   *loss of cold sensation:
   Cf.* cryoanesthesia;
   Brit. ·an′·aes·

cry′·es·the′·sia   *Brit.*
   ·aes·
cry′·mo·
cry′·mo·ther′·a·py
   var. of cryotherapy
cry′o·
cry′o·an′·es·the′·sia
   *local anesthesia by
   freezing: Cf.* cryanes-
   thesia; *Brit.* ·an′·aes·
cry′o·bi·ol′·o·gy
cry′o·cau′·tery
cry′·o·crit
cry′o·ex·trac′·tion
cry′o·ex·trac′·tor
cry′o·fi·brin′·o·gen
cry′·o·gen
cry′·o·gen′·ic
cry′o·glob′·u·lin
cry′o·glob′·u·lin·e′·mia
   Brit. ·ae′·mia
cry′o·hy·poph′·y·sec′·
   to·my
cry′·o·lite
cry·om′·e·ter
cry′o·pal′·li·dec′·to·my
cry′·o·phake
cry′o·pre·cip′·i·tate
cry′o·pre·cip′·i·ta′·tion
cry′o·pres′·er·va′·tion
cry′o·probe
cry′o·pro′·tein
cry′·o·scope
cry′·o·scop′·ic
cry·os′·co·py
cry′·o·stat
cry′o·sur′·gery
cry′o·thal·a·mec′·to·my
cry′o·ther′·a·py
crypt
cryp′·ta   *pl.* ·tae
crypt·ec′·to·my [cryp·
   tec′·]
cryp·ten′·a·mine
cryp′·tic
cryp·tic′·i·ty
cryp·ti′·tis
cryp′·to·

cryp′·to·bi·o′·sis
cryp′·to·ceph′·a·lus
Cryp′·to·coc·ca′·ce·ae
cryp′·to·coc′·cal
cryp′·to·coc·co′·ma
cryp′·to·coc·co′·sis
Cryp′·to·coc′·cus
  C. ne′o·for′·mans
cryp′·to·de·ter′·mi·nant
cryp′·to·did′·y·mus
cryp′·to·ge·net′·ic
cryp′·to·gen′·ic
cryp′·to·leu·ke′·mia
  Brit. ·kae′·mia
cryp′·to·men′·or·rhe′a
  Brit. ·rhoe′a
cryp′·tom·ne′·sia
cryp′·toph·thal′·mia
cryp′·toph·thal′·mos
  also ·mus
cryp′·to·plas′·mic
crypt·or′·chid [cryp·tor′·]
crypt·or′·chi·dec′·to·my [cryp·tor′·]
crypt·or′·chi·dis′m [cryp·tor′·] also ·or′·chism
crypt·or′·chi·do·pex′y [cryp·tor′·]
cryp′·to·spo·rid′·i·o′·sis
Cryp′·to·spo·rid′·i·um
Cryp′·to·stro′·ma
cryp′·to·stro·mo′·sis
cryp·to′·tia
cryp′·to·tox′·ic
cryp′·to·zo′·ite
cryp′·to·zy′·gous
crys′·tal solid with regular atomic pattern: Cf. cristal
crys·tal′·lin
crys·tal·li′·na
crys′·tal·line
crys·tal·li′·tis
crys′·tal·li·za′·tion
crys′·tal·log′·ra·phy

crys′·tal·loid
crys′·tal·lu′·ria
Cte′·no·ce·phal′·i·des
cte′·noid
cu′·beb
cu′·beb·is′m
cu′·bi·tal
cu′·bi·ta′·le neut. of cubitalis
cu′·bi·ta′·lis pl. ·les
cu′·bi·to·car′·pal
cu′·bi·tus pl. & gen. sg. ·ti
cu′·boid
cu·boi′·dal
cu·boi′·deo·na·vic′·u·lar
cu·boi′·deo·na·vic′·u·la′·re
cu·boi′·des
cu·boi′·de·um gen. ·dei
cu′·bo·na·vic′·u·lar
cu·cur′·bi·ta′·cin
cu·cur′·bo·cit′·rin
cud′·bear
cuff
cuff′·ing
cui·rass′
cul′-de-sac′
cul′·do·cen·te′·sis
cul′·do·plas′·ty
cul′·do·scope
cul·dos′·co·py
cul·dot′·o·my
Cu′·lex
  C. pi′·pi·ens
  C. quin′·que·fas′·ci·a′·tus
  C. tar·sa′·lis
  C. tri′·tae′·nio·rhyn′·chus
Cu·lic′·i·dae
cu′·li·cid′·al [·ci′·dal]
cu′·li·cide
cu′·li·cine
Cu′·li·coi′·des
cu′·li·co′·sis

Cu′·li·se′·ta
  C. mel′·a·nu′·ra
cull′·ing
cul′·men pl. ·mi·na
cul′·mi·nal
cul′·ti·va′·tion
cul′·tur·a·ble
cul′·ture
cu′·mu·la·tive
cu′·mu·lus pl. ·li
cu′·ne·ate
cu′·ne·a′·tum neut. of cuneatus
cu′·ne·a′·tus gen. ·ti
cu′·nei gen. of cuneus
cu·ne′·iform [cu′·ne·]
cu·ne′·ifor′·mis neut. ·ifor′·me
cu′·neo·cu′·boid
cu′·neo·cu·boi′·de·us
  fem. ·dea, neut. ·de·um
cu′·neo·me′·ta·tar·sa′·lia
cu′·neo·na·vic′·u·lar
cu′·neo·na·vic′·u·la′·ris
  neut. pl. ·la′·ria
cu′·ne·us pl. & gen. sg. ·nei
cu·nic′·u·lar
cu·nic′·u·la′·tum
cu·nic′·u·lus pl. ·li
cun′·ni·lin′·gus also ·linc′·tus
cun′·nus
cup′·ping
cu′·pric
cu′·pro·
cu′·pro·pro′·tein
cu′·prous
cu′·pu·la pl. ·lae
cu′·pu·lar
cu′·pu·la′·ris neut. ·la′·re
cu′·pu·late
cu′·pu·li·form
cur′·a·ble
cu·rage′
cu·ra′·re also ·ri

cu·ra′′·ri·form
cu·ra′′·rine
cu′′·ra·tive
cure cured, cur′·ing
cu·ret·tage′ [·ret′·tage]
cu·rette′ also cu·ret′
cu′·rie
cu′·ri·um
cur′·rens
cur′·rent
cur′·va·tu′·ra
cur′·va·ture
curve
cur′·vi·lin′·e·ar
cush′·ing·oid
cush′·ion
cusp
cus′·pid
cus′·pi·date
cus′·pis pl. cus′·pi·des
cu′·sums
cu·ta′·nea fem. of cutaneus
cu·ta′·neo·mu′·co·u′ve·al
cu·ta′·ne·ous
cu·ta′·ne·um neut. of cutaneus
cu·ta′·ne·us gen. sg. ·nei, gen. pl. cu·ta′·ne·o′·rum
cut′·down
cu′·ti·cle
cu·tic′·u·la pl. ·lae
cu·tic′·u·lar
cu·tic′·u·lar·i·za′·tion
cu′·ti·re·ac′·tion
cu′·tis gen. cutis, accusative cu′·tem
cu·vette′
cy·an′·a·mide
cy′·a·nate
cy′·an·he′·mo·glo′·bin Brit. ·hae′·mo·glo′·
cy′·a·nide
cy′·an·met·he′·mo·glo′·bin Brit. ·hae′·mo·glo′·

cy′·an·met·my′·o·glo′·bin
cy′·a·no·
cy′·a·no·ac′·e·tate
cy′·a·no·ac′·ry·late
cy′·a·no·bac·te′·ria sg. ·ri·um
cy′·a·no·co·bal′·a·min
cy·an′·o·gen
cy′·a·no·met·he′·mo·glo′·bin Brit. ·hae′··mo·glo′·; var. of cyanmethemoglobin
cy′·a·no·met·my′·o·glo′·bin var. of cyanmetmyoglobin
cy′·a·nop′·sia also cy′·a·no′·pia
cy′·a·nop′·sin
cy′·a·nosed
cy′·a·no′·sis
cy′·a·not′·ic
cy′·a·nu′·ric
cy′·cla·mate
cy·clam′·ic
cy·clan′·de·late
cy′·clase
cy·clec′·to·my
cy′·clen·ceph′·a·ly
cy′·clic also cy′·cli·cal
cy′·cli′·tis
cy′·cli·za′·tion
cy′·cli·zine
cy′·clo·
cy′·clo·bar′·bi·tal
cy′·clo·di·al′·y·sis
cy′·clo·di′·a·ther′·my
cy′·clo·duc′·tion
cy′·clo·hex′·i·mide
cy′·cloid
cy′·clo·isom′·er·ase
cy′·clo·ker′·a·ti′·tis
cy′·clo·meth′·y·caine
cy′·clo·ox′·y·gen·ase
cy′·clo·pe′·an [cy·clo′·pe·an]
cy′·clo·pen′·ta·mine
cy′·clo·pen′·to·late

cy′·clo·pen′·tyl·pro′·pi·o·nate
cy′·clo·pho′·ria
cy′·clo·phos′·pha·mide
Cy′·clo·phyl·lid′·e·a
cy·clo′·pia
cy·clo′·pic
cy′·clo·ple′·gia
cy′·clo·ple′·gic
cy′·clo·pro′·pane
cy′·clops
cy′·clo·ser′·ine
cy·clo′·sis
cy′·clo·spas′m
cy′·clo·spo′·rin
cy′·clo·spo′·rine
cy′·clo·thi′·a·zide
cy′·clo·thy′·mia
cy′·clo·thy′·mic
cy′·clo·tome
cy·clot′·o·my
cy′·clo·tor′·sion
cy′·clo·tron
cy′·clo·tro′·pia
cy′·clo·zo′·o·no′·sis
cy′·cri·mine
cy·e′·sis
cy·et′·ic
cyl′·in·der
cyl′·in·drar·thro′·sis
cy·lin′·dric also ·dri·cal
cy·lin′·dri·form
cyl′·in·dro·cel′·lu·la′·re
cyl′·in·droid [cy·lin′·droid]
cyl′·in·dro′·ma pl. ·mas or ·ma·ta
cyl′·in·dro′·ma·tous [·drom′a·]
Cy·lin′·dro·tho′·rax
C. mel′·a·no·ceph′·a·la
cyl′·in·dru′·ria
cy′·ma·rin
cym′·ba
cym′·bi·form
cym′·bo·

cym′·bo·ce·phal′·ic
cym′·bo·ceph′·a·lous
cym′·bo·ceph′·a·lus
cym′·bo·ceph′·a·ly
cy′·mo·graph   *var. of*
   kymograph
cyn′·ic
cy′·no·
cy′·no·ce·phal′·ic
cy′·no·ceph′·a·lus
cy′·no·ceph′·a·ly
cy′·no·dont
cy′·no·don′·tism
cy′·no·mol′·gus
Cy′·no·my′·ia
cy·oc′·tol
cyp′·i·o·nate
cyp′·ri·pe′·di·um
cy′·pro·hep′·ta·dine
cyr′·toid
cyr·tom′·e·ter
cyst
cyst·ad′·e·no·car′·ci·no′·ma   *pl.* ·mas *or* ·ma·ta
cyst·ad′·e·no·fi·bro′·ma   *pl.* ·mas *or* ·ma·ta
cyst′·ad′·e·no′·ma   *pl.* ·mas *or* ·ma·ta
cys·tal′·gia
cys′·ta·mine
cys′·ta·thi′·o·nine
cys′·ta·thi′·o·nin·u′·ria [·ni·nu′·ria]
cyst′·atro′·phia
cyst′·ec·ta′·sia
cys·tec′·to·my
cys·te′·ic
cys′·te·ine
cyst′·en·ceph′·a·lus
cys′·ti·
cys′·tic
cys′·ti·ca   *fem. of* cysticus
cys′·ti·cer·ci′·a·sis
cys′·ti·cer′·coid
cys′·ti·cer·co′·sis
Cys′·ti·cer′·cus

C. bo′·vis
C. cel′·lu·lo′·sae
cys′·ti·cer′·cus   *pl.* ·ci
cys′·ti·co·du′·o·de′·nal
cys′·ti·cor′·rha·phy
cys′·ti·cot′·o·my
cys′·ti·cus   *fem.* ·ca, *neut.* ·cum
cys′·ti·do·
cys′·ti·do·trach′·e·lot′·o·my
cys′·ti·form
cys′·tine
cys′·tin·e′·mia [·ti·ne′·mia]   *Brit.* ·ae′·mia
cys′·ti·no′·sis
cys′·ti·not′·ic
cys′·tin·u′·ria [·ti·nu′·ria]
cys′·tin·u′·ric [·ti·nu′·ric]
cys′·tir·rha′·gia   *var. of* cystorrhagia
cys′·tir·rhe′a   *Brit.* ·rhoe′a; *var. of* cystorrhea
cys·ti′·tis
cys′·ti·tome
cys′·to·
cys′·to·ad′·e·no′·ma   *var. of* cystadenoma
cys′·to·cele
cys′·to·co·los′·to·my
cys′·to·dyn′·ia
cys′·to·en′·ter·o·cele
cys′·to·epip′·lo·cele
cys′·to·fi·bro′·ma
cys′·to·gas·tros′·to·my
cys′·to·gen′·e·sis
cys′·to·gram
cys·tog′·ra·phy
cys′·toid
cys′·to·je′·ju·nos′·to·my
cys′·to·lith
cys′·to·li·thec′·to·my
cys′·to·li·thi′·a·sis
cys′·to·li·thot′·o·my

cys·to′·ma   *pl.* ·mas *or* ·ma·ta
cys·to′·ma·tous [·tom′a·]
cys′·to·me′·ro·cele
cys·tom′·e·ter
cys′·to·met′·ro·gram
cys′·to·me·trog′·ra·phy
cys·tom′·e·try
cys′·to·pex′y
cys′·to·ple′·gia
cys′·to·proc·tos′·to·my
cys′·to·pros′·ta·tec′·to·my
cys′·to·py′·e·lo·ne·phri′·tis
cys′·tor·rha′·gia
cys·tor′·rha·phy
cys′·to·sar·co′·ma   *pl.* ·mas *or* ·ma·ta
cys′·to·scope
cys′·to·scop′·ic
cys·tos′·co·py
cys·tos′·to·my
cys′·to·tome
cys·tot′·o·my
cys′·to·ure′·ter·i′·tis
cys′·to·ure′·ter·o·cele
cys′·to·u′re·thri′·tis
cys′·to·ure′·thro·cele
cys′·to·ure′·thro·gram
cys′·to·u′re·throg′·ra·phy
cys′·to·ure′·thro·scope
cys′·tous
cyt′·apher·e′·sis [·apher′·e·]
cyt·ar′·a·bine
cyt′·as·ter
cy′·ti·dine
cy′·ti·dyl′·ic
cy′·ti·sine
cy′·to·
cy′·to·ar′·chi·tec·ton′·ic
cy′·to·ar′·chi·tec′·tur·al
cy′·to·ar′·chi·tec′·ture
cy′·to·blast

cy′·to·chal′·a·sin
cy′·to·chem′·is·try
cy′·to·chrome
cy′·to·cid′·al [·ci′·dal]
cy′·to·cide
cy·toc′·la·sis
cy′·to·clas′·tic
cy′·tode
cy′·to·derm
cy′·to·di′·ag·no′·sis
cy′·to·di·er′·e·sis
cy′·to·dif′·fer·en′·ti·a′·tion
cy′·to·gene
cy′·to·gen′·e·sis
cy′·to·ge·net′·ic
cy′·to·gen′·ic
cy·tog′·e·ny   var. of cytogenesis
cy′·toid
cy′·to·kine
cy′·to·ki·ne′·sis
cy′·to·ki′·nin
cy′·to·log′·ic   also ·log′·i·cal
cy·tol′·o·gy
cy·tol′·y·sate
cy′·to·ly′·sin [cy·tol′·y·sin]
cy·tol′·y·sis
cy′·to·lyt′·ic
cy′·to·me·gal′·ic
cy′·to·meg′·a·lo·vi′·rus
cy′·to·meg′·a·ly
cy′·to·mem′·brane
cy·tom′·e·ter
cy·tom′·e·try
cy′·to·mor·phol′·o·gy
cy′·to·mor·pho′·sis
cy′·to·path′·ic
cy′·to·path′o·gen′·e·sis
cy′·to·path′·o·gen′·ic
cy′·to·path′·o·ge·nic′·i·ty
cy′·to·path′·o·log′·ic   also ·log′·i·cal
cy′·to·pa·thol′·o·gy
cy′·to·pe′·nia

cy′·to·phag′·ic
cy′·to·phag′·o·cy·to′·sis
cy′·to·phil
cy′·to·phil′·ic
cy′·to·pho·tom′·e·try
cy′·to·phys′·i·ol′·o·gy
cy′·to·pi·pette′
cy′·to·plas′m
cy′·to·plas′·mic
cy′·to·prep′·a·ra′·tion
cy·tos′·co·py
cy′·to·sine
cy′·to·skel′·e·ton
cy′·to·smear
cy′·to·sol
cy′·to·some
cy′·to·stat′·ic
cy′·to·stome
cy′·to·tac′·tic
cy′·to·tax′·is
cy′·to·tech·nol′·o·gist
cy′·to·tech·nol′·o·gy
cy′·to·tox′·ic
cy′·to·tox·ic′·i·ty
cy′·to·tox′·in
cy′·to·tro′·pho·blast
cy′·to·tro′·pic [·trop′·ic]
cy·tot′·ro·pis′m [cy′·to·tro′·pism]
cy′·to·zo′·ic
cy′·to·zo′·on   pl. ·zo′a

D

da·car′·ba·zine
dac′·ry·ad′·e·ni′·tis
dac′·ry·a·gog′·ic
dac′·ry·a·gogue
dac′·ryo·
dac′·ryo·ad′·e·nal′·gia
dac′·ryo·ad′·e·nec′·to·my
dac′·ryo·ad′·e·ni′·tis
dac′·ryo·cyst
dac′·ryo·cys·tec′·to·my

dac′·ryo·cys·ti′·tis
dac′·ryo·cys′·to·
dac′·ryo·cys′·to·blen·nor·rhe′a   Brit. ·rhoe′a
dac′ryo·cys′·to·cele
dac′·ryo·cys·tog′·ra·phy
dac′·ryo·cys′·to·rhi·nos′·to·my
dac′·ryo·cys·tos′·to·my
dac′·ryo·cys′·to·syr′·in·got′·o·my
dac′·ryo·cys′·to·tome
dac′·ryo·cys·tot′·o·my
dac′·ry·o·cyte
dac′·ry·o·gen′·ic
dac′·ry·o·lith
dac′·ry·o·li·thi′·a·sis
dac·ry·o′·ma   pl. ·mas   or ·ma·ta
dac′·ry·on   pl. ·rya
dac′·ry·or·rhe′a   Brit. ·rhoe′a
dac′·ryo·so′·le·ni′·tis
dac′·ryo·ste·no′·sis
dac′·ti·no·my′·cin
dac′·tyl
dac·tyl′·i·on
dac′·ty·li′·tis
dac′·ty·lo·
dac′·ty·lo·dys′·tro·phy
dac′·ty·lo·gram
dac′·ty·log′·ra·phy
dac′·ty·lol′·y·sis
dac′·ty·los′·co·py
dac′·ty·lo·spas′m
dac′·ty·lus
dal′·ton
dan′·der
dan′·druff
dan′·syl
dap′·sone
dark′·field
darm′·brand
dar·to′·ic
dar′·toid
dar′·tos

dar·win′·i·an
dar′·win·is′m *also* Darwinism
Das′·y·proc′·ta
da′·ta *sg.* da′·tum
da′·ta·base
Da·tu′·ra
da′·tur·is′m
dau′·no·my′·cin
dau′·no·ru′·bi·cin
de·ac′·ti·va′·tion
de·ac′·yl·ase
de·af′·fer·en·tate′
de·af′·fer·en·ta′·tion
deaf′-mute′
deaf′-mut′·ism
deaf′·ness
de·am′·i·nase
de′·ami′·no-ox′y·to′·cin
de·an′·i·mate
de′·a·nol
de′·aqua′·tion
death′·cap *also* ·cup
de·bil′·i·tant
de·bil′·i·tate ·tat′·ed, ·tat′·ing
de·bil′·i·ty
de·bouch′
dé′·bouche·ment′ [·bouche′·ment]
de·branch′·er
de·branch′·ing
dé·bride′ *also* de·bride′
dé′·bride·ment′ *also* de·bride′·ment
de·bris′
de·bug′ ·bugged′, ·bug′·ging
dec′a·
de′·cal′·ci·fi·ca′·tion
de·cal′·ci·fy′·ing
de·cal′·vans
dec′a·me·tho′·ni·um
dec′·ane
de′·can′·nu·la′·tion
de′·ca·pac′·i·ta′·tion

de·cap′·i·tate ·tat′·ed, ·tat′·ing
de·cap′·i·ta′·tion
de·cap′·su·la′·tion
de·car′·bon·a′·tion
de′·car·box′·yl·ase
de′·car·box′·yl·a′·tion
de·cay′
de·ce′·dent
de·cel′·er·a′·tion
de·cen′·tered
de·cen′·ter·ing
de′·cen·tra′·tion
de·cer′·e·bel·la′·tion
de·cer′·e·brate *adj. & v.* ·brat′·ed, ·brat′·ing
de·cer′·e·bra′·tion
de·cer′·e·bra′·tor
de·cer′·e·brize ·brized, ·briz′·ing; *var. of verb* decerebrate
de·chlo′·ri·na′·tion
de·chlor′·u·rant
de′·cho·les′·te·rol·i·za′·tion
dec′i·
dec′i·bel
de·cid′·ua *fem. of* deciduus
de·cid′·u·al
de·cid′·u·ate
de·cid′·u·a′·tion
de·cid′·u·i′·tis
de·cid′·uo·cel′·lu·lar
de·cid′·u·o′·ma *pl.* ·mas *or* ·ma·ta
de·cid′·u·ous
de·cid′·u·us *fem.* ·ua
dec′i·gram
dec′i·li′·ter *Brit.* ·li′·tre
dec′i·me′·ter *Brit.* ·me′·tre
dec′i·mo′·lar
dec′i·nor′·mal
de·ci′·sion
deck′·plat·te
dec′·li·na′·tion

de·clive′
de′·co·ag′·u·lant
de·coc′·tion
de·coc′·tum
de′·col′·or·a′·tion *Brit. also* ·col′·our·
de·col′·or·ize ·ized, ·iz′·ing; *Brit. also* ·col′·our·
de′·com·bus′·tion
de·com′·pen·sat′·ed
de·com′·pen·sa′·tion
de′·com·pose′ ·posed′, ·pos′·ing
de′·com·pos′·er
de·com′·po·si′·tion
de′·com·pres′·sion
de′·con·den·sa′·tion
de′·con·di′·tion·ing
de′·con·ges′·tant [·gest′·ant]
de′·con·ges′·tive
de′·con·tam′·i·na′·tion
de·cor′·ti·cate
de·cor′·ti·ca′·tion
dec′·re·ment
dec′·re·men′·tal
de′·cu·ba′·tion
de·cu′·bi·tal
de·cu′·bi·tus *pl. & gen. sg.* ·ti
de·cus′·sate *adj. & v.* ·sat·ed, ·sat·ing
de′·cus·sa′·tio *pl.* ·sa′·ti·o′·nes
de′·cus·sa′·tion
de′·dif′·fer·en′·ti·a′·tion
de·duct′·i·ble
de·duc′·tion
de-ef′·fer·en·ta′·tion
de·fat′·i·ga′·tion
de·fat′ fat′·ted, fat′·ting
de·fau′·nate ·nat·ed, ·nat·ing
def′·e·ca′·tion *Brit. also* def′·ae·

de′·fect
de·fec′·tive
de·fem′·i·ni·za′·tion
de·fense′ Brit. de·fence′
de·fen′·sive
def′·er·ens gen. sg.
 def′·er·en′·tis, masc. &
 fem. pl. def′·er·en′·tes,
 neut. pl. def′·er·en′·tia
def′·er·ent
def′·er·en·tec′·to·my
def′·er·en′·tial
def′·er·en′·ti·a′·lis
def′·er·en·ti′·tis
def′·er·ves′·cence
def′·er·ves′·cent
de·fib′·ril·la′·tion [·fi′·bril·]
de·fib′·ril·la′·tor [·fi′·bril·]
de·fi′·brin·at′·ed
de·fi′·brin·a′·tion
de·fi′·cien·cy
de·fic′·i·ens
def′·i·cit
de·fin′·ing
def′·i·ni′·tion
de·fin′·i·tive
de·flec′·tion
de′·flo·ra′·tion
de′·flo·res′·cence
de·flu′·vi·um
de·flux′·ion
de·form′·a·bil′·i·ty
de·for′·mans
de′·for·ma′·tion
de′·for·ma′·tum
de·for′·mi·ty
de·gan′·gli·on·ate
de·gen′·er·a·cy
de·gen′·er·ate adj. & v.
 ·at′·ed, ·at′·ing
de·gen′·er·a′·tion
de·gen′·er·a·tive
de·gen′·er·a·ti′·vus
de·germ′
de·glu′·ti·ble

de′·glu·ti′·tion
de·glu′·ti·to′·ry
de·grad′·a·bil′·i·ty
de·grad′·a·ble
deg′·ra·da′·tion
de·gran′·u·la′·tion
de·gree′
de·his′·cence
de′·hu·mid′·i·fi′·er
de·hy′·drant
de·hy′·dra·tase
de·hy′·drate ·drat·ed,
 ·drat·ing
de′·hy·dra′·tion
de·hy′·dro·
de·hy′·dro·ascor′·bic
de·hy′·dro·cho′·late
de·hy′·dro·cho·les′·ter·ol
de·hy′·dro·cho′·lic
de·hy′·dro·cor′·ti·cos′·ter·one [·co·ste′·rone]
de·hy′·dro·em′·e·tine
de·hy′·dro·ep′i·an·dros′·ter·one
de·hy′·dro·gen·ase′
 [de′·hy·drog′·e·nașe]
de·hy′·dro·ge·nate
 ·nat′·ed, ·nat′·ing
de·hy′·dro·i′so·an·dros′·ter·one
de·hyp′·no·tize ·tized,
 ·tiz′·ing
de·i′on·i·za′·tion
dé′·jà vé·cu′
dé′·jà vu′
dé′·jà fait′
de·jec′·ta
de·jec′·tion
dek′a· var. of deca-
de·lam′·i·na′·tion
de·lead′
del′·e·te′·ri·ous
de·le′·tion
de·lic′·ti
de·lip′·i·da′·tion
del′·i·ques′·cent

de·lir′·i·ant
de·lir′·i·fa′·cient
de·lir′·i·ous
de·lir′·i·um pl. de·lir′·ia
del′·i·tes′·cence
de·liv′·er
de·liv′·ery
del′·le pl. ·len
de′·lo·mor′·phic also ·phous
del′·ta
del′·toid
del·toi′·de·us fem.
 ·dea, neut. ·de·um
del′·to·pec′·to·ral
de·lu′·sion
de·lu′·sion·al
de′·mar·ca′·tion
de·mas′·cu·lin·i·za′·tion
dem′·e·car′·i·um
dem′·e·clo·cy′·cline
de·ment′·ed
de·men′·tia
de·meth′·yl·a′·tion
dem′i·
dem′i·fac′·et
dem′i·gaunt′·let
dem′i·lune
de·min′·er·al·i·za′·tion
dem′·o·dec′·tic
Dem′·o·dex
 D. fol·lic′·u·lo′·rum
dem′·o·di·ci′·a·sis
dem′·o·di·co′·sis
de·mog′·ra·pher
dem′·o·graph′·ic
de·mog′·ra·phy
de·mon′·stra·ti′·vus
de·mul′·cent
de·my′·e·lin·ate ·at′·ed, ·at′·ing
de·my′·e·lin·a′·tion
 also ·lin·i·za′·tion
de·my′·e·lin·ize ·ized,
 ·iz′·ing; var. of demyelinate

de·nar′·co·tize ·tized,
·tiz′·ing
de·na′·tur·a′·tion
de·na′·ture ·tured,
·tur·ing
Den·dras′·pis
den·drax′·on
den′·dric
den′·dri·form
den′·drite
den·drit′·ic
den·dri′·tum
den′·dro·
den′·dro·den·drit′·ic
den′·droid
de′·ner·vate [de·ner′·
vate] ·vat′·ed, ·vat′·
ing
de′·ner·va′·tion
den′·gue
de·ni′·al
den′·i·da′·tion
Den′·i·so′·nia
de·ni′·tri·fi·ca′·tion
de·ni′·tro·gen·a′·tion
[de′·ni·trog′·e·na′·
tion]
dens *pl.* den′·tes, *gen.
sg.* den′·tis, *gen. pl.*
den′·ti·um
den′·sa
den·sim′·e·ter
den′·si·tom′·e·ter
den′·si·tom′·e·try
den′·si·ty
den·sog′·ra·phy
den′·tal
den·ta′·le *neut. of*
dentalis
den·tal′·gia
den·ta′·lis *pl.* ·les
den′·ta·ry
den·ta′·ta *fem. of*
dentatus
den′·tate
den·ta′·to·ru′·bral
den·ta′·to·tha·lam′·ic

den·ta′·tus *gen.* ·ti
den′·tes *pl. of* dens
den′·ti·
den′·ti·cle
den·tic′·u·lar
den·tic′·u·late
den·tic′·u·la′·tion
den·tic′·u·la′·tum
den′·ti·frice
den·tig′·er·ous
den′·tin *Brit.* ·tine
den′·tin·al
den′·ti·no·blast
den′·ti·no·ce·men′·tal
den′·ti·no·enam′·el
den′·ti·no·gen′·e·sis
den′·tin·oid [·ti·noid]
den′·ti·no′·ma *pl.*
·mas *or* ·ma·ta
den·ti′·num
den′·tis *gen. sg. of*
dens
den′·tist
den′·tist·ry
den·ti′·tion
den′·ti·um *gen. pl. of*
dens
den′·to·
den′·to·al·ve′·o·lar
den′·to·enam′·el
den′·to·fa′·cial
den′·to·form
den′·toid
den′·to·la′·bi·al
den′·tu·lous
den′·ture
den′·tur·ist
de′·nu·da′·tion [den′·
u·]
de·o′·dor·ant
de·o′·dor·iz′·er
de′··on·tol′·o·gy
de·or′·sum·duc′·tion
de·or′·sum·ver′·sion
de·ox′·y·
de·ox′·y·ad′·e·nyl′·ic
de·ox′·y·cho′·lic

de·ox′·y·cor′·ti·cos′·ter·
one [·co·ste′·rone]
de·ox′·y·cy′·ti·dyl′·ic
de·ox′·y·gen·ate ·at′·
ed, ·at′·ing
de·ox′·y·nu′·cle·o·side
de·ox′·y·ri′·bo·nu′·cle·
ase
de·ox′·y·ri′·bo·nu·cle′·
ic
de·ox′·y·ri′·bo·side
de·pan′·cre·a·tize
·tized, ·tiz′·ing
de·pat′·tern·ing
de·pend′
de·pen′·dence [·pend′·
ence] *var. of* dependency
de·pen′·den·cy [·pend′·
en·cy]
de·pen′·dent [·pend′·
ent]
de·per′·son·al·i·za′·tion
de′·pig′·men·ta′·tion
dep′·i·late ·lat′·ed,
·lat′·ing
dep′·i·la′·tion
de·pil′·a·to·ry
de·plete′ ·plet′·ed,
·plet′·ing
de·ple′·tion
de·po′·lar·i·za′·tion
de·po′·lar·ize
de·po′·lar·iz′·er
de′·por·ta′·tion
de·pos′·it
dep′·o·si′·tion
de′·pot [dep′·ot]
de·press′
de·pres′·sant
de·pres′·sion
de·pres′·sive
de·pres′·so·mo′·tor
de·pres′·sor
dep′·ri·va′·tion
de·pro′·tein·i·za′·tion
dep′·si·pep′·tide
dep′·u·ra′·tion

dep'·u·ra'·tive
de·pu'·ri·na'·tion
de·range'·ment
de·re'·al·i·za'·tion
de·re'·ism [de'·re·]
de'·re·is'·tic
der'·en·ceph'·a·ly
de'·re·pres'·sion
derm'·a·brad'·er
derm'·abra'·sion
Der'·ma·cen'·tor
  D. an'·der·so'·ni
  D. mar'·gi·na'·tus
  D. var'·i·a'·bi·lis
Der'·ma·cen·trox'·e·nus [·cen'·trox·e'·]
der'·ma·chal'·a·sis
  var. of dermatochalasis
der'·mal
der·mal'·gia var. of dermatalgia
der'·ma·my·i'·a·sis
  var. of dermatomyiasis
Der'·ma·nys'·sus
  D. gal·li'·nae
der'·ma·tal'·gia
der'·ma·tan
der·mat'·i·ca
der'ma·ti'·tis pl. ·tit'·i·des
der'·ma·to·
der'·ma·to·ar·thri'·tis
Der'·ma·to'·bia
der'·ma·to·bi'·a·sis
der'·ma·to·chal'·a·sis
  also ·cha·la'·sia
der'·ma·to·fi·bro'·ma
  pl. ·mas or ·ma·ta
der'·ma·to·fi'·bro·sar·co'·ma
der'·ma·to·fi·bro'·sis
der'·ma·to·gen'·ic
der'·ma·to·glyph'

der'·ma·to·glyph'·ic
der'·ma·to·graph'·ia
  var. of dermographia
der'·ma·tog'·ra·phis'm
  var. of dermographism
der'·ma·toid
der'·ma·to·log'·ic
  also ·i·cal
der'·ma·tol'·o·gy
der'·ma·tol'·y·sis
der'·ma·tom'·al [·to'·mal]
der'·ma·tome
der'·ma·to·mere
der'·ma·to'·mic
der'·ma·to·my·co'·sis pl. ·ses
der'·ma·to·my·i'·a·sis
der'·ma·to·my'·o·si'·tis
der'·ma·to·no·sol'·o·gy
der'·ma·to·path'·ic
der'·ma·to·pa·thol'·o·gy
der'·ma·top'·a·thy
Der'·ma·to·pha·goi'·des
der'·ma·to·phyte [der·mat'·o·]
der'·ma·to·phy'·tid
  also ·tide
der'·ma·to·phy·to'·sis pl. ·ses
der'·ma·to·plas'·ty [der·mat'·o·]
der'·ma·to·pol'·y·neu·ri'·tis
der'·ma·to·scle·ro'·sis
der'·ma·to'·sis pl. ·ses
der'·ma·to·some
der'·ma·to·sto'·ma·to·oph·thal'·mic
der'·ma·to·tro'·pic [·trop'·ic]

der'·ma·to·zo·i'·a·sis
der'ma·to·zo'·on pl. ·zo'a
der'·ma·to·zo'·o·no'·sis
der'·mic
der'·mis gen. der'·mi·dis
der'·mo·
der'·mo·blast
der'·mo·ep'·i·der'·mal
der'·mo·gen'·e·sis
der'·mo·glyph'·ic var. of dermatoglyphic
der'·mo·graph'·ia
der'·mo·graph'·ic
der·mog'·ra·phis'm
der'·mo·hy·grom'·e·ter
der'·moid
der'·mo·li·po'·ma pl. ·mas or ·ma·ta
der·mom'·e·ter
der'·mo·my·co'·sis
  var. of dermatomycosis
der'·mo·my'·o·tome
der'·mo·ne·crot'·ic
der'·mo·neu'·ro·tro'·pic [·trop'·ic]
der·mop'·a·thy var. of dermatopathy
der'·mo·phy'·ma
der'·mo·phy·to'·sis
  var. of dermatophytosis
der'·mo·plas'·ty var. of dermatoplasty
der'·mo·syn'·o·vi'·tis [·sy'·no·]
der'·mo·tome[19] var. of dermatome
der'·mo·tox'·in
der'·mo·tro'·pic [·trop'·ic]
der'·mo·tu·ber'·cu·lin
der·ren'·ga·der'a

---

19 The spelling *dermotome* is used only in its embryological meaning (cutis plate) by some authorities who wish to reserve the spelling *dermatome* for the cutaneous areas innervated by segmental nerves. However, *dermatome* is the usual spelling in all contexts.

de·sat'·u·ra'·tion
des'·ce·me·ti'·tis
des'·ce·met'·o·cele
des·cen'·dens *gen.*
  des'·cen·den'·tis
des·cen'·sus
des·cent'
de·sen'·si·ti·za'·tion
de·sen'·si·tize   ·tized,
  ·tiz'·ing
de·ser'·pi·dine
de·sex'
de·sex'·u·al·i·za'·tion
de·sex'·u·al·ize   ·ized,
  ·iz'·ing
des'·ic·cant
des'·ic·cate   ·cat'·ed,
  ·cat'·ing
des'·ic·ca'·tion
des'·ic·ca'·tive
des'·ic·ca'·tor
de·sick'·le   ·led, ·ling
de·sign'
de·sip'·ra·mine
des·lan'·o·side
des·mec'·ta·sis
des·mi'·tis
des'·mo·
des'·mo·cra'·ni·um
des·mog'·e·nous
des'·moid
des'·mo·lase
des·mo'·ma
des'·mon
des'·mo·pex'·ia
des'·mo·pla'·sia
des'·mo·plas'·tic
des'·mo·pres'·sin
des'·mor·rhex'·is
des'·mo·sine
des'·mo·some
des·ox'·i·met'·a·sone
des·ox'y·   *var. of*
  deoxy-
des·ox'y·cor'·ti·cos'·te·
  rone [·co·ste'·rone]
des·ox'y·ri'·bo·nu·cle'·
  ic

des·ox'y·ri'·bose
de·spe'·ci·at'·ed
de·spe'·ci·a'·tion
des'·qua·mate   ·mat'·
  ed, ·mat'·ing
des'·qua·ma'·tion
des'·qua·ma'·tive [de·
  squam'·a·]
des'·qua·ma·to'·ry [de·
  squam'·a·]
des'·thi'o·bi'·o·tin
de·stru'·ens [de'·stru·]
de'·sulf·hy'·drase
de'·syn·ap'·sis
de·syn'·chro·ni·za'·tion
de·syn'·chro·nize
  ·nized, ·niz'·ing
de·tach'·ment
de·tec'·tor
de·ter'·gent
de·te'·ri·o·ra'·tion
de·ter'·mi·nant
de·ter'·mi·na'·tion
de·ter'·mi·na·tive
de·ter'·min·is'm
de·tor'·sion
de·tox'·i·cate   ·cat'·ed,
  ·cat'·ing
de·tox'·i·fi·ca'·tion
  also de·tox'·i·ca'·tion
de·tox'·i·fy   ·fied, ·fy'·
  ing
det'·ri·ment
de·tri'·tion
de·tri'·tus
de·tru'·sion
de·tru'·sor
de'·tu·ba'·tion
de'·tu·mes'·cence
de'·tu·mes'·cent
deu'·ter·   *var. of*
  deutero-
deu'·ter·anom'·a·lous
deu'·ter·anom'·a·ly
deu'·ter·an·ope'
deu'·ter·an·o'pia
deu'·ter·an·o'·pic
deu'·ter·an·op'·sia

deu'·ter·ate   ·at'·ed,
  ·at'·ing
deu'·ter·a'·tion
deu·te'·ri·um
deu'·ter·ize   ·ized, ·iz'·
  ing
deu'·tero·
Deu'·ter·o·my·ce'·tes
deu'·ter·on
deu'·ter·o·path'·ic
deu'·ter·op'·a·thy
deu'·ter·o·plas'm   *var.*
  of deutoplasm
deu'·ter·o·plas·mol''·y·
  sis *var. of* deutoplas-
  molysis
deu'·ter·o·to'·cia   *also*
  ·ter·ot'·o·ky
deu'·to·
deu'·to·plas'm
deu'·to·plas·mol''·y·sis
de'·vas·a'·tion
de·vas'·cu·lar·i·za'·tion
de·vel'·op·ment
de·vel'·op·men'·tal
de'·vi·ance
de'·vi·ant
de'·vi·ate   ·at'·ed, ·at'·
  ing
de'·vi·a'·tion
de'·vi·a'·tion·al
de·vice'
de·vi'·tal
de·vi'·tal·i·za'·tion
de·vi'·tal·ize   ·ized,
  ·iz'·ing
dev'·o·lu'·tion [de'·vo·]
dev'·o·lu'·tive [de'·vo·]
dex'·a·meth'·a·sone
dex·chlor'·phen·ir'·a·
  mine
dex'·ter   *gen.* ·tri
dex'·tra   *fem. of*
  dexter; *gen.* ·trae
dex'·trad
dex'·tral
dex·tral'·i·ty
dex'·tran

dex′·tri *gen. of* dexter
dex′·trin
dex′·tro·
dex′·tro·car′·dia
dex′·tro·car′·di·o·gram
dex′·tro·cer′·e·bral
[·ce·re′·]
dex·troc′·u·lar
dex·troc′·u·lar′·i·ty
dex′·tro·duc′·tion
dex′·tro·meth·or′·phan
dex′·tro·posed′
dex′·tro·po·si′·tion
dex′·tro·ro′·ta·to′·ry
dex′·trose
dex′·tro·tor′·sion
dex′·tro·ver′·sion
dex′·trum *neut. of* dexter
di′·a·
di′·a·be′·tes
di′·a·bet′·ic
di′·a·bet′·i·cus *gen. pl.* ·bet′·i·co′·rum
di′·a·bet′·o·gen′·ic [·be′·to·]
di·ac′·e·tate
di′·ac′·e·tu′·ria
di′·ace′·tyl
di′·ace′·tyl·dap′·sone
di′·ace′·tyl·mor′·phine
di′·ace′·ty·na·lor′·phine
di′·a·clast
di·ac′·ri·nous
di·ac′·yl·glyc′·er·ol
di′·a·der′·mic
di·ad′·o·cho·ki·ne′·sia [di′·a·do′·cho·]
also ·ki·ne′·sis
di·ad′·o·cho·ki·net′·ic [di′·a·do′·cho·]
di′·ag·nose′ [di′·ag·nose] ·nosed′, ·nos′·ing
di′·ag·no′·sis *pl.* ·ses
di′·ag·nos′·tic
di′·ag·nos·ti′·cian

di′·a·gram *n. & v.* ·gramed *or* ·grammed, ·gram′·ing *or* ·gram′·ming
di′·a·gram·mat′·ic
di′·a·graph
di·ag′·ra·phy
di′a·ki·ne′·sis
di′·a·lu′·ric
di·al′·y·sance
di·al′·y·sate
di·al′·y·sis *pl.* ·ses
di′·a·lyz′·a·ble *Brit.* ·lys′·
di′·a·lyze ·lyzed, ·lyz′·ing; *Brit.* ·lyse, ·lysed, ·lys′·ing
di′·a·lyz′·er *Brit.* ·lys′·
di·am′·e·ter
di′·a·mine [di·am′·ine]
di′·ami′·no·pim′·e·late
di′·ami′·no·py·rim′·i·dine
di′a·mor′·phine
di·am′·tha·zole
di′a·pause
di′·a·pe·de′·sis
di′·a·pe·det′·ic
di·aph′·a·nom′·e·ter
di·aph′·a·nom′·e·try
di·aph′·a·no·scope
di·aph′·a·nos′·co·py
di·aph′·o·rase
di′·a·pho·re′·sis
di′·a·pho·ret′·ic
di′·a·phragm
di′·a·phrag′·ma *pl.* ·ma·ta, *gen. sg.* ·ma·tis
di′·a·phrag·mat′·ic
di′·a·phrag·mat′·i·ca *pl.* ·cae
di′·a·phys′·e·al [di·aph′·y·se′·al] *var. of* diaphysial
di′·a·phy·sec′·to·my [di·aph′·y·]
di′·a·phys′·i·al

di·aph′·y·sis *pl.* ·ses
di′·a·phy·si′·tis [di·aph′·y·]
di′·a·plex′·us
di′·apoph′·y·sis *pl.* ·ses
di′·ar·rhe′a *Brit.* ·rhoe′a
di′·ar·rhe′·al *Brit.* ·rhoe′·al
di′·ar·rhe′·ic *Brit.* ·rhoe′·ic
di·ar′·thric
di′·ar·thro′·di·al
di′·ar·thro′·sis *pl.* ·ses
di′·ar·tic′·u·lar
di·as′·chi·sis
di′·a·scop′·ic
di·as′·co·py
di′·a·stase
di′·a·stas·e′·mia [·sta·se′·] *Brit.* ·ae′·mia
di·as′·ta·sis *pl.* ·ses
di′·a·stat′·ic
di′·a·ste′·ma
di′·a·ste′·ma·ta [·stem′·a·] *pl. of* diastema
di′·a·ste′·ma·to·my·e′·lia [·stem′·a·to·]
di′·as′·ter [di·as′·ter]
di′a·ste′·reo·i′so·mer
di·as′·to·le
di′·a·stol′·ic
di·as′·to·my·e′·lia
di′·a·ther′·mic
di′·a·ther′·mo·co·ag′·u·la′·tion
di′·a·ther′·my
di·ath′·e·sis *pl.* ·ses
di′·a·thet′·ic
di′·a·tom
di′·a·to·ma′·ceous
di·at′·o·mite
di′·a·tri·zo′·ate
di′·a·tri·zo′·ic
di·au′·che·nos
di·aux′·ic

di′·aux′y [di·aux′y]
   also di·aux′·ie
di·az′·e·pam
di′·a·zine
di·az′o·
di·az′o
di·az′o·meth′·ane
di′·a·zo′·ni·um
di·az′·o·ti·za′·tion
di′·az·ox′·ide
di·ben′·zyl·chlor·eth′·a·mine
di·both′·rio·ceph′·a·li′·a·sis
Di·both′·rio·ceph′·a·lus
di·bra′·chi·us
di·bro′·mide
di′·bu·caine
di·bu′·to·line
di·bu′·tyr·yl
di·cal′·ci·um
di·ce′·lous *var. of*
   dicoelous
di·cen′·tric
di·ceph′·a·lous
di·ceph′·a·lus
di·ceph′·a·ly
di·chei′·lia
di′·chlor·al·phen′·a·zone
di′·chlor·eth′·yl·ar′·sine
di·chlo′·ri·sone
di·chlo′·ro·ace′·tic
di·chlo′·ro·di·eth′·yl
di·chlo′·ro·di·phen′·yl·tri′·chlo·ro·eth′·ane
di·chlo′·ro·ni′·tro·ben·zene′ [·ben′·zene]
di·chlo′·ro·phen·ox′y·ace′·tic
di·chlo′·ro·xy′·le·nol
di′·chlor·phen′·a·mide
di·chog′·a·mous
di·cho′·ri·al
di′·cho·ri·on′·ic
di·chot′·o·my
di·chro′·ic

di′·chro·is′m
di·chro′·ma·sy
di′·chro·mat [di·chro′·]
di′·chro·mat′·ic
di·chro′·ma·tis′m
   also di′·chro·mis′m
di′·chro′·ma·top′·sia
di·chro′·mic
dic′·ing
di·clox′·a·cil′·lin
di·coe′·lous
di·co′·ria
di·cou′·ma·rol *var. of*
   dicumarol
di·crot′·ic
di′·cro·tis′m
dic′·tyo·ki·ne′·sis
dic′·ty·o·some
dic′·ty·o·tene
di·cu′·ma·rol
di·cy′·clo·hex′·yl·car′·bo·di·im′·ide
di·dac′·tic
di·dac′·tyl·is′m
di·dac′·ty·lous
di·del′·phia
di·del′·phic
di′·de·ox′y·aden′·o·sine
di′·de·ox′y·cy′·ti·dine
di′·de·ox′y·hex′·ose
di′·de·ox′y·in′·o·sine
di·der′·mal
did′·y·mi′·tis
did′·y·mous
die died, dy′·ing
diel′·drin
di′·elec′·tric
di′·elec·trol′·y·sis
di·em′·bry·o·ny
di′·en·ce·phal′·ic
di′·en·ceph′·a·lo·hy′·po·phys′·i·al
di′·en·ceph′·a·lon
die′·ner
di′·en·es′·trol *Brit.*
   ·oes′·trol

Di·ent′·amoe′·ba frag′·i·lis
di·er′·e·sis
di·es′·ter·ase
di·es′·trus *also* ·trum;
   Brit. di·oes′·
di′·et
di′·etar′y
di′·etet′·ic
di′·eth′·a·nol′·a·mine
di·eth′·yl
di·eth′·yl·am′·ide
di·eth′·yl·amine′ [·am′ine]
di′·eth′·yl·ami′·no·eth′·yl
di′·eth′·yl·car·bam′·a·zine
di·eth′·yl·ene
di·eth′·yl·mal′·o·nyl·ure′a
di·eth′·yl·pro′·pi·on
di·eth′·yl·stil·bes′·trol
   Brit. ·stil·boes′·
di·eti′·cian
di′·eto·ther′·a·py
dif′·fer·en′·tia
dif′·fer·en′·tial
dif′·fer·en′·ti·ate ·at′·ed, ·at′·ing
dif′·fer·en′·ti·a′·tion
dif·frac′·tion
dif·fu′·sa *fem. of*
   diffusus
dif·fu′·sate
dif·fuse′ ·fused′, ·fus′·ing
dif·fus′·i·ble
dif·fu′·sion
dif·fu′·sus *fem.* ·sa,
   neut. ·sum
di′·ga·met′·ic
di·gas′·tric
di·gas′·tri·ca *fem. of*
   digastricus
di·gas′·tri·cus *pl. & gen. sg.* ·ci
Di·ge′·nea

di·gen′·e·sis
di′·ge·net′·ic
di·gen′·ic
di·gest′ v.
di′·gest n.
di·ges′·tant
di·ges′·ter
di·gest′·i·bil′·i·ty
di·gest′·i·ble
di·ges′·tion
di·ges′·tive
di′·ges·to′·ri·us neut.
 ·ri·um
dig′·it
dig′·i·tal
dig′·i·tal′·gia
dig′·i·tal′·in
dig′·i·tal′·is cardio-
 tonic drug
dig′·i·ta′·lis Latin
 word for digital; pl.
 ·les
dig′·i·tal·i·za′·tion
dig′·i·tal′·ose
dig′·i·ta′·ta pl. ·tae
dig′·i·ta′·tio pl. ·ta′·ti·
 o′·nes
dig′·i·ta′·tion
dig′·i·ti pl. & gen. sg.
 of digitus
dig′·i·ti·grade′
dig′·i·to·fib′·u·lar
dig′·i·to′·nin
dig′·i·to·plan′·tar
dig′·i·to·ra′·di·al
dig′·i·to′·rum gen. pl.
 of digitus
dig′·i·to·tib′·i·al
dig′·i·to·ul′·nar
dig′·i·tox′·i·gen′·in
dig′·i·tox′·in
dig′·i·tox′·ose
dig′·i·tus pl. & gen.
 sg. ·ti, gen. pl. dig′·i·
 to′·rum
di·glos′·sia
di·glyc′·er·ide
di·gox′·in

di·het′·er·ox·en′·ic
di·het′·ero·zy′·gote
di·hy′·brid
di·hy′·drate
di·hy′·dric
di·hy′·dro·chlo′·ride
di′·hy′·dro·co′·deine
di′·hy′·dro·cor′·ti·sol
di′·hy′·dro·cor′·ti·sone
di′·hy′·dro·er′·go·cor′·
 nine
di′·hy′·dro·er·got′·
 amine
di′·hy′·dro·fo′·late
di′·hy′·dro·fo′·lic
di′·hy′·dro·lip′o·am′·
 ide
di′·hy′·dro·or′·o·tate
di′·hy′·dro·orot′·ic
di′·hy′·dro·ta·chys′·ter·
 ol
di′·hy′·dro·tes·tos′·ter·
 one
di′·hy·drox′y·ac′·e·
 tone
di′·hy·drox′y·alu′·mi·
 num
di′·hy·drox′y·cho′·le·
 cal·cif′·er·ol
di′·hy·drox′y·phen′·yl·
 al′·a·nine
di·i′o·do·hy·drox′y·
 quin
di′·i′o·do·sal′·i·cyl′·ic
di′·i′o·do·ty′·ro·sine
di′·i′so·cy′·a·nate
di′·i′so·pro′·pyl
di·kar′·y·on
di′·ke′·to·pi·per′·a·zine
dik′·ty·o′·ma
di·lac′·er·a′·tion
di·lat′·a·ble
di·la′·tan·cy
di·la′·tant
dil′·a·ta′·tion
dil′·a·ta′·tor
di·late′ [di′·late] ·lat′·
 ed, ·lat′·ing

di·la′·tion
dil′·a·tom′·e·ter
di·la′·tor [di′·la·]
di·lev′·a·lol
di·lox′·a·nide
dil′·u·ent
di·lute′ ·lut′·ed, ·lut′·
 ing
di·lu′·tion
di′·men·hy′·dri·nate
di′·mer
di′·mer·cap′·rol
di·mer′·ic
di·meth′·i·cone
di′·me·this′·ter·one
di·meth′·yl
di′·meth′·yl·amine′
 [·am′ine]
di′·meth′·yl·ni·tro′·sa·
 mine [·tros′·a·]
di·me′·tria
di·mid′·i·a′·ta
di·mor′·phic
di·mor′·phism
di·mor′·phous
di·mox′·y·line
dim′·ple
dim′·pling
di·ner′·ic
di·ni′·tro·ami′·no·phe′·
 nol
di·ni′·tro·ben·zene′
 [·ben′·zene]
di·ni′·tro·chlo′·ro·ben·
 zene′ [·ben′·zene]
di·ni′·tro·gen
di·ni′·tro·phe′·nol
di·ni′·tro·phen′·yl·hy′·
 dra·zine
di′·no·flag′·el·late
Di′·no·fla·gel′·li·da
 also ·flag′·el·la′·ta
di·nu′·cle·o·tide′
Di·oc′·to·phy′·ma
 D. re·na′·le
di·oc′·tyl
di′·ode
di′·o·don′·tic

di·oes′·trus Brit. spel.
  of diestrus
di·op′·ter [di′·op·]
  Brit. ·tre
di′·op·tom′·e·ter also
  ·trom′·e·ter
di′·op·tom′·e·try also
  ·trom′·e·try
di·op′·tric
di′·op·tros′·co·py
di·op′·try [di′·op·]
  var. of diopter
di′·os·gen′·in
di·ov′u·lar [·o′vu·]
di·ov′u·la·to′·ry
  [·o′vu·]
di·ox′·ane
di·ox′·ide
di·ox′·in
di·ox′·y·gen·ase
di·ox′·y·line
di·pen′·tene
di·pep′·ti·dase
di·pep′·tide
Di·pet′·a·lo·ne′·ma
di·phal′·lia
di′·phal·lus
di·pha′·sic
di·phe′·ma·nil
di·phen′·a·di′·one
di′·phen·hy′·dra·mine
di·phen′·yl·amine′
  [·am′·ine]
di·phen′·yl·amine′·ar′·
  sine
di·phen′·yl·chlor·ar′·
  sine
di·phen′·yl·hy·dan′·to·
  in
di·phen′·yl·py′·ra·line
di·phos′·gene
di·phos′·phate
di·phos′·pho·di·glyc′·
  er·ide
di·phos′·pho·ga·lac′·
  tose
di·phos′·pho·glu′·cose
di·phos′·pho·ki′·nase

di·phos′·pho·pyr′·i·dine
diph′·tha·mide
diph·the′·ria
diph·the′·ri·al
diph′·the·rin
diph′·the·rit′·ic also
  diph·the′·ric
diph′·the·roid
diph′·the·ro·tox′·in
diph′y·ge·net′·ic
di·phyl′·lo·both·ri′·a·sis
Di·phyl′·lo·both′·ri·um
  D. la′·tum
diph′y·o·dont [di·phy′·
  o·dont]
dip′·la·cu′·sis
di·plas′·tic
di·ple′·gia
di·ple′·gic
dip′·lo·
dip′·lo·bac′·il·lar′y
dip′·lo·ba·cil′·lus pl.
  ·li
dip′·lo·blas′·tic
dip′·lo·car′·dia
dip′·lo·car′·di·ac
dip′·lo·ceph′·a·lus
dip′·lo·ceph′·a·ly
dip′·lo·coc′·cus pl. ·ci
dip′·lo·co′·ria
dip′·loë also dip′·loe
dip′·lo·gen′·e·sis
dip·lo′·ic [dip·lo′·]
  also dip′·lo·et′·ic
di·plo′·ica fem. of
  diploicus; pl. ·icae
di·plo′·icus pl. ·ici
dip′·loid
dip′·loi·dy
dip′·lo·kar′y·on
dip′·lo·mate
dip′·lo·my·e′·lia
dip′·lo·neu′·ral
dip′·lont
dip·lop′·a·gus
dip′·lo·phase
dip′·lo·pho′·nia
dip·lo′·pia

dip′·lo·po′·dia
dip·lo′·sis pl. ·ses
dip′·lo·some
dip′·lo·so′·mia
dip′·lo·tene
Di·plu′·ri·dae
di·po′·dia
di·po′·lar
di′·pole
di·po·tas′·si·um
di·pro′·pi·o·nate
di′·pro·so′·pus [di·
  pros′·o·pus]
dip′·so·gen
dip′·so·gen′·ic
dip′·so·ma′·nia
dip′·stick
Dip′·tera
dip′·ter·an
dip′·ter·ous
Di′·pus
di′·pus
di·py′·gus
Di′·py·lid′·i·um
  D. ca·ni′·num
di′·py·rid′·a·mole
di·py′·rone
di·rec′·tion
di·rec′·tive
di·rec′·tor
Di′·ro·fi·lar′·ia
  D. im·mi′·tis
  D. re′·pens
di′·ro·fil′·a·ri′·a·sis
dis negative prefix: Cf.
  dys-
dis′·abil′·i·ty
dis·a″ble ·a″bled,
  ·a″bling
dis·a″ble·ment
di·sac′·cha·ri·dase
di·sac′·cha·ride
dis·ag′·gre·ga′·tion
dis′·ar·tic′·u·la′·tion
dis′·as·sim′·i·late
  ·lat″ed, ·lat″ing
dis′·as·sim′·i·la′·tion
dis′·as·so′·ci·a′·tion

dis'·as·sor'·ta·tive
dis·az'o· *var. of* diazo-
disc *var. of* disk
dis'·cal
disc·ec'·to·my *var. of* diskectomy
dis'·charge
dis'·ci *pl. & gen. sg. of* discus
dis'·ci·form
dis·cis'·sion
dis·ci'·tis *var. of* diskitis
dis'·co·
dis'·co·blas'·tu·la
dis·cob'·o·lus
dis'·co·gas'·tru·la
dis'·co·gen'·ic
dis'·co·gram *var. of* diskogram
dis·cog'·ra·phy *var. of* diskography
dis'·coid
dis·coi'·dal
dis·coi'·dea
dis'·con·tin'·u·ous
dis·cop'·a·thy *var. of* diskopathy
dis·cor'·dance
dis·cot'·o·my
dis·crete'
dis·crim'·i·nant
dis·crim'·i·na'·tion
dis·crim'·i·na·tive
dis·crim'·i·na'·tor
dis'·cus *pl. & gen. sg.* ·ci
dis·cus'·sive
dis·cu'·tient
dis·ease'
dis'·equil'·i·bra'·tion
dis'·equi·lib'·ri·um
  imbalance: Cf. dysequilibrium
dis'·fa·cil'·i·ta'·tion
dis·fig'·ure ·fig'·ured, ·fig'·ur·ing

dis·func'·tion *var. of* dysfunction
dis·har'·mo·ny
dis'·im·pact'
dis'·in·fect'
dis'·in·fec'·tant
dis'·in·fec'·tion
dis'·in·fes·ta'·tion
dis'·in·hi·bi'·tion
dis'·in·ser'·tion
dis·in'·te·grant
dis·in'·te·gra'·tion
dis·in'·te·gra'·tor
dis'·in·tox'·i·ca'·tion
dis'·ju·gate
dis·junc'·tion
dis·junc'·tive
disk *also* disc
disk·ec'·to·my
dis·ki'·tis
dis'·ko· *var. of* disco-
dis'·ko·gram
dis·kog'·ra·phy
dis·kop'·a·thy
dis·lo'·cate [dis'·lo·] ·cat·ed, ·cat·ing
dis'·lo·ca'·tio *pl.* ·lo·ca'·ti·o'·nes
dis'·lo·ca'·tion
dis·mem'·ber
dis·mem'·ber·ment
dis·mu'·tase [dis'·mu·]
dis'·mu·ta'·tion
dis'·oc·clude'
di·so'·di·um
di·so'·mic
di'·so·my
di'·so·pyr'·a·mide
dis·or'·der
dis·or'·i·en·ta'·tion
dis'·pa·rate
dis·par'·i·ty
dis·pen'·sa·ry
dis·pen'·sa·to'·ry
di'·sper·my
dis·per'·sal
dis'·per·sate

dis·perse' ·persed', ·pers'·ing
dis·per'·sion
dis·per'·sive
di·spi'·reme
dis·pos'·a·ble
dis·rup'·tion
dis·rup'·tive
dis·sect'
dis·sec'·tion
dis·sec'·tor
dis·sem'·i·nate ·nat'· ed, ·nat'·ing
dis·sem'·i·na'·tus *fem.* ·ta, *neut.* ·tum
dis·sep'·i·ment
dis·sim'·i·late
dis·sim'·i·la'·tion
  breakdown or catabolism: Cf. dissimulation
dis·sim'·u·la'·tion *act of feigning: Cf.* dissimilation
dis·so'·ci·a·ble
dis·so'·ci·ate
dis·so'·ci·a'·tion
dis·so'·ci·a·tive
dis'·so·lu'·tion
dis·solve' ·solved', ·solv'·ing
dis'·so·nance
dis'·sym·met'·ric
dis'·tad
dis'·tal
dis·ta'·lis *m. & f. pl.* ·les, *neut. pl.* ·lia
dis·tem'·per
dis·tend'
dis·ten'·si·bil'·i·ty
dis·ten'·si·ble
dis·ten'·sion *also* ·tion
dis·tich'·ia
dis'·ti·chi'·a·sis
dis·till' *Brit.* dis·til', ·tilled', ·til'·ling
dis'·til·land
dis'·til·late
dis'·til·la'·tion

dis′·to·
dis′·to·cep′·tor
dis′·to·clu′·sal *also*
  dis′·to-oc·clu′·sal
dis′·to·clu′·sion *also*
  dis′·to-oc·clu′·sion
Dis′·to·ma
di·sto′·ma·to′·sis
dis′·to·mi′·a·sis
dis·tor′·tion
dis·tor′·tum
dis′·to·ver′·sion
dis·tract′·i·bil′·i·ty
dis·trac′·tion
dis·tress′
dis′·tri·bu′·tion
dis·trib′·u·tive
dis′·tri·chi′·a·sis
dis·tur′·bance [·turb′·ance]
dis·turbed′
di·sul′·fide *Brit.* ·phide
di·sul′·fi·ram *Brit.* ·phi·ram
di·sym′·me·tros
di′·syn·ap′·tic
di·ter′·pene
di·thi′·ol
di·thi′·o·nate
di·thi′·o·nite
dith′·ra·nol
di′·ure′·sis *pl.* ·ses
di′·uret′·ic
di·u′·ria
di·ur′·nal
di·ur′·nule
di·va′·lent
di·ver′·gence
di·ver′·gent
di·ver′·sion
di·ver′·si·ty
di′·ver·tic′·u·la *pl. of* diverticulum
di′·ver·tic′·u·lar
di′·ver·tic′·u·lec′·to·my
di′·ver·tic′·u·li′·tis
di′·ver·tic′·u·lo·esoph′·a·gos′·to·my *Brit.*
  ·u·lo-oe·soph′·

di′·ver·tic′·u·lo·pex′y
di′·ver·tic′·u·lo′·sis
di′·ver·tic′·u·lum *pl.* ·la
di·vi′·cine
di·vi′·sion
di·vulse′ ·vulsed′, ·vuls′·ing
di·vul′·sion
di·vul′·sor
di′·zy·got′·ic
diz′·zi·ness
doc′·i·ma′·sy [do′·ci·]
  also doc′·i·ma′·sia
doc′·tor
doc′·trine
doc′·u·ment
do′·deca· [do·dec′a·]
do′·de·cane
do′·dec·yl [do·dec′·yl]
dog′·ma
doigt′ mort′
dol′·i·cho·
dol′·i·cho·ce·phal′·ic
  also ·ceph′·a·lous
dol′·i·cho·ceph′·a·ly
dol′·i·cho·co′·lon
dol′·i·cho·cra′·ni·al
dol′·i·cho·fa′·cial
dol′·i·cho·mor′·phic
dol′·i·cho·pel′·lic *also* ·pel′·vic
dol′·i·cho·pro·so′·pic
dol′·i·chu·ran′·ic
do′·lor *pl.* do·lo′·res
do′·lo·rif′·ic
do′·lo·rim′·e·ter
do′·lo·rim′·e·try
do′·lo·ro′·sus *fem.* ·sa, *neut.* ·sum
do·main′
dom′·i·nance
dom′·i·nant
dom′·i·na′·tor
do′·mi·phen
do·nee′
do′·nor

Don′·o·va′·nia gran′·u·lo′·ma·tis
don′·o·va·no′·sis
do′·pa *also* DOPA
do′·pa·mine
do′·pa·mi·ner′·gic
Dop′·pler
dor′·man·cy
dor′·mant
dor′·mi·fa′·cient
dor′·nase
dor′·sa *pl. of* dorsum
dor′·sad
dor′·sal
dor·sa′·le *neut. of* dorsalis; *pl.* ·lia
dor·sal′·gia
dor·sa′·lis *pl.* ·les, *gen. pl.* ·li·um
dor′·si *gen. of* dorsum
dor′·si·
dor′·si·cum′·bent
dor′·si·duct
dor′·si·flex′·ion
dor′·si·flex′·or
dor′·si·spi′·nal
dor′·so·
dor′·so·an·te′·ri·or
dor′·so·ceph′·a·lad
dor′·so·cu·boi′·dal
dor′·so·lat′·er·al
dor′·so·lat′·er·a′·lis
dor′·so·lum′·bar
dor′·so·me′·di·al
dor′·so·me′·di·an
dor′·so·me′·si·al
dor′·so·pos·te′·ri·or
dor′·so·ven′·trad
dor′·so·ven′·tral
dor′·sum *pl.* ·sa, *gen. sg.* ·si
dos′·age
dose
do·sim′·e·ter
do′·si·met′·ric
do·sim′·e·try
do′·sis
dou′·ble-blind′

dou'·ble-masked'
dou'·ble-strand'·ed
douche
dou·rine'
dow'·el
down'·gaze
dox'·a·pram
dox'·e·pin
dox'y·cy'·cline
drachm
drac'·on·ti'·a·sis
dra·cun'·cu·lar
dra·cun'·cu·li'·a·sis
Dra·cun'·cu·lus
   D. med'·i·nen'·sis
draft
dra·gée
drain'·age
dram
draught   *Brit. spel. of* draft
drep'·a·no·cyte
dress'·ing
dro'·mic
dro'·mo·   [drom'o·]
dro'·mo·graph   [drom'·o·]
dro'·mo·stan'·o·lone
dro'·mo·tro'·pic
   [drom'·o·, ·trop'·ic]
dro·mot'·ro·pis'm
dro·per'·i·dol
drop'·let
dropped
drop'·per
drop'·si·cal
drop'·sy
Dro·soph'·i·la
dro·stan'·o·lone
drown'·ing
drug'-fast
drug'·gist
drug'-re·sis'·tant   [-re·sist'·ant]
drum'·head
drum'·stick
drunk'·en·ness
dru'·sen   *sg.* dru'·se

du'·al·is'm
du'·al·ist
du·az'·o·my'·cin
duct
duc'·tal
duc'·ti·bus   *ablative pl. of* ductus
duc'·tile
duc·til'·i·ty
duc'·tion
duct'·less
duc'·tu·lar
duc'·tule
duc'·tu·lus   *pl.* ·li
duc'·tus   *pl. & gen. sg.* ductus
dul'·cin
dul'·ci·tol
dull'·ness   *also* dul'·ness
dulse
dumb
dumb'·bell
dumb'·ness
du'·o·de'·nal
du·o'·de·na'·lis   *pl.* ·les
du'·o·de·nec'·to·my
du'·o·de'·ni   *gen. of* duodenum
du'·o·de·ni'·tis
du'·o·de'·no·   [du·od'e·no·]
du'·o·de'·no·cho'·le·cys·tos'·to·my
du'·o·de'·no·cho·led'·o·chot'·o·my
du'·o·de'·no·gas'·tric
du'·o·de·nog'·ra·phy
du'·o·de'·no·he·pat'·ic
du'·o·de'·no·il'·e·os'·to·my
du'·o·de'·no·je·ju'·nal
du'·o·de'·no·je'·ju·na'·lis
du'·o·de·nol'·y·sis
du'·o·de'·no·mes'o·co'·lic

du'·o·de'·no·plas'·ty
du'·o·de·nor'·rha·phy
du'·o·de'·no·scope
du'·o·de·nos'·co·py
du'·o·de·nos'·to·my
du'·o·de·not'·o·my
du'·o·de'·num   *gen.* ·ni
du'·plex
du'·pli·ca'·tion
du'·pli·ca·ture
du·plic'·i·tas
du'·ra   *fem. of* durus;   *gen.* ·rae
du'·ral
du'·ra·plas'·ty
du·ra'·tion
du·ri'·tis
du'·ro·ar'ach·ni'·tis
du'·rus   *fem.* ·ra, *neut.* ·rum
dwarf
dwarf'·ish
dwarf'·ism
dy'·ad
dy·ad'·ic
dy'·as·ter   [dy·as'·ter]
   var. of diaster
dy'·clo·nine
dy'·dro·ges'·ter·one
dy·nam'·ic
dy'·na·mis'm
dy'·na·mo·
dy'·na·mo·gen'·e·sis
dy'·na·mo·gen'·ic
dy'·na·mog'·e·ny
dy'·na·mom'·e·ter
dy'·na·mo·met'·ric
dy·nam'·o·path'·ic
dy·nam'·o·scope
dyne
dy'·nein
dy·phyl'·line
dys   *faulty: Cf.* dis-
dys'·acou'·sis   *also*
   ·acou'·sia; *var. of* dysacusis
dys'·acu'·sis

dys·ad′·ap·ta′·tion
dys′·aes·the′·sia *Brit.*
  spel. of dysesthesia
dys·a′phia
dys·a′phic
dys·ar′·thria
dys·ar′·thric
dys′·ar·thro′·sis
dys′·au·to·no′·mia
dys′·bar·is′m
dys·ba′·sia
dys′·be′·ta·lip′o·pro′·
  tein·e′·mia [·li′po·]
  Brit. ·ae′·mia
dys′·cal·cu′·lia
dys·chei′·ria *also*
  ·chi′·ria
dys·che′·zia *also* ·sia
dys·chon′·dro·pla′·sia
dys′·chon·dros′·te·o′·
  sis
dys·chro′·mia
dys·chro′·mi·cum
dys′·chro·nous
dys·cra′·sia
dys·cras′·ic
dys·crat′·ic
dys′·di·ad′·o·cho·ki·
  ne′·sia [·di′·a·do′·
  cho·]
dys′·di·ad′·o·cho·ki·
  net′·ic [·di′·a·do′·
  cho·]
dys′·en·ce·pha′·lia
dys·en′·do·crin·is′m
dys′·en·ter′·ic
dys′·en·ter′y
dys·e′qui·lib′·ri·um
  faulty balance: Cf.
  disequilibrium
dys′·er·ga′·sia
dys·er′·gia
dys′·eryth′·ro·poi·e′·sis
dys′·eryth′·ro·poi·et′·ic
dys′·es·the′·sia *Brit.*
  ·aes-
dys′·fi·brin′·o·gen·e′·
  mia *Brit.* ·ae′·mia

dys·func′·tion
dys·func′·tion·al
dys′·ga·lac′·tia
dys·gam′·ma·glob′·u·
  lin·e′·mia *Brit.* ·ae′·
  mia
dys·gen′·e·sis
dys′·ge·net′·ic
dys·gen′·ic
dys·ger′·mi·no′·ma
  pl. ·mas *or* ·ma·ta
dys·geu′·sia
dys·gnath′·ia
dys·gon′·ic
dys·gram′·ma·tis′m
dys·graph′·ia
dys′·hi·dro′·sis
dys′·hi·drot′·ic
dys·im′·mu·no·glob′·u·
  lin·e′·mia *Brit.* ·ae′·
  mia
dys·kar′y·o′·sis
dys·kar′y·ot′·ic
dys·ker′·a·to′·ma
dys·ker′·a·to′·sis
dys·ker′·a·tot′·ic
dys′·ki·ne′·sia
dys′·ki·net′·ic
dys·la′·lia
dys·lex′·ia
dys·lex′·ic *also* dys·
  lec′·tic
dys·lip′·i·do′·sis
dys·lo′·gia
dys′·ma·tur′·i·ty
dys·me′·lia
dys·men′·or·rhe′a
  Brit. ·rhoe′a
dys·men′·tia
dys·met′·ria
dys′·me·trop′·sia
dys·mne′·sia
dys·mne′·sic
dys·mor′·phia
dys·mor′·phic
dys·mor′·phism
dys·mor′·pho·gen′·e·sis
dys·mor′·pho·pho′·bia

dys·my′·e·lin·a′·tion
dys·my′·e·li·na′·tus
dys·my′·e·li·ni·sa′·tus
dys·my′·e·lin·o·gen′·ic
dys·my′·e·lo·poi·et′·ic
dys·no′·mia
dys′·o·dyn′·ia
dys·on′·to·gen′·e·sis
dys·on′·to·ge·net′·ic
dys′·orex′·ia
dys′·os·to′·sis
dys′·pa·reu′·nia
dys·pep′·sia
dys·pep′·tic
dys·pha′·gia
dys·pha′·gic
dys·pha′·sia
dys·pha′·sic
dys·phe′·mia
dys·pho′·nia
dys·phon′·ic
dys·pho′·ria
dys·phra′·sia
dys′·pi·tu′·i·tar·is′m
dys·pla′·sia
dys·plas′·tic
dys·pne′a *Brit.*
  ·pnoe′a
dys·pne′·ic *Brit.*
  ·pnoe′·ic
dys′·poi·e′·sis
dys′·poi·et′·ic
dys′·po·ne′·sis
dys·prax′·ia
dys·pro′·si·um
dys·pros′·o·dy
dys·pro′·tein·e′·mia
  Brit. ·ae′·mia
dys′·pro·throm′·bin·e′·
  mia *Brit.* ·ae′·mia
dys·ra′·phia *also*
  ·rha′·
dys·ra′·phic *also*
  ·rha′·
dys·ra′·phi·cus *also*
  ·rha′·
dys·ra′·phism *var. of*
  dysraphia

dys·rhyth′·mia
dys′·se·ba′·cia *also*
 ·ba′·cea
dys·so′·cial
dys·so′·ma·tog·no′·sia
dys·som′·nia
dys·sper′·ma·to·gen′·ic
 [dys′·sper·mat′o·]
dys·sper′·mia
dys·sta′·sia *also* dys·
 ta′·sia
dys·stat′·ic
dys′·sym·bo′·lia *also*
 dys·sym′·bo·ly
dys·sym′·me·try
dys·sy·ner′·gia *also*
 dys·syn′·er·gy
dys·ta′·sia *var. of*
 dysstasia
dys·tax′·ia
dys·thy′·mia
dys·thy′·mic
dys·to′·cia
dys·to′·nia
dys·ton′·ic
dys·to′·pia
dys·top′·ic
dys·tro′·phia
dys·tro′·phic [·troph′·
 ic]
dys·tro′·phi·ca
 [·troph′·i·ca]
dys·tro′·pho·neu·ro′·sis
dys′·tro·phy
dys·u′·ria
dys·u′·ric
dys·vi′·ta·min·o′·sis

E

ear′·ache
ear′·drum
ear′·lobe
ear′·phone
ear′·wax
E′ber·thel′·la [Eb′er·]
ebri′·ety

e′bur·nat′·ed [eb′ur·]
e′bur·na′·tion [eb′ur·]
ec·bol′·ic
ec·cen′·tric
ec′·chon·dro′·ma *pl.*
 ·mas *or* ·ma·ta
ec·chon′·dro·tome
ec′·chy·mosed
ec′·chy·mo′·sis *pl.*
 ·ses
ec′·chy·mot′·ic
ec′·crine
ec′·cri·nol′·o·gy
ec·dem′·ic
ec′·dy·sis
ec′·dy·sone
ec′·go·nine
Ech′·id·noph′·a·ga
echi′·no·
echi′·no·coc·co′·sis
 also ·coc·co′·sis
Echi′·no·coc′·cus
echi′·no·cyte
echi′·no·derm
Echi′·no·lae′·laps
Ech′·i·nos′·to·ma
 E. ma′·lay·a′·num
echin′·u·late
Ech′is [E′chis]
ech′·no·thi′·o·phate
ech′o *pl.* ech′·oes
ech′o·car′·di·o·gram
ech′o·car′·di·og′·ra·phy
ech′o·en·ceph′·a·lo·
 gram
ech′o·en·ceph′·a·lo·
 graph
ech′o·en·ceph′·a·log′·
 ra·phy
ech′o·gram
echog′·ra·phy
ech′o·ki·ne′·sis
ech′o·la′·lia
ech′o·prax′·ia
ech′o·vi′·rus *also*
 ECHO virus
ec·lamp′·sia
ec·lamp′·tic

ec·lamp′·to·gen′·ic
eclipse′
ec·mne′·sia
ec·mne′·sic
ec′·mo·vi′·rus
e′co· [ec′o·]
e′co·log′·ic *also* ·i·cal
ecol′·o·gy
é′cor·ché′
e′co·site
e′co·sphere
e′co·sys′·tem
e′co·tro′·pic [·trop′·ic]
écrase·ment′
écra·seur′
ec′·so·vi′·rus
ec′·stro·phy *var. of*
 exstrophy
ec′·ta·co′·lia
ec′·tad
ec′·tal
ec·ta′·sia
ec·tat′·ic
ect·eth′·moid
ec·thy′·ma
ec·thy′·ma·tous
ec′·to·
ec′·to·bat′·ic
ec′·to·bi·ol′·o·gy
ec′·to·blast
ec′·to·blas′·tic
ec′·to·car′·dia
ec′·to·car′·di·al *also*
 ·car′·di·ac
ec′·to·cer′·vi·cal
ec′·to·cho·roi′·dea
ec′·to·co′·lon
ec′·to·co·los′·to·my
ec′·to·con′·dy·lar
ec′·to·con′·dyle
ec′·to·cor′·nea
ec′·to·cra′·ni·al
ec′·to·cyst
ec′·to·derm
ec′·to·der′·mal *also*
 ·mic
ec′·to·der′·ma·to′·sis
ec′·to·der·moi′·dal

ec′·to·der·mo′·sis
ec′·to·en′·tad
ec′·to·en′·zyme
ec′·to·gen′·ic
ec·tog′·e·nous
ec·tog′·lia
ec′·to·hor′·mone
ec′·to·me′·ninx
ec′·to·mere
ec′·to·morph
ec′·to·mor′·phic
ec′·to·mor′·phy
ec′·to·pa′·gia
ec·top′·a·gus
ec′·to·par′·a·site
ec′·to·par′·a·sit·is′m
ec′·to·per′·i·to·ne′·al
ec·to′·pia
ec·top′·ic
ec′·to·pla·cen′·tal
ec′·to·plas′m
ec′·to·plas·mat′·ic
ec′·to·plas′·tic
ec′·to·py *var. of* ectopia
ec′·to·ret′·i·na
ec′·to·sarc
ec′·to·skel′·e·ton *var. of* exoskeleton
ec′·to·sphere
ect·os′·te·al
ect′·os·to′·sis
ec′·to·therm
ec′·to·ther′·mic
ec′·to·ther′·my
ec′·to·thrix
ec′·to·tox·e′·mia *Brit.* ·ae′·mia
ec′·to·tox′·in *var. of* exotoxin
ec′·to·zo′·ic *also* ·zo′·al
ec′·to·zo′·on *pl.* ·zo′a
ec′·tro·
ec′·tro·chei′·ry *also* ·chi′·ry
ec′·tro·dac′·ty·ly *also* ·dac·tyl′·ia *or* ·dac′·tyl·is′m

ec′·tro·me′·lia
ec′·tro·mel′·ic [·me′·lic]
ec·trom′·e·lus
ec·tro′·pi·on
ec·tro′·pi·on·ize ·ized, ·iz′·ing
ec′·tyl·ure′a
ec′·type
ec·typ′·ia
ec′·ze·ma
ec·zem′·a·ti·form [·ze·mat′i·]
ec·zem′·a·ti·za′·tion [·ze′ma·]
ec·zem′·a·toid [·ze′ma·]
ec·zem′·a·tous [·ze′ma·]
edath′·a·mil
ede′·ma *Brit.* oe·de′·
edem′·a·tous [ede′·ma·] *Brit.* oe·dem′·
eden′·tate
eden′·tu·late
eden′·tu·lous
edes′·tin
ed′·e·tate
edet′·ic
ed′·i·ble
edis′·y·late
ed′·ro·pho′·ni·um
ed′·u·ca·ble
ed′·u·ca′·tion
ed′·u·ca′·tor
e′duct
edul′·co·rant
edul′·co·rate ·rat′·ed, ·rat′·ing
ef·face′·ment
ef·fect′
ef·fec′·tive
ef·fec′·tor
ef·fem′·i·na′·tion
ef′·fer·ens *masc. & fem. pl.* ef′·fer·en′·tes, *neut. pl.* ·en′·tia
ef′·fer·ent *conveying away from the center:* Cf. afferent

ef′·fer·vesce′ ·vesced′, ·vesc′·ing
ef′·fer·ves′·cent
ef′·fi·ca·cy
ef′·fleu·rage′
ef′·flo·resce′
ef′·flo·res′·cence
ef′·flo·res′·cent
ef′·flu·ent
ef·flu′·vi·um *pl.* ·via
ef·fu′·sion
egest′
eges′·ta
eges′·tion
e′go [eg′o]
e′go·cen′·tric
e′go·cen′·trism
e′go-dys·ton′·ic
e′go·is′m
e′go·ma′·nia
e′go·phon′·ic *Brit.* ae′·go·
egoph′·o·ny *Brit.* ae·goph′·
e′go-syn·ton′·ic
e′go·tis′m
ei·co′·sa· *var. of* icosa-
ei·det′·ic
ei′·do·
ei′·do·gen
ei′·ko·nom′·e·ter *also* ei′·co·
Ei·me′·ria
Ei′·me·ri′·idae
ein·stein′·i·um [·stei′·ni·]
ei′·weiss·milch′
ejac′·u·late ·lat′·ed, ·lat′·ing
ejac′·u·la′·tio
ejac′·u·la′·tion
ejac′·u·la·to′·ri·us
ejac′·u·la·to′·ry
ejac·u·lum *pl.* ·la
ejec′·ta
ejec′·tion
ek′a·

elab'·o·ra'·tion
elai'o· *also* e'laeo·; *var. of* eleo-
e'lai·op'·a·thy
elai'·o·plast
elap'·id
Elap'·i·dae
elas'·tance
elas'·tase
elas'·tic
e'las·tic'·i·ty
elas'·ti·cus *fem.* ·ca, *neut.* ·cum
elas'·tin
elas'·to·
elas'·to·blast
elas'·to·fi·bro'·ma *pl.* ·mas *or* ·ma·ta
elas'·toid
elas'·toi·do'·sis
e'las·to'·ma *pl.* ·mas *or* ·ma·ta
e'las·tom'·e·ter
e'las·tom'·e·try
elas·to'·sis
elas·tot'·ic
elec'·tive
elec'·tro·
elec'·tro·an'·al·ge'·sia
elec'·tro·an'·es·the'·sia *Brit.* ·aes·the'·
elec'·tro·aug'·men·ta'·tion
elec'·tro·bi·os'·co·py
elec'·tro·cap'il·lar'·i·ty
elec'·tro·car'·di·o·gram
elec'·tro·car'·di·o·graph
elec'·tro·car'·di·og'·ra·phy
elec'·tro·cau'·ter·i·za'·tion
elec'·tro·cau'·tery
elec'·tro·chem'·i·cal
elec'·tro·co·ag'·u·la'·tion
elec'·tro·coch'·le·og'·ra·phy
elec'·tro·co'·ma
elec'·tro·con'·trac·til'·i·ty
elec'·tro·con·vul'·sive
elec'·tro·cor'·ti·co·gram
elec'·tro·cor'·ti·cog'·ra·phy
elec'·tro·cys·tog'·ra·phy
elec'·trode
elec'·tro·der'·mal
elec'·tro·des'·ic·ca'·tion
elec'·tro·di'·ag·no'·sis
elec'·tro·di'·ag·nos'·tic
elec'·tro·di·al'·y·sis
elec'·tro·di'·a·lyz'·er
elec'·tro·en·ceph'·a·lo·gram
elec'·tro·en·ceph'·a·lo·graph
elec'·tro·en·ceph'·a·lo·graph'·ic
elec'·tro·en·ceph'·a·log'·ra·phy
elec'·tro·end'·os·mo'·sis
elec'·tro·ex·ci'·sion
elec'·tro·gen'·ic
elec'·tro·go'·ni·om'·e·ter
elec'·tro·gram
elec'·tro·graph
elec'·trog'·ra·phy
elec'·tro·hy·drau'·lic
elec'·tro·hys'·ter·o·gram
elec'·tro·hys'·ter·o·graph
elec'·tro·hys'·ter·og'·ra·phy
elec'·tro·im'·mu·no·as·say' [·as'·say]
elec'·tro·im'·mu·no·dif·fu'·sion
elec'·tro·ky'·mo·gram
elec'·tro·ky'·mo·graph
elec'·tro·ky·mog'·ra·phy
elec'·tro·la·ryn'·go·gram
elec'·tro·la·ryn'·go·graph
elec'·tro·lar'·yn·gog'·ra·phy
elec'·trol'·y·sis
elec'·tro·lyte
elec'·tro·lyt'·ic
elec'·tro·lyz'·er
elec'·tro·mag'·net
elec'·tro·mag·net'·ic
elec'·tro·mag'·net·is'm [·ne·tis'm]
elec'·tro·ma·nom'·e·ter
elec'·tro·ma·nom'·e·try
elec'·tro·mas·sage'
elec'·trom'·e·ter
elec'·tro·met'·ric
elec'·tro·morph
elec'·tro·mo'·tive
elec'·tro·my'·o·gram
elec'·tro·my'·o·graph
elec'·tro·my·og'·ra·phy
elec'·tron
elec'·tro·nar·co'·sis
elec'·tron-dense'
elec'·tro·neg'·a·tive
elec'·tro·neg'·a·tiv'·i·ty
elec'·tron'·ic
elec'·tron·volt'
elec'·tro·nys·tag'·mo·graph
elec'·tro·nys'·tag·mog'·ra·phy
elec'·tro-oc'·u·log'·ra·phy
elec'·tro-os·mo'·sis
elec'·tro·phile
elec'·tro·phil'·ic
elec'·tro·pho·re'·sis
elec'·tro·pho·ret'·ic
elec'·tro·pho·ret'·o·gram
elec'·tro·pho·tom'·e·ter
elec'·tro·phren'·ic

elec'·tro·phys'·i·ol'·o·gy
elec'·tro·pos'·i·tive
elec'·tro·pros·the'·sis *pl.* ·ses
elec'·tro·py·rex'·ia
elec'·tro·ra'·di·om'·e·ter
elec'·tro·ret'·i·no·gram
elec'·tro·ret'·i·no·graph
elec'·tro·ret'·i·nog'·ra·phy
elec'·tro·scis'·sion
elec'·tro·scope
elec'·tro·shock
elec'·tro·sleep
elec'·tro·stat'·ic
elec'·tro·stim'·u·la'·tion
elec'·tro·sur'·gery
elec'·tro·tax'·is
elec'·tro·ther'·a·peu'·tic
elec'·tro·ther'·a·py
elec'·tro·throm·bo'·sis
elec'·tro·tome
elec'·trot'·o·my
elec'·tro·ton'·ic
elec'·trot'·o·nus
elec'·tro·tro'·pism
elec'·tro·ver'·sion
elec'·tro·vert
elec'·tu·ar'y
ele'·idin
el'·e·ment
el'·e·men'·tal
el'·e·men'·ta·ry
e'le·o·
e'le·o'ma
e'le·om'·e·ter
el'·e·phan'·ti·ac
el'·e·phan'·ti·as'·ic
el'·e·phan·ti'·a·sis
el'·e·phan'·toid
el'·e·va'·tion
el'·e·va'·tor
elim'·i·nant
elim'·i·na'·tion

el'·i·nin
elix'·ir
el·lag'·ic
el·lip'·soid
el·lip'·soi'·dal
el'·lip·soi·dea *pl.* ·deae
el·lip'·ti·cus
el·lip'·to·cyte
el·lip'·to·cyt'·ic
el·lip'·to·cy·to'·sis
el·lip'·to·cy·tot'·ic
el'·u·ate
el'·u·ent
elute' elut'·ed, elut'·ing
elu'·tion
elu'·tri·a'·tion
el'·y·tro·
el'·y·tro·ce'·li·ot'·o·my
el'·y·tro·plas'·ty
ema'·ci·at'·ed
ema'·ci·a'·tion
em'·a·na'·tion
eman'·ci·pa'·tion
emas'·cu·la'·tion
Em'·ba·dom'·o·nas
em·balm'
em·bed' ·bed'·ded, ·bed'·ding
em'·bo·la'·lia *var. of* embolalia
em'·bo·lec'·to·my
em'·bo·li *pl. of* embolus
em·bol'·ic
em·bol'·i·form
em'·bo·lis'm
em'·bo·li·za'·tion
em'·bo·lo·la'·lia
em'·bo·lo·phra'·sia
em'·bo·lo·ther'·a·py
em'·bo·lus *pl.* ·li
em'·bo·ly
em'·bo·nate
em'·bouche·ment'
em·bra'·sure
em'·bro·ca'·tion

em'·bry·ec'·to·my
em'·bryo
em'bryo·
em'·bry·o·car'·dia
em'·bry·o·cid'·al [·ci'·dal]
em'·bry·o·gen'·e·sis
em'·bry·o·ge·net'·ic
em'·bry·o·gen'·ic
em'·bry·og'·e·ny
em'·bry·oid
em'·bry·o·log'·ic *also* ·i·cal
em'·bry·ol'·o·gy
em'·bry·o'·ma *pl.* ·mas *or* ·ma·ta
em'·bry·o·mor'·phous
em'·bry·o·nal
em'·bry·o·nate
em'·bry·on'·ic
em'·bry·o·path'·ia
em'·bry·op'·a·thy
em'·bry·ot'·o·my
em'·bryo·tox'·ic
em'·bryo·tox·i'·ci·ty
em'·bry·o·tox'·on
em'·bry·o·troph *also* ·trophe
em'·bry·o·tro'·phic [·troph'·ic]
emed'·ul·late ·lat'·ed, ·lat'·ing
emer'·gen·cy
emer'·gent
em'·e·sis [eme'·sis]
emet'·ic
em'·e·tine
em'·i·nence
em'·i·nen'·tia
em'·is·sa'·ria *pl.* ·ri·ae
em'·is·sar'y
emis'·sion
em'is·siv'·i·ty [e'mis·]
em·men'·a·gog'·ic
em·men'·a·gogue
em'·me·trope
em'·me·tro'·pia

em'·me·tro'·pic [·trop'·
ic]
Em'·mon·si·el'·la
em'·o·din
emol'·li·ent
emo'·tion
emo'·tion·al
emo'·tio·vas'·cu·lar
em·pas'·ma
em·path'·ic *also* em'·
pa·thet'·ic
em'·pa·thize ·thized,
·thiz·ing
em'·pa·thy
em·per'·i·po·le'·sis
em'·phy·se'·ma
em'·phy·sem'a·tous
[·se'ma·]
em·pir'·ic *also* ·i·cal
em·plas'·tic
em'·pros·thot'·o·nos
em'·py·e'·ma
em'·py·e'·mic
em'·py·e'·sis
em'·py·reu·mat'·ic
emul'·gent
emul'·si·fi·ca'·tion
emul'·si·fy ·fied, ·fy'·
ing
emul'·sin
emul'·sion
emunc'·to·ry
emyl'·ca·mate [em'yl·
cam'·ate]
enal'·a·pril
enam'·el
enam'·e·lo·gen'·e·sis
enam'·e·lo·ma
enam'·e·lum
en'·a·mine
en'·an·thal'·de·hyde
en·an'·thate
en·an'·them *var. of*
enanthema
en'·an·the'·ma *pl.*
·mas *or* ·ma·ta
en'·an·them'·a·tous
[·the'·ma·]

en·an'·ti·o·mer
en·an'·ti·o·morph
en·an'·ti·o·mor'·phic
en·an'·ti·o·mor'·phism
en'·ar·thri'·tis
en'·ar·thro'·di·al
en'·ar·thro'·sis *pl.*
·ses
en·cap'·si·date ·dat'·
ed, ·dat'·ing
en·cap'·su·late ·lat'·
ed, ·lat'·ing
en·cap'·su·la'·tion
en·cap'·suled
en'·car·di'·tis
en'·ca·tar'·rha·phy
en·ceinte'
en·ceph'·a·lal'·gia
en·cé·phale' i·so·lé'
en·ceph'·a·li *gen. of*
encephalon
en'·ce·phal'·ic
en·ceph'·a·lit'·ic
en·ceph'·a·li'·tis *pl.*
·lit'·i·des
en·ceph'·a·lit'·o·gen
en·ceph'·a·lit'·o·gen'·ic
En'·ce·phal'·i·to·zo'·on
[*En·ceph'·a·li'·to·*]
en·ceph'·a·li·za'·tion
en·ceph'·a·lo·
en·ceph'·a·lo·cele
brain herniation: Cf.
encephalocoele
en·ceph'·a·lo·clas'·tic
en·ceph'·a·lo·coele
brain cavity: Cf.
encephalocele
en·ceph'·a·lo·dys·pla'·
sia
en·ceph'·a·lo·fa'·cial
en·ceph'·a·lo·gram
en·ceph'·a·log'·ra·phy
en·ceph'·a·loid
en·ceph'·a·lo·lith
en·ceph'·a·lo·ma·la'·cia
en·ceph'·a·lo·men'·in·
gi'·tis

en·ceph'·a·lo·me·nin'·
go·cele
en·ceph'·a·lo·mere
en·ceph'·a·lo·my'·e·li'·
tis
en·ceph'·a·lo·my'·e·lo·
cele
en·ceph'·a·lo·my'·e·lo·
neu·rop'·a·thy
en·ceph'·a·lo·my'·e·
lop'·a·thy
en·ceph'·a·lo·my'·e·lo·
ra·dic'·u·li'·tis
en·ceph'·a·lo·my'·e·lo·
ra·dic'·u·lo·neu·ri'·tis
en·ceph'·a·lo·my'·e·lo·
ra·dic'·u·lop'·a·thy
en·ceph'·a·lo·my'·o·
car·di'·tis
en·ceph'·a·lon *gen.* ·li
en·ceph'·a·lo-oph·thal'·
mic
en·ceph'·a·lo·path'·ic
en·ceph'·a·lop'·a·thy
en·ceph'·a·lo·punc'·
ture
en·ceph'·a·lo·ra·dic'·u·
li'·tis
en·ceph'·a·lor·rha'·gia
en·ceph'·a·los'·chi·sis
en·ceph'·a·lo'·sis
en·ceph'·a·lo·tome
en·ceph'·a·lot'·o·my
en·ceph'·a·lo·tri·gem'·i·
nal
en·chon'·dral
en'·chon·dro'·ma *pl.*
·mas *or* ·ma·ta
en'·chon·dro'·ma·to'·
sis
en'·chon·dro'·ma·tous
[·drom'·a·]
en'·chon·dro'·sis
en'·clave
en·clo'·sure
en'·col·pis'·mus
en'·co·pre'·sis
en·coun'·ter

en'·crus·ta'·tion
en' cui·rasse'
en·cyst'·ed
en·cyst'·ment
End'·amoe'·ba [En'·da·moe'·ba]
End'·amoe'·bi·dae [En'·da·moe'·]
end·an'·gi·i'tis
end·a'or·ti'·tis
end·ar'·ter·ec'·to·mize
·mized, ·miz'·ing
end·ar'·ter·ec'·to·my
end'·ar·te'·ri·al
end·ar'·ter·i'·tis
end·au'·ral
end'·brain
end'-brush *also* end brush
end'-bulb *also* end bulb
end'-di'·a·stol'·ic
en·dem'·ic
en'·de·mic'·i·ty
en·dem'·i·cum
en'·de·mo·ep'·i·dem'·ic
end·ep'·i·der'·mis
end'·er·gon'·ic
en·der'·mic *also* en'·der·mat'·ic
end'·ing
en'·do·
en'·do·ab·dom'·i·nal
en'·do·am'·y·lase
en'·do·an'·eu·rys'·mo·plas'·ty
en'·do·an'·eu·rys·mor'·rha·phy
en'·do·a'or·ti'·tis *var. of* endaortitis
en'·do·ar·te'·ri·al *var. of* endarterial
en'·do·ar'·ter·i'·tis *var. of* endarteritis
en'·do·bi·ot'·ic
en'·do·blast
en'·do·bron'·chi·al
en'·do·car'·di·al
en'·do·car'·di·og'·ra·phy
en'·do·car·di'·tis
en'·do·car'·di·um gen. ·dii
en'·do·cel'·lu·lar
en'·do·cer'·vi·cal
en'·do·cer'·vi·ci'·tis
en'·do·cer'·vix
en'·do·chon'·dral
en'·do·chon·dro'·ma
en'·do·chrome
en'·do·coch'·le·ar
en'·do·com·men'·sal
en'·do·cor·pus'·cu·lar
en'·do·cra'·nial
en'·do·cra'·ni·um
en'·do·cri'·na *pl.* ·nae
en'·do·crine
en'·do·crin'·ic
en'·do·cri'·no·log'·ic *also* ·i·cal
en'·do·cri·nol'·o·gy
en'·do·cri'·no·path'·ic
en'·do·cri·nop'·a·thy
en'·do·cyst
en'·do·cys·ti'·tis
en'·do·cyt'·ic
en'·do·cy'·tize ·tized, ·tiz·ing; *var. of* endocytose
en'·do·cy'·tose ·tosed, ·tos·ing
en'·do·cy·to'·sis
en'·do·derm
en'·do·der'·mal *also* ·der'·mic
en'·do·di'·a·scope
en'·do·don'·tia
en'·do·don'·tic
en'·do·don'·tist
en'·do·don'·ti·um
en'·do·don·tol'·o·gy
en'·do·du'·ral
en'·do·dy·og'·e·ny
en'·do·ec'·to·thrix
en'·do·en'·zyme
en'·do·ep'·i·the'·li·al
en·dog'·a·mous
en·dog'·a·my
en'·do·gas'·tric
en'·do·gen'·ic
en·dog'·e·nous
en·dog'·e·ny
en'·do·gnath'·ic
en'·do·gna'·thi·on
en'·do·in·tox'·i·ca'·tion
En'·do·li'·max
en'·do·lymph
en'·do·lym'·pha
en'·do·lym·phat'·ic
en'·do·lym·phat'·i·cus
en·dol'·y·sin
en'·do·me·nin'·ges sg. ·me'·ninx
en'·do·mes'o·derm
en'·do·mes'o·gnath'·ic
en'·do·me·trec'·to·my
en'·do·me'·tri·al
en'·do·me'·tri·o'·ma *pl.* ·mas *or* ·ma·ta
en'·do·me'·tri·o'·sis
en'·do·me'·tri·ot'·ic
en'·do·me·tri'·tis
en'·do·me'·tri·um gen. ·me'·trii
en'·do·mi·to'·sis
en'·do·mix'·is
en'·do·morph
en'·do·mor'·phic
en'·do·mor'·phy
en'·do·my'·e·log'·ra·phy
en'·do·my'·o·car'·di·al
en'·do·my'·o·car·di'·tis
en'·do·my'·o·me·tri'·tis
en'·do·mys'·i·al
en'·do·mys'·i·um
en'·do·neu'·ral
en'·do·neu'·ri·al
en'·do·neu'·ri·um
en'·do·nu'·cle·ase
en'·do·par'·a·site
en'·do·par'·a·sit'·ic
en'·do·pep'·ti·dase
en'·do·per'i·car'·di·al

endoperineuritis / *Enterobius*   90

en'·do·per'i·neu·ri'·tis
en'·do·per·ox'·ide
en'·do·phle·bi'·tis
en'·doph·thal·mi'·tis
en'·do·phyt'·ic
en'·do·phy'·tum
en'·do·plas'm
en'·do·plas'·mic
en'·do·pol'y·ploid
en'·do·pol'y·ploi·dy
en'·do·py'·e·lot'·o·my
en'·do·ra'·dio·sonde'
en'·do·ra'·dio·ther'·a·py
end'-or'·gan *also* end organ
en·dor'·phin
en'·do·sal'·pin·gi'·tis
en'·do·sal'·pin·go'·sis
en'·do·sal'·pinx
en'·do·scope
en'·do·scop'·ic
en·dos'·co·py
en'·do·skel'·e·tal
en'·do·skel'·e·ton
end'·os·mom'·e·ter
end'·os·mo'·sis
end'·os·mot'·ic
en'·do·some
en'·do·spore
en'·do·spo'·ri·um
end·os'·te·al
end·os'·te·i'tis *also* end'·os·ti'·tis
end·os'·te·um
en'·do·sym'·bi·ont
en'·do·sym'·bi·o'·sis
en'·do·the'·lia *pl. of* endothelium
en'·do·the'·li·al
en'·do·the'·li·al·i·za'·tion
en'·do·the'·lio·
en'·do·the'·li·o·blas·to'·ma *pl.* ·mas *or* ·ma·ta
en'·do·the'·lio·cho'·ri·al

en'·do·the'·li·oid
en'·do·the'·lio·ly'·sin
en'·do·the'·li·o·lyt'·ic
en'·do·the'·li·o'·ma
pl. ·mas *or* ·ma·ta
en'·do·the'·li·o'ma·tous [·om'a·]
en'·do·the'·li·o'·sis
en'·do·the'·lio·tox'·in
en'·do·the'·li·um *pl.* ·the'·lia
en'·do·ther'·mic
en'·do·ther'·my
en'·do·tho·rac'·i·ca
en'·do·thrix
en'·do·thy·roi'·do·pex'y *var. of* endothyropexy
en'·do·thy'·ro·pex'y
en'·do·tox·e'·mia
Brit. ·ae'·mia
en'·do·tox'·ic
en'·do·tox'·i·co'·sis
en'·do·tox'·in
en'·do·tox'·oid
en'·do·tra'·che·al
en'·do·ure'·thral
en'·do·ves·tib'·u·lar
end'·plate *also* end plate
en'·e·ma
en'·er·get'·ics
en'·er·gid
en'·er·giz'·er
en'·er·gy
en'·er·vate ·vat'·ed.
·vat'·ing
en'·er·va'·tion
en'·flu·rane
en·globe' globed',
·glob'·ing
en·globe'·ment
en·gorge' gorged',
·gorg'·ing
en·gorge'·ment
en'·gram
en·graft'·ment
en' grappe'

en·hance'·ment
en·hanc'·er
en·keph'·a·lin
en·keph'·a·lin·ase
en·keph'·a·lin·er'·gic
e'nol
e'nol·i·za'·tion
en'·oph·thal'·mos
also ·mus
en'·os·to'·sis *pl.* ·ses
en' plaque'
en·sheathe'
·sheathed', ·sheath'·ing
en'·si·form
en'·tad
en'·tal
en'·ta·la·ção'
Ent'·amoe'·ba
E. co'·li
E. gin'·gi·va'·lis
E. his'·to·lyt'·i·ca
ent'·amoe·bi'·a·sis
also ent'·ame'·
en'·ter·al *var. of* enteric
en'·ter·al'·gia
en'·ter·ec'·to·my
en·ter'·ic
en·ter'·i·coid
en·ter'·i·cus *fem.* ·ca
en'·ter·i'·tis
en'·tero·
en'·tero·anas'·to·mo'·sis
en'·tero·ap'·o·klei'·sis
also ·clei'·sis
En'·ter·o·bac'·ter
E. aer·og'·e·nes
E. ag·glom'·er·ans
E. clo·a'·cae
En'·tero·bac·te'·ri·a'·ce·ae
en'·tero·bac·te'·ri·um
pl. ·te'·ria
en'·ter·o·bac'·tin
en'·ter·o·bi'·a·sis
En'·ter·o'·bi·us

en′·ter·o·cele *intestinal hernia: Cf.* enterocoele
en′·ter·o·cen·te′·sis
en′·ter·o·cep′·tive
en′·ter·o·che′·lin
en′·tero·chro′·maf·fin
en′·ter·o·clei′·sis
en′·tero·coc·ce′·mia *Brit.* ·cae′·
en′·tero·coc′·cus *pl.* ·coc′·ci
en′·ter·o·coele *also* ·coel; *embryonic gut cavity: Cf.* enterocele
en′·ter·o·coe′·lic
en′·tero·co′·lic
en′·tero·co·li′·tis
en′·tero·co·los′·to·my
en′·ter·o·cri′·nin
en′·tero·cu·ta′·ne·ous
en′·tero·cyst
en′·tero·cys′·to·cele
en′·ter·o·cyte
en′·tero·en·ter′·ic
en′·tero·en·te·ros′·to·my
en′·tero·gas′·tric
en′tero·gas′·trone
en′·te·rog′·e·nous
en′·ter·og′·ra·phy
en′·tero·he·pat′·ic
en′·tero·hep′·a·ti′·tis
en′·tero·hep′·a·to·cele
en′·tero·hep′·a·to·pex′y
en′·ter·oi′·dea
en′·tero·in·tes′·ti·nal
en′·tero·ki′·nase
en′·ter·o·lith
en′·ter·o·li·thi′·a·sis
en′·ter·ol′·o·gy
en′·tero·meg′·a·ly
en′·ter·o·me′·nia
en′·tero·me′·ro·cele
en′·tero·my·co′·sis *pl.* ·ses
en′·tero·my·i′·a·sis
en′·ter·on
en·ter·o·path′·ic
en′·tero·path′·o·gen′·ic
en′·ter·op′·a·thy
en′·tero·pep′·ti·dase
en′·ter·o·pex′y
en′·ter·o·plas′·ty
en′·ter·o·proc′·tia
en′·ter·op·to′·sis
en′·ter·op·tot′·ic
en′·ter·or·rha′·gia
en′·ter·or′·rha·phy
en′·ter·or·rhex′·is
en′·ter·o·scope
en′·tero·sta′·sis
en′·tero·ste·no′·sis
en′·ter·o·sto′·mal [·os′·to·mal]
en′·ter·os′·to·my
en′·ter·o·tome
en′·ter·ot′·o·my
en′·tero·tox·e′·mia *Brit.* ·ae′·mia
en′·tero·tox′·i·gen′·ic
en′·tero·tox′·in
en′·tero·vag′·i·nal
en′·tero·ves′·i·cal
en′·tero·vi′·rus
en′·ter·o·zo′·ic
en′·ter·o·zo′·on *pl.* ·zo′a
en′·thal·py
en·thal′·sis
en′ thyrse′
en′·to·
en′·to·blast *var. of* endoblast
en′·to·cho·roi′·dea
en′·to·con′·dyle
en′·to·cone
en′·to·co′·nid
en′·to·derm *var. of* endoderm
en′·to·der′·mal *var. of* entodermal
en′·to·mere
en′·to·mo·
en′·to·mog′·e·nous
en′·to·mo·log′·i·cal
en′·to·mol′·o·gist
en′·to·mol′·o·gy
en′·to·moph′·a·gous
en′·to·mo·pho′·bia
En′·to·moph′·tho·ra
en·to·moph′·tho·ro·my·co′·sis
en′·to-oc·cip′·i·tal
en·top′·ic
en′·to·plas′m *var. of* endoplasm
ent·op′·tic
ent·op′·to·scop′·ic
ent′·op·tos′·co·py
ent·or′·bit·al
en′·to·ret′·i·na
en′·to·rhi′·nal
ent′·os·to′·sis *var. of* enostosis
en′·to·zo′·al
en′·to·zo′·ic
en′·to·zo′·on *pl.* ·zo′a
en·train′·ment
en·trap′·ment
en·tro′·pi·on
en·tro′·pi·on·ize ·ized, ·iz′·ing
en′·tro·py
en′·ty·py
enu′·cle·ate ·at′·ed, ·at′·ing
enu′·cle·a′·tion
en′·ure′·sis
en′·uret′·ic
en′·ve·lope
en·ven′·om
en·ven′·om·a′·tion
en·vi′·ron·ment
en′·vy
en′·zo·ot′·ic
en′·zy·got′·ic
en′·zy·mat′·ic *also* en·zy′·mic

en′·zyme[20]
en′·zy·mo·im′·mu·no·
  elec′·tro·pho·re′·sis
en′·zy·mol′·o·gy
en′·zy·mop′·a·thy
e′o·sin
e′o·sin′·o·blast
e′o·sin′·o·cyte
e′o·sin′·o·pe′·nia
e′o·sin′·o·phil
e′o·sin′·o·phil′·ia
e′o·sin′·o·phil′·ic
epac′·tal
ep′·ar·te′·ri·al
ep·ax′·i·al
ep·en′·dy·ma
ep·en′·dy·mal
ep·en′·dy·mi′·tis
ep·en′·dy·mo·blas·to′·
  ma
ep·en′·dy·mo·cyte
ep·en′·dy·mo·cy·to′·ma
  var. of ependymoma
ep·en′·dy·mo′·ma pl.
  ·mas or ·ma·ta
Ep′·eryth′·ro·zo′·on
ep′·eryth′·ro·zo′·o·no′·
  sis
eph′·apse
eph·ap′·tic
ephe′·bi·at′·rics
ephed′·rine
ephe′·lis pl. ephel′·i·
  des
ephem′·er·al
ep′i·
ep′i·an·dros′·ter·one
ep′·i·blast
ep′·i·bol′·ic
epib′·o·ly also epib′·
  o·le
ep′i·bran′·chi·al
ep′i·bul′·bar
ep′i·cal·lo′·sus

ep′i·can′·thic
ep′i·can′·thus pl. ·thi
ep′·i·car′·dia
ep′·i·car′·di·al
ep′·i·car′·di·ec′·to·my
ep′·i·car′·di·um
ep′i·cen′·tral
ep′i·chor′·dal [·chord′·
  al]
ep′·i·cil′·lin
ep′i·con′·dy·lar
ep′i·con′·dyle
ep′i·con′·dy·li′·tis
ep′i·con′·dy·lus pl. &
  gen. sg. ·li
ep′i·cos′·tal
ep′i·cra′·ni·al
ep′i·cra′·ni·um
ep′i·cra′·ni·us
ep′i·cri′·sis second
  crisis in a disease
epic′·ri·sis postdisease
  analysis
ep′·i·crit′·ic
ep′i·cu·ta′·ne·ous
ep′·i·cyte
ep′·i·dem′·ic
ep′·i·de·mic′·i·ty
ep′·i·dem′·i·cus fem.
  ·ca, neut. ·cum
ep′·i·de′·mi·o·log′·ic
ep′·i·de′·mi·ol′·o·gy
ep′·i·der′·mal also
  ·mic
ep′·i·der·mat′·ic
ep′·i·der′·ma·ti′·tis
ep′·i·der′·ma·to·
ep′·i·der′·mi·dal·i·za′·
  tion
ep′·i·der′·mis pl.
  ·der′·mi·des, gen. sg.
  ·der′·mi·dis
ep′·i·der·mi′·tis
ep′·i·der′·mi·za′·tion

ep′·i·der′·mo·
ep′·i·der′·moid
ep′·i·der·mol′·y·sis
ep′·i·der′·mo·lyt′·ic
ep′·i·der′·mo·my·co′·
  sis
Ep′·i·der·moph′·y·ton
ep′·i·der′·mo·phy·to′·
  sis
ep′·i·did′·y·mal
ep′·i·did′·y·mec′·to·my
ep′·i·did′·y·mis pl. ·di·
  dym′·i·des, gen. sg.
  ·di·dym′·i·dis
ep′·i·did′·y·mi′·tis
ep′·i·did′·y·mo·
ep′·i·did′·y·mo·def′·er·
  en·tec′·to·my
ep′·i·did′·y·mo·or·chi′·
  tis
ep′·i·did′·y·mot′·o·my
ep′·i·did′·y·mo·va·sec′·
  to·my
ep′·i·did′·y·mo·va·sos′·
  to·my
ep′i·du′·ral
ep′i·du·ra′·lis neut.
  ·le
ep′i·du·rog′·ra·phy
ep′i·es′·tri·ol
ep′i·fas′·ci·al
ep′i·fol·lic′·u·li′·tis
epig′·a·mous
ep′i·gas′·ter
ep′i·gas·tral′·gia
ep′i·gas′·tric
ep′i·gas′·tri·ca fem.
  of epigastricus; pl. ·cae
ep′i·gas′·tri·cus pl. ·ci
ep′i·gas′·tri·um
ep′i·gas′·tri·us
ep′i·gen′·e·sis
ep′i·ge·net′·ic
ep′i·glot′·tal

ep′i·glot·tec″·to·my
ep′i·glot′·tic
ep′i·glot′·ti·cus   fem.
 ·ca, neut. ·cum
ep′i·glot·tid″·e·an
ep′i·glot′·ti·dec″·to·my
  var. of epiglottectomy
ep′i·glot″·tis   gen. ·ti·
  dis
ep′i·glot·ti′·tis
ep′i·gna″·thus
ep′i·hy″·al
ep′i·hy″·oid
ep′i·ker′·a·to·mi·leu″·
  sis
ep′i·la·mel″·lar
ep″·i·late   ·lat′·ed, ·lat′·
  ing
ep″·i·la″·tion
epil″·a·to′·ry
ep″·i·lep′·sia
ep″·i·lep′·sy
ep″·i·lep′·tic
ep″·i·lep″·ti·cus   fem.
  ·ca, neut. ·cum
ep″·i·lep″·ti·form
ep″·i·lep′·to·gen″·ic
ep″·i·lep·tog′·e·nous
ep″·i·lep′·toid
ep″·i·lep·tol″·o·gy
ep″·i·loi′a
ep′i·mas″·ti·gote
ep″·i·mer   a type of
  isomer: Cf. epimere
ep″·i·mer·ase
ep″·i·mere   embryonic
  segment: Cf. epimer
ep″·i·mer·i·za′·tion
ep″·i·mor′·pho·sis
  [·mor·pho″·sis]
ep′i·my′·o·car″·di·um
ep″·i·mys″·i·um
ep″·i·neph″·rine
ep′i·neph″·ros
ep′i·neu′·ral
ep″·i·neu″·ri·al
ep″·i·neu″·ri·um
ep″·i·no″·sic

ep′i·o′tic
ep′i·per″·i·car″·di·al
ep′i·phe·nom″·e·non
  pl. ·na
epiph″·o·ra
ep′i·phren″·ic
ep″·i·phys″·e·al [epiph″·
  y·se″·al]   var. of
  epiphysial
epiph″·y·sec″·to·my
ep″·i·phys″·i·al
ep″·i·phys″·i·a″·lis
ep″·i·phys″·i·od″·e·sis
  [·o·de″·sis]
ep″·i·phys″·i·oid
ep″·i·phys″·i·o·lis·the″·
  sis
ep″·i·phys″·i·ol″·y·sis
ep″·i·phys″·i·op″·a·thy
  also ·phys″·e·
epiph″·y·sis   pl. ·ses
epiph″·y·si″·tis
ep′i·pi″·al
epip″·lo·
epip″·lo·cele
epip″·lo·ec″·to·my
ep″·i·plo″·ic
ep″·i·plo″·ica   fem. of
  epiploicus; pl. ·icae
ep″·i·plo″·icus   pl. ·ici
epip″·lo·on   pl. ·loa
ep″·i·pter″·ic
ep″·i·py″·gus
ep′i·scle″·ra
ep′i·scle″·ral
ep′i·scle·ra″·le   neut.
  of episcleralis
ep′i·scle·ra″·lis   pl.
  ·les
ep′i·scle·ri″·tis   also
  ·scle″·ro·ti″·tis
epis″·io·
epis″·io·per″·i·ne″·o·
  plasty
epis″·i·o·plas′·ty
epis″·i·or″·rha·phy
epis″·i·ot″·o·my
ep″·i·sode

ep″·i·sod″·ic
ep″·i·some
ep″·i·spa″·di·ac   also
  ·di·al
ep″·i·spa″·di·as
ep″·i·spas″·tic
ep′i·spi″·nal
ep′i·sple·ni″·tis
epis″·ta·sis
ep″·i·stat″·ic
ep″·i·stax″·is
ep′i·ster″·nal
ep″·i·stro″·phe·us
ep′i·tar″·sus
ep″·i·ten·din″·e·um
ep″·i·ten″·on
ep″·i·tha·lam″·ic
ep″·i·thal″·a·mus
ep″·i·the″·lia   pl. of
  epithelium
ep″·i·the″·li·al
ep″·i·the″·li·al·i·za″·tion
ep″·i·the″·li·al·ize
  ·ized, ·iz′·ing
ep″·i·the″·lio·
ep″·i·the″·lio·cho″·ri·al
ep″·i·the″·li·o·cy″·tus
ep″·i·the″·li·oid
ep″·i·the″·lio·ly″·sin
ep″·i·the″·li·ol″·y·sis
ep″·i·the″·li·o·lyt″·ic
ep″·i·the″·li·o″·ma   pl.
  ·mas or ·ma·ta
ep″·i·the″·li·o″·ma·to″·
  sis
ep″·i·the″·li·o″ma·tous
  [·om′a·]
ep″·i·the″·lio·se·ro″·sa
ep″·i·the″·li·o·tro″·pic
  [·trop″·ic]
ep″·i·the″·li·um   pl. ·lia
ep″·i·the″·li·za″·tion
  var. of epithelialization
ep″·i·the″·lize   ·lized,
  ·liz′·ing; var. of epithe-
  lialize
ep″·i·thet
ep′i·ton″·ic

ep′·i·tope
ep′·i·trich′·i·al
ep′·i·trich′·i·um
ep′i·troch′·lea
ep′i·troch′·le·ar
ep′i·troch′·le·i′tis
ep′i·tu·ber′·cu·lo′·sis
ep′i·tu·ber′·cu·lous
ep′i·tym·pan′·ic
ep′i·tym·pan′·i·cus *gen.* ·ci
ep′i·typh·li′·tis
ep′·i·zo′·ic
ep′i·zo·ol′·o·gy
ep′·i·zo′·on *pl.* ·zo′a
ep′·i·zo′·o·no′·sis
ep′·i·zo·ot′·ic
ep′·i·zo·ot′·i·ol′·o·gy
ep′·o·nych′·i·um *pl.* ·nych′·ia
ep′·o·nym
ep′·o·nym′·ic
epon′·y·mous
ep′·ooph′·o·rec′·to·my
ep′·oöph′·o·ron *also* ·ooph·; *gen.* ·ri *or* ·oöph′·o·ron′·tis
ep·ox′·ide
ep·ox′·y
ep·ox′·y·meth′·a·mine
ep′·si·lon
Ep′·som
epu′·lis *pl.* epu′·li·des
ep′·u·lo·fi·bro′·ma *pl.* ·mas *or* ·ma·ta
ep′·u·loid
equa′·tion
equa′·tor
e′qua·to′·ri·al
e′qui·ax′·i·al
e′qui·ca·lo′·ric
equil′·i·brat′·ed
equil′·i·bra′·tion
e′qui·lib′·ra·to′·ry
e′qui·lib′·ri·um *pl.* ·ria
e′qui·mo′·lar

equi′·na *fem. of* equinus
e′quine [eq′·uine]
equi′·no·ca′·vus
equi′·no·val′·gus
equi′·no·va′·rus
equi′·nus *fem.* ·na, *neut.* ·num
e′qui·pha′·sic
e′qui·po·ten′·tial
e′qui·po·ten′·ti·al′·i·ty
equiv′·a·lence
equiv′·a·lent
erad′·i·ca′·tion
era′·sion
erec′·ta
erec′·tile
e′rec·til′·i·ty
erec′·tion
erec′·tor
er′·e·mo·pho′·bia
er′·e·this′m
er′·e·this′·mic *also* ·this′·tic
er·ga′·sia
er·gas′·tic
er·gas′·to·plas′m
er′·go·
er′·go·cal·cif′·er·ol
er′·go·cor′·nine
er′·go·cryp′·tine
er′·go·gram
er′·go·graph
er′·go·graph′·ic
er·gom′·e·ter
er·gom′·e·try
er′·go·nom′·ics
er′·go·no′·vine
er·gos′·ter·ol
er′·got
er·got′·amine
er′·go·ther′·a·py
er′·go·thi′·o·ne′·ine [·thi·o′·ne·ine]
er·got′·i·ca
er′·got·is′m
er′·got·ize ·ized, ·iz′·ing

er′·go·tox′·ine
er′·go·tro′·pic [·trop′·ic]
er′·i·gens
er′·i·o·dic′·ty·on
eris′·i·phake *var. of* erysiphake
Er′·i·sta′·lis ten′·ax [Eris′·ta·]
erode′ erod′·ed, erod′·ing
er′·o·ge·ne′·i·ty
erog′·e·nous
e′ros
ero′·sio
ero′·sion
e′ro·si′·va
ero′·sive
erot′·ic
erot′·i·cis′m
erot′·i·cize ·cized, ·ciz′·ing
erot′·i·co·
erot′·i·co·ma′·nia *var. of* erotomania
er′·o·tis′m *var. of* eroticism
er′·o·ti·za′·tion
er′·o·tize
ero′·to· [erot′o·]
ero′·to·gen′·ic
ero′·to·ma′·nia
er′·rhine
e′ruc·ta′·tion
erup′·tion
erup′·tive
e′rup·ti′·vus *fem.* ·va, *neut.* ·vum
er′·y·sip′·e·las
er′·y·si·pel′·a·tous
er′·y·sip′·e·loid
Er′·y·sip′·e·lo·thrix rhu′·si·o·path′·i·ae
erys′·i·phake
er′·y·the′·ma
er′·y·the′·ma·to′·sus
er′·y·the′·ma·tous [·them′·a·]

er′·y·thras′·ma
eryth′·re·de′·ma   Brit.
 ·roe·de′·ma
er′·y·thre′·mia   Brit.
 ·thrae′·
er′·y·thris′m
er′·y·thris′·tic
eryth′·ri·tol
eryth′·ri·tyl
eryth′·ro·
eryth′·ro·blast
eryth′·ro·blas·te′·mia
 Brit. ·tae′·
eryth′·ro·blas′·tic
eryth′·ro·blas·to′·ma
 pl. ·mas or ·ma·ta
eryth′·ro·blas·to′·ma·
 to′·sis
eryth′·ro·blas′·to·pe′·
 nia
eryth′·ro·blas·to′·sis
eryth′·ro·blas·tot′·ic
eryth′·ro·chro′·mia
eryth′·ro·cy′·a·no′·sis
eryth′·ro·cyte
eryth′·ro·cy·the′·mia
 Brit. ·thae′·
eryth′·ro·cyt′·ic
eryth′·ro·cy·tom′·e·ter
eryth′·ro·cy·tom′·e·try
eryth′·ro·cy′·to·pe′·nia
eryth′·ro·cy′·to·poi·e′·
 sis
eryth′·ro·cy′·tor·rhex′·
 is
eryth′·ro·cy·to′·sis
eryth′·ro·der′·ma
 also ·der′·mia
eryth′·ro·der′·mic
eryth′·ro·don′·tia
eryth′·ro·gen′·e·sis
eryth′·ro·gen′·ic
eryth′·roid
eryth′·ro·ka·tal′·y·sis
eryth′·ro·ker′·a·to·der′·
 ma also ·der′·mia
eryth′·ro·ki·net′·ics

eryth′·ro·leu·ke′·mia
 Brit. ·kae′·
eryth′·ro·mel·al′·gia
eryth′·ro·my′·cin
er′·y·thron
eryth′·ro·par′·a·site
eryth′·ro·pe′·nia
eryth′·ro·phage
eryth′·ro·pha′·gia
eryth′·ro·phag′·o·cyte
eryth′·ro·phag′·o·cy·
 to′·sis
er′·y·throph′·a·gous
er′·y·throph′·a·gy
eryth′·ro·phil
er′·y·throph′·i·lous
er′·y·thro′·pia also
 ·throp′·sia
eryth′·ro·pla′·sia
eryth′·ro·poi·e′·sis
eryth′·ro·poi·et′·ic
eryth′·ro·poi′·e·tin
eryth′·ro·pyk·no′·sis
eryth′·ror·rhex′·is
eryth′·ro·sar·co′·ma
 pl. ·mas or ·ma·ta
er′·y·throse [eryth′·
 rose]
eryth′·ro·sin
er′·y·thro′·sis
es·cape′
es·cap′·ism
es′·char
es′·cha·rot′·ic
es′·cha·rot′·o·my
Esch′·er·ich′·ia
 E. co′·li
es′·cu·lent
es′·cu·lin
es·cutch′·eon
es′·er·ine
es′o· [e′so·]
es′o·de′·vi·a′·tion
esod′·ic
esoph- Words
 beginning thus have
 the British spelling
 oesoph-

esoph′·a·gal′·gia
e′so·phag′·ea [esoph′·
 a·ge′a] pl. ·phag′·e·
 ae; fem. of esophageus
esoph′·a·ge′·al
e′so·phag′·e·a′·lis pl.
 ·les
esoph′·a·gec·ta′·sia
 also ·gec′·ta·sis
esoph′·a·gec′·to·my
e′so·phag′·e·us
 [esoph′·a·ge′·us]
 pl. ·phag′·ei
esoph′·a·gi gen. of
 esophagus
esoph′·a·gis′·mus
esoph′·a·gi′·tis
esoph′·a·go· Brit. oe·
 soph′·a·go·
esoph′·a·go·cele
esoph′·a·go·ec′·ta·sis
 var. of esophagectasia
esoph′·a·go·fun′·do·
 pex′y
esoph′·a·go·gas·trec′·
 to·my
esoph′·a·go·gas′·tric
esoph′·a·go·gas′·tro·
 plas′·ty
esoph′·a·go·gas·tros′·
 co·py
esoph′·a·gog′·ra·phy
esoph′·a·go·je·ju′·nal
esoph′·a·go·je·ju′·no·
 gas′·tro·sto·mo′·sis
 also ·gas·tros′·to·my
esoph′·a·go·je·ju′·no·
 plas′·ty
esoph′·a·go·je′·ju·nos′·
 to·my
esoph′·a·go·my·ot′·o·
 my
esoph′·a·go·pha·ryn′·
 go·lar′·yn·gec′·to·my
esoph′·a·go·plas′·ty
esoph′·a·go·pli·ca′·tion
esoph′·a·go·sal′·i·var′y
esoph′·a·go·scope

esoph′·a·gos′·co·py
esoph′·a·go·ste·no′·sis
esoph′·a·gos′·to·my
esoph′·a·got′·o·my
esoph′·a·go·tome
esoph′·a·go·tra′·che·al
esoph′·a·gus *Brit.* oe·soph′·; *pl. & gen. sg.* ·gi
es′o·pho′·ria
es′o·pho′·ric
es′o·tro′·pia
es′o·tro′·pic
es·pun′·dia
es′·sence
es·sen′·tial
es′·ter
es′·ter·ase
es·ter′·i·fy ·fied, ·fy′·ing
es·the′·ma·tol′·o·gy *Brit.* aes·the′·
es·the′·sia *Brit.* aes·the′·
es·the′·sio· *Brit.* aes·the′·sio·
es·the′·si·o·gen
es·the′·si·o·gen′·ic
es·the′·si·ol′·o·gy
es·the′·si·om′·e·ter
es·the′·si·om′·e·try
es·the′·si·o·neure
es·the′·sio·phys′·i·ol′·o·gy
es·thet′·ic
es′·thi·om′·e·ne [es·thi′·o·mene]
es′·ti·ma′·tion
es′·ti·val *Brit.* aes′·
es′·ti·va′·tion
es′·to·late
es′·tra·di′·ol
es′·trane
es′·trin
es′·trin·i·za′·tion
es′·tri·ol
es′·tro·gen *Brit.* oes′·
es′·tro·gen′·ic

es′·tro·ge·nic′·i·ty
es′·trone
es′·trous *Brit.* oes′·
es′·tru·a′·tion
es′·trus *Brit.* oes′·
es′·y·late
état′
eth′·a·cryn′·ic
eth·am′·bu·tol
eth·am′·i·van
eth′·am·ox′y·tri·phe′·tol
eth′·a·nal
eth′·ane
eth′·a·no′·ic
eth′·a·nol
eth′·a·nol′·a·mine
eth′·a·ver′·ine [eth·av′·er·ine]
eth·chlor′·vy·nol
eth′·ene
e′ther
ethe′·re·al
ether′·i·fi·ca′·tion
e′ther·i·za′·tion
eth′·i·cal
eth′·ics
eth′·i·nyl
eth′·i·on′·a·mide
ethi′·o·nine
ethis′·ter·one
eth′·mo·
eth′·mo·fron′·tal
eth′·moid
eth·moi′·dal
eth′·moi·da′·le *neut.* *of* ethmoidalis; *pl.* ·lia
eth′·moi·da′·lis *pl.* ·les
eth′·moid·ec′·to·my
eth′·moid·i′·tis
eth·moi′·do·fron′·tal *var. of* ethmofrontal
eth·moi′·do·lac′·ri·ma′·lis
eth·moi′·do·max′·il·la′·ris

eth′·moid·ot′·o·my [·moi·dot′·]
eth′·mo·lac′·ri·mal *also* eth·moi′·do·
eth′·mo·max′·il·lar′y
eth′·mo·pal′·a·tal
eth′·mo·sphe′·noid
eth′·mo·tur′·bi·nal
eth′·mo·vo′·mer·ine
eth′·nic
eth′·no·bi·ol′·o·gy
eth·nog′·ra·phy
eth′·no·log′·ic *also* ·i·cal
eth·nol′·o·gy
eth′·no·psy·chi′·a·try
eth′o·hep′·ta·zine
e′tho·log′·i·cal
ethol′·o·gy
eth′o·pro′·pa·zine
eth′o·sux′·i·mide
eth′·o·to′·in
ethox′·a·zene
eth·ox′·ide
ethox′y·
eth′·ox·zol′·a·mide
eth′·yl
eth′·yl·a′·tion
eth′·yl·car′·bon·ate
eth′·yl·ene
eth′·yl·ene·di′·a·mine
eth′·yl·ene·di′·a·mine·tet′·ra·ace′·tic
eth′·yl·ene·di′·a·mine·tet′·ra·ac′·e·tate
eth′·yl·i·dene
eth′·yl·ni·tro′·so·ure′a
eth′·yl·suc′·ci·nate
eth′·y·nyl
eti′·do·caine
e′tio· *Brit.* ae′·tio·
e′tio·cho′·lane
e′tio·chol·an′·o·lone
e′ti·o·gen′·ic
e′ti·o·la′·ted
e′ti·o·la′·tion
e′ti·o·log′·ic *also* ·i·cal; *Brit.* ae′·ti·o·

e'ti·ol'·o·gy *Brit.* ae'·ti·
e'ti·o·path'·ic
e'tio·por'·phy·rin
e'ti·o·tro'·pic [·trop'·ic]
etor'·phine
etrot'·o·my
eu'·adre'·no·cor'·ti·cal
Eu'·bac·te'·ri·um
eu'·bac·te'·ri·um *pl.*
·te'·ria
eu'·caine
eu'·ca·lyp'·tol
eu'·ca·lyp'·tus
eu·cap'·nia
eu·car'y·ote *var. of*
eukaryote
eu'·cary·ot'·ic *var. of*
eukaryotic
Eu'·ces·to'·da
eu'·chlor·hy'·dria
eu·cho'·lia
eu'·chro·mat'·ic
eu·chro'·ma·tin
eu'·di·om'·e·ter
eu·gen'·ic
eu·gen'·i·cist
eu'·ge·nol
Eu·gle'·na
eu·gle'·noid
eu·glob'·u·lin
eu'·gly·ce'·mia *Brit.*
·cae'·
eu·kar'y·ote
eu'·kary·ot'·ic
eu'·ki·net'·ic
eu·lam'·i·nate
eu'·men·or·rhe'a *Brit.*
·rhoe'a
eu·mor'·phics
eu'·nuch
eu'·nuch·is'm
eu'·nuch·oid
eu'·nuch·oid·is'm
eu·on'·y·min
eu'·pa·ral
eu·path'·e·o·scope'
eu'·pa·to'·rin

eu·pep'·sia
eu·pep'·tic
eu·phen'·ics [·phe'·nics]
eu·phor'·bism
eu·pho'·ria
eu·pho'·ri·ant
eu·pho'·ri·gen'·ic
eu·pla'·sia
eu·plas'·tic
eu'·ploid
eu'·ploi·dy
eu·pne'a *Brit.* ·pnoe'a
eu·prax'·ia
eu·prax'·ic *also* ·prac'·tic
eu·rhyth'·mia
eu·ro'·pi·um
eu·rox'·e·nous
eu'·ry·
eu'·ry·ce·phal'·ic
eu·ryg'·a·mous
eu'·ry·gnath'·ic [·ryg·nath'·]
eu·ryg'·na·this'm
eu'·ry·me'·ric
eu'·ry·on
eu'·ry·o'·pia
eu'·ry·ther'·mal
eu'·ry·ther'·mic
eu'·ry·tro'·phic [·troph'·ic]
Eu·scor'·pi·us ital'·i·cus
eu·sta'·chi·an
eu·stron'·gy·li·di'·a·sis
eus·the'·nia
eu·tec'·tic
eu'·tha·na'·sia
eu·then'·ics
eu·ther'·mic
eu'·thy·pho'·ria
eu·thy'·roid
eu·thy'·roid·is'm
eu·to'·cia
eu·top'·ic
evac'·u·ant

evac'·u·ate ·at'·ed, ·at'·ing
evac'·u·a'·tion
evag'·i·na'·tion
ev'·a·nes'·cent
evap'·o·rate ·rat'·ed, ·rat'·ing
evap'·o·ra'·tion
even'·om·a'·tion
e'ven·tra'·tion
ever'·sion
evert'
ever'·tor
évide·ment'
évi·deur'
e'·vi·ra'·tion
evis'·cer·ate ·at'·ed, ·at'·ing
evis'·cer·a'·tion
evis'·cero·neu·rot'·o·my
ev'o·ca'·tion [e'vo·]
ev'o·ca'·tor [e'vo·]
evoked'
ev'o·lu'·tion [e'vo·]
evulse' evulsed', evuls'·ing
evul'·sio
evul'·sion
ex·ac'·er·ba'·tion
ex'·al·ta'·tion
ex·am'·i·na'·tion
ex·am'·in·ee'
ex·am'·in·er
ex·an'·i·ma'·tion
ex·an'·them *var. of*
exanthema
ex·an·the'·ma *pl.*
·mas *or* ·ma·ta
ex'·an·them'·a·tous [·the'·ma·]
ex'·an·throp'·ic
ex'·ar·tic'·u·la'·tion
ex'·car·na'·tion
ex'·ca·va'·tio *pl.* ·va'·ti·o'·nes
ex'·ca·va'·tion
ex'·ca·va'·tor

ex'·ce·men·to'·sis
ex·cer'·nent
ex·cess' [ex'·cess]
ex·change'
ex·change'·able
ex·chang'·er
ex·cip'·i·ent
ex·cise'   ·cised', ·cis'·ing
ex·ci'·sion
ex·cit'·a·bil'·i·ty
ex·cit'·a·ble
ex·cit'·ant
ex'·ci·ta'·tion
ex·cit'·a·tive
ex·cit'·a·to'·ry
ex·cite'·ment
ex·ci'·to·mo'·tor
ex·ci'·to·tox'·in
ex'·clave
ex·clu'·sion
ex·coch'·le·a'·tion
ex·con'·ju·gant
ex·co'·ri·a'·tion
ex'·cre·ment
ex'·cre·men'·tal
ex'·cre·men·ti'·tious
ex·cres'·cence
ex·cres'·cent
ex·cre'·ta
ex·crete'   ·cret'·ed, ·cret'·ing
ex·cret'·er
ex·cre'·tion
ex'·cre·to'·ri·us   pl. ·rii
ex'·cre·to'·ry [ex·cre'·to·ry]
ex·cur'·sion
ex·cur'·sive
ex·cy'·clo·de'·vi·a'·tion
ex·cy'·clo·pho'·ria
ex·cy'·clo·tro'·pia
ex·cyst'
ex'·cys·ta'·tion
ex·cyst'·ment
ex'·en'·ce·phal'·ic
ex'·en·ceph'·a·lo·cele
ex'·en·ceph'·a·ly

ex·en'·ter·ate   ·at'·ed, ·at'·ing
ex·en'·ter·a'·tion
ex'·er·cise
ex·er'·e·sis   pl. ·ses
ex'·er·gon'·ic
ex·flag'·el·la'·tion
ex·fo'·li·ate   ·at'·ed, ·at'·ing
ex·fo'·li·a'·tion
ex·fo'·li·a·ti'·va
ex·fo'·li·a·tive
ex'·ha·la'·tion
ex·hale'   ·haled', ·hal'·ing
ex·haus'·tion
ex'·hi·bi'·tion
ex'·hi·bi'·tion·is'm
ex·hil'·a·rant
ex'·hu·ma'·tion
ex'·i·tus
ex'·o·
ex'·o·bi·ol'·o·gy
ex'·o·cho'·ri·al
ex'·oc·cip'·i·tal
ex'·o·coe'·lom
ex'·o·cra'·ni·al
ex'·o·crine
ex'·o·cy'·clic
ex'·o·cy·to'·sis
ex'·o·de'·vi·a'·tion
ex·od'·ic
ex'·o·don'·tia
ex'·o·don'·tics
ex'o·en'·zyme
ex'o·eryth'·ro·cyt'·ic
ex·og'·a·mous
ex·og'·a·my
ex'o·gas'·tru·la'·tion
ex·og'·e·nous   also ex'·o·gen'·ic
ex'·o·hor'·mone
ex·om'·pha·los
ex'·on
ex'·o·nu'·cle·ase
ex'·o·pep'·ti·dase
ex'·o·pho'·ria
ex'·o·pho'·ric
ex'·oph·thal'·mic

ex'·oph·thal'·mo·gen'·ic
ex'·oph·thal·mom'·e·ter
ex'·oph·thal'·mos
ex'·o·phyt'·ic
ex'·o·phy'·tum
ex'·o·plas'm
ex'o·skel'·e·tal
ex'o·skel'·e·ton
ex'·os·mo'·sis
ex'·os·mot'·ic
ex'·os·tec'·to·my
ex'·os·to'·sis   pl. ·ses
ex'·os·tot'·ic
ex'·o·ter'·ic
ex'o·ther'·mal
ex'o·ther'·mic
ex'o·thy'·mo·pex'y
ex'o·thy'·ro·pex'y
ex·ot'·ic
ex'o·tox'·ic
ex'o·tox'·in
ex'o·tro'·pia
ex'o·tro'·pic
ex·pand'·er
ex·pan'·sile
ex·pan'·sion
ex·pec'·tan·cy
ex·pec'·tant
ex'·pec·ta'·tion
ex·pec'·to·rant
ex·pec'·to·rate   ·rat'·ed, ·rat'·ing
ex·pec'·to·ra'·tion
ex·pel'·lent
ex·per'·i·ment
ex·per'·i·men'·tal
ex'·pert
ex'·pi·ra'·tion
ex·pi'·ra·to'·ry [ex'·pi·]
ex·pire'   ·pired', ·pir'·ing
ex'·plant   n.
ex·plant'   v.
ex'·plo·ra'·tion
ex·plor'·a·to'·ry
ex·po'·nent [ex'·po·]
ex'·po·nen'·tial

ex·pose′ ·posed′, ·pos′·ing
ex·po′·sure
ex·press′
ex·press′·er
ex·pres′·sion
ex′·pres·siv′·i·ty
ex·pul′·sion
ex·pul′·sive
ex·san′·gui·nate ·nat′·ed, ·nat′·ing
ex·san′·gui·na′·tion
ex·san′·guine
ex′·san·guin′·i·ty
ex·sect′
ex·sec′·tion
ex″·sic·cant
ex″·sic·cate ·cat′·ed, ·cat′·ing
ex′·sic·ca′·tion
ex′·sic·co′·sis
ex·sorp′·tion
ex′·stro·phy
ex·tend′
ex·tend′·er
ex·ten′·sa *fem. of* extensus
ex·ten′·si·bil′·i·ty
ex·ten′·sion
ex′·ten·som′·e·ter
ex·ten′·sor *pl.* ex′·ten·so′·res, *gen. sg.* ex′·ten·so′·ris, *gen. pl.* ex′·ten·so′·rum
ex·ten′·sus *fem.* ·sa, *neut.* ·sum
ex·te′·ri·or
ex·te′·ri·or·i·za′·tion
ex·te′·ri·or·ize ·ized. ·iz′·ing
ex′·tern *also* ·terne
ex·ter′·na *fem. of* externus; *pl. & gen. sg.* ·nae
ex·ter′·nal
ex·ter′·nal·i·za′·tion
ex·ter′·nal·ize ·ized, ·iz′·ing

ex·ter′·num *neut. of* externus
ex·ter′·nus *pl. & gen. sg.* ·ni
ex′·ter·o·
ex″·ter·o·cep′·tive
ex″·ter·o·cep′·tor
ex″·ter·o·fec′·tion
ex″·ter·o·fec′·tive
ex·tinc′·tion
ex·tin′·guish
ex′·tir·pate ·pat′·ed, ·pat′·ing
ex′·tir·pa′·tion
ex·tor′·sion
ex·tor′·tor
ex′·tra·
ex′·tra-adre′·nal
ex′·tra-am′·ni·ot′·ic
ex′·tra-ar·tic′·u·lar
ex′·tra·bul′·bar
ex′·tra·can′·thic
ex′·tra·cap′·il·lar′y
ex′·tra·cap′·su·lar
ex′·tra·cap′·su·la′·re *pl.* ·ria
ex′·tra·car′·ti·lag′·i·nous
ex′·tra·cel′·lu·lar
ex′·tra·chro′·mo·som′·al [·so′·mal]
ex′·tra·cor·po′·re·al *also* ·cor′·po·ral
ex′·tra·cor·pus′·cu·lar
ex′·tra·cor′·ti·co·spi′·nal
ex′·tra·cra′·ni·al
ex·tract′ *v.*
ex″·tract *n.*
ex·trac′·tant [·tract′·ant]
ex·trac′·tion
ex·trac′·tor
ex·trac′·tum
ex′·tra·cys′·tic
ex′·tra·du′·ral
ex′·tra·em′·bry·on′·ic
ex′·tra·fu′·sal
ex′·tra·mac′·u·lar

ex′·tra·mam′·ma·ry
ex′·tra·mas′·toid·i′·tis
ex′·tra·med′·ul·lar′y
ex′·tra·mu′·ral
ex·tra″·ne·ous
ex′·tra·nu′·cle·ar
ex′·tra·oc′·u·lar
ex′·tra·o′ral
ex′·tra·os″·se·ous
ex′·tra·per′·i·ne′·al
ex′·tra·per′·i·to·ne′·al
ex′·tra·per′·i·to′·ne·a′·lis
ex′·tra·phys′·i·o·log′·ic *also* ·i·cal
ex′·tra·pla·cen′·tal
ex′·tra·pleu″·ral
ex·trap′·o·late ·lat′·ed, ·lat′·ing
ex·trap′·o·la′·tion
ex′·tra·pul′·mo·nar′y
ex′·tra·pu′·ni·tive
ex′·tra·py·ram′·i·dal
ex′·tra·re′·nal
ex′·tra·sen′·so·ry
ex′·tra·so·mat′·ic
ex′·tra·spi′·nal
ex′·tra·stri′·ate
ex′·tra·sys′·to·le
ex′·tra·tub′·al [·tu′·bal]
ex′·tra·tym·pan′·ic
ex′·tra·u′ter·ine
ex′·tra·vag′·i·nal
ex·trav′·a·sate ·sat′·ed, ·sat′·ing
ex·trav′·a·sa′·tion
ex′·tra·vas′·cu·lar
ex′·tra·ven·tric′·u·lar
ex′·tra·ver′·sion *var. of* extroversion
ex′·tra·vert *var. of* extrovert
ex′·tra·ves′·i·cal
ex′·tra·vi′·su·al
ex·tre′·ma
ex·trem′·i·tas *pl.* ex·trem′·i·ta′·tes, *gen. sg.* ex·trem′·i·ta′·tis
ex·trem′·i·ty

ex·trin′·sic
ex′·tro·
extrophy *misspelling of*
 exstrophy
ex·tror′·sum
ex′·tro·ver′·sion
ex′·tro·vert
ex·trude′ ·trud′·ed,
 ·trud′·ing
ex·tru′·sion
ex′·tu·bate [ex·tu′·
 bate] ·bat′·ed, ·bat′·
 ing
ex′·tu·ba′·tion
ex·u′·ber·ant
ex′·u·date
ex′·u·da′·tion
ex′·u·da′·tive [ex·u′·
 da·tive]
ex·ude′ ·ud′·ed, ·ud′·
 ing
ex ul′·ce·re
ex·u′·vi·ae
ex·u′·vi·a′·tion
eye′·ball
eye′·brow
eye′·cup
eye′·glass′·es
eye′·ground
eye′·lash
eye′·lid
eye′·piece
eye′·spot
eye′·strain
eye′·wash *also* eye
 wash

F

fa·bel′·la *pl.* ·lae
fa′·bism *var. of* favism
fab′·ri·ca′·tion
face′-lift
face′-bow

fac′·et
fac′·et·ec′·to·my
fa′·cial
fa′·ci·a′·le *neut. of*
 facialis; *pl.* ·lia
fa′·ci·a′·li *ablative of*
 facialis
fa′·ci·a′·lis *pl.* ·les
fa′·ci·es *pl.* facies,
 gen. sg. fa′·ci·e′i
fa·cil′·i·ta′·tion
fa·cil′·i·ta·to′·ry
fa·cil′·i·ty
fac′·ing
fa′·cio·
fa′·cio·bra′·chial
fa′·cio·hy′·po·glos′·sal
fa′·cio·lin′·gual
fa′·ci·o·ple′·gia
fa′·ci·o·ple′·gic
fa′·cio·scap′·u·lo·hu′·
 mer·al
fac·ti′·tial
fac·ti′·tious
fac′·tor[21]
fac·to′·ri·al
fac′·ul·ta′·tive
fac′·ul·ty
fae′·cal *Brit. spel. of*
 fecal
fae′·ca·lith *Brit. spel.
 of* fecalith
fae′·cal·u′·ria *Brit.
 spel. of* fecaluria
fae′·ces *Brit. spel. of*
 feces
fag′·o·py′·rism
Fahr′·en·heit
fail′·ure
faint′·ing
fal′·cate
fal′·ces *pl. of* falx
fal′·cial
fal′·ci·form

fal′·ci·for′·mis *neut.*
 ·me
fal·cip′·a·rum
fal′·cu·lar
fal′·la·cy
fal·lo′·pi·an
Fal·lo′·pii *gen. of*
 Fallopius
fall′·out
fal′·si·fi·ca′·tion
falx *pl.* fal′·ces
fa′·mes
fa·mil′·i·al
fam′·i·ly
fam′·ine
fan′·go
Fan′·nia
fan′·ning
fan′·ta·sy
far′·ad
far′·a·day
fa·rad′·ic
far′·a·dis′m
far′·a·di·za′·tion
far′·a·dize ·dized,
 ·diz′·ing
far′·a·do·con′·trac·til′·
 i·ty
far′·a·do·mus′·cu·lar
far′·a·do·ther′·a·py
far′·cy
far′·fa·ra
fa·ri′·na
far′·i·na′·ceous
far′·i·na′·ta
far′·ne·sol
far′·ne·syl
far′·sight′·ed
far′·sight′·ed·ness
fas′·cia *pl. & gen. sg.*
 ·ci·ae
fas′·cial
fas′·ci·cle
fas·cic′·u·lar

---

[21] Blood coagulation factors are written with Roman numerals I–XII. Blood platelet factors are written with Arabic numerals 1–7.

fas·cic′·u·la′·ta
fas·cic′·u·lat′·ed
fas·cic′·u·la′·tion
fas·cic′·u·li′·tis
fas·cic′·u·lus *pl. & gen. sg.* ·li
fas′·ci·ec′·to·my
fas′·ci·i′tis
Fas·ci′·o·la
fas·ci′·o·la *pl.* ·lae
fas·ci′·o·lar
fas′·ci·o·la′·ris
fas′·ci·o·li′·a·sis
Fas′·ci·ol′·i·dae
fas′·ci·o·loi·di′·a·sis
fas′·ci·o·lop·si′·a·sis
Fas′·ci·o·lop′·sis
  F. *busk′i*
fas′·ci·or′·rha·phy
fas′·ci·ot′·o·my
fas·ci′·tis *var. of* fasciitis
fas·tid′·i·ous
fas·tig′·i·al
fas·tig′·io·bul′·bar
fas·tig′·io·per′i·ven·tric′·u·lar
fas·tig′·io·ves·tib′·u·lar
fas·tig′·i·um
fa′·tal
fa·tal′·i·ty
fat′·i·ga·bil′·i·ty
fa·tigue′
fat′·ty
fau′·ces *gen.* fau′·ci·um
fau′·cial
fau′·na
faun′·tail
fa·ve′·o·lar
fa·ve′·o·late
fa·ve′·o·lus *pl.* ·li
fa′·vic
fa′·vid
fa′·vi·form
fa′·vism
fa′·vus
fax′·en-psy·cho′·sis

F-duc′·tion
fea′·tur·al
feb′·ri·fa′·cient
fe·brif′·ic
fe·brif′·u·gal
feb′·ri·fuge
fe′·brile [feb′·rile]
fe·bri′·lis
fe′·bris
fe′·cal *Brit.* fae′·
fe′·ca·lith
fe′·ca·loid
fe′·cal·u′·ria
fe′·ces *Brit.* fae′·
fe′·cun·date ·dat′·ed, ·dat′·ing
fe′·cun·da′·tion
fe·cun′·di·ty
fee′·ble·mind′·ed
feed′·back
feel′·ing
fel
fe′·line
fel′·lea *gen.* ·le·ae
fel·la′·tio
fel′·on
felt′·work
fe′·male
fem′·i·ni′·na *fem. of* femininus; *gen.* ·nae
fem′·i·nine
fem′·i·nin′·i·ty
fem′·i·ni′·nus *neut.* ·num
fem′·i·ni·za′·tion
fem′·i·nize ·nized, ·niz′·ing
fem′·o·ra *pl. of* femur
fem′·o·ral
fem′·o·ra′·lis *neut.* ·ra′·le
fem′·o·ris *gen. of* femur
fem′·o·ro·ab·dom′·i·nal
fem′·o·ro·cele
fem′·o·ro·pa·tel′·lar
fem′·o·ro·pop·lit′·e·al [·pop′·li·te′·al]

fem′·o·ro·tib′·i·al
fem′·to·
fe′·mur *pl.* fem′·o·ra, *gen. sg.* fem′·o·ris
fe·nes′·tra *pl. & gen. sg.* ·trae, *accusative* ·tram
fen′·es·trate ·trat′·ed, ·trat′·ing
fen′·es·tra′·tion
fe′·no·pro′·fen
fen′·ta·nyl
fer′·ment *n.*
fer·ment′ *v.*
fer′·men·ta′·tion
fer′·mi·um
fern′·ing
fer′·rate
fer′·re·dox′·in
fer′·ri·
fer′·ric
fer′·ri·cy′·a·nide
fer′·ri·he′·mo·glo′·bin *Brit.* ·hae′·mo·glo′·
fer′·ri·por′·phy·rin
fer′·ri·pro′·to·por′·phy·rin
fer′·ri·tin
fer′·ro·
fer′·ro·che′·la·tase
fer′·ro·cy′·a·nide
fer′·rous
fer·ru′·gi·nous
fer′·tile
fer·til′·i·ty
fer′·til·i·za′·tion
fer′·til·ize ·ized, ·iz′·ing
fer·til′·i·zin
fes′·ter
fes′·ti·nans
fes′·ti·nate ·nat′·ed, ·nat′·ing
fes′·ti·na′·tion
fes·toon′
fe′·tal *Brit. also* foe′·tal
fe·ta′·lis

fe′·tal·is′m
fe·ta′·tion
fe′·ti·cide
fet′·id Brit. foe′·tid
fet′·ish
fet′·ish·is′m
fet′·ish·ist
fe′·to· Brit. also foe′·to·
fe′·to·am′·ni·ot′·ic
fe·tol′·o·gist
fe·tol′·o·gy
fe′·to·ma·ter′·nal
fe·tom′·e·try
fe′·to·pla·cen′·tal
fe′·to·pro′·tein
fe′·tor Brit. foe′·
fe′·to·scope
fe·tos′·co·py
fe′·to·tox′·ic
fe′·tus[22] gen. fetus; Brit. also foe′·tus
Feul′·gen-pos′·i·tive
fe′·ver
fe′·ver·ish
fi′·at
fi′·ber Brit. ·bre
fi′·ber·co·lon′·o·scope
fi′·ber·gas′·tro·scope
fi′·ber·op′·tic
fi′·ber·op′·tics
fi′·ber·scope also fi′·bre·
fi′·bra pl. ·brae
fi·bra′·tion
fi′·bre Brit. spel. of fiber
fi·bre′·mia Brit. ·brae′·
fi′·bri·form
fi′·bril
fi·bril′·la pl. ·lae
fi′·bril·lar
fi′·bril·lar′y
fib′·ril·late [fi′·bril·] ·lat′·ed, ·lat′·ing

fib′·ril·la′·tion [fi′·bril·]
fi′·bril·lo·gen′·e·sis
fi′·brin
fi′·brin·ase
fi′·bri·no·cel′·lu·lar
fi·brin′·o·gen
fi′·bri·no·gen′·e·sis
fi′·bri·no·gen′·ic
fi′·bri·no·gen′·o·pe′·nia
fi′·bri·no·hem′·or·rhag′·ic Brit. ·haem′·
fi′·bri·noid
fi′·bri·no·li′·gase
fi′·bri·no·ly′·sin
fi′·bri·nol′·y·sis [·no·ly′·sis]
fi′·bri·no·lyt′·ic
fi′·bri·no·pe′·nia
fi′·bri·no·pep′·tide
fi′·bri·no·pu′·ru·lent
fi′·bri·nous
fi′·brin·u′·ria [·bri·nu′·]
fi′·bro·
fi′·bro·ad′·e·no′·ma
fi′·bro·an′·gi·o′·ma
fi′·bro·are′·o·lar
fi′·bro·blast
fi′·bro·blas′·tic
fi′·bro·cal·cif′·ic
fi′·bro·car′·ti·lage
fi′·bro·car′·ti·la·gin′·e·us
fi′·bro·car′·ti·lag′·i·nous
fi′·bro·car′·ti·la′·go pl. ·lag′·i·nes
fi′·bro·ca′·se·ous
fi′·bro·cav′·i·tar′y
fi′·bro·cel′·lu·lar
fi′·bro·con·ges′·tive
fi′·bro·cys′·tic
fi′·bro·cyte
fi′·bro·dys·pla′·sia
fi′·bro·elas′·tic
fi′·bro·elas′·ti·ca

fi′·bro·elas′·to′·sis
fi′·bro·en′·do·the′·li·o′·ma
fi′·bro·ep′·i·the′·li·al
fi′·bro·ep′·i·the′·li·o′·ma
fi′·bro·gen′·e·sis
fi′·bro·gen′·ic
fi·brog′·lia
fi′·bro·hy′·a·line
fi′·broid
fi′·bro·ker′·a·to′·ma
fi′·bro·lei′o·my·o′·ma
fi′·bro·li·po′·ma
fi·bro′·ma pl. ·mas or ·ma·ta
fi·bro′·ma·to·gen′·ic
fi·bro′·ma·toid
fi·bro′·ma·to′·sis
fi·bro′·ma·tous
fi′·bro·my·al′·gia
fi′·bro·mus′·cu·lar
fi′·bro·my′·e·lin′·ic
fi′·bro·my·o′·ma pl. ·mas or ·ma·ta
fi′·bro·my′·o·mec′·to·my
fi′·bro·my′·o·si′·tis
fi′·bro·my·ot′·o·my
fi′·bro·myx·o′·ma pl. ·mas or ·ma·ta
fi′·bro·myx′o·sar·co′·ma
fi′·bro·nec′·tin
fi′·bro·neu·ro′·ma pl. ·mas or ·ma·ta
fi′·bro·neu′·ro·sar·co′·ma
fi′·bro·nu′·cle·ar
fi′·bro-o′·don·to′·ma
fi′·bro·os′·se·ous
fi′·bro·os′·te·o′·ma
fi′·bro·pla′·sia
fi′·bro·plas′·tic

22 See note at *foetus*.

fi·bro′·sa *fem. of*
   fibrosus; *pl. & gen. sg.*
   ·sae
fi′·bro·sar·co′·ma
fi′·bro·scle·ro′·sis
fi′·brose *adj. & v.*
   ·brosed, ·bros·ing
fi′·bro·se′·rous
fi·bro′·sis
fi′·bro·sit′·ic
fi′·bro·si′·tis
fi′·bro·sple′·no·meg′·a·ly
fi·bro′·sum *neut. of*
   fibrosus
fi·bro′·sus *pl. & gen.*
   sg. ·si
fi′·bro·tho′·rax
fi·brot′·ic
fi′·brous
fi′·bro·vas′·cu·lar
fib′·u·la *pl. & gen. sg.*
   ·lae
fib′·u·lar
fib′·u·la′·re *neut. of*
   fibularis
fib′·u·la′·ris *pl.* ·res
fib′·u·lo·cal·ca′·ne·al
fi′·cin
fig′·u·ra′·tus *fem.* ·ta,
   neut. ·tum
fi′·la *pl. of* filum
fil′·a·ment
fil′·a·men·ta′·tion
fil′·a·men′·tous
fil′·a·men′·tum *pl.* ·ta
fi′·lar
Fi·lar′·ia
fi·lar′·ia *pl.* ·i·ae
fi·lar′·i·al
fil′·a·ri′·a·sis
fi·lar′·i·cid′·al [·ci′·dal]
fi·lar′·i·cide
fi·lar′·i·form
Fi·lar′·i·oi′·dea
fi·lar′·i·ous
fil′·i·al
fil′·i·form [fi′·li·]

fi′·li·for′·mis *pl.* ·les
fil′·let
fil′·o·pod
fil′·o·po′·di·um *pl.*
   ·dia
fil′·ter
fil′·ter·a·ble *also* fil′·tra·ble
fil′·trate
fil·tra′·tion
fil′·trum
fi′·lum *pl.* ·la
fim′·bria *pl.* ·bri·ae
fim′·bri·al
fim′·bri·ate *also* ·at′·ed
fim′·bri·a′·tion
fim′·bri·a′·tus *fem.*
   ·ta, *neut.* ·tum
fim′·bri·ec′·to·my
fim′·brio·den′·tate
fin′·ger
fin′·ger·drop
fin′·ger·nail
fin′·ger·stall
fire′·damp
fis′·sion
fis·sip′·a·rous
fis′·su·la *pl.* ·lae
fis·su′·ra *pl.* ·rae
fis′·sur·al
fis′·su·ra′·tion
fis′·su·ra′·tum
fis′·sure
fis′·tu·la
fis′·tu·lec′·to·my
fis′·tu·li·za′·tion *also*
   fis′·tu·la′·tion
fis′·tu·lize ·lized, ·liz′·ing
fis′·tu·lo·en′·ter·os′·to·my
fis′·tu·log′·ra·phy
fis′·tu·lous
fix′·ate
fix·a′·tion
fix′·a·tive
fix′·a·tor

flac′·cid
flac′·ci·da
flac·cid′·i·ty
fla·gel′·la *pl. of*
   flagellum
fla·gel′·lar
flag′·el·late *v. & adj.*
   ·lat′·ed, ·lat′·ing
fla′·gel·la′·tion
fla·gel′·li·form
fla·gel′·lin
fla·gel′·lum *pl.* ·la
flash′·blind·ness *also*
   flash blindness
flat′·foot
flat′·u·lence
flat′·u·lent
fla′·tus
flat′·worm
fla′·va
fla′·va·none
fla′·vi·an′·ic
fla′·vi·mac′·u·la′·tus
fla′·vin
fla′·vi·vi′·rus
fla′·vo·
Fla′·vo·bac·te′·ri·um
fla′·vo·noid
fla′·vo·nol
fla′·vo·pro′·tein
fla′·vor *Brit.* ·vour
fla·vox′·ate
flax′·seed
flay
flea
flec′·tion *var. of*
   flexion
fleece
flesh
fletch′·er·is′m
flex
flex′a *fem. of* flexus
flex′·i·bil′·i·tas
flex′·i·bil′·i·ty
flex′·i·ble
flex′·ion
flex′·or *L. pl.* flex·o′·res, *gen. sg.* ·ris, *gen.*
   pl. ·rum

flexura / follow-up 104

flex·u′·ra
flex′·ur·al
flex′·ure
flex′·us *fem.* flex′a
flick′·er
flight
float′·ers
float′·ing
floc
floc′·cil·la′·tion
floc′·cu·lar
floc′·cu·la′·tion
floc′·cule
floc′·cu·lent
floc′·cu·lo·nod′·u·lar
floc′·cu·lus *pl. & gen. sg.* ·li
flood′·ing
flo′·ra
flor′·id
flo′·ri·form
floss
flow′·ers
flow′·me′·ter
flox·u′·ri·dine
flu
flu′·cry·late
fluc′·tu·ans
fluc′·tu·a′·tion
flu·cy′·to·sine
flu′·dro·cor′·ti·sone
flu′·ence
flu′·fe·nam′·ic
flu′·id
flu′·id·ex′·tract *also* fluid extract
flu′·id·ex·trac′·tum
flu′·id·glyc′·er·ate
flu·id′·i·ty
flu′·id·ounce′ *also* fluid ounce
flu′·i·dram′ *also* flu′·i·drachm′
flu′·i·tans *pl.* flu′·i·tan′·tes

fluke
fluk′·i·cide
flu′·men *pl.* flu′·mi·na
flu·meth′·a·sone
flu·nar′·i·zine
flu′·o·cin′·o·line
flu′·or
flu′·or·ap′·a·tite
fluo·res′·ce·in
fluo·res′·cence
fluo·res′·cent
flu′o·ri·date ·dat′·ed, ·dat′·ing
flu′o·ri·da′·tion
flu′o·ride
flu′o·ri·di·za′·tion
flu′o·ri·dize ·dized, ·diz′·ing
flu′o·rine
flu′o·ro·
flu′o·ro·ace′·tic
flu′o·ro·car′·bon
flu′o·ro·chrome
flu′o·ro·cit′·ric
fluo·rog′·ra·phy
fluo·rom′·e·ter
flu′o·ro·meth′·o·lone
flu′o·ro·phos′·phate
flu′o·ro·roent′·gen·og′·ra·phy
flu′o·ro·scope
flu′o·ro·scop′·ic
fluo·ros′·co·py
fluo·ro′·sis
flu′o·ro·u′ra·cil
flu′o·sil′·i·cate
flu·ox′·e·tine
flu·ox′y·mes′·ter·one
flu·phen′·a·zine
flu′·pred·nis′·o·lone
flur′·an·dren′·o·lide
flur·az′·e·pam
flur·ox′·ene
flu·spi′·ri·lene

flut′·ter
flut′·ter-fib′·ril·la′·tion
flux
flux′·ion
flux′·ion·ar′y
foam
fo′·cal
fo·cim′·e·ter
fo′·cus *n. & v.* ·cused *or* ·cussed, ·cus·ing *or* cus·sing; *pl.* ·ci
foe′·tal *Brit. spel. of* fetal
foe′·to- *Brit. spel. of* feto-
foe′·tor *Brit. spel. of* fetor
foe′·tus[23] *Brit. spel. of* fetus
fog′·ging
fo′·go sel·va′·gem
fo′·la·cin
fo′·late
fo′·lia *pl. of* folium
fo′·li·a′·ceous
fo′·li·a′·ce·us
fo′·li·a′·ta *pl.* ·tae
fo′·li·ate ·at′·ed, ·at′·ing
fo′·lic
fo·lie′
fo·lin′·ic
fo′·li·um *pl.* fo′·lia
fol′·li·cle
fol·lic′·u·lar
fol·lic′·u·la′·ris
fol·lic′·u·li′·tis
fol·lic′·u·lo·gen′·e·sis
fol·lic′·u·lo′·ma
fol·lic′·u·lo′·sis
fol·lic′·u·lus *pl. & gen. sg.* ·li, *gen. pl.* fol·lic′·u·lo′·rum
fol′·low-up *n.*

---

[23] In this word the simplified spelling restores the classical Latin form *fetus*, preferred over *foetus* (a medieval variant) not only in America but often in Britain as well.

fo'·men·ta'·tion
fo'·mes *pl.* ·mi·tes
fon'·ta·nel' *also* ·nelle'
fon·tic'·u·lus *pl.* ·li
foot'·drop
foot'·ling
foot'·plate
fo·rage'
fo·ra'·men *pl.* fo·ram'·i·na, *gen. sg.* fo·ram'·i·nis
fo·ram'·i·nal
fo·ram'·i·na'·lis
fo'·ram·i·not'·o·my [fo·ram'·]
fo·ram'·i·nous
for'·ceps *pl.* forceps
for'·ci·pate
for·cip'·i·tal
for'·ci·pres'·sure
fore'·arm
fore'·brain
fore'·fin·ger
fore'·foot
fore'·gut
fore'·head
for'·eign
fore'·leg
fore'·milk
fo·ren'·sic
fore'·quar·ter
fore'·skin
fore'·wa·ters
for·mal'·de·hyde
for'·ma·lin
for'·mate
for·ma'·tio *pl.* for·ma'·ti·o'·nes
for·ma'·tion
for'·ma·tive
form'·board
forme' fruste' *pl.* formes' frustes'
forme' tar·dive'
form'·ge'·nus
for'·mic
for'·mi·ca'·tion

for·mim'·i·no
for·mim'·i·no·glu·tam'·ic
for·mim'·i·no·glu·tam'·ic·ac'·id·u'·ria
for'·mol
for'·mu·la *pl.* ·las *or* ·lae
for'·mu·lar'y
for'·mu·la'·tion
for'·myl
for'·myl·a'·tion
for'·myl·me·thi'·o·nine
for'·ni·cal
for'·ni·cate *adj.*
for'·ni·ca'·tus
for'·nix *pl.* ·ni·ces, *gen. sg.* ·ni·cis
fos·car'·net
fos'·sa *pl. & gen. sg.* ·sae
fos'·su·la *pl.* ·lae
fou·droy'·ant [·droy·ant']
four·chette'
fo'·vea *pl.* fo'·ve·ae
fo'·ve·al
fo'·ve·ate
fo'·ve·a'tion
fo·ve'·o·la *pl.* ·lae
fo·ve'·o·lar
fo·ve'·o·late [fo'·ve·]
fox'·glove
frac'·tion
frac'·tion·al
frac'·tion·ate ·at'·ed, ·at'·ing
frac'·tion·a'·tion
frac·tog'·ra·phy
frac'·ture *n. & v.* ·tured, ·tur·ing
frag'·ile
fra·gil'·i·tas
fra·gil'·i·ty
fra·gil'·o·cyte
fra·gil'·o·cy·to'·sis
frag'·ment
frag'·men·ta'·tion

fraise
fram·be'·sia *also* ·boe'·
frame'·work
Fran'·ci·sel'·la tu'·la·ren'·sis
fran'·ci·um
frank
frank'·in·cense
fra·ter'·nal
frat'·ri·cide
freck'·le
free'·liv'·ing
freeze froze, fro'·zen, freez'·ing
freeze'·dry' ·dried', ·dry'·ing
freeze'·etch'
frem'·i·tus *pl.* fremitus
fre'·na *pl. of* frenum
fre'·nal
fre·nec'·to·my
fre'·no·plas'·ty
fre·not'·o·my
fren'·u·lum *pl.* ·la
fre'·num *pl.* ·na
fren'·zy
fre'·quen·cy
fre'·tum *pl.* ·ta
freud'·i·an
fri'·a·ble
frig'·i·da
fri·gid'·i·ty
frig'o·la'·bile
frig'·o·ris'm
frig'o·sta'·ble *also* ·sta'·bile
fringe
fron'·dose
fron·do'·sum
frons *pl.* fron'·tes, *gen. sg.* fron'·tis
fron'·tad
fron'·tal
fron·ta'·le *neut. of* frontalis
fron·ta'·lis *pl.* ·les
fron·tip'·e·tal

fron'·to·
fron'·to·an·te'·ri·or
fron'·to·ba·sa'·lis
fron'·to·cer'·e·bel'·lar
fron'·to·cor'·ti·cal
fron'·to·eth'·moid
   also ·eth·moi'·dal
fron'·to·eth'·moi·da'·lis
fron'·to·eth'·moid·ec'·
   to·my
fron'·to·lac'·ri·mal
fron'·to·lac'·ri·ma'·lis
fron'·to·lat'·er·al
fron'·to·max'·il·la'·ris
fron'·to·max'·il·lar'y
fron'·to·men'·tal
fron'·to·na'·sal
fron'·to·na·sa'·lis
fron'·to-oc·cip'·i·tal
fron'·to·or'·bi·tal
fron'·to·pa·ri'·etal
fron'·to·pon'·tine
   also ·pon'·tile
fron'·to·pon·ti'·nus
fron'·to·pos·te'·ri·or
fron'·to·sphe'·noid
   also ·sphe·noi'·dal
fron'·to·tem'·po·ral
fron'·to·tem'·po·ra'·le
fron'·to·trans·verse'
fron'·to·zy'·go·mat'·ic
fron'·to·zy'·go·mat'·i·ca
frost'·bite
froth
frot·tage'
frot·teur'
fruc·tiv'·o·rous
fruc'·to·
fruc'·to·fu'·ra·nose
fruc'·to·ki'·nase
fruc'·tose
fruc'·tos·u'·ri·a [·to·su'·ria]
fruc'·to·syl
fru·giv'·o·rous

fruit·ar'·i·an
fruit·ar'·i·an·is'm
fuch'·sin
fuch·sin'·o·phil
fuch'·sin·o·phil'·ic
fu'·cose
fu'·co·side
fu'·co·si·do'·sis
fu'·gax
fu'·gu
fugue
ful'·gu·rant
ful'·gu·rate   ·rat'·ed, ·rat'·ing
ful'·gu·ra'·tion
ful'·mi·nans
ful'·mi·nant
ful'·mi·nat'·ing
fu'·ma·rase
fu'·ma·rate
fu·mar'·ic
fu·mig'·a·cin
fu'·mi·gant
fu'·mi·gate   ·gat'·ed, ·gat'·ing
fu'·mi·ga'·tion
fu'·mi·ga'·tor
func'·tio
func'·tion
func'·tion·al
func'·ti·o·na'·le
fun'·da
fun'·dal
fun'·da·ment
fun·dec'·to·my
fun'·di   pl. & gen. sg.
   of fundus
fun'·dic
fun'·di·form
fun'·di·for'·mis   neut. ·me
fun'·do·plas'·ty
fun'·do·pli·ca'·tion
Fun'·du·lus
fun'·dus   pl. & gen. sg. ·di
fun'·du·scope

fun·dus'·co·py   also ·dos'·co·py
fun'·dus·ec'·to·my
fun'·gal
fun'·gate   ·gat'·ed, ·gat'·ing
fun·ge'·mia   Brit. ·gae'·mia
fun'·gi   pl. of fungus
fun'·gi·cid'·al
fun'·gi·cide
fun'·gi·ci'·din
fun'·gi·form
fun'·gi·for'·mis
Fun'·gi Im'·per·fec'·ti
fun'·gi·my'·cin
fun'·gi·stat
fun'·gi·stat'·ic
fun'·goid
fun·goi'·des
fun·go'·sus
fun'·gous
fun·gu'·ria
fun'·gus   pl. fun'·gi
fu'·nic
fu'·ni·cle   var. of funiculus
fu·nic'·u·lar
fu·nic'·u·late
fu·nic·u·li'·tis
fu·nic'·u·lo·pex'y
fu·nic'·u·lus   pl. & gen. sg. ·li
fu'·ni·form
fu'·nis
fu'·ni·si'·tis
fu'·ran
fu'·ra·nose
fu·ran'·o·side
fu'·ra·zol'·i·done
fu'·ra·zo'·li·um
fur'·ca
fur'·cal
fur'·cate
fur·ca'·tion
fur'·cu·la
fur'·fur   pl. fur'·fu·res
fur'·fu·ra'·ceous

fu′·ro·ate
fu·ro′·se·mide *also*
　fur′·se·mide
fu′·run·cle
fu·run′·cu·lar
fu·run′·cu·loid
fu·run′·cu·lo′·sis
fu·run′·cu·lous
fu·run′·cu·lus *pl.* ·li
fu·sar′·i·al
Fu·sar′·i·um
fus′·ca
fus′·cin
fu′·si *pl. of* fusus
fus′·i·ble
fu′·si·date
fu′·si·form
fu′·si·for′·mis
fu′·si·mo′·tor
fu′·sio *gen.* fu′·si·o′·nis
fu′·sion
Fu′·so·bac·te′·ri·um
　F. fu′·si·for′·mis
fu′·so·cel′·lu·lar
　also fu′·si·
fu′·so·spi′·ril·lo′·sis
fu′·so·spi′·ro·chet′·al
　[·che′·tal] *also*
　·chaet′·
fu′·so·spi′·ro·chet·o′·sis [·che·to′·] *also*
　·chaet·
fu′·sus *pl.* fu′·si

G

gad′·o·lin′·i·um
gage *var. of* gauge
ga·lac′·ta·gogue
ga·lac′·tan
ga·lac′·tin
ga·lac′·ti·tol
ga·lac′·to·
ga·lac′·to·cele
ga·lac′·to·cer′·e·bro·side

galactogogue *misspelling of* galactagogue
ga·lac′·to·ki′·nase
ga·lac′·to·lip′·id
gal′·ac·tom′·e·ter
ga·lac′·to·phore
gal′·ac·toph′·o·rous
ga·lac′·to·poi·e′·sis
ga·lac′·to·poi·et′·ic
ga·lac′·tor·rhe′a *Brit.*
　·rhoe′a
ga·lac·tos′·amine
ga·lac′·tose
ga·lac′·tos·e′·mia [·to·se′·] *Brit.* ·ae′·mia
ga·lac′·to·si′·dase
ga·lac′·to·side
ga·lac′·tos·u′·ria [·to·su′·]
ga·lac′·to·syl
ga·lact′·uron′·ic
ga′·lea [gal′·ea]
gal′·e·a′·tum
ga·len′·ic *also* ·i·cal
gall
gal′·la·mine
gal′·late
gall′·blad·der *also* gall bladder
gal′·le·in
gal′·li·um
gal′·lo·cy′·a·nin
gal′·lop
gal′·lo·tan′·nic
gall′·stone
gal·van′·ic
gal′·van·is′m [·va·nis′m]
gal′·va·ni·za′·tion
gal′·va·no·
gal′·va·no·cau′·tery
gal′·va·nom′·e·ter
gal′·va·no·tax′·is
gal′·va·no·ther′·a·py
gal′·va·no·ton′·ic
gal′·va·no·to′·nus
gal′·va·not′·ro·pis′m

gam′·a·sid
Ga·mas′·i·dae
gam′·bir
gam′·ble·gram
gam·boge′
gam′·e·tan′·gi·um *pl.*
　·gia
gam′·ete [ga·mete′]
ga·met′·ic
ga·me′·ti·cid′·al [gam′·e·ti·, ·ci′·dal] *var.*
　of gametocidal
ga·me′·to· [gam′·e·to·]
ga·me′·to·cid′·al [gam′·e·, ·ci′·dal]
ga·me′·to·cide [gam′·e·to·] *also* ·ti·cide
ga·me′·to·cyte
ga·me′·to·cyt·e′·mia
　Brit. ·ae′·mia
ga·me′·to·gen′·e·sis
　[gam′·e·to·]
ga·me′·to·gen′·ic
　[gam′·e·to·]
gam′·e·tog′·e·ny
　production of gametes:
　Cf. gametogony
gam′·e·tog′·o·ny
　reproduction by
　gametes: Cf.
　gametogeny
gam′·e·toid
ga·me′·to·phyte
ga·me′·to·tro′·pic
　[·trop′·ic]
gam′·ic
gam′·ma
gam′·ma·cis′m
gam′·ma·glob′·u·lin·op′·a·thy
gam·mex′·ane
gam·mop′·a·thy
gam′o·
gam·o′·bi·um
gam′o·gen′·e·sis
gam′o·ge·net′·ic
gam′·on *also* ·one
gam′·ont

gan·cy′·clo·vir
gan′·glia   *pl. of*
   ganglion
gan′·gli·al
gan′·gli·at′·ed
gan′·gli·ec′·to·my
   var. of ganglionectomy
gan′·gli·form
gan′·glii   *gen. of*
   ganglion
gan′·gli·i′·tis
gan′·glio·
gan′·gli·o·blast
gan′·gli·o·cyte
gan′·gli·o·cy·to′·ma
gan′·gli·o·lyt′·ic
gan′·gli·o′·ma
gan′·gli·on   *pl.* ·glia,
   gen. sg. ·glii
gan′·gli·o·na′·ris
   neut. ·re
gan′·gli·on·at′·ed
gan′·gli·on·ec′·to·my
gan′·glio·neu′·ro·blas·
   to′·ma   *pl.* ·mas *or*
   ·ma·ta
gan′·glio·neu′·ro·fi·
   bro′·ma   *pl.* ·mas *or*
   ·ma·ta
gan′·glio·neu·ro′·ma
   pl. ·mas *or* ·ma·ta
gan′·gli·on′·ic
gan′·gli·on·i′·tis
gan′·gli·on·os′·to·my
gan′·gli·o·ple′·gic
gan′·gli·o·side
gan′·gli·o·si·do′·sis
   pl. ·ses
gan′·gli·o′·sus   *neut.*
   ·sum
gan·go′·sa
gan′·grene
gan′·gre·no′·sus   *fem.*
   ·sa, *neut.* ·sum
gan′·gre·nous
gan′·ja
gan′·try
gar′·a·pat′a

gar′·ga·lan′·es·the′·sia
   Brit. ·aes·the′·
gar′·ga·les·the′·sia
   Brit. ·laes·the′·
gar′·gle   ·gled, ·gling
gar′·goyl·is′m
gar′·lic
gar′·rot [gar·rot′]
gar·rot′·ing
gas   *pl.* gas′·es *or* gas′·
   ses
gas′·e·ous
gas·om′·e·ter
gas′·o·met′·ric
gas·om′·e·try
gas′·ser·ec′·to·my
gas·se′·ri·an
gas′·ser·i′·tis
gas′·ter   *gen.* gas′·tris
gas′·tero·
Gas′·ter·oph′·i·lus in·
   tes′·ti·na′·lis
gas′·tral
gas·tral′·gia
gas·trec′·to·my
gas′·tric
gas′·tri·ca   *fem. of*
   gastricus; *pl.* ·cae
gas′·tri·cum   *neut. of*
   gastricus
gas′·tri·cus   *pl. & gen.*
   sg. ·ci
gas′·trin
gas′·trin·o′·ma [·tri·
   no′·ma]   *pl.* ·mas *or*
   ·ma·ta
gas′·tris   *gen. of* gaster
gas·trit′·ic
gas·tri′·tis
gas′·tro·
gas′·tro·aceph′·a·lus
gas′·tro·anas′·to·mo′·
   sis   *pl.* ·ses
gas′·tro·cele   *gastric*
   hernia: Cf. gastrocoele
gas′·tro·cne′·mi·us
   [·troc·ne′·]   *gen.* ·mii

gas′·tro·coele   *also*
   ·coel; *gastrula cavity:*
   Cf. gastrocele
gas′·tro·co′·lic
gas′·tro·co′·li·cum
gas′·tro·co·los′·to·my
gas′·tro·co·lot′·o·my
gas′·tro·dis·ci′·a·sis
Gas′·tro·dis·coi′·des
gas′·tro·du′·o·de′·nal
gas′·tro·du·o′·de·na′·lis
gas′·tro·du′·o·de·nec′·
   to·my
gas′·tro·du′·o·de·ni′·tis
gas′·tro·du′·o·de′·no·
   en′·ter·os′·to·my
gas′·tro·du′·o·de·nos′·
   co·py
gas′·tro·du′·o·de·nos′·
   to·my
gas′·tro·dyn′·ia
gas′·tro·en·ter′·ic
gas′·tro·en·ter·i′·tis
gas′·tro·en′·tero·co·li′·
   tis
gas′·tro·en′·tero·co·
   los′·to·my
gas′·tro·en′·ter·o·log′·
   ic   *also* ·i·cal
gas′·tro·en′·ter·ol′·o·
   gist
gas′·tro·en′·ter·ol′·o·gy
gas′·tro·en′·ter·op′·a·
   thy
gas′·tro·en′·ter·os′·to·
   my
gas′·tro·en′·ter·ot′·o·
   my
gas′·tro·ep′·i·plo′·ic
gas′·tro·ep′·i·plo′·ica
gas′·tro·esoph′·a·ge′·al
gas′·tro·esoph′·a·gi′·tis
gas′·tro·esoph′·a·go·
   plas′·ty
gas′·tro·esoph′·a·gos′·
   to·my
gas′·tro·fi′·ber·scope
gas′·tro·gas·tros′·to·my

gas′·tro·ga·vage′
gas′·tro·gen′·ic
gas′·tro·graph
gas′·tro·he·pat′·ic
gas′·tro·hy′·dror·rhe′a *Brit.* ·rhoe′a
gas′·tro·il′e·al
gas′·tro·il′e·os′·to·my
gas′·tro·in·tes′·ti·nal
gas′·tro·in·tes′·ti·na′·lis
gas′·tro·je·ju′·nal
gas′·tro·je·ju′·no·esoph′·a·gos′·to·my *Brit.* ·no-oe·soph′·
gas′·tro·je′·ju·nos′·to·my
gas′·tro·ki·ne′·so·graph
gas′·tro·la·vage′
gas′·tro·li′·enal
gas′·tro·lith
gas′·tro·li·thi′·a·sis
gas·trol′·o·gy
gas·trol′·y·sis
gas′·tro·ma·la′·cia
gas′·tro·me′·nia
gas′·tro·my·ot′·o·my
gas′·tro-oe·soph′·a·ge′·al *Brit. spel. of* gastroesophageal
gas′·tro-oe·soph′·a·gi′tis *Brit. spel. of* gastroesophagitis
gas′·tro-oe·soph′·a·go·plas′·ty *Brit. spel. of* gastroesophagoplasty
gas′·tro-oe·soph′·a·gos′·to·my *Brit. spel. of* gastroesophagostomy
gas′·tro-omen′·tal
gas′·tro-o′men·ta′·lis
gas·trop′·a·gus
gas′·tro·pan′·cre·at′·ic
gas′·tro·pan′·cre·at′·i·ca
gas′·tro·pa·re′·sis
gas·trop′·a·thy
gas′·tro·pex′y

Gas·troph′·i·lus var. *of Gasterophilus*
gas′·tro·phore
gas′·tro·phren′·ic
gas′·tro·phren′·i·cum
gas′·tro·pli·ca′·tion
gas′·tro·pod
gas′·trop·to′·sis
gas′·tro·py′·lo·rec′·to·my
gas′·tro·py·lo′·ric
gas′·tror·rhag′·ia
gas·tror′·rha·phy
gas′·tror·rhe′a *Brit.* ·rhoe′a
gas′·tro·sal′·i·var′y
gas·tros′chi·sis
gas′·tro·scope
gas′·tro·scop′·ic
gas·tros′·co·py
gas′·tro·splen′·ic
gas′·tro·splen′·i·cum
gas·tros′·to·my
gas′·tro·suc′·cor·rhe′a *Brit.* ·rhoe′a
gas′·tro·tho′·ra·cop′·a·gus
gas·trot′·o·my
gas′·tro·to·nom′·e·ter
gas′·tro·to·nom′·e·try
gas′·tro·tro′·pic [·trop′·ic]
gas′·tru·la *pl.* ·lae *or* ·las
gas′·tru·la′·tion
gat′·ing
gat′·ism
gauge *also* gage
gaunt′·let
gauss′·i·an
gauze
ga·vage′
ge′·gen·hal′·ten
gel
ge·las′·mus
ge·las′·tic
gel′·a·tin
ge·lat′·i·noid

ge·lat′·i·no′·sa
ge·lat′·i·nous
ge·la′·tion
gel′·se·mine
gel·sem′·i·nine
gel′·se·mis′m
ge·mel′·lus *pl.* ·li
gem·fi′·bro·zil
gem′·i·nate
gem′·i·na′·tion
ge·mis′·to·cyte
ge·mis′·to·cyt′·ic
ge·mis′·to·cy·to′·ma *pl.* ·mas *or* ·ma·ta
gem′·ma *pl.* ·mae
gem·ma′·tion
gem′·mule
ge′·na *pl. & gen. sg.* ge′·nae
ge′·nal
gen′·der
gene
gen′·era *pl. of* genus (*taxon*)
gen′·er·al′·i·sa′·tus *fem.* ·ta
gen′·er·al·ize
gen′·er·a′·tion
gen′·er·a·tive
gen′·er·a′·tor
ge·ner′·ic
gen′·e·sis
gene′-splic′·ing
ge·net′·ic
ge·net′·i·cist
ge·net′·ics
ge·net′·o·tro′·phic [·troph′·ic]
ge′·ni·al [ge·ni′·al]
gen′·ic
ge·nic′·u·lar
ge·nic′·u·la′·ris *pl.* ·res
ge·nic′·u·late
ge·nic′·u·la′·tum
ge·nic′·u·lo·cal′·ca·rine
ge·nic′·u·lo·stri′·ate
ge·nic′·u·lo·tem′·po·ral

ge·nic′·u·lum pl. ·la,
   gen. sg. ·li
gen′·in
ge′·nio· [ge·ni′o·]
ge′·nio·chei′·lo·plas′·ty
ge′·ni·o·glos′·sal
ge′·ni·o·glos′·sus
ge′·nio·hy′·o·glos′·sus
ge′·nio·hy′·oid
ge′·nio·hy·oi′·de·us
ge′·ni·o·plas′·ty [ge·ni′·o·]
gen′·i·tal
gen′·i·ta′·lia also gen′·i·tals
gen′·i·ta′·lis
gen′·i·tal′·i·ty
gen′·i·to·
gen′·i·to·cru′·ral
gen′·i·to·fem′·o·ral
gen′·i·to·fem′·o·ra′·lis
gen′·i·to·in′·gui·nal
gen′·i·to·in′·gui·na′·le
gen′·i·to·mes′·en·ter′·ic
gen′·i·to·spi′·nal
gen′·i·to·u′·ri·nar′y
ge′·nius
gen′·o· [ge′no·]
gen′·o·cide
gen′·o·cop′y [ge′no·]
gen′·o·der′·ma·to′·sis [ge′no·]
ge′·nome
ge·no′·mic
gen′·o·type [ge′no·]
gen′·o·typ′·ic [ge′no·] also ·i·cal
gen′·ta·mi′·cin also ·my′·sin
gen′·tian
gen·tis′·ic
gen′u [ge′nu] pl. gen′·ua
gen′·u·al
gen′u·cu′·bi·tal

gen′u·fa′·cial
gen′u·pec′·to·ral
ge′·nus[24] taxon; pl. gen′·era
ge′·nus [gen′·us] knee; pl. gen′·ua, gen. sg. genus
gen′y·chei′·lo·plas′·ty var. of geniocheiloplasty; also ·chi′·lo·
gen′y·plas′·ty var. of genioplasty
ge′o·
ge′·ode
ge′o·med′·i·cine
ge·om′·e·try
ge′o·pa·thol′·o·gy
ge·oph′·a·gy also ·gis′m or ge′·o·pha′·gia
ge′o·tax′·is
ge′·o·tri·cho′·sis
Ge·ot′·ri·chum
ge′·o·tro′·pic [·trop′·ic]
ge·ot′·ro·pis′m
ge·ra′·ni·ol
ge·ra′·nyl
ger′·i·at′·ric
ger′·i·a·tri′·cian
ger′·i·at′·rics
ger′·i·at′·rist
ger′·i·o·don′·tics var. of gerodontics
ger′·io·psy·cho′·sis pl. ·ses
ger·ma′·ni·um
germ′-free
ger′·mi·cid′·al [·ci′·dal]
ger′·mi·cide
ger′·mi·fuge
ger′·mi·nal
ger′·mi·na′·tion
ger′·mi·na·tive
ger′·mi·na·ti′·vus fem. ·va, neut. ·vum
ger′·mi·no·blast

ger′·mi·no·cyte
ger′·mi·no′·ma
ger′·o·
ger′·o·der′·ma also ·der′·mia
ger′·o·don′·tia
ger′·o·don′·tics
ger′·o·mor′·phism
ge·ron′·to·
ger′·on·tol′·o·gist
ger′·on·tol′·o·gy
ge·ron′·to·phil′·ia
ge·ron′·to·pho′·bia
ger′·on·to′·pia
ge·rüst′·mark
ge·stalt′ pl. ge·stalt′·en
ge·stalt′·ism
ge·stalt′·ist
ges′·tant
ges·ta′·tio gen. ges·ta′·ti·o′·nis
ges·ta′·tion
ges·ta′·tion·al
ges·to′·sis
ghost
gi′·ant
gi′·ant·is′m
Gi·ar′·dia
   G. lam′·blia
gi′·ar·di′·a·sis
gib′·ber
gib′·bus
gi′·ga·
gi′·ga·hertz
gi·gan′·tis′m [gi′·gan·]
gi·gan′·to·
Gi·gan′·to·bil·har′·zia
gill
gin·gi′·va [gin′·gi·]
   pl. & gen. sg. ·vae
gin′·gi·val [gin·gi′·]
gin′·gi·vec′·to·my
gin′·gi·vi′·tis
gin′·gi·vo·

---

[24] A genus name is always capitalized and printed in italics (underlined when typewritten).

gin'·gi·vo·buc'·cal
gin'·gi·vo·den'·tal
gin'·gi·vo·lin'·gual
gin'·gi·vo·plas'·ty
gin'·gi·vo·sto'·ma·ti'·tis
gin'·gly·mo·ar·thro'·di·al
gin'·gly·moid
gin'·gly·mus *pl.* ·mi
gin'·seng
gir'·dle
git'·a·lin
git'·ter
git'·ter·fa'·sern
gla·bel'·la
gla·bel'·lar
gla·bro'·sa
gla'·brous
gla·di'·o·lus [glad'·i·o'·lus] *gen.* ·li
glair'y   glair'·i·er, glair'·i·est
gland
glan'·ders
glan'·du·la *pl. & gen. sg.* ·lae
glan'·du·lar
glan'·du·la'·ris *pl.* ·ris
glans *gen.* glan'·dis
gla·se'·ri·an
glau·co'·ma
glau·co'·ma·to'·sus
glau·co'·ma·tous
gleet
gle'·no·hu'·mer·al
gle'·no·hu'·mer·a'·le *pl.* ·lia
gle'·noid
gle'·noi·da'·lis
gli'a
gli'a·cyte *var. of* gliocyte
gli'·a·din
gli'·al
gli'·o·
gli'·o·blas·to'·ma *pl.* ·mas *or* ·ma·ta
Gli'·o·cla'·di·um

gli'·o·cyte
gli'·o·cy·to'·ma
gli'·o·cy'·tus *pl.* ·ti
gli'o·fi·bril'·la *pl.* ·lae
gli'o·fi'·bril·lar'y
gli'o·fi'·bro·sar·co'·ma
gli·o'·ma *pl.* ·mas *or* ·ma·ta
gli·o'·ma·to'·sis
gli·om'a·tous [·o'ma·]
gli'·o·pha'·gia
gli'·o·pil
gli'o·sar·co'·ma *pl.* ·mas *or* ·ma·ta
gli·o'·sis
gli·ot'·ic
gli'o·tox'·in
glis'·son·i'·tis
glob'·al [glo'·bal]
glo·ba'·ta
glo'·bate
globe'·fish
glo'·bi *pl. & gen. sg. of* globus
glo·bid'·i·o'·sis
Glo·bid'·i·um
glo'·bin
glo'·boid
glo'·bose
glo'·bo·side
glo·bo'·sus *fem.* ·sa
glob'·u·lar
glob'·ule
glob'·u·lin
glob'·u·lin·u'·ria [·li·nu'·]
glob'·u·lus *pl.* ·li
glo'·bus *pl.* ·li
glo·man'·gi·o'·ma
glo·man'·gi·o'·sis
glome
glo·mec'·to·my
glom'·era *pl. of* glomus
glom'·er·ate
glo·mer'·u·lar
glo·mer'·u·la'·ris

glo·mer'·u·li *pl. & gen. sg. of* glomerulus
glo·mer'·u·li'·tis
glo·mer'·u·lo·ne·phri'·tis
glo·mer'·u·lop'·a·thy
glo·mer'·u·lo'·sa
glo·mer'·u·lo·scle·ro'·sis
glo·mer'·u·lo·tu'·bu·lar
glo·mer'·u·lus *pl. & gen. sg.* ·li
glo'·mic
glom'·i·form
glom'·i·for'·mis *pl.* ·mes
glo'·mus *pl.* glom'·era
glos'·sa
glos'·sal
glos·sal'·gia
glos·sec'·to·my
Glos·si'·na
glos·si'·tis
glos'·so·
glos'·so·dy'·na·mom'·e·ter
glos'·so·dyn'·ia
glos'·so·ep'i·glott'·ti·ca
glos'·so·graph
glos'·so·kin'·es·thet'·ic *Brit.* ·aes·thet'·
glos'·so·la'·bi·al
glos'·so·la'·lia
glos'·so·pal'·a·tine
glos'·so·pal'·a·ti'·nus
glos·sop'·a·thy
glos'·so·pex'y
glos'·so·pha·ryn'·gea *fem. of* glossopharyngeus
glos'·so·pha·ryn'·ge·al
glos'·so·pha·ryn'·geo·la'·bi·al *also* ·pha·ryn'·go·
glos'·so·pha·ryn'·ge·us *pl. & gen. sg.* ·gei, *ablative* ·geo
glos'·so·ple'·gia

glos'·sop·to'·sis
glos·sor'·rha·phy
glot'·tal
glot'·tic
glot·tid'·e·an
glot'·tis *pl.* ·ti·des,
  gen. sg. ·ti·dis
glot'·to·
glu'·ca·gon
glu'·ca·gon·o'·ma
glu'·co·
glu'·co·ascor'·bic
glu'·co·cer'·e·bro·si'·
  dase
glu'·co·cer'·e·bro·si·
  do'·sis
glu'·co·cor'·ti·coid
glu'·co·cor'·ti·co·ste'·
  roid
glu'·co·gen'·e·sis
glu'·co·ki'·nase
glu'·co·nate
glu'·co·ne'o·gen'·e·sis
glu·con'·ic
glu'·co·no·lac'·tone
glu'·co·pe'·nia
glu'·co·phos'·pha·te'·
  mic
glu'·co·py'·ra·nose
glu·cos'·amine
glu·cos'·amine·phos'·
  phate
glu'·cose
glu·co'·si·dase
glu'·co·side
glu'·co·sin'·o·late
glu'·co·ste'·roid
glu'·co·sul'·fone
glu'·cos·u'·ria [·co·
  su'·]
glu'·co·syl
gluc·u'ro·nate
gluc'·uron'·ic
gluc'·uron'·i·dase
gluc·u'ro·nide
glu'·ta·mate
glu·tam'·ic
glu'·ta·mi·nase [glu·
  tam'·i·nase]
glu'·ta·mine
glu·tam'·i·nyl
glu'·ta·myl
glu'·tar·al'·de·hyde
glu'·ta·re·dox'·in
glu·tar'·ic
glu'·ta·ryl
glu'·ta·thi'·one
glu'·tea *fem. of*
  gluteus; *pl. & gen. sg.*
  ·te·ae
glu'·te·al
glu'·te·a'·lis *neut.* ·le
glu'·ten
glu'·te·nin
glu'·teo·fem'·o·ral
glu·teth'·i·mide
glu'·te·us *pl. & gen.*
  sg. ·tei, *gen. pl.* glu'·te·
  o'·rum
glu'·ti·nous
gly'·ca·no·hy'·dro·lase
gly·ce'·mia *Brit.*
  ·cae'·
glyc'·er·al'·de·hyde
gly·cer'·ic
glyc'·er·ide
glyc'·er·in *also* ·ine
glyc'·er·in·at'·ed
glyc'·er·ite
glyc'·er·ol
glyc'·er·one
glyc'·ero·phos'·phate
glyc'·er·ose
glyc'·er·yl
gly'·cine
gly'·cin·u'·ria [·ci·nu'·]
gly'·co·
gly'·co·bi·ar'·sol
gly'·co·ca'·lyx
gly'·co·cho'·lic
gly'·co·gen
gly'·co·gen'·e·sis
  formation of glycogen:
  Cf. glycogenosis
gly'·co·gen'·ic
gly'·co·ge·nol'·y·sis
gly'·co·gen'·o·lyt'·ic
gly'·co·ge·no'·sis
  storage disease: Cf.
  glycogenesis
gly'·col
gly'·col·al'·de·hyde
gly·col'·ic
gly'·co·lip'·id
gly·col'·y·sis *pl.* ·ses
gly·co·lyt'·ic
gly'·co·ne'o·gen'·e·sis
gly'·co·pep'·tide
gly'·co·pho'·rin
gly'·co·pro'·tein
gly·cos'·ami'·no·gly'·
  can
gly·co'·si·dase
gly'·co·side
gly'·cos·u'·ria [·co·
  su'·]
gly'·cos·u'·ric [·co·
  su'·]
gly'·co·syl
gly·co'·sy·lat'·ed [gly'·
  co·syl·at'·ed]
gly'·co·syl·a'·tion
gly'·co·syl·trans'·fer·
  ase
gly'·co·tro'·pic [·trop'·
  ic]
gly'·cyl
Gly·cyph'·a·gus
glyc'·yr·rhi'·za
glyc'·yr·rhi'·zin
gly·ox'·al
gly·ox'·a·lase
gly'·ox·al'·ic
gly·ox'·y·late
gly'·ox·yl'·ic
gly·ox'·y·some
gnath'·ic
gna'·thi·on
gnath'o·
gnath'o·dy'·na·mom'·e·
  ter
gna·thol'·o·gy

gnath'o·pal'·a·tos'·chi·sis pl. ·ses
gna·thos'·chi·sis pl. ·ses
Gna·thos'·to·ma
gna·thos'·to·mi'·a·sis
gnos'·tic
gno'·to·bi·ol'·o·gy
gno'·to·bi'·ote
gno'·to·bi·ot'·ic
goi'·ter also goi'·tre
goi'·tro·gen
goi'·tro·gen'·ic
goi'·trous
go·mit'·o·li
gom·pho'·sis pl. ·ses
go'·nad
go·nad'·al also go·nad'·i·al
go'·nad·ec'·to·mize ·mized, ·miz'·ing
go'·nad·ec'·to·my [gon'·ad·]
gon'·a·do·blas·to'·ma [go·nad'·o·]
go·nad'·o·gen'·e·sis [gon'·a·do·]
go·nad'·o·trope [gon'·a·do·]
go·nad'·o·tro'·phic [gon'·a·do·, ·troph'·ic] var. of gonadotropic
go·nad'·o·tro'·pic [gon'·a·do·, ·trop'·ic]
go·nad'·o·tro'·pin [gon'·a·do·] also ·tro'·phin
gon'a·duct
gon·an'·gi·ec'·to·my
gon'·ar·thro'·sis
gon'·ar·throt'·o·my
gon'e·cys'·tic

gon'e·cys·ti'·tis
gon'e·cys'·to·lith
Gon'·gy·lo·ne'·ma
G. pul'·chrum
go'·ni·al
go·nid'·i·al
go'·nio·
go'·nio·lens'
go'·ni·om'·e·ter
go'·ni·on pl. go'·nia
go'·nio·pris'm
go'·nio·punc'·ture
go'·ni·o·scope
go'·ni·os'·co·py
go'·ni·ot'·o·my
go·ni'·tis
gon'o·
gon'·o·cele
gon'o·coc'·cal
gon'o·coc·ce'·mia Brit. ·cae'·mia
gon'o·coc'·co·cide also ·coc'·cide
gon'o·coc'·cus pl. ·ci
gon'·o·cyte
gon'o·duct
gon'·or·rhe'a Brit. ·rhoe'a
gon'·or·rhe'·al Brit. ·rhoe'·al
gon·os'·che·o·cele
gon'o·tox·e'·mia Brit. ·ae'·mia
Gon'y·au'·lax
gon'y·camp'·sis
gon'y·on'·cus
goose'·flesh also goose flesh
Gor'·di·a'·cea
Gor'·di·us
gor'·get
gos'·sy·pol
gouge

goun'·dou
gout
gout'·i·ness
gout'y
graaf'·i·an
grac'·ile
grac'·i·lis neut. ·le
gra·da'·tim
gra'·di·ent
gra'·do·col
grad'·u·ate
grad'·u·at'·ed
graft
grain
gram[25] Brit. also gramme
Gram'-am'·pho·phil'·ic also gram-
gram'-at'·om
gram'-cal'·o·rie
gram'·i·cid'·in [·ci'·din]
gram'-mole'
gram'-mol'·e·cule
Gram'-neg'·a·tive also gram-
Gram'-pos'·i·tive also gram-
gram'-rad'
grand' mal'
gran'·u·lar
gran'·u·la'·ris
gran'·u·late v. & adj. ·lat'·ed, ·lat'·ing
gran'·u·la'·tio pl. ·la'·ti·o'·nes
gran'·u·la'·tion
gran'·ule
gran'·u·lo·
gran'·u·lo·blast
gran'·u·lo·blas·to'·sis
gran'·u·lo·cyt'·apher·e'·sis [·apher'·e·]
gran'·u·lo·cyte

---

[25] In British medical and scientific writing the spelling *gramme* has largely given way to *gram*, especially with prefixes as in *kilogram, milligram*. In any case, use of the abbreviation g (kg, mg, etc.) often makes it unnecessary to choose between the full spellings.

gran'·u·lo·cy'·to·pe'·nia
gran'·u·lo·cy'·to·poi·e'·sis
gran'·u·lo·cy'·to·poi·et'·ic
gran'·u·lo·cy·to'·sis
gran'·u·lo'·ma   pl. ·mas or ·ma·ta
gran'·u·lo·ma·to'·sis
gran'·u·lom'a·tous [·lo'ma·]
gran'·u·lo·pe'·nia
gran'·u·lo·poi·e'·sis
gran'·u·lo·poi·et'·ic
gran'·u·lo'·sa   fem. of granulosus
gran'·u·lose
gran'·u·lo'·sis
gran'·u·los'·i·ty
gran'·u·lo'·sus
gran'·u·lo·vac'·u·o'·lar
graph
graph'·ic
graph'·ite
graph'o·
graph'o·ki·net'·ic
gra·phol'·o·gy
graph'o·ma'·nia
graph'o·mo'·tor
graph'·or·rhe'a   Brit. ·rhoe'a
graph'o·spas'm
grat·tage'
grav'·id
grav'·i·da[26]   pl. ·dae or ·das, gen. pl. grav'·i·da'·rum
gra·vid'·i·ty
gra·vim'·e·ter
grav'·i·met'·ric
grav'·is [gra'·vis]
grav'·i·stat'·ic

grav'·i·ta'·tion
grav'·i·tom'·e·ter
grav'·i·ty
gray[27]   also grey
gray'·out
grip'·pal
grippe
gris'·e·in
gris'·e·o·ful'·vin
gris'·e·us   fem. ·ea
groin
gross
gru'·mous   also ·mose
gry'·o·chrome
gry·po'·sis
guai'·ac
guai'·a·col
guai'·a·cum
guai·fen'·e·sin
gua'·nase
gua·neth'·i·dine
gua'·ni·dine
gua'·ni·di'·no
gua'·ni·di'·no·ace'·tic
gua'·ni·di'·no·suc·cin'·ic
gua'·nine
gua'·no·sine
gua'·nyl
gua'·ny·late
gua·nyl'·ic
gua·nyl'·yl
guard
gu'·ber·nac'·u·lar
gu'·ber·nac'·u·lum
guid'·ance
guide
guide'·line
guil'·lo·tine
guilt
guin'·ea pig'
gul'·let
gu'·lose

gul'·uron'·ic
gum'·boil
gum'·ma   pl. ·mas or ·ma·ta
gum'·ma·tous
gum'·my   ·mi·er, ·mi·est
gur'·ney   pl. gur'·neys
gus·ta'·tion
gus'·ta·to'·ria   fem. of gustatorius; pl. ·ri·ae
gus'·ta·to'·ri·us   pl. ·rii
gus'·ta·to'·ry
gus'·to·lac'·ri·mal
gus·tom'·e·try
gus'·tus   gen. gustus
gut'·ta   pl. ·tae
gut'·ta-per'·cha
gut·ta'·ta
gut'·tate
gut'·ter
gut'·ter·ing
gut'·tur
gut'·tur·al
gym·nas'·tics
gym'·no·
gym'·no·cyte
gym'·no·plast
Gym'·no·tho'·rax
gy'·nae·co·   Brit. spel. of gyneco-
gy'·nae·col'·o·gy   Brit. spel. of gynecology
gy'·nae·co·mas'·tia   Brit. spel. of gynecomastia
gyn·an'·drism
gyn·an'·dro·blas·to'·ma
gyn·an'·droid
gyn·an'·dro·morph
gyn·an'·dro·mor'·phism

---

[26] This term is ordinarily followed by a numeral (usually Roman) indicating the number of times a woman has been pregnant: gravida I (primigravida), gravida II (secundigravida).

[27] When denoting a color, *gray* has the variant spelling *grey*, but not when denoting the measurement.

gyn·an'·dro·mor'·phous
gyn'·an·dry *var. of*
  gynandrism
gyn'·atre'·sia
gynec- *Words beginning thus have the British spelling* gynaec-
gy·ne'·cic
gy'·ne·co· *Brit.* gy'·nae·co·
gy'·ne·co·gen'·ic
gy'·ne·cog'·ra·phy
gy'·ne·coid
gy'·ne·co·log'·ic *also* ·i·cal
gy'·ne·col'·o·gist
gy'·ne·col'·o·gy
gy'·ne·co·mas'·tia
gy'·ne·co·pho'·ric *also* gy'·ne·coph'·o·ral
gy'·ne·pho'·bia
gy'·ne·plas'·ty *var. of* gynoplasty
gy'·no·
gy'·no·gen'·e·sis
gy·nog'·ra·phy *var. of* gynecography
gy'·noid *var. of* gynecoid
gy'·no·mer'·o·gon *also* ·gone
gy'·no·mer·og'·o·ny
gy'·no·plas'·tic
gy'·no·plas'·ty
gyp'·sum
gy'·ral
gy'·rase
gy·ra'·ta
gy'·rate
gy·rec'·to·my
gyr'·en'·ce·phal'·ic
gy'·ro·
gy'·ro·mag·net'·ic
gy'·rose
gy'·ro·spas'm
gy'·rus *pl. & gen. sg.* ·ri

H

ha·be'·na
ha·be'·nal *also* ·nar
ha·ben'·u·la *pl. & gen. sg.* ·lae, *gen. pl.* ha·ben'·u·la'·rum
ha·ben'·u·lar
ha·ben'·u·lo·in'·ter·pe·dun'·cu·lar
ha·bil'·i·ta'·tion
hab'·it
hab'·i·tat
ha·bit'·u·a'·tion
hab'·i·tus *pl.* habitus
Hab'·ro·ne'·ma
hab'·ro·ne·mi'·a·sis
ha'·bu
hache·ment'
Ha·dru'·rus
haem *Brit. spel. of* heme
haem- *See also words beginning* hem-
Hae'·ma·dip'·sa
Hae'·ma·go'·gus
hae·man'·gi·o'·ma *Brit. spel. of* hemangioma
Hae'·ma·phy'·sa·lis
  H. cin'·na·bar'·i·na
  H. lep'·o·ris·pa·lus'·tris
hae'·ma·to· *Brit. spel. of* hemato-
Hae'·ma·to'·bia
hae·mat'·o·crit [hae'·ma·to·]
hae'·ma·tol'·o·gy
hae'·ma·to'·ma *pl.* ·mas *or* ·ma·ta
Hae'·ma·to·pi'·nus
  H. su'·is
Hae'·ma·to·si'·phon
hae'·ma·tu'·ria *Brit. spel. of* hematuria
Hae'·men·ter'·ia

hae'·mo· *Brit. spel. of* hemo-
Hae'·mo·bar'·to·nel'·la
hae'·mo·di·al'·y·sis
hae'·mo·glo'·bin *Brit. spel. of* hemoglobin
hae'·mo·glo'·bin·ae'·mia *Brit. spel. of* hemoglobinemia
hae'·mo·glo'·bin·u'·ria [·bi·nu'·]
hae·mol'·y·sis
hae'·mo·lyt'·ic
Hae·mon'·chus
hae'·mo·phil'·ia
Hae·moph'·i·lus
  H. ae·gyp'·ti·us
  H. du·crey'i
  H. hae'·mo·lyt'·i·cus
  H. in'·flu·en'·zae
haem'·or·rhage *Brit. spel. of* hemorrhage
haem'·or·rhag'·i·ca
haem'·or·rhoid
hae'·mo·sid·er·o'·sis
Hae'·mo·spo·rid'·ia
hae'·mo·spo·rid'·i·an
hae'·mo·spo·rid'·i·um *pl.* ·rid'·ia
hae'·mo·sta'·sis [hae·mos'·ta·sis]
hae'·mo·stat'·ic
hae'·mo·tho'·rax
hae'·mo·zo'·in
Haf'·nia al''·vei
haf'·ni·um
hahn'·e·mann·is'm
hair'·ball
hair'·worm
hair'y hair'·i·er, hair'·i·est
hal·cin'·o·nide
half-lay'·er
half'-life
half'-thick'·ness
ha'·lide
hal'·i·ste·re'·sis
hal'·i·to'·sis

halitus / hellebore

hal′·i·tus
hal′·lex   pl.   ·li·ces,
   gen. sg.   ·li·cis; var. of
   hallux
hal′·lu·ces   pl.   of
   hallux
hal·lu′·ci·na′·tion
hal·lu′·ci·na·to′·ry
hal·lu′·ci·no·gen
hal·lu′·ci·no·gen′·ic
hal·lu′·ci·no′·sis
hal·lu′·ci·not′·ic
hal′·lux   pl.   ·lu·ces,
   gen. sg.   ·lu·cis
ha′·lo
hal′o·
hal′·o·der′·mia
hal′·o·gen
hal′·o·gen·a′·tion
ha·lom′·e·ter
ha·lom′·e·try
hal′·o·per′·i·dol
hal′·o·phile   also   ·phil
hal′·o·phil′·ic
hal′·o·thane
hal·zoun′
ham′·ar·ti′a [ha·mar′·
   tia]
ham′·ar·to′·ma   pl.
   ·mas or ·ma·ta
ham′·ar·tom′a·tous
   [·to′ma·]
ha′·mate
ha·ma′·tum
ham′·mer
ham′·mer·toe′   also
   hammer toe
ha′·mose
ham′·string
ham′·u·lar
ham′·u·late
ham′·u·lose
ham′·u·lus   pl. & gen.
   sg.   ·li
ha·my′·cin
hand′·ed·ness
hand′·i·cap
hand′·i·capped
hand′·piece
hang′·ing
hang′·nail
hang′·o′ver
hap′·a·lo·nych′·ia
haph′·al·ge′·sia
haph′e·pho′·bia
hap′·lo·
hap′·lo·dip′·loi·dy
hap′·lo·dont
hap′·loid
hap′·loi·dy
hap′·lont
hap′·lo·phase
hap′·lo·scope
hap′·lo·scop′·ic
hap′·lo·spo·ran′·gin
hap′·lo·type
hap′·ten   also   ·tene or
   ·tin
hap·ten′·ic
hap′·tic
hap′·to·
hap′·to·glo′·bin
ha·ra′·ra
hard′·en·ing
hare′·lip
har′·le·quin
har′·ma·line
har′·mine
har·mon′·ic
har·poon′
Hart′·man·nel′·la
har′·vest
ha·shish′ [hash′·ish]
hatch′·et
haunch
haus′·tral
haus·tra′·tion
haus′·trum   pl.   ·tra
haus′·tus   pl.   haustus
haut′ mal′
ha·ver′·sian
hay′ fe′·ver   also hay′·
   fe′ver
hay′·rake
haz′·ard
head′·ache
head′·gear
head′·gut
heal′·er
heal′·ing
health
health′y   health′·i·er,
   health′·i·est
hear′·ing
heart
heart′·beat
heart′·burn
heart′·worm
heat′·stroke
he′·be·phre′·nia
he′·be·phren′·ic
heb′·e·tude
he′·bi·at′·rics
he′·boid
hec′·tic
hec′·to·
he·don′·ic
He′La   also   he′la
hel′·coid
hel·co′·ma   pl.   ·mas or
   ·ma·ta
he′·li·an′·thin
hel′·i·cal
hel′·i·ces   pl.   of helix
hel′·i·ci′·na   fem. of
   helicinus;   pl.   ·nae
hel′·i·cine
hel′·i·ci′·nus   pl.   ·ni
hel′·i·cis   gen. of helix
hel′·i·co·
Hel′·i·co·bac′·ter py·
   lo′·ri
hel′·i·coid
hel′·i·co·po′·dia
hel′·i·co·tre′·ma
he′·lio·
he′·lio·tax′·is
he′·lio·ther′·a·py
he′·li·ot′·ro·pis′m [·o·
   tro′·]
he′·li·um
he′·lix   pl.   hel′·i·ces,
   gen. sg.   hel′·i·cis
hel′·le·bore

hel′·minth
hel·min′·tha·gogue
hel′·min·thi′′·a·sis
hel′·min·thol′′·o·gy
hel·min′·tic *also*
·min′·thic
he′·lo-
He′·lo·der′·ma
He·loph′·i·lus
hel·vel′·lic
hel·vol′·ic
he′·ma· *Brit.* hae′·ma·
he′·ma·chro′·ma·to′·sis
var. of hemochromatosis
he′·ma·chrome *var.*
of hemochrome
he′·ma·chro′·sis
he′·ma·cyte *var. of*
hemocyte
he′·ma·cy·tom′·e·ter
var. of hemocytometer
hem′·ad·sor′·bent
[·sorb′·ent]
hem′·ad·sorb′·ing
hem′·ad·sorp′·tion
he′·ma·dy′·na·mom′·e·ter
he′·ma·dy′·na·mom′·e·try
hem′·ag·glu′·ti·nat′·ing
hem′·ag·glu′·ti·na′·tion
hem′·ag·glu′·ti·na·tive
hem′·ag·glu′·ti·nin
he′·ma·gog′·ic
he′·mal
hem·al′·um
hem′·anal′·y·sis
he·man′·gi·ec·ta′·sia
also ·ec′·ta·sis
he·man′·gi·ec·tat′·ic
he·man′·gio· *Brit.*
hae-
he·man′·gi·o·blast
he·man′·gi·o·blas′·tic
he·man′·gi·o·blas·to′·ma
he·man′·gi·o·en′·do·the·li·o′·ma
he·man′·gi·o′·ma *pl.*
·mas *or* ·ma·ta
he·man′·gi·o′·ma·to′·sis
he·man′·gio·per′·i·cyt′·ic
he·man′·gio·per′·i·cy·to′·ma
hem′·a·phe′·in [he′·ma·]
hem′·apher·e′·sis
[·apher′·e·]
he′·ma·poi·e′·sis *var.*
of hematopoiesis
he′·ma·poi·et′·ic *var.*
of hematopoietic
hem′·apoph′·y·sis
hem′·ar·thro′·sis
hem′·a·te′·in
he′·ma·tem′·e·sis
he′·ma·ther′·a·py
he′·ma·ther′·mal
he′·ma·tho′·rax *var.*
of hemothorax
he·mat′·ic
hem′·a·tid [he′·ma·]
he′·ma·ti·dro′·sis
[hem′·a·] *also* he′·mat·hi·
he′·ma·tin [hem′·a·]
he′·ma·ti·ne′·mia
Brit. ·nae′·
he′·ma·tin′·ic
he′·ma·to· *Brit.* hae′·
he′·ma·to·bil′·ia
he′·ma·to′·bi·um *pl.*
·bia
he′·ma·to·cele′ [he·mat′o·]
he′·ma·to·che′·zia
he′·ma·to·chy·lu′·ria
he′·ma·to·col′·pos
he·mat′·o·crit [he′·ma·to·]
he′·ma·to·cyst [hem′·a·]
he′·ma·to·cyte [hem′·a·] *var. of* hemocyte
he′·ma·to·cy·tom′·e·ter
var. of hemocytometer
he′·ma·to·cy′·to·pe′·nia
he′·ma·to·gen′·e·sis
he′·ma·to·gen′·ic
he′·ma·tog′·e·nous
he′·ma·to·gone
he′·ma·toid
he′·ma·toi′·din
he′·ma·tol′·o·gist
he′·ma·tol′·o·gy
he′·ma·tol′·y·sis *var.*
of hemolysis
he′·ma·to·lyt′·ic *var.*
of hemolytic
he′·ma·to′·ma *pl.*
·mas *or* ·ma·ta
he′·ma·to′ma·tous
[·tom′a·]
he′·ma·tom′·e·ter
he′·ma·to·me′·tra
he′·ma·to·my·e′·lia
he′·ma·to·my′·e·li′·tis
he′·ma·to·my′·e·lo·pore
he′·ma·to·pa·thol′·o·gy
he′·ma·to·per′·i·car′·di·um *var. of*
hemopericardium
he′·ma·to·per′·i·to·ne′·um *var. of*
hemoperitoneum
he′·ma·to·pha′·gia
also he′·ma·toph′·a·gy
he′·ma·toph′·a·gous
he′·ma·to·phyte
he′·ma·to·phyt′·ic
he′·ma·to·poi·e′·sis
[hem′·a·]
he′·ma·to·poi·et′·ic
[hem′·a·]
he′·ma·to·por′·phy·rin
he′·ma·to·por′·phy·rin·is′m
he′·ma·to·por′·phy·rin·u′·ria

he′·ma·tor·rha′·chis
he′·ma·to·sal′·pinx
he′·ma·to·sper·mat′·o·cele [·sper′·ma·to·]
he′·ma·to·ther′·mal
he′·ma·to·tho′·rax
  var. of hemothorax
he′·ma·tox′·y·lin
he′·ma·to·zo′·ic
he′·ma·to·zo′·on pl.
  ·zo″a
he′·ma·tu′·ria
he′·ma·tu′·ric
heme Brit. haem
hem′·er·a·lope′
hem′·er·a·lo′·pia
Hem′·er·o·cam′·pa
  H. leu′·ko·stig′·ma
hem′·i·
hem′·i·acar′·dius
hem′·i·ac′·e·tal
hem′·i·a′chro′·ma·top′·sia
hem′·i·agen′·e·sis
hem′·i·ag·no′·sia
hem′·i·al·ge′·sia
hem′·i·an′·es·the′·sia
  Brit. ·an′·aes·
hem′·i·an·o′·pia also
  ·op′·sia
hem′·i·an·o′·pic
hem′·i·an·op′·tic
hem′·i·an·os′·mia
hem′·i·aso′·ma·tog·no′·sia
hem′·i·ato′·nia
hem′·i·at′·ro·phy
hem′·i·az′·y·gos
hem′·i·bal·lis′·mus
  also ·bal′·lism
hem′·i·block
he′·mic Brit. hae′·mic
hem′·i·car′·dia
hem′·i·cel′·lu·lose
hem′·i·ceph′·a·ly
hem′·i·cer′·e·brum [·ce·re′·brum] pl. ·bra
hem′·i·cho·re′a

hem′·i·chro′·ma·top′·sia
hem′·i·co·lec′·to·my
hem′·i·cra′·nia
hem′·i·cra′·ni·ec′·to·my
hem′·i·cra′·ni·o′·sis
hem′·i·cra′·ni·ot′·o·my
hem′·i·de·cor′·ti·ca′·tion
hem′·i·des′·mo·some
hem′·i·di′·a·phragm
hem′·i·fa′·cial
hem′·i·field
hem′·i·gas·trec′·to·my
hem′·i·glos·sec′·to·my
hem′·i·glos′·so·ple′·gia
hem′·i·hep′·a·tec′·to·my
hem′·i·hi·dro′·sis
hem′·i·hy′·per·es·the′·sia Brit. ·aes·the′·
hem′·i·hy′·per·hi·dro′·sis
hem′·i·hy·per′·tro·phy
hem′·i·hyp′·es·the′·sia Brit. ·aes·the′·
hem′·i·hy′·po·es·the′·sia Brit. ·aes·; var. of hemihypesthesia
hem′·i·hy′·po·geu′·sia
hem′·i·kar′·y·on
hem′·i·lam′·i·nec′·to·my
hem′·i·lar′·yn·gec′·to·my
hem′·i·lar′·ynx
hem′·i·lat′·er·al
hem′·i·man′·di·ble
hem′·i·man·dib′·u·lec′·to·my
hem′·i·me′·lia
hem′·i·mel′·i·ca [·me′·li·]
hem′·i·me′·lus
hem′·i·me·tab′·o·lous
he′·min Brit. hae′·min
hem′·i·ne·phrec′·to·my
hem′·i·o′·pia
hem′·i·pa·ral′·y·sis pl. ·ses
hem′·i·par′·a·ple′·gic

hem′·i·pa·re′·sis pl. ·ses
hem′·i·par′·es·the′·sia Brit. ·aes·; pl. ·si·ae or ·sias
hem′·i·pa·ret′·ic
hem′·i·pel·vec′·to·my
hem′·i·pel′·vis
hem′·i·ple′·gia
hem′·i·ple′·gic
He·mip′·tera
he·mip′·ter·ous
hem′·i·ret′·i·na
hem′·i·sac′·ral·i·za′·tion
hem′·i·sec′·tion
hem′·i·sep′·tum pl. ·sep′·ta
hem·i·so·ton′·ic Brit. haem·
hem′·i·spas′m
hem′·i·sphae′·ri·um
  var. of hemispherium
hem′·i·sphere
hem′·i·spher·ec′·to·my
hem′·i·spher′·ic
hem′·i·sphe′·ri·um pl. ·ria, gen. sg. ·rii
hem′·i·ter′·pene
hem′·i·ther′·mo·an′·es·the′·sia Brit. ·an′·aes·
hem′·i·tho′·rax
hem′·i·thy′·roid·ec′·to·my
hem′·i·ver′·te·bra pl. ·brae
hem′·i·zy·gos′·i·ty
hem′·i·zy′·gote
hem′·i·zy′·gous
hem′·lock
he′·mo· Brit. hae′·mo·
he′·mo·ag·glu′·ti·na′·tion var. of hemagglutination
he′·mo·ag·glu′·ti·nin var. of hemagglutinin
he′·mo·bil′·ia
he′·mo·blast

he′·mo·blas′·tic
he′·mo·blas·to′·sis
he′·mo·cele var. of hemocoel
he′·mo·che′·zia
he′·mo·cho′·le·cys·ti′·tis
he′·mo·cho′·ri·al
he′·mo·chro′·ma·to′·sis
he′·mo·chro′·ma·tot′·ic
he′·mo·chrome
he′·mo·chro′·mo·gen
he′·mo·chro·mom′·e·ter
he′·mo·chro·mom′·e·try
he′·mo·clas′·tic
he′·mo·clip
he′·mo·co·ag′·u·la′·tion
he′·mo·co·ag′·u·lin
he′·mo·coel
he′·mo·con′·cen·tra′·tion
he′·mo·crine
he′·mo·cul′·ture
he′·mo·cy′·a·nin
he′·mo·cyte
he′·mo·cy′·to·blast
he′·mo·cy′·to·blas′·tic
he′·mo·cy·tol′·y·sis
he′·mo·cy′·to·lyt′·ic
he′·mo·cy·tom′·e·ter
he′·mo·cy′·to·pha′·gia
he′·mo·cy′·to·phag′·ic
he′·mo·di′·ag·no′·sis
he′·mo·di′·al′·y·sis
he′·mo·di′·a·lyz′·er
he′·mo·di′·a·pe·de′·sis
he′·mo·di·lu′·tion
he′·mo·dy·nam′·ic
he′·mo·dy·nam′·ics
he′·mo·dys′·tro·phy

he′·mo·en′·do·the′·li·al
he′·mo·fil·tra′·tion
he′·mo·flag′·el·late
he′·mo·fus′·cin
he′·mo·glo′·bin[28]
 Brit. hae′·mo·glo′·
he′·mo·glo′·bin·e′·mia [·bi·ne′·mia]
he′·mo·glo′·bin·om′·e·ter
he′·mo·glo′·bin·om′·e·try
he′·mo·glo′·bin·op′·a·thy
he′·mo·glo′·bi·nous
he′·mo·glo′·bin·u′·ria [·bi·nu′·]
he′·mo·glo′·bin·u′·ric [·bi·nu′·]
he′·mo·gram
he′·mo·his′·ti·o·blast
he·mol′·o·gy var. of hematology
he′·mo·lymph
he′·mo·lym·phan′·gi·o′·ma
he′·mo·lym′·pho·cy′·to·tox′·in
he·mol′·y·sate
he·mol′·y·sin [he′·mo·ly′·sin]
he·mol′·y·sis
he′·mo·lyt′·ic
he′·mo·lyz′·a·ble
he′·mo·lyze ·lyzed, ·lyz′·ing; Brit. ·lyse, ·lysed, ·lys′·ing
he′·mo·ma·nom′·e·try
he·mom′·e·ter
he·mom′·e·try
he′·mo·my′·e·lo·gram
he′·mo·pa·thol′·o·gy

he·mop′·a·thy
he′·mo·per·fu′·sion
he′·mo·per′·i·car′·di·um
he′·mo·per′·i·to·ne′·um
he′·mo·pex′·in
he′·mo·pha′·gia
he′·mo·phag′·o·cyt′·ic
he′·mo·phil
he′·mo·phil′·ia
he′·mo·phil′·i·ac
he′·mo·phil′·ic
He·moph′·i·lus[29] var. of Haemophilus
he′·mo·pho·re′·sis
he·moph′·thi·sis [·moph·thi′·sis]
he′·mo·plas·mop′·a·thy
he′·mo·plas′·tic
he′·mo·plas′·ty
he′·mo·pleu′·ro·pneu·mon′·ic
he′·mo·pneu′·mo·per′·i·car′·di·um
he′·mo·pneu′·mo·tho′·rax
he′·mo·poi·e′·sis var. of hematopoiesis
he′·mo·poi·et′·ic var. of hematopoietic
he′·mo·po′·sia
he′·mo·pro′·tein
he′·mo·pro′·to·zo′a
he′·mop·tys′·ic [·ty′·sic]
he·mop′·ty·sis
he′·mo·re·pel′·lant
he′·mo·rhe·ol′·o·gy also ·mor·rhe·
hem′·or·rhage
hem′·or·rhag′·ic
hem′·or·rhag′·i·cus
 fem. ·ca, neut. ·cum

---

[28] The name of a specific hemoglobin is written last: *hemoglobin Bart's, hemoglobin Zürich.*

[29] This was formerly a common American spelling for *Haemophilus,* but it has been generally abandoned in conformity with international usage.

hemorrhagin / hepatomalacia

hem'·or·rha'·gin [·rhag'·in]
hem'·or·rhoid *Brit.* haem'·
hem'·or·rhoi'·dal
hem'·or·rhoi·da'·lis
hem'·or·rhoid·ec'·to·my
hem'·or·rhoi·dol'·y·sis
he'·mo·sal'·pinx
he'·mo·sid'·er·in
he'·mo·sid'·er·o'·sis
he'·mo·sper'·mia
he'·mo·spo·rid'·i·um *pl.* ·rid'·ia; *var. of* haemosporidium
he'·mo·spo'·rine
he'·mo·sta'·sis [he·mos'·ta·sis]
he'·mo·stat
he'·mo·stat'·ic
he'·mo·ther'·a·py
he'·mo·tho'·rax
he'·mo·tox'·ic
he'·mo·tox·ic'·i·ty
he'·mo·tox'·in
he'·mo·troph *also* ·trophe
he'·mo·tro'·pic [·trop'·ic]
he'·mo·tym'·pa·num
he'·mo·zo'·in
hem'·ure'·sis
Hen'·der·son'·u·la
hen'·der·son'·u·lo'·sis
hen·pu'e *also* ·pu'·ye
hen'·ry *pl.* ·rys *or* ·ries
he'·par *gen.* hep'·a·tis
hep'·a·ran
hep'·a·rin
hep'·a·rin·ize ·ized, ·iz'·ing
hep'·a·rit'·in·u'·ria [·i·nu'·ria]
hep'·a·tal'·gia
hep'·a·taux'e
hep'·a·tec'·to·my
he·pat'·ic

he·pat'·i·ca *fem. of* hepaticus; *pl. & gen. sg.* ·cae
he·pat'·i·co·
he·pat'·i·co·cho·lan'·gio·je'·ju·nos'·to·my
he·pat'·i·co·cho·led'·o·chos'·to·my
he·pat'·i·co·do·chot'·o·my
he·pat'·i·co·du'·o·de·nos'·to·my
he·pat'·i·co·en'·ter·os'·to·my
he·pat'·i·co·je'·ju·nos'·to·my
he·pat'·i·co·li·thot'·o·my
he·pat'·i·co·lith'·o·trip'·sy
he·pat'·i·cos'·to·my
he·pat'·i·cot'·o·my
he·pat'·i·cus *pl. & gen. sg.* ·ci
hep'·a·tis *gen. of* hepar
hep'·a·tit'·ic
hep'·a·ti'·tis *pl.* ·tit'·i·des
hep'·a·ti·za'·tion
hep'·a·tized
hep'·a·to· [he·pat'o·]
hep'·a·to·bil'·i·ar'y
hep'·a·to·blast
hep'·a·to·blas·to'·ma
hep'·a·to·can'·a·lic'·u·lar
hep'·a·to·car'·ci·no·gen'·ic
hep'·a·to·car'·ci·no'·ma *pl.* ·mas *or* ·ma·ta
hep'·a·to·cele [he·pat'·o·]
hep'·a·to·cel'·lu·lar
hep'·a·to·cho·lan'·ge·i'tis *var. of* hepatocholangitis

hep'·a·to·cho·lan'·gio·du'·o·de·nos'·to·my
hep'·a·to·cho·lan'·gio·en'·ter·os'·to·my
hep'·a·to·cho·lan'·gio·gas·tros'·to·my
hep'·a·to·cho·lan'·gio·je'·ju·nos'·to·my
hep'·a·to·cho·lan'·gi·os'·to·my
hep'·a·to·cho'·lan·gi'·tis
hep'·a·to·co'·lic
hep'·a·to·co'·li·cum
hep'·a·to·cys'·tic
hep'·a·to·cys'·to·co'·lic
hep'·a·to·cyte [he·pat'·o·]
hep'·a·to·du'·o·de'·nal
hep'·a·to·du·o'·de·na'·le
hep'·a·to·du'·o·de·nos'·to·my
hep'·a·to·en·ter'·ic
hep'·a·to·en'·ter·os'·to·my
hep'·a·to·esoph'·a·ge'·al *Brit.* ·to-oe·soph'·
hep'·a·tof'·u·gal
hep'·a·to·gas'·tric
hep'·a·to·gas'·tri·cum
hep'·a·to·gas'·tro·du'·o·de'·nal
hep'·a·tog'·e·nous *also* hep'·a·to·gen'·ic
hep'·a·to·gram
hep'·a·tog'·ra·phy
hep'·a·to·jug'·u·lar
hep'·a·to·len·tic'·u·lar
hep'·a·to·li'·enal
hep'·a·to·li'·enog'·ra·phy
hep'·a·to·li·thi'·a·sis
hep'·a·tol'·o·gy
hep'·a·to'·ma *pl.* ·mas *or* ·ma·ta
hep'·a·to·ma·la'·cia

hep'·a·to·meg'·a·ly
 also ·me·ga'·lia
hep'·a·to·neph'·ric
hep'·a·to·ne·phri'·tis
hep'·a·to·pan'·cre·at'·ic
hep'·a·to·pan'·cre·at'·i·ca gen. ·cae
hep'·a·top'·a·thy
hep'·a·top'·e·tal
hep'·a·to·pex'y
hep'·a·to·phle·bog'·ra·phy
hep'·a·to·phos·pho'·ry·lase
hep'·a·to·pleu'·ral
hep'·a·to·por'·tal
hep'·a·to·re'·nal
hep'·a·to·re·na'·lis neut. ·le
hep'·a·tor'·rha·phy
hep'·a·to·splen'·ic
hep'·a·to·sple·nog'·ra·phy
hep'·a·to·sple'·no·meg'·a·ly
hep'·a·tos'·to·my
hep'·a·tot'·o·my
hep'·a·to·tox'·ic
hep'·a·to·tox·ic'·i·ty
hep'·a·to·tox'·in
hep'·a·to·tro'·pic [·trop'·ic]
hep'·ta·
hep'·ta·bar'·bi·tal
her'·bal
her'·bal·ist
her'·bi·cide
her'·bi·vore
her·biv'·o·rous
he·red'·i·ta·ble
he·red'·i·ta'·ria
he·red'·i·tar'y
he·red'·i·ty
her'·e·do·
her'·e·do·de·gen'·er·a'·tion
her'·e·do·de·gen'·er·a·tive

her'·e·do·fa·mil'·i·al
her'·e·do·in·fec'·tion
her'·e·do·mac'·u·lar
her'·e·do·path'·ia
her'·e·do·syph'·i·lit'·ic
her'·i·ta·bil'·i·ty
her'·i·ta·ble
her·maph'·ro·dite
her·maph'·ro·dit'·ic
her·maph'·ro·dit·is'm
 also her·maph'·ro·dis'm
her·maph'·ro·di·tis'·mus
her·met'·ic
her'·nia
her'·ni·al
her'·ni·at'·ed
her'·ni·a'·tion
her'·nio·
her'·nio·en'·ter·ot'·o·my
her'·nio·lap'·a·rot'·o·my
her'·ni·o·plas'·ty
her'·nio·punc'·ture
her'·ni·or'·rha·phy
her'·ni·ot'·o·my
he·ro'·ic
her'·o·in
He·roph'·i·li gen. of Herophilus
her'·pan·gi'·na
her'·pes
Her'·pes·vi'·rus
her·pes·vi'·rus
her·pet'·ic
her·pet'·i·form
her·pet'·i·for'·mis
her'·pe·tol'·o·gy
her'·pe·to·pho'·bia
Her'·pe·to·vi'·ri·dae
her·sage'
hertz
hes·per'·i·din
het'·er·aux·e'·sis
het'·er·e'·cious
het'·er·e'·cism
het'·er·er'·gic

het'·er·es·the'·sia
 Brit. ·aes·the'·
het'·ero·
het'·ero·ag·glu'·ti·nin
het'·ero·al·lele'
het'·ero·al·le'·lic
het'·ero·at'·om
het'·ero·aux'·in
Het'·ero·bil·har'·zia
 H. amer'·i·ca'·na
het'·er·o·blas'·tic
het'·ero·car'·y·on var. of heterokaryon
het'·ero·cel'·lu·lar
het'·ero·chro'·ma·tin
het'·ero·chro'·ma·tin·i·za'·tion
het'·ero·chro'·ma·to'·sis
het'·er·o·chro'·mia
het'·er·o·chro'·mic
het'·er·o·chro'·mo·some
het'·er·o·chro'·nia
 also het'·er·och'·ro·ny
het'·er·och'·ro·nous
het'·er·o·clad'·ic
het'·er·o·crine
het'·ero·cy'·cle
het'·ero·cy'·clic
het'·ero·cy'·to·tox'·in
het'·er·o·dont
het'·er·o·du'·plex
het'·er·oe'·cious var. of heterecious
het'·er·oe'·cism var. of heterecism
het'·ero·fer·men'·ta·tive
het'·ero·gam'·ete [·ga·mete']
het'·ero·ga·met'·ic
het'·er·og'·a·mous
het'·er·og'·a·my
het'·er·o·ge·ne'·ic
het'·er·o·ge·ne'·ity
het'·er·o·ge'·ne·ous
het'·ero·gen'·e·sis
het'·ero·ge·net'·ic

heterogenic / hieric 122

het'·er·o·gen'·ic
het'·er·o·ge·nic'·i·ty
het'·er·o·ge'·note
het'·er·og'·e·nous
het'·er·o·gon'·ic
het'·ero·graft
het'·ero·he·mol'·y·sin
[·he'·mo·ly'·sin]
Brit. ·hae·
het'·ero·im·mu'·ni·ty
het'·ero·in·fec'·tion
het'·ero·kar'y·on
het'·ero·kar'y·o'·sis
het'·ero·ki·ne'·sia
het'·ero·lat'·er·al
het'·er·ol'·o·gous
het'·ero·ly'·sin
het'·ero·ly'·sis [het'·er·ol'·y·sis]
het'·ero·ly'·so·some
het'·er·o·lyt'·ic
het'·er·o·met'·ric
het'·er·o·me·tro'·pia
het'·er·o·mor·pho'·sis
het'·er·o·mor'·phous
also ·mor'·phic
het'·er·on'·y·mous
het'·er·oph'·a·gous
het'·er·o·phil *also* ·phile
het'·er·o·pho'·nia
also het'·er·oph'·o·ny
het'·ero·pho'·ria
het'·ero·pho'·ric
Het'·er·oph'·y·es [·o·phy'·es]
H. het'·er·oph'·y·es
H. ka·tsu'·ra·da'i
het'·er·o·phy·i'·a·sis
Het'·er·o·phy'·i·dae
het'·er·o·pla'·sia
het'·er·o·plas'm
het'·er·o·plas'·tic
het'·er·o·plas'·ty
het'·er·o·ploid
het'·er·o·ploi'·dy
het'·er·op'·sia
Het'·er·op'·tera

het'·ero·pyk·no'·sis
het'·ero·pyk·not'·ic
het'·ero·scope
het'·er·os'·co·py
het'·ero·sex'·u·al
het'·ero·sex'·u·al'·i·ty
het'·er·o'·sis
het'·er·o·tax'·ia *also* ·tax'·is
het'·er·o·ther'·mic
het'·er·o·ther'·my
het'·er·o·to'·pia *also* ·ot'·o·py
het'·er·o·top'·ic
het'ero·tox'·ic
het'·ero·tox'·in
het'·ero·trans'·plant
het'·ero·trans'·plan·ta'·tion
het'·ero·tri·cho'·sis
het'·er·ot'·ri·chous
het'·er·o·troph
het'·er·o·tro'·phic [·troph'·ic]
het'·er·o·tro'·pia
het'·er·o·tro'·pic [·trop'·ic]
het'·er·o·type
het'·er·o·typ'·ic *also* ·i·cal
het'·ero·vac·cine' [·vac'·cin·]
het'·er·ox'·e·nous
het'·er·ox'·e·ny
het'·ero·zy·go'·sis
het'·ero·zy·gos'·i·ty
het'·ero·zy'·gote
het'·ero·zy·got'·ic
het'·er·o·zy'·gous
hex'a·
hex'·a·canth
hexacetonide
hex'a·chlo'·ride
hex'a·chlo'·ro·ben'·zene
hex'a·chlo·ro·cy'·clo·hex'·ane

hex'a·chlo'·ro·phene
also ·phane
hex'a·dac'·ty·ly
hex'a·di·meth'·rine
hex'a·me·tho'·ni·um
hex'a·meth'·yl
hex'·a·mine
hex'·ane
hex'·a·no'·ic
hex'·a·ploid
hex'·a·ploi'·dy
hex·ax'·i·al
hex'·es·trol *Brit.* ·oes·trol
hex·et'·i·dine
hex'o·bar'·bi·tal
hex'·o·cy'·cli·um
hex'o·ki'·nase
hex·os'·a·mine
hex·os'·a·min'·i·dase
hex'·ose
hex'·ose·phos·pho'·ric
hex'·yl·caine
hex'·yl·re·sor'·ci·nol
hi·a'·tal
hi·a'·to·pex'y
hi·a'·tus *L. pl. & gen. sg.* hiatus
hi'·ber·na'·tion
hi'·ber·no'·ma *pl.* ·mas *or* ·ma·ta
hic'·cup ·cuped *or* ·cupped, ·cup·ing *or* ·cup·ping
hide'·bound
hi·drad'·e·ni'·tis
hi·drad'·e·no'·ma
also hi'·dro·ad'·e·no'·ma; *pl.* ·mas *or* ·ma·ta
hi'·dro·
hi·dro'a *var. of* hydroa
hi'·dro·cys·to'·ma *pl.* ·mas *or* ·ma·ta
hi·dro'·sis
hi·drot'·ic
hi'·emal
hi'·ema·lis
hi·er'·ic

hi′·er·o·lis·the′·sis
hi′·lar
hill′·ock
hi′·lum *pl.* ·la, *gen. sg.*
·li
hi′·lus *var. of* hilum;
pl. & gen. sg. ·li
hind′·brain
hind′·foot *posterior of human foot; Cf.* hind foot
hind foot′ *rear foot of quadruped; Cf.* hindfoot
hind′·gut
hind′·wa·ter
hinge′-bow
Hip′·pe·la′·tes
Hip′·po·bos′·ca
Hip′·po·bos′·ci·dae
hip′po·cam′·pal
hip′·po·cam·pa′·lis
hip′·po·cam′·pus *gen.* ·pi
hip′·po·crat′·ic
hip′·po·crat′·i·ca
hip′·pu·rate
hip·pu′·ric
hip′·pus
hir′·ci *sg.* ·cus
hir′·sute [hir·sute′]
hir·su′·ti·es *var. of* hirsutism
hir′·sut·is′m
hir′·su·toid
hi·ru′·din [hir′·u·din]
Hir′·u·din′·ea
hi·ru′·di·ni′·a·sis [hir′·u·]
hi·ru′·din·i·za′·tion [hir′·u·]
hi·ru′·din·ize [hir′·u·] ·ized, ·iz′·ing
Hi·ru′·do
H. ja·pon′·i·ca
H. ja·van′·i·ca
H. me·dic′·i·na′·lis

his′·ta·mi·nase [his·tam′·i·nase]
his′·ta·mine
his′·ta·min·e′·mia [·mi·ne′·mia] *Brit.* ·ae′·mia
his′·ti·dine
his′·ti·din·e′·mia [·di·ne′·mia] *Brit.* ·ae′·mia
his′·ti·din·u′·ria [·di·nu′·ria]
his′·tio·
his′·ti·o·blast
his′·ti·o·cyte
his′·ti·o·cyt′·ic
his′·ti·o·cy·to′·ma
his′·ti·o·cy·to′·sis
his′·ti·o·gen′·ic *var. of* histogenous
his′·ti·o·typ′·ic
his′·to-
his′·to·au′·to·ra′·di·og′·ra·phy
his′·to·blast
his′·to·chem′·i·cal
his′·to·chem′·is·try
his′·to·che′·mo·ther′·a·py
his′·to·com·pat′·i·bil′·i·ty
his′·to·com·pat′·i·ble
his′·to·cyte *var. of* histiocyte
his′·to·cy·to′·sis *var. of* histiocytosis
his′·to·di′·ag·no′·sis
his′·to·dif′·fer·en′·ti·a′·tion
his′·to·fluo·res′·cence
his′·to·gen′·e·sis
his·tog′·e·nous
his·tog′·e·ny
his′·to·gram
his′·toid
his′·to·in′·com·pat′·i·bil′·i·ty

his′·to·in′·com·pat′·i·ble
his′·to·ki·ne′·sis
his′·to·log′·ic *also* ·i·cal
his·tol′·o·gist
his·tol′·o·gy
his·tol′·y·sate
his·tol′·y·sis
his′·to·lyt′·ic
his′·to·mor·phol′·o·gy
his′·tone
his′·ton·u′·ria
his′·to·path′o·gen′·e·sis
his′·to·pa·thol′·o·gy
his′·to·phys′·i·ol′·o·gy
His′·to·plas′·ma
his′·to·plas′·min
his′·to·plas·mo′·ma
his′·to·plas·mo′·sis
his′·to·ra′·di·o·graph
his′·to·ra′·di·og′·ra·phy
his′·to·ry
his′·to·tox′·ic
his′·to·troph *also* ·trophe
his′·to·tro′·pic [·trop′·ic]
his′·to·zo′·ic
hives
hoarse hoars′·er, hoars′·est
hoarse′·ness
ho′·do·graph
ho·dol′·o·gy
ho′·do·pho′·bia
hof
hol·an′·dric
hold′·fast
ho′·lism
ho·lis′·tic
hol′·mi·um
ho′lo [hol′o·]
ho′lo·acar′·di·us
ho′lo·blas′·tic
ho′lo·crine
ho′lo·di′·a·stol′·ic
ho′lo·en·dem′·ic

ho′lo·en′·zyme
ho·log′·a·mous
ho·log′·a·my
ho′lo·gram
ho·log′·ra·phy
ho′lo·gyn′·ic
ho′lo·me·tab′·o·lous
ho′lo·phyt′·ic
ho′lo·pros′·en·ceph′·a·ly
ho′lo·sys·tol′·ic
ho′lo·tel′·en·ceph′·a·ly
ho·lot′·ri·chous
ho′lo·type
ho′lo·zo′·ic
hom′·a·lu′·ria
hom·at′·ro·pine
hom·ax′·i·al
ho·me′·cious *also* ·moe′·
ho′·meo· *also* ho′··moeo·
ho′·meo·graft
ho′·me·o·mor′·phous
ho′·me·o·path
ho′·me·o·path′·ic
ho′·me·op′·a·thy
ho′·me·o·pla′·sia
ho′·me·o·plas′·tic
ho′·me·o′·sis *also* ·moe·o′·
ho′·meo·sta′·sis [ho′··me·os′·ta·sis]
ho′·meo·stat′·ic
ho′meo·ther′·a·py
ho′·me·o·therm
ho′·me·o·ther′·mal
ho′·me·o·ther′·mic
ho′·me·o·ther′·my
ho′·me·ot′·ic *also* ·moe·
ho′·meo·tox′·ic
ho′·meo·tox′·in
ho′meo·trans′·plant
ho′·meo·trans′·plan·ta′·tion
ho′·me·o·typ′·ic
hom·er′·gic

hom′·i·nid
Ho·min′·i·dae
Hom′·i·noi′·dea
Ho′·mo
H. sa′·pi·ens
ho′·mo· [hom′o·]
ho′·mo·blas′·tic
ho′·mo·clad′·ic
ho′·mo·cys′·te·ine
ho′·mo·cys′·tine
ho′·mo·cys′·tin·u′·ria [·ti·nu′·]
ho′·mo·cys′·tin·u′·ric [·ti·nu′·]
ho′·mo·cy′·to·tro′·pic [·trop′·ic]
ho·mod′·ro·mous
ho′·mo·dy·nam′·ic
ho·moe′·cious *var. of* homecious
ho′·moeo· *var. of* homeo-
ho′·moe·op′·a·thy *var. of* homeopathy
ho′·moeo·o′·sis *var. of* homeosis
ho′·moeo·sta′·sis *var. of* homeostasis
ho′·moeo·tox′·in *var. of* homeotoxin
ho′·mo·erot′·ic
ho′·mo·erot′·i·cis′m *also* ·er′·o·tis′m
ho′·mo·fer·men′·ta·tive
ho′·mo·ga·met′·ic
ho·mog′·a·mous
ho·mog′·a·my
ho·mog′·e·nate
ho′·mo·ge·ne′·ity
ho′·mo·ge′·ne·ous
ho′·mo·gen′·ic
ho·mog′·e·ni·za′·tion
ho·mog′·e·nize ·nized, ·niz′·ing
ho·mog′·e·nous
ho′·mo·gen·tis′·ic
ho′·mo·gon′·ic
ho′·mo·graft

ho′·moio·[ho·moi′o′·]
ho′·moi·o·pla′·sia *var. of* homeoplasia
ho′·moi·op′·o·dal
ho′·moi·os·mot′·ic
ho′·moio·sta′·sis *var. of* homeostasis
ho′·moi·o·ther′·mal *var. of* homeothermal
ho′·moi·o·ther′·mic *var. of* homeothermic
ho′·mo·kar′y·on
ho′·mo·lac′·tic
ho′·mo·lat′·er·al
ho·mol′·o·gous
hom′·o·logue [ho′·mo·]
ho·mol′·o·gy
ho′·mo·ly′·sin
ho′·mo·ly′·sis [ho·mol′·y·sis]
ho′·mo·mor′·phic *also* ·phous
ho·mon′·o·mous *being in a series of similar structures: Cf.* homonymous
ho·mon′·y·mous *uncrossed, as a double visual image: Cf.* homonomous
ho′·mo·phile
ho′·mo·plas′·tic
ho′·mo·plas′·ty
ho′·mo·pla′·sy
ho′·mo·pol′·y·mer
ho′·mo·ser′·ine
ho′·mo·sex′·u·al
ho′·mo·sex′·u·al′·i·ty
ho′·mo·som′·al [·so′·mal]
ho′·mo·spo′·rous
ho′·mo·therm *var. of* homeotherm
ho′·mo·ther′·mal *var. of* homeothermal; *also* ·ic
ho′·mo·ton′·ic
ho′·mo·top′·ic

ho'·mo·trans'·plant
ho'·mo·trans'·plan·ta'·tion
ho'·mo·type
ho'·mo·typ'·ic *also* ·i·cal
ho'·mo·va·nil'·lic
ho'·mo·zy·go'·sis
ho'·mo·zy·gos'·i·ty
ho'·mo·zy'·gote
ho'·mo·zy'·gous
ho·mun'·cu·lus *pl.* ·li
hon'·ey·comb
hook'·let
hook'·worm
hor'·de·nine
hor·de'·o·lum
hore'·hound
hor'·i·zon'·tal
hor'·i·zon·ta'·lis
hor·me'·sis
hor·mo'·nal [hor'·mon·al]
hor'·mone
hor'·mo·no·gen'·e·sis
hor'·mo·no·gen'·ic
hor'·mo·nol'·o·gy
hor'·mo·no·poi·e'·sis
hor'·mo·no·poi·et'·ic
hor'·mo·no·ther'·a·peu'·tic
hor'·mo·no·ther'·a·py
horn'·i·fi·ca'·tion
horn'·skin
horn'y horn'·i·er, horn'·i·est
ho·rop'·ter
hor'·ror
horse'·fly
horse'·pox
horse'·shoe
hor'·tungs·kör'·per
hos'·pice

hos'·pi·tal
hos'·pi·tal·is'm
hos'·pi·tal·i'·tis
hos'·pi·tal·i·za'·tion
hos'·pi·tal·ize ·ized, ·iz'·ing
house'·bound
house'·fly
hous'·ing
house'·man *pl.* ·men
house'·man·ship
huck'·le·bone
hue
hu'·man
hu·mec'·tant
hu'·mec·ta'·tion
hu'·mer·al *of the humerus: Cf.* humoral
hu'·mer·a'·le
hu'·mero·ra'·di·al
hu'·mero·ra'·di·a'·lis
hu'·mero·ul'·nar
hu'·mero·ul·na'·ris *neut.* ·re
hu'·mer·us *pl. & gen. sg.* ·meri
hu·mid'·i·fi·ca'·tion
hu·mid'·i·fi'·er
hu·mid'·i·fy ·fied, ·fy'·ing
hu·mid'·i·stat
hu·mid'·i·ty
hu'·min
hum'·ming
hu'·mor[30] *Brit.* ·mour
hu'·mor·al *of certain body fluids: Cf.* humeral
hu'·mor·al·is'm *also* hu'·mor·is'm
hump'·back
hunch'·back
hun'·ger

hun·te'·ri·an
huy·ge'·ni·an
hy'·al
hy'·a·lin
hy'·a·line
hy'·a·lin·i·za'·tion
hy'·a·li·no'·sis
hy'·a·li'·tis
hy'·a·lo·
hy'·a·loid
hy'·a·loid·e'·us *fem.* ·dea
hy'·a·loid·i'·tis
hy'·a·loi·dop'·a·thy
Hy'·a·lom'·ma
hy'·a·lo·mu'·coid
hy'·a·lo·nyx'·is
hy'·a·lo·plas'm
hy'·a·lo·se'·ro·si'·tis
hy'·a·lo'·sis
hy'·a·lu'·ro·nate
hy'·a·lu·ron'·ic
hy'·a·lu·ron'·i·dase
hy'·brid
hy'·brid·is'm
hy'·brid·i·za'·tion
hy'·brid·ize ·ized, ·iz'·ing
hy'·brid·o'·ma
hy·can'·thone
hy'·clate
hy·dan'·to·in
hy'·da·tid
hy'·da·tid'·i·form
hy'·da·ti·do'·sis
hy'·da·ti·dos'·to·my
hy'·da·toid
hy·drae'·mia *Brit. spel. of* hydremia
hy'·dra·gogue
hy·dral'·a·zine
hy·dram'·ni·os *also* ·ni·on

---

[30] While the British spelling *humour* is limited to English-language contexts, *humor* is used in Latin as well as in American English. For example, British *vitreous humour*, American *vitreous humor*, Latin *humor vitreus*.

hy·dran'·en·ceph'·a·ly
hy'·drar·gyr'·ia
hy·drar'·gy·ris'm
hy·drar'·gy·rum
hy'·drar·thro'·di·al
hy'·drar·thro'·sis
hy·dras'·tine
hy'·dra·tase
hy'·drate
hy'·drat·ed
hy·dra'·tion
hy·drau'·lic
hy'·dra·zide
hy'·dra·zine
hy'·dra·zi·nol'·y·sis
hy'·dra·zo'·ic
hy'·dra·zone
hy·dre'·mia *Brit.* ·drae'·
hy·dre'·mic *Brit.* ·drae'·
hy'·dren·ceph'·a·lo·cele
hy'·dren·ceph'·a·lus
hy'·dren·ceph'·a·ly
hy'·dride
hy'·dri·od'·ic
hy'·dro·
hy·dro'a
hy'·dro·bleph'·a·ron
hy'·dro·bro'·mic
hy'·dro·bro'·mide
hy'·dro·cal'·i·co'·sis
hy'·dro·car'·bon
hy'·dro·cele
hy'·dro·ce·lec'·to·my
hy'·dro·ce·phal'·ic
hy'·dro·ceph'·a·lo·cele
hy'·dro·ceph'·a·loid
hy'·dro·ceph'·a·lus
  also ·ceph'·a·ly
hy'·dro·chlo'·ric
hy'·dro·chlo'·ride
hy'·dro·chlo'·ro·thi'·a·zide
hy'·dro·cho'·le·ret'·ic
hy'·dro·co'·done
hy'·dro·col'·loid

hy'·dro·col'·po·cele
hy'·dro·col'·pos
hy'·dro·cor'·ta·mate
hy'·dro·cor'·ti·sone
hy'·dro·cy·an'·ic
hy'·dro·cy'·a·nis'm
hy'·dro·cys·to'·ma
  var. of hidrocystoma
hy'·dro·di'·a·scope
hy'·dro·dy·nam'·ic
hy'·dro·en·ceph'·a·lo·cele
hy'·dro·en·ceph'·a·lo·me·nin'·go·cele
hy'·dro·flu'o·ric
hy'·dro·gen
hy·drog'·e·nase [hy'·dro·gen·ase]
hy'·dro·gen·ate [hy·drog'·e·nate] ·at'·ed, ·at'·ing
hy'·dro·gen·a'·tion [hy·drog'·e·na'·tion]
hy'·dro·gen·ly'·ase
hy'·dro·hem'·ar·thro'·sis *Brit.* ·haem'·
hy'·dro·he'·ma·to·sal'·pinx *Brit.* ·hae'·ma·
hy'·dro·ki·net'·ic
hy'·dro·kol'·lag
hy'·dro·lase
hy·drol'·o·gy
hy'·dro·ly'·ase
hy·drol'·y·sate
hy·drol'·y·sis
hy·drol·yt'·ic
hy'·dro·lyze ·lyzed, ·lyz'·ing; *Brit.* ·lyse, ·lysed, ·lys'·ing
hy·dro'·ma
hy'·dro·mas·sage'
hy'·dro·me·nin'·go·cele
hy·drom'·e·ter
hy'·dro·me'·tra
hy'·dro·me'·tro·col'·pos
hy·drom'·e·try

hy'·dro·mi'·cro·ceph'·a·ly
hy'·dro·mor'·phone
hy'·dro·my·e'·lia
hy'·dro·my'·e·lo·cele
hy'·dro·my'·e·lo·me·nin'·go·cele
hy'·dron
hy'·dro·ne·phro'·sis
hy'·dro·ne·phrot'·ic
hy·dro'·ni·um
hy·dro·path'·ic
hy·drop'·a·thy
hy'·dro·pe'·nia
hy'·dro·pe'·nic
hy'·dro·per'·i·car'·di·um
hy'·dro·per'i·ne·phro'·sis
hy'·dro·per'·i·on
hy'·dro·per'·i·to·ne'·um
hy'·dro·pex'·ic
hy'·dro·phil'·ic
hy'·dro·pho'·bia
hy'·dro·pho'·bic
hy'·droph·thal'·mia
hy'·droph·thal'·mos *also* ·mus
hy·drop'·ic
hy'·dro·plas'·mia *also* hy'·dro·plas'·my
hy'·dro·pleu'·ra
hy'·dro·pneu'·ma·to'·sis
hy'·dro·pneu'·mo·tho'·rax
hy'·drops
hy'·dro·quin'·ol
hy'·dro·qui·none' [·quin'·one]
hy'·dror·rhe'a *Brit.* ·rhoe'a
hy'·dro·sal'·pinx
hy'·dro·sar'·co·cele
hy·dros'·che·o·cele
hy'·dro·sol
hy'·dro·stat'·ic

hy'·dro·sul·fu"·ric
hy'·dro·tax"·is
hy'·dro·ther'·a·peu"·tic
hy'·dro·ther"·a·pist
hy'·dro·ther"·a·py
hy'·dro·ther"·mal
hy'·dro·thi"·o·ne"·mia *Brit.* ·nae"·
hy'·dro·tho·rac"·ic
hy'·dro·tho"·rax
hy·drot"·o·my
hy'·dro·tro"·pic [·trop"·ic]
hy'·dro·tro"·pism
hy'·dro·tym"·pa·num
hy'·dro·ure"·ter
hy"·drous
hy'·dro·var"·i·um
hy'·drox·am"·ic
hy·drox"·ide
hy·drox'o·
hy·drox'o·co·bal"·a·min
hy·drox'y·
hy·drox'y·ac"·yl
hy·drox'y·ac"·yl·glu'·ta·thi"·one
hy·drox'y·am·phet"·a·mine
hy·drox'y·an"·dro·stene"·di·one
hy·drox'y·ap"·a·tite
hy·drox'y·ben"·zene [·ben·zene"]
hy·drox'y·bu"·ty·rate
hy·drox'y·bu·tyr"·ic
hy·drox'y·chlo"·ro·quine
hy·drox'y·cho"·le·cal·cif"·er·ol
hy·drox'y·cor"·ti·co·ste"·roid
hy·drox'y·di·hy"·dro·ta·chys"·ter·ol
hy·drox'y·di"·one
hy·drox'y·er"·go·cal·cif"·er·ol
hy·drox'y·es"·tra·di"·ol

hy·drox'y·eth"·yl·apo·cu"·pre·ine
hy·drox'y·in"·dole·ace"·tic
hy·drox"·yl
hy·drox"·yl·amine"
hy·drox"·yl·ase
hy·drox"·yl·a"·tion
hy·drox'y·ly"·sine
hy·drox'y·meth"·yl
hy·drox'y·meth"·yl·glu"·ta·ryl
hy·drox'y·phen"·yl·u"·ria
hy·drox'y·pro·ges"·ter·one
hy·drox'y·pro"·line
hy·drox'y·pro"·lin·e"·mia [·li·ne"·mia] *Brit.* ·ae"·mia
hy·drox'y·pro"·lin·u"·ria [·li·nu"·ria]
hy·drox'y·quin"·o·line
hy·drox'y·ste"·roid [·ster"·oid]
hy·drox'y·stil·bam"·i·dine
hy·drox'y·tryp"·ta·mine
hy·drox'y·tryp"·to·phan
hy·drox'y·ure"a
hy·drox'y·zine
hy"·giene
hy'·gi·en"·ic
hy·gien"·ist
hy"·gric
hy"·grine
hy'·gro·
hy'·gro·ble·phar"·ic
hy·gro"·ma *pl.* ·mas *or* ·ma·ta
hy·grom"·a·tous
hy·grom"·e·ter
hy'·gro·met"·ric
hy·grom"·e·try
hy'·gro·scop"·ic
hy'·lo·
hy"·men
hy"·men·al

hy'·men·ec"·to·my
hy'·men·i"·tis
hy'·me·no·le·pi"·a·sis
Hy'·me·no·le·pid"·i·dae
Hy·me·nol'·e·pis
H. di'·mi·nu"·ta
H. na"·na
hy'·me·nol"·o·gy
Hy'·me·nop"·tera
hy'·me·nop"·ter·an
hy'·men·ot"·o·my
hy'o·
hy'o·bran"·chi·al
hy'o·ep'i·glot"·tic
hy'o·ep'i·glot"·ti·cum
hy'o·ep'i·glot·tid"·e·an
hy'o·glos"·sal
hy'o·glos"·sus
hy"·oid
hy·oi'·de·um *gen.* ·dei
hy'o·man·dib"·u·lar
hy'·o·scine
hy'·o·scy"·a·mine
hy'·o·scy"·a·mus
hy'o·thy"·roid
hyp'·acu"·sis *also* ·sia; *var. of* hypoacusis
hyp'·al·ge"·sia
hyp'·al·ge"·sic
hyp'·al·get"·ic
hyp·aph'·ro·dis"·ia
hyp'·ar·te"·ri·al
hyp·ax"·i·al
hyp·en'·ce·phal"·ic
hy'·per
hy'·per·acid"·i·ty
hy'·per·ac"·tive
hy'·per·ac·tiv"·i·ty
hy'·per·acu"·i·ty
hy'·per·acu"·sis *also* ·sia
hy'·per·acute"
hy'·per·ad'·i·pos"·i·ty
hy'·per·adre"·nal
hy'·per·adre"·nal·is"m
hy'·per·adre"·no·cor"·ti·cis"m *also* ·cor"·ti·cal·is"m

hy'·per·adre'·no·cor'·ti·cal
hy'·per·ae'·mia *Brit. spel. of* hyperemia
hy'·per·aer·a'·tion
hy'·per·aes·the'·sia *Brit. spel. of* hyperesthesia
hy'·per·al·bu'·min·e'·mia *Brit.* ·ae'·mia
hy'·per·al·dos'·ter·on·e'·mia [·al'·do·ster'·] *Brit.* ·ae'·mia
hy'·per·al·dos'·ter·on·is'm [·al'·do·ster'·]
hy'·per·al·dos'·ter·on·u'·ria [·al'·do·ster'·]
hy'·per·al·ge'·sia
hy'·per·al·ge'·sic
hy'·per·al'·i·men·ta'·tion
hy'·per·al'·i·ment·ed
hy'·per·ami'·no·ac'·id·e'·mia *Brit.* ·ae'·mia
hy'·per·ami'·no·ac'·id·u'·ria
hy'·per·am·mo·ne'·mia *also* ·am·mo'·ni·e'mia; *Brit.* ·ae'·mia
hy'·per·am'·mo·nu'·ria
hy'·per·am'·y·las·e'·mia *Brit.* ·ae'·mia
hy'·per·a'·phia
hy'·per·ap'o·be'·ta·lip'o·pro'·tein·e'·mia *Brit.* ·ae'·mia
hy'·per·az'o·te'·mia *Brit.* ·tae'·mia
hy'·per·bar'·ic
hy'·per·bar'·ism
hy'·per·be'·ta·al'·a·nin·e'·mia *Brit.* ·ae'·mia
hy'·per·be'·ta·lip'o·pro'·tein·e'·mia *Brit.* ·ae'·mia
hy'·per·bil'·i·ru'·bin·e'·mia *Brit.* ·ae'·mia

hy'·per·cal·ce'·mia *Brit.* ·cae·mia
hy'·per·cal'·ci·to'·nin·e'·mia *Brit.* ·ae'·mia
hy'·per·cal'·ci·u'·ria
hy'·per·cap'·nia
hy'·per·cap'·nic
hy'·per·car'·o·ten·e'·mia [·te·ne'·] *Brit.* ·ae'·mia
hy'·per·cat'·a·bol'·ic
hy'·per·ca·tab'·o·lis'm
hy'·per·ca·thex'·is
hy'·per·cel'·lu·lar'·i·ty
hy'·per·ce'·men·to'·sis
hy'·per·chlo·re'·mia *Brit.* ·rae'·mia
hy'·per·chlo·re'·mic *Brit.* ·re'·mic
hy'·per·chlor·hy'·dria
hy'·per·chlo'·ri·da'·tion
hy'·per·chlor·u'·ria
hy'·per·cho·les'·ter·ol·e'·mia *Brit.* ·ae'·mia
hy'·per·cho·les'·ter·ol·e'·mic *Brit.* ·ae'·mic
hy'·per·cho'·lia
hy'·per·chro·maf'·fin·is'm [·chro'·maf·]
hy'·per·chro·ma'·sia
hy'·per·chro'·ma·tin
hy'·per·chro'·ma·top'·sia
hy'·per·chro'·mia
hy'·per·chro'·mic
hy'·per·chro·mic'·i·ty
hy'·per·chy'·lo·mi'·cro·ne'·mia *Brit.* ·nae'·
hy'·per·cit·ru'·ria
hy'·per·co·ag'·u·la·bil'·i·ty
hy'·per·co·ag'·u·la·ble
hy'·per·co'·ria
hy'·per·cor'·ti·cis'm *also* ·cor'·ti·cal·is'm
hy'·per·cor'·ti·sol·is'm
hy'·per·cry'·al·ge'·sia

hy'·per·cry'·es·the'·sia *Brit.* ·aes·the'·
hy'·per·cu·pre'·mia *Brit.* ·prae'·
hy'·per·cu'·pri·u'·ria
hy'·per·cy·the'·mia *Brit.* ·thae'·
hy'·per·di·as'·to·le
hy'·per·dip'·loid
hy'·per·dip'·loi·dy
hy'·per·dip'·sia
hy'·per·don'·tia
hy'·per·dy·nam'·ia
hy'·per·dy·nam'·ic
hy'·per·elas'·ti·ca
hy'·per·em'·e·sis
hy'·per·emet'·ic
hy'·per·e'·mia *Brit.* ·ae'·mia
hy'·per·en·dem'·ic
hy'·per·en'·de·mic'·i·ty
hy'·per·ep'·i·neph'·rin·e'·mia [·ri·ne'·] *Brit.* ·ae'·mia
hy'·per·e'·qui·lib'·ri·um
hy'·per·er'·gia
hy'·per·er'·gic
hy'·per·er'·gy
hy'·per·es·o·pho'·ria
hy'·per·es·the'·sia *Brit.* ·aes·the'·
hy'·per·es·thet'·ic *Brit.* ·aes·thet'·
hy'·per·es'·tro·gen·e'·mia *Brit.* ·oes'·tro·gen·ae'·mia
hy'·per·es'·tro·gen·is'm *Brit.* ·oes'·tro·
hy'·per·ex·o·pho'·ria
hy'·per·ex·ten'·si·ble
hy'·per·ex·ten'·sion
hy'·per·fer·re'·mia *Brit.* ·rae'·
hy'·per·fer·re'·mic *Brit.* ·rae'·
hy'·per·fer'·ri·ce'·mia *Brit.* ·cae'·

hy'·per·fi·brin'·o·gen·e'·mia Brit. ·ae'·mia
hy'·per·fi'·bri·nol'·y·sis
hy'·per·flex'·ion
hy'·per·frac'·tion·a'·tion
hy'·per·func'·tion
hy'·per·ga·lac'·tia
hy'·per·gam'·ma·glob'·u·lin·e'·mia Brit. ·ae'·mia
hy'·per·gen'·i·tal·is'm
hy'·per·geu'·sia
hy'·per·glob'·u·lin·e'·mia Brit. ·ae'·mia
hy'·per·gly·ce'·mia Brit. ·cae'·
hy'·per·gly·ce'·mic Brit. ·cae'·
hy'·per·glyc'·er·i·de'·mia [·id·e'·] Brit. ·dae'·mia
hy'·per·gly'·ci·ne'·mia [·cin·e'·] Brit. ·nae'·
hy'·per·gly'·cor·rha'·chia
hy'·per·gly'·cos·e'·mia Brit. ·ae'·mia
hy'·per·gly·ox'·yl·e'·mia Brit. ·ae'·mia
hy'·per·go'·nad·is'm
hy'·per·go·nad'·o·tro'·phic [·gon'·a·do·, ·troph'·ic]
hy'·per·go·nad'·o·tro'·pic [·gon'·a·do·, ·trop'·ic]
hy'·per·gran'·u·la'·tion
hy'·per·hep'·a·rin·e'·mia Brit. ·ae'·mia
hy'·per·hi·dro'·sis also ·idro'·sis
hy'·per·hi·drot'·ic
hy'·per·hy·dra'·tion
hy·per'·i·cin
hy'·per·im·mune'
hy'·per·im·mu'·ni·ty

hy'·per·im'·mu·ni·za'·tion
hy'·per·in·fla'·tion
hy'·per·in'·ner·va'·tion
hy'·per·in'·su·lin·e'·mia Brit. ·ae'·mia
hy'·per·in'·su·lin·is'm
hy'·per·in'·vo·lu'·tion
hy'·per·i'·o·de'·mia Brit. ·dae'·
hy'·per·ir'·ri·ta·bil'·i·ty
hy'·per·ka·le'·mia Brit. ·lae'·mia
hy'·per·ka·le'·mic Brit. ·lae'·mic
hy'·per·kal'·i·e'·mia var. of hyperkalemia; Brit. ·ae'·mia
hy'·per·ker'·a·tin·i·za'·tion
hy'·per·ker'·a·to'·sis
hy'·per·ker'·a·tot'·ic
hy'·per·ke'·to·ne'·mia Brit. ·nae'·
hy'·per·ki·ne'·mia Brit. ·nae'·
hy'·per·ki·ne'·mic Brit. ·nae'·mic
hy'·per·ki·ne'·sia
hy'·per·ki·ne'·sis
hy'·per·ki·net'·ic
hy'·per·le'·thal
hy'·per·ley'·dig·is'm
hy'·per·li·pe'·mia Brit. ·pae'·
hy'·per·lip'·id·e'·mia Brit. ·ae'·mia
hy'·per·lip'o·pro'·tein·e'·mia [·li'po·] Brit. ·ae'·mia
hy'·per·lu'·cen·cy
hy'·per·lu'·cent
hy'·per·lu'·tein·i·za'·tion
hy'·per·ly·sin·e'·mia Brit. ·ae'mia
hy'·per·ly·sin·u'·ria

hy'·per·mag'·ne·se'·mia Brit. ·sae'·
hy'·per·ma'·nia
hy'·per·ma·ture'
hy'·per·men'·or·rhe'a Brit. ·rhoe'a
hy'·per·met'·a·bol'·ic
hy'·per·me·tab'·o·lis'm
hy'·per·me'·tria
hy'·per·met'·rope
hy'·per·me·tro'·pia
hy'·per·me·tro'·pic
hy'·per·mne'·sia
hy'·per·mo·bil'·i·ty
hy'·per·mo·til'·i·ty
hy'·per·my'·o·to'·nia
hy'·per·na·sal'·i·ty
hy'·per·na·tre'·mia Brit. ·trae'·
hy'·per·na·tre'·mic Brit. ·trae'·
hy'·per·ne·phro'·ma pl. ·mas or ·ma·ta
hy'·per·ni·da'·tion
hy'·per·nu·tri'·tion
hy'·per·oc·clu'·sion
hy'·per·oes'·tro·gen·is'm Brit. spel. of hyperestrogenism
hy'·per·onych'·ia
hy'·per·ope
hy'·per·o'·pia
hy'·per·o'·pic
hy'·per·or'·chi·dis'm
hy'·per·or'·ni·the'·mia Brit. ·thae'·
hy'·per·os'·mia
hy'·per·os·mo'·lal
hy'·per·os·mo·lal'·i·ty
hy'·per·os·mo'·lar
hy'·per·os·mo·lar'·i·ty
hy'·per·os·mot'·ic
hy'·per·os·to'·sis
hy'·per·os·tot'·ic
hy'·per·ox'·a·lu'·ria
hy'·per·ox'·ia
hy'·per·ox'·ic
hy'·per·par'·a·site

hyperparasitic / hypervitaminosis — 130

hy′·per·par′·a·sit′·ic
hy′·per·par′·a·sit·is′m
hy′·per·par′a·thy′·roid
hy′·per·par′a·thy′·roid·is′m
hy′·per·path′·ia
hy′·per·path′·ic
hy′·per·pep′·sia
hy′·per·pep′·sin·e′·mia *Brit.* ·ae′·mia
hy′·per·per′·i·stal′·sis
hy′·per·per′·i·stal′·tic
hy′·per·pha′·gia
hy′·per·phag′·ic
hy′·per·pha·lan′·gism
hy′·per·phen′·yl·al′·a·nin·e′·mia *Brit.* ·ae′·mia
hy′·per·pho′·ria
hy′·per·phos′·pha·tas·e′·mia *Brit.* ·ae′·mia
hy′·per·phos′·pha·ta′·sia
hy′·per·phos′·pha·te′·mia *Brit.* ·tae′·
hy′·per·phos′·pha·tu′·ria
hy′·per·pi·e′sis *also* ·pi·e′sia
hy′·per·pi·et′·ic
hy′·per·pig′·men·ta′·tion
hy′·per·pi·tu′·i·tar·is′m
hy′·per·pi·tu′·i·tar′y
hy′·per·pla′·sia
hy′·per·plas′·mia
hy′·per·plas′·min·e′·mia *Brit.* ·ae′·mia
hy′·per·plas′·tic
hy′·per·ploid
hy′·per·ploi′·dy
hy′·per·pne′a *Brit.* ·pnoe′a
hy′·per·pne′·ic *Brit.* ·pnoe′·ic
hy′·per·po·lar·i·za′·tion
hy′·per·po·ne′·sis

hy′·per·po·tas′·se′·mia [·pot′·as·] *Brit.* ·sae′·
hy′·per·pre·be′·ta·lip′o·pro′·tein·e′·mia [·li′po·] *Brit.* ·ae′·mia
hy′·per·pro·lac′·tin·e′·mia *Brit.* ·ae′·mia
hy′·per·pro′·lin·e′·mia *Brit.* ·ae′·mia
hy′·per·pro·sex′·ia
hy′·per·pro′·tein·e′·mia *Brit.* ·ae′·mia
hy′·per·py·ret′·ic
hy′·per·py·rex′·ia
hy′·per·re·ac′·tive
hy′·per·re·ac′·tiv′·i·ty
hy′·per·re·flex′·ia
hy′·per·res′·o·nance
hy′·per·sa′·line
hy′·per·sal′·i·va′·tion
hy′·per·se·cre′·tion
hy′·per·seg′·ment·ed
hy′·per·sen′·si·tive
hy′·per·sen′·si·tiv′·i·ty
hy′·per·sen′·si·ti·za′·tion
hy′·per·se′·ro·to·ne′·mia *Brit.* ·nae′·
hy′·per·sex′·u·al′·i·ty
hy′·per·so′·ma·to·tro′·pism
hy′·per·som′·nia
hy′·per·splen′·ic
hy′·per·sple′·nism [·splen′·ism]
hy′·per·spon′·gi·o′·sis
hy′·per·ste′·a·to′·sis
hy′·per·sthe′·nia
hy′·per·sthen′·ic
hy′·per·sthen·u′·ria
hy′·per·sus·cep′·ti·bil′·i·ty
hy′·per·syn′·chro·nous
hy′·per·tel′·o·ris′m
hy′·per·ten′·sin
hy′·per·ten′·sin·ase

hy′·per·ten·sin′·o·gen
hy′·per·ten′·sion
hy′·per·ten′·sive
hy′·per·ten′·sor
hy′·per·tes·tos′·te·ron·is′m
hy′·per·the·co′·sis
hy′·per·the′·lia
hy′·per·ther′·mal
hy′·per·ther′·mia
hy′·per·ther′·mic
hy′·per·throm′·bin·e′·mia *Brit.* ·ae′·mia
hy′·per·thy′·mia
hy′·per·thy′·mism
hy′·per·thy′·roid
hy′·per·thy′·roid·is′m
hy′·per·thy·rox′·in·e′·mia [·i·ne′·mia] *Brit.* ·ae′·mia
hy′·per·to′·nia
hy′·per·ton′·ic
hy′·per·to·nic′·i·ty
hy′·per·to′·nus
hy′·per·tri·cho′·sis
hy′·per·tri·glyc′·er·i·de′·mia [·id·e′·mia] *Brit.* ·dae′·
hy′·per·tro′·phic [·troph′·ic]
hy′·per·tro′·phi·cum [·troph′·i·cum]
hy·per′·tro·phy
hy′·per·tro′·pia
hy′·per·u′·ri·ce′·mia *Brit.* ·cae′·
hy′·per·u′·ri·co·su′·ria
hy′·per·u′·ric·u′·ria
hy′·per·vac′·ci·na′·tion
hy′·per·val′·in·e′·mia *Brit.* ·ae′·mia
hy′·per·var′·i·a·ble
hy′·per·vas′·cu·lar
hy′·per·ven′·ti·late ·lat′·ed, ·lat′·ing
hy′·per·ven′·ti·la′·tion
hy′·per·vis·cos′·i·ty
hy′·per·vi′·ta·min·o′·sis

hy'·per·vol·e'·mia [·vo·le'·mia] *Brit.* ·ae'··mia
hy'·per·vol·e'·mic [·vo·le'·mic] *Brit.* ·ae'·mic
hyp'·es·the'·sia *Brit.* ·aes·the'·; *var. of* hypoesthesia
hyp'·es·thet'·ic *Brit.* ·aes·thet'·
hy'·pha
hy'·phal
hyp'·he·do'·nia
hy·phe'·ma *Brit.* ·phae'·
hy'·phyl·line
hyp'·na·gog'·ic
hyp'·na·gogue
hyp'·nic
hyp'·no·
hyp'·no·anal'·y·sis
hyp'·no·an'·es·the'·sia *Brit.* ·an'·aes·
hyp'·no·cin'·e·mat'·o·graph
hyp'·no·gen'·ic
hypnogogic *misspelling of* hypnagogic
hyp'·noid
hyp·nol'·o·gy
hyp'·no·pom'·pic
hyp·no'·sis
hyp'·no·ther'·a·py
hyp·not'·ic
hyp'·no·tis'm
hyp'·no·tize ·tized, ·tiz'·ing
hy'·po·
hy'·po·ac'·tive
hy'·po·ac·tiv'·i·ty
hy'·po·acu'·sis
hy'·po·adre'·nal·is'm
hy'·po·adre'·no·cor'·ti·cal
hy'·po·adre'·no·cor'·ti·cis'm

hy'·po·aes·the'·sia *Brit. spel. of* hypoesthesia
hy'·po·al·bu'·min·e'·mia *Brit.* ·ae'·mia
hy'·po·al·dos'·ter·on·e'·mia [·al'··do·ster'·] *Brit.* ·ae'·mia
hy'·po·al·dos'·ter·on·is'm [·al'··do·ster'·on·]
hy'·po·al·ge'·sia *var. of* hypalgesia
hy'·po·al'·i·men·ta'·tion
hy'·po·al'·ler·gen'·ic
hy'·po·ami'·no·ac'·id·e'·mia *Brit.* ·ae'·mia
hy'·po·an'·dro·gen·is'm
hy'·po·ar·te'·ri·al *var. of* hyparterial
hy'·po·bar'·ic
hy'·po·bar'·ism
hy'·po·be'·ta·lip'o·pro'·tein·e'·mia *Brit.* ·ae'·mia
hy'·po·blast
hy'·po·bou'·lia *also* ·bu'·lia
hy'·po·bran'·chi·al
hy'·po·cal·ce'·mia *Brit.* ·cae'·
hy'·po·cal'·cia
hy'·po·cal'·ci·fi·ca'·tion
hy'·po·cal'·ci·pex'y
hy'·po·cal'·ci·to·ne'·mia *Brit.* ·nae'·; *var. of* hypocalcitoninemia
hy'·po·cal'·ci·to'·nin·e'·mia *Brit.* ·ae'·mia
hy'·po·cal'·ci·u'·ria
hy'·po·cap'·nia
hy'·po·cap'·nic
hy'·po·cat'·a·las·e'·mia *Brit.* ·ae'·mia
hy'·po·cel'·lu·lar
hy'·po·cel'·lu·lar'·i·ty

hy'·po·ce·ru'·lo·plas'·min·e'·mia *Brit.* ·ae'·mia
hy'·po·chlo·re'·mia *Brit.* ·rae'·
hy'·po·chlor·hy'·dria
hy'·po·chlor·hy'·dric
hy'·po·chlo'·rite
hy'·po·chlo'·rous
hy'·po·chlor·u'·ria
hy'·po·cho·les'·ter·ol·e'·mia *Brit.* ·ae'·mia
hy'·po·chon'·dria
hy'·po·chon'·dri·ac
hy'·po·chon·dri'·a·ca
hy'·po·chon·dri'·a·cal
hy'·po·chon·dri'·a·sis
hy'·po·chon·dri·um *pl.* ·dria
hy'·po·chor'·dal [·chord'·al]
hy'·po·chro·ma'·sia
hy'·po·chro·mat'·ic
hy'·po·chro'·mia
hy'·po·chro'·mic
hy'·po·chy'·lia
hy'·po·cit·ru'·ria
hy'·po·co·ag'·u·la·bil'·i·ty
hy'·po·co·ag'·u·la·ble
hy'·po·com'·ple·men·te'·mia [·ment·e'·mia] *Brit.* ·tae'·mia
hy'·po·cu·pre'·mia *Brit.* ·prae'·mia
hy'·po·cy·clo'·sis
hy'·po·derm
Hy'·po·der'·ma
hy'·po·der'·ma
hy'·po·der'·mal
hy'·po·der·mat'·ic
hy'·po·der·mi'·a·sis
hy'·po·der'·mic
hy'·po·der'·mis
hy'·po·der·moc'·ly·sis *pl.* ·ses
hy'·po·der'·mo·my·co'·sis *pl.* ·ses

hypodiploid / hypophosphatemia

hy′·po·dip′·loid
hy′·po·dip′·loi·dy
hy′·po·don′·tia
hy′·po·dy·nam′·ia
hy′·po·dy·nam′·ic
hy′·po·ep′·i·neph′·rin·e′·mia *Brit.* ·ae′·mia
hy′·po·er′·gia
hy′·po·er′·gic
hy′·po·er′·gy
hy′·po·es′o·pho′·ria
hy′·po·es·the′·sia *Brit.* ·aes·hy′·po·es′·tro·gen·e′·mia *Brit.* hy′·po·oes′·tro·gen·ae′·mia
hy′·po·es′·tro·gen·is′m *Brit.* hy′·po·oes′·tro·hy′·po·ex·cit′·a·bil′·i·ty
hy′·po·ex·cit′·a·ble
hy′·po·ex′o·pho′·ria
hy′·po·fer·re′·mia *Brit.* ·rae′·mia
hy′·po·fi·brin′·o·gen·e′·mia *Brit.* ·ae′·mia
hy′·po·fun′·ction
hy′·po·ga·lac′·tia
hy′·po·gam′·ma·glob′·u·lin·e′·mia *Brit.* ·ae′·mia
hy′·po·gas′·tric
hy′·po·gas′·tri·cus *fem.* ·ca
hy′·po·gas′·tri·um
hy′·po·gas·trop′·a·gus
hy′·po·gas·tros′·chi·sis
hy′·po·gen′·e·sis
hy′·po·gen′·i·tal·is′m
hy′·po·geu′·sia
hy′·po·glos′·sal
hy′·po·glos′·si·ca
hy′·po·glos′·sus *gen.* ·si, *ablative* ·so
hy′·po·glot′·tis
hy′·po·gly·ce′·mia *Brit.* ·cae′·
hy′·po·gly·ce′·mic *Brit.* ·cae′·

hy′·po·go·nad′·al
hy′·po·go′·nad·is′m
hy′·po·go·nad′·o·tro′·phic [·troph′·ic] *var. of* hypogonadotropic
hy′·po·go·nad′·o·tro′·phism *var. of* hypogonadotropism
hy′·po·go·nad′·o·tro′·pic [·gon′·a·do·, ·trop′·ic]
hy′·po·go·nad′·o·tro′·pism [·gon′·a·do·]
hy′·po·hi·dro′·sis
hy′·po·hi·drot′·ic
hy′·po·hy′·al
hy′·po·hy·dra′·tion
hy′·po·hyp·not′·ic
hy′·po·idro′·sis *var. of* hypohidrosis
hy′·po·in′·su·lin·e′·mia *Brit.* ·ae′·mia
hy′·po·in′·su·lin·is′m
hy′·po·ka·le′·mia *Brit.* ·lae′·
hy′·po·ka·le′·mic *Brit.* ·lae′·
hy′·po·kal′·i·e′·mia *var. of* hypokalemia; *Brit.* ·ae′·mia
hy′·po·ki·ne′·mia *Brit.* ·nae′·
hy′·po·ki·ne′·sia *also* ·ne′·sis
hy′·po·ki·net′·ic
hy′·po·lem′·mal
hy′·po·le′·thal
hy′·po·ley′·dig·is′m
hy′·po·li·pe′·mia *Brit.* ·pae′·mia
hy′·po·lip′o·pro′·tein·e′·mia [·li′po·] *Brit.* ·ae′·mia
hy′·po·lu·te′·mia *Brit.* ·tae′·
hy′·po·mag′·ne·se′·mia *Brit.* ·sae′·

hy′·po·ma′·nia
hy′·po·man′·ic
hy′·po·mas′·tia
hy′·po·mel′·a·nis′m
hy′·po·mel′·a·no′·sis
hy′·po·men′·or·rhe′a *Brit.* ·rhoe′a
hy′·po·mere
hy′·po·mer′·ic
hy′·po·met′·a·bol′·ic
hy′·po·me·tab′·o·lis′m
hy′·po·me′·tria
hy′·po·min′·er·al·i·za′·tion
hy′·po·morph
hy′·po·mo·til′·i·ty
hy′·po·na·sal′·i·ty
hy′·po·na·tre′·mia *Brit.* ·trae′·
hy′·po·na·tru′·ria
hy′·po·nych′·i·al
hy′·po·nych′·i·um *pl.* ·ia
hy·pon′·y·chon
hy′·po-on·cot′·ic
hy′·po-os·mo′·lar
hy′·po-os·mo′·sis
hy′·po-os·mot′·ic
hy′·po-ovar′·i·an·is′m
hy′·po·pal′·les·the′·sia *Brit.* ·laes·the′·
hy′·po·pan′·cre·a·tis′m
hy′·po·par′a·thy′·roid
hy′·po·par′a·thy′·roid·is′m
hy′·po·pep′·sia
hy′·po·pep′·tic
hy′·po·pex′·ia *also* hy′·po·pex′y
hy′·po·pha·lan′·gism
hy′·po·pha·ryn′·ge·al
hy′·po·phar′·ynx
hy′·po·pho′·nia
hy′·po·pho′·ria
hy′·po·phos′·pha·ta′·sia
hy′·po·phos′·pha·te′·mia *Brit.* ·tae′·

hy'·po·phos'·pha·tu'·
ria
hy'·po·phos'·phite
hy'·po·phre'·nia
hy'·po·phren'·ic
hy'·po·phys'·e·al
[hy·poph'·y·se'·al]
var. of hypophysial
hy·poph'·y·sec'·to·
mize
hy·poph'·y·sec'·to·my
also hy'·po·phys'·i·ec'·
to·my
hy'·po·phys'·eo·por'·
tal also ·phys'·io·
hy'·po·phys'·i·al
hy'·po·phys'·i·a'·lis
hy·poph'·y·sin
hy'·po·phys'·io·di'·en·
ce·phal'·ic
hy'·po·phys'·i·o·pri'·va
hy'·po·phys'·i·o·tro'·
pic [·trop'·ic]
hy·poph'·y·sis pl. ·ses
hy·poph'·y·si'·tis
hy'·po·pig'·men·ta'·
tion
hy'·po·pi·tu'·i·tar·is'm
hy'·po·pi·tu'·i·tar'y
hy'·po·pla'·sia
hy'·po·plas'·tic
hy'·po·ploid
hy'·po·ploi'·dy
hy'·po·pne'a [hy·pop'·
nea] Brit. ·pnoe'a
hy'·po·po·tas'·se'·mia
[·pot'·as·] Brit.
·sae'·
hy'·po·po·tas'·se'·mic
[·pot'·as·] Brit.
·sae'·
hy'·po·pro'·ac·cel'·er·
in·e'·mia Brit. ·ae'·
mia
hy'·po·pro'·con·ver'·
tin·e'·mia Brit. ·ae'·
mia
hy'·po·pro·ges'·ter·one

hy'·po·pro'·tein·e'·mia
Brit. ·ae'·mia
hy'·po·pro'·tein·e'·mic
Brit. ·ae'·mic
hy'·po·pro·throm'·bin·
e'·mia Brit. ·ae'·mia
hy'·po·psel'·a·phe'·sia
hy·po'·pus [hy'·po·]
pl. ·pi
hy·po'·py·on
hy'·po·re·ac'·tive
hy'·po·re·flex'·ia
hy'·po·ren'·in·e'·mic
Brit. ·ae'·mic
hy'·po·ri'·bo·fla'·vin·
o'·sis
hy'·po·sar'·ca
hy·pos'·che·ot'·o·my
hy'·po·scle'·ral
hy'·po·se·cre'·tion
hy'·po·sen'·si·tive
hy'·po·sen'·si·tiv'·i·ty
hy'·po·sen'·si·ti·za'·
tion
hy'·po·sen'·si·tize
·tized, ·tiz'·ing
hy·pos'·mia
hy'·po·so'·ma·to·tro'·
pism
hy'·po·so'·mia
hy'·po·som'·nia
hy'·po·spa'·di·ac
hy'·po·spa'·di·as also
·spa'·dia
hy'·pos·phre'·sia
hy·pos'·ta·sis
hy'·po·stat'·ic
hy'·po·sthe'·nia
hy'·po·sthe'·ni·ant
hy'·po·sthen'·ic
hy'·po·sthen·u'·ria [hy·
pos'·then·]
hy'·po·stome
hy'·po·sul'·fite
hy'·po·su'·pra·re'·nal·
is'm
hy'·po·tel'·o·ris'm
hy'·po·ten'·sion

hy'·po·ten'·sive
hy'·po·thal'·a·mi pl.
& gen. sg. of hypo-
thalamus
hy'·po·tha·lam'·ic
hy'·po·tha·lam'·i·cus
fem. ·ca
hy'·po·thal'·a·mo·hy'·
po·phys'·i·al
hy'·po·thal'·a·mo·neu'·
ro·hy'·po·phys'·i·al
hy'·po·thal'·a·mot'·o·
my
hy'·po·thal'·a·mus pl.
& gen. sg. ·mi
hy'·po·the'·nar [hy·
poth'·e·nar]
hy'·po·ther'·mal
hy'·po·ther'·mia also
hy'·po·ther'·my
hy·poth'·e·sis pl. ·ses
hy'·po·throm'·bo·plas·
tin·e'·mia Brit. ·ae'·
mia
hy'·po·thy'·mia
hy'·po·thy'·roid
hy'·po·thy'·roid·is'm
hy'·po·to'·nia
hy'·po·ton'·ic
hy'·po·to·nic'·i·ty
hy'·po·to'·nus
hy·pot'·o·ny var. of
hypotonia
hy'·po·trans'·fer·rin·e'·
mia Brit. ·ae'·mia
hy'·po·tri·cho'·sis
also ·chi'·a·sis
hy·pot'·ro·phy
hy'·po·tro'·pia
hy'·po·tym·pan'·ic
hy'·po·tym'·pa·num
hy'·po·u'·ri·co·su'·ria
var. of hypouricuria
hy'·po·u'·ric·u'·ria
hy'·po·va'·so·pres'·sin·
e'·mia Brit. ·ae'·mia
hy'·po·ven'·ti·la'·tion
hy'·po·vi·gil'·i·ty

hy'·po·vi'·ta·min·o'·sis
hy'·po·vol·e'·mia [·vo·
 le'·] *Brit.* ·ae'·mia
hy'·po·vol·e'·mic [·vo·
 le'·] *Brit.* ·ae'·mic;
 *with low blood volume:
 Cf.* hypovolumic
hy'·po·vo'·lia
hy'·po·vol·u'·mic [·vo·
 lu'·] *with low
 volume: Cf.* hypovo-
 lemic
hy'·po·xan'·thine
hy'·pox·e'·mia *Brit.*
 ·ae'·mia
hy·pox'·ia
hy·pox'·ic
hyps·ar·rhyth'·mia
hyp'·si· *var. of* hypso-
hyp'·si·ce·phal'·ic
hyp'·si·loid
hyp'·si·loid
hyp'·so·
hyp'·so·chro'·mic
hys'·ter·atre'·sia
hys'·ter·ec'·to·mize
 ·mized, ·miz'·ing
hys'·ter·ec'·to·my
hys'·ter·e'·sis
hys'·ter·et'·ic
hys'·ter·eu·ryn'·ter
hys'·ter·eu'·ry·sis
hys·te'·ria
hys·ter'·ic
hys·ter'·i·cal
hys·ter'·i·cus
hys·ter'·i·form
hys'·tero·
hys'·tero·col·pec'·to·
 my
hys'·tero·col'·po·scope
hys'·tero·cys'·to·clei'·
 sis
hys'·tero·ep'·i·lep'·sy
hys'·ter·o·gen'·ic
hys'·ter·o·gram
hys'·ter·o·graph
hys'·ter·og'·ra·phy

hys'·ter·oid
hys'·ter·om'·e·ter
hys'·ter·om'·e·try
hys'·tero-o'o·pho·rec'·
 to·my
hys'·ter·o·pex'y
hys'·ter·o'·pia
hys'·ter·o·plas'·ty
hys'·ter·or'·rha·phy
hys'·tero·sal'·pin·gec'·
 to·my
hys'·tero·sal'·pin·gog'·
 ra·phy
hys'·tero·sal'·pin·go-
 o'o·pho·rec'·to·my
hys'·tero·sal'·pin·gos'·
 to·my
hys'·tero·sal'·pinx *pl.*
 ·sal·pin'·ges
hys'·ter·o·scope
hys'·ter·os'·co·py
hys'·tero·sto·mat'·o·my
hys'·ter·ot'·o·my
hys'·tero·trach'·e·lo·
 plas'·ty
hys'·trix

I

i'a·ma·tol'·o·gy
i'a·tra·lip'·tic
iat'·ric
iat'·ro· [i'a·tro·]
iat'·ro·chem'·is·try
iat'·ro·gen'·e·sis
iat'·ro·gen'·ic
iat'·ro·tech'·ni·cal
ibo'·ga·ine
i'bu·pro'·fen
i'chor
i'chor·ous
ich'·tham·mol
ich'·thyo·
ich'·thy·oid
ich'·thyo·sar'·co·tox'·
 in

ich'·thyo·sar'·co·tox'·
 ism
ich'·thy·o'·si·form
ich'·thy·o'·sis
ich'·thyo·sul'·fo·nate
 Brit. ·sul'·pho·
ich'·thy·ot'·ic *also*
 ·o'·sic
ich'·thyo·tox'·i·col'·o·
 gy
ich'·thyo·tox'·in
ico'·sa·
ico'·sa·he'·dral
ico'·sa·noid
ic'·tal
ic·ter'·ic
ic'·tero·
ic'·tero·ane'·mia *Brit.*
 ·anae'·
ic'·ter·o·gen'·ic
ic'·tero·hem'·or·rhag'·
 ic *Brit.* ·haem'·
ic'·ter·oid
ic'·ter·us
ic·tom'·e·ter
ic'·tus *pl.* ictus
i'de·a'·tion
idée' fixe' *pl.* idées'
 fixes'
i'deo·
i'deo·ge·net'·ic
i'deo·ki·net'·ic
i'deo·mo'·tor
i'deo·mus'·cu·lar *of
 mentally activated
 muscle movement: Cf.*
 idiomuscular
id'·io·
id'·io·chro'·mo·some
id'·i·o·cy
id'·i·o·glos'·sia
id'·i·o·glot'·tic
id'·i·o·gram
id'·i·o·graph'·ic
id'·io·mus'·cu·lar
 *exclusive to muscular
 tissue: Cf.* ideomus-
 cular

id′·io·nod′·al [·no′·dal]
id′·i·o·path′·ic
id′·i·op′·a·thy
id′·i·o·plas′m
id′·io·ret′·i·nal
id′·i·o·some
id′·i·o·syn′·cra·sy
id′·i·o·syn·crat′·ic
id′·i·ot
id′·i·o·tope
id′·i·ot sa·vant′ *pl.*
 idiots savants
id′·i·o·type
id′·io·ven·tric′·u·lar
i′di·tol
i′dose
i′dox·u′ri·dine
i′du·ro·nate
i′du·ron′·ic
ig·na′·tia
ig′·ni·ex′·tir·pa′·tion
ig′·ni·op′·er·a′·tion
ig′·ni·pe·di′·tes
ig′·ni·punc′·ture
il′·e·al *also* ·ac
il′·e·a′lis *pl.* ·a″les
il′e·ec′·to·my
il′e·i′tis
il′·eo *denoting the ileum of the intestine: Cf.* ilio-
il′·eo·cae·ca′·lis *neut.*
 ·le; *also* ·ce·ca′·
il′·eo·ce′·cal Brit.
 ·cae′·cal
il′·eo·ce·cos′·to·my
 Brit. ·cae·cos′·
il′·eo·co′·lic
il′·eo·co′·li·ca *fem. of* ileocolicus; *pl. & gen. sg.* ·cae
il′·eo·co′·li·cus *pl.* ·ci
il′·eo·co·li′·tis
il′·eo·co·lon′·ic
il′·eo·co·los′·to·my
il′·eo·co·lot′·o·my
il′·eo·cys′·to·plas′·ty
il′·eo·cys·tos′·to·my

il′·eo·gas′·tric
il′·eo·il′·e·os′·to·my
il′·eo·je·ju′·nal
il′·eo·je′·ju·ni′·tis
il′·e·o·pex′y
il′·eo·proc·tos′·to·my
il′·e·or′·rha·phy
il′·eo·sig′·moid
il′·eo·sig′·moid·os′·to·my
il′·e·os′·to·my
il′·e·ot′·o·my
il′·eo·trans·verse′
il′·eo·trans′·vers·os′·to·my
il′·eo·typh·li′·tis
il′·e·um *part of small intestine: Cf.* ilium
il′·e·us
il′·ia *pl. of* ilium
il′·i·ac
ili′·a·ca *fem. of* iliacus; *pl. & gen. sg.* ·cae
ili′·a·cus *pl. & gen. sg.* ·ci
i′li·cin
il′·ii *gen. of* ilium
il′·io *denoting part of the hip bone: Cf.* ileo-
il′·io·coc·cyg′·e·al
il′·io·coc·cyg′·e·us
il′·io·cos′·tal
il′·io·cos·ta′·lis
il′·io·cos′·to·cer′·vi·ca′·lis
il′·io·fem′·o·ral
il′·io·fem′·o·ra′·le
il′·io·fem′·o·ro·plas′·ty
il′·io·hy′·po·gas′·tric
il′·io·hy′·po·gas′·tri·cus *pl. & gen. sg.* ·ci
il′·io·in′·gui·nal
il′·io·in′·gui·na′·lis
il′·io·lum·ba′·lis *neut.* ·le
il′·io·lum′·bar
il′·i·op′·a·gus

il′·io·par′·a·si′·tus
il·io·pec·tin′·ea
il′·io·pec·tin′·e·al
il′·io·pec·tin′·e·a′lis *neut.* ·a″le
il′·io·pec·tin′·e·us *fem.* ·tin′·ea
il′·io·pso′·as
il′·io·pu′·bic
il′·io·pu′·bi·ca
il′·io·sa′·cral
il′·io·spi′·nal
il′·io·tho′·ra·cop′·a·gus
il′·io·tib′·i·al
il′·io·tib′·i·a′·lis
il′·io·tro′·chan·ter′·ic
il′·i·um *part of hip bone: Cf.* ileum; *pl.* il′·ia, *gen. sg.* il′·ii
ill′·ness
il·lu′·mi·nant
il·lu′·mi·na′·tion
il·lu′·mi·na′·tor
il·lu′·sion
i′ma *fem. of* imus; *pl.* i′mae
im′·age
im′·age·ry
im′·ag·ing
ima′·go *pl.* ·gi·nes *or* ·gos *or* ·goes
im·bal′·ance
im′·be·cile
im′·be·cil′·ic
im′·be·cil′·i·ty
im·bed′ ·bed′·ded, ·bed′·ding; *var. of* embed
im′·bi·bi′·tion
im′·bri·cate ·cat′·ed, ·cat′·ing
im′·bri·ca′·tion
im′·id·am′·ine
im′·id·az′·ole
im′·id·az′·o·line
im′·ide
im′·i·do·
im′·i·do·suc′·ci·nate

im′·ine
im′·i·no
im′·i·no·gly′·cin·u′·ria
imip′·ra·mine
im′·ma·ture′
im′·ma·tu′·ri·ty
im·med′·i·ca·ble
im·mer′·sion
im·mis′·ci·ble
im·mo′·bi·li·za′·tion
im·mo′·bi·lize ·lized,
·liz′·ing
im·mune′
im·mu′·ni·fa′·cient
im·mu′·ni·ty
im′·mu·ni·za′·tion
im′·mu·nize ·nized,
·niz′·ing
im′·mu·no [im·mu′·no·]
im′·mu·no·ad′·ju·vant
im′·mu·no·ad·sor′·bent
[·sorb′·ent]
im′·mu·no·ad·sorp′·tion
im′·mu·no·ag·glu′·ti·na′·tion
im′·mu·no·as·say′
[·as′·say]
im′·mu·no·bi·ol′·o·gy
im′·mu·no·blast
im′·mu·no·blas′·tic
im′·mu·no·chem′·i·cal
im′·mu·no·chem′·is·try
im′·mu·no·com′·pe·tence
im′·mu·no·com′·pe·tent
im′·mu·no·com′·pro·mised
im′·mu·no·con·glu′·ti·nin
im′·mu·no·cyte
im′·mu·no·cy′·to·ad·her′·ence
im′·mu·no·cy′·to·chem′·is·try
im′·mu·no·cy·tol′·o·gy

im′·mu·no·de·fi′·cien·cy
im′·mu·no·de·fi′·cient
im′·mu·no·de·pres′·sant
im′·mu·no·de·pres′·sion
im′·mu·no·de·pres′·sive
im′·mu·no·di′·ag·no′·sis *pl.* ·ses
im′·mu·no·dif·fu′·sion
im′·mu·no·dom′·i·nant
im′·mu·no·elec′·tro·pho·re′·sis
im′·mu·no·fer′·ri·tin
im′·mu·no·fil·tra′·tion
im′·mu·no·fluo·res′·cence
im′·mu·no·fluo·res′·cent
im′·mu·no·gen
im′·mu·no·ge·net′·ics
im′·mu·no·gen′·ic
im′·mu·no·ge·nic′·i·ty
im′·mu·no·glob′·u·lin
im′·mu·no·he′·ma·tol′·o·gy *Brit.* ·hae′·ma·
im′·mu·no·he′·mo·lyt′·ic *Brit.* ·hae′·
im′·mu·no·his′·to·chem′·i·cal
im′·mu·no·log′·ic *also* ·i·cal
im′·mu·nol′·o·gist
im′·mu·nol′·o·gy
im′·mu·no·path′·o·log′·ic *also* ·i·cal
im′·mu·no·pa·thol′·o·gy
im′·mu·no·per·ox′·i·dase
im′·mu·no·pho·re′·sis
im′·mu·no·pre·cip′·i·ta′·tion
im′·mu·no·pro·lif′·er·a·tive

im′·mu·no·pro′·phy·lax′·is
im′·mu·no·re·ac′·tion
im′·mu·no·re·ac′·tive
im′·mu·no·re′·ac·tiv′·i·ty
im′·mu·no·se·lec′·tion
im′·mu·no·se·nes′·cence
im′·mu·no·sor′·bent
im′·mu·no·sup·pres′·sant
im′·mu·no·sup·pres′·sion
im′·mu·no·sup·pres′·sive
im′·mu·no·sur·veil′·lance
im′·mu·no·sym′·pa·thec′·to·my
im′·mu·no·ther′·a·py
im′·pact
im·pact′·ed
im·pac′·tion
im·pac′·tor
im·paired′
im·pair′·ment
im·pal′·pa·ble
im′·par
im·pa′·ten·cy
im·pa′·tent
im·ped′·ance
im·per′·a·tive
im′·per·cep′·tion
im′·per·fec′·ta
im·per′·fo·rate
im·per′·me·a·ble
im′·pe·tig′·i·ni·za′·tion
im′·pe·tig′·i·noid
im′·pe·tig′·i·nous
im·pe·ti′·go *pl.* im′·pe·tig′·i·nes
im′·plant *n.*
im·plant′ *v.*
im′·plan·ta′·tion
im′·plan·tol′·o·gist
im′·plan·tol′·o·gy
im·plo′·sion

im·plo′·sive
im′·po·tence *also*
  ·ten·cy
im·preg′·nate ·nat·ed,
  ·nat·ing
im′·preg·na′·tion
im·pres′·sio *pl.* im·
  pres′·si·o′·nes
im·pres′·sion
im·pres′·sum
im·print′·ing
im·pro′·cre·ance
im′·pulse
im·pul′·sion
im·pul′·sive
i′mu
i′mus
in·ac′·ti·vate ·vat′·ed,
  ·vat′·ing
in·ac′·ti·va′·tion
in·ac′·ti·va′·tor
in′·ag·glu′·ti·na·ble
in·an′·i·mate
in′·a·ni′·tion
in′·ap·par′·ent
in·ap′·pe·tence *also*
  ·ten·cy
in ar·tic′·u·lo mor′·tis
in′·as·sim′·i·la·ble
in′·at·ten′·tion
in′·born
in′·bred
in′·breed·ing
in′·ca *also* In′·ca
in·cap′·a·ri′·na
in·car′·cer·at′·ed
in·car′·cer·a′·tion
in·car′·i·al
in·car′·na·tive
in′·car·na′·tus
in·cep′·tus *pl.*
  inceptus
in·cer′·ta *gen.* ·tae
in·cer′·tae se′·dis

in′·cest
in·ces′·tu·ous
in′·ci·dence
in′·ci·dent
in·cin′·er·ate ·at′·ed,
  ·at′·ing
in·cin′·er·a′·tion
in·cip′·i·ent
in·ci′·sal
in·cise′ ·cised′, ·cis′·
  ing
in·ci′·sion
in′·ci·si′·va *fem. of*
  incisivus
in·ci′·sive
in′·ci·si′·vum *neut. of*
  incisivus
in′·ci·si′·vus *pl.* ·vi
in·ci′·sor
in′·ci·su′·ra *pl. & gen.*
  sg. ·rae
in·ci′·su·ral [·ci·su′·]
in·ci′·sure
in·cit′·ant
in′·cli·na′·tio
in·cli·na′·tion
in′·cli·nom′·e·ter
in·clu′·sion
in′·co·ag′·u·la·bil′·i·ty
in′·co·ag′·u·la·ble
in·com′·i·tance
in·com′·i·tant
in′·com·pat′·i·bil′·i·ty
in′·com·pat′·i·ble
in′·com·pe·tence *also*
  ·ten·cy
in·com′·pe·tent
in′·con·gru′·ence
in·con′·ti·nence
in·con′·ti·nent
in′·con·ti·nen′·tia
in′·co·or′·di·na′·tion
in′·cre·ment
in′·cre·men′·tal

in′·cross
in′·crus·ta′·tion
in·crust′·ed
in′·cu·bate ·bat′·ed,
  ·bat′·ing
in′·cu·ba′·tion
in′·cu·ba′·tor
in′·cu·bus *pl.* ·bi *or*
  ·bus·es
in′·cu·dal
in·cu′·dis *gen. of*
  incus
in·cu′·di·us
in′·cu·do·mal′·le·ar
  also ·mal′·le·al, ·mal·
  le′·o·lar
in′·cu·do·mal′·le·a′ris
in′·cu·do·sta·pe′·dia
in′·cu·do·sta·pe′·di·al
in·cur′·a·ble
in′·cur·va′·tion
in′·cus *pl.* in·cu′·des,
  gen. sg. in·cu′·dis
in·cy′·clo·de′·vi·a′·tion
in·cy′·clo·pho′·ria
in·cy′·clo·tro′·pia
in·cy′·clo·ver′·gence
in′·den·ta′·tion
in′·de·ter′·mi·nate
in′·dex[31] *pl.* in′·di·ces,
  gen. sg. in′·di·cis
in′·di·can
in′·di·can·e′·mia *Brit.*
  ·ae′·mia
in′·di·cant
in′·di·can·u′·ria
in′·di·cate ·cat′·ed,
  ·cat′·ing
in′·di·ca′·tion
in′·di·ca′·tor
in′·di·ces *pl. of* index
in′·di·cis *gen. of* index
in·dig′·e·nous
in′·di·gest′·i·ble

---

[31] When referring to the index of a book, the plural form *indexes* is more common, but in disciplines such as anatomy or statistics, only *indices* is used.

in'·di·ges'·tion
in·dig'·i·ta'·tion
in'·di·go
in'·di·go'·tin [in·dig'·o·tin]
in'·di·ru'·bin
in'·di·ru'·bin·u'·ria
in·dis'·po·si'·tion
in'·di·um
in'·di·vid'·u·al·i·za'·tion
in'·di·vid'·u·a'·tion
in'·do·cy'·a·nine
in'·dole
in'·do·lent
in'·do·lyl·acryl'·o·yl·gly'·cine
in'·do·meth'·a·cin
in'·do·phe'·nol
in·dox'·yl
in·dox'·yl·e'·mia *Brit.* ·ae'·mia
in·dox'·yl·u'·ria
in·duce' ·duced', ·duc'·ing
in·duc'·er
in·duc'·i·ble
in·duc'·tance [·duct'·ance]
in·duc'·tion
in·duc'·tive
in·duc'·tor
in·duc'·to·therm
in·duc'·to·ther'·my
in'·du·lin *also* ·line
in'·du·rat'·ed
in'·du·ra'·tion
in'·du·ra·tive
in'·du·ra'·tum
in·du'·si·um
in'·dwell·ing
in·e'·bri·ant
in·e'·bri·a'·tion
in'·e·bri'·ety
in'·elas'·tic
in·ert'
in·er'·tia
in'·ex·cit'·a·bil'·i·ty
in'·ex·cit'·a·ble
in ex·tre'·mis
in'·fan·cy
in'·fans *gen. pl.* in·fan'·tum
in'·fant
in·fan'·ti·cide
in'·fan·tile
in'·fan·ti'·lis
in'·fan·til·is'·m [in·fan'·]
in·fan'·tum *gen. pl. of* infans
in'·farct
in·farc'·tion
in·fect'
in·fec'·tion
in·fec'·ti·o'·sus *fem.* ·sa, *neut.* ·sum
in·fec'·tious
in·fec'·tious·ness
in·fec'·tive
in'·fec·tiv'·i·ty
in'·fe·cun'·di·ty
in·fe'·ri·or *pl.* in·fe'·ri·o'·res, *gen. sg.* ·o'·ris, *ablative* ·o'·ri
in·fe'·ri·or'·i·ty
in·fe'·ri·us *neut. of* inferior
in'·fero·
in'·fero·cos'·tal
in'·fero·fron'·tal
in'·fero·lat'·er·al
in'·fero·lat'·er·a'·lis
in'·fero·me'·di·al
in'·fero·me'·di·an
in'·fero·pa·ri'·etal
in'·fero·pos·te'·ri·or
in·fer'·tile
in'·fer·til'·i·ty
in·fest'
in'·fes·ta'·tion
in·fib'·u·la'·tion
in·fil'·trate [in'·fil·] ·trat·ed, ·trat·ing
in'·fil·tra'·tion
in·firm'
in·fir'·ma·ry
in·fir'·mi·ty
in·flame' ·flamed', ·flam'·ing
in'·flam·ma'·tion
in·flam'·ma·to'·ria
in·flam'·ma·to·ry
in·fla'·tion
in·fla'·tor
in·flec'·tion *also* in·flex'·ion
in'·flu·en'·za
in'·flu·en'·zal
in'·flux
in·fold' [in'·fold]
in'·fra·
in'·fra·al·ve'·o·lar
in'·fra·au·ric'·u·la'·ris *pl.* ·res
in'·fra·ax'·il·lar'y
in'·fra·cal'·ca·ri'·nus
in'·fra·car'·di·ac
in'·fra·class'
in'·fra·cla·vic'·u·lar
in'·fra·cla·vic'·u·la'·ris
in'·fra·cli'·noid
in'·fra·clu'·sion
in'·fra·cos'·tal
in'·fra·cot'·y·loid
in·frac'·tion
in'·fra·den·ta'·le
in'·fra·duc'·tion
in'·fra·gle'·noid
in'·fra·gle'·noi·da'·lis *neut.* ·le
in'·fra·glot'·tic
in'·fra·glot'·ti·cus *fem.* ·ca, *neut.* ·cum
in'·fra·gran'·u·lar
in'·fra·hy'·oid
in'·fra·hy·oi'·dea *fem. of* infrahyoideus
in'·fra·hy·oi'·de·us *pl. & gen. sg.* ·dei
in'·fra·mam·ma'·ria
in'·fra·mam'·ma·ry
in·fra·man·dib'·u·lar
in'·fra·na'·tant

in'·fra·nod'·al [·no'·dal]
in'·fra·nu'·cle·ar
in'·fra·oc·cip'·i·tal
in'·fra·or'·bi·tal
in'·fra·or'·bi·ta'·lis
in'·fra·pa·tel'·lar
in'·fra·pat'·el·la'·ris *neut.* ·re
in'·fra·pop·lit'·e·al [·pop'·li·te'·al]
in'·fra·red'
in'·fra·scap'·u·la'·ris
in'·fra·seg·men'·tal
in'·fra·son'·ic
in'·fra·sound
in'·fra·spe·cif'·ic
in'·fra·spi·na'·ta *fem. of* infraspinatus
in'·fra·spi·na'·tus *gen.* ·ti
in'·fra·spi'·nous
in'·fra·ster'·nal
in'·fra·ster·na'·lis
in'·fra·tem'·po·ral
in'·fra·tem'·po·ra'·lis
in'·fra·ten·to'·ri·al
in'·fra·troch'·le·ar
in'·fra·troch'·le·a'·ris
in'·fra·um·bil'·i·cal
in'·fra·ver'·sion
in'·fun·dib'·u·lar
in'·fun·dib'·u·lec'·to·my
in'·fun·dib'·u·li·form
in'·fun·dib'·u·lo·hy'·po·phys'·i·al
in'·fun·dib'·u·lo-ovar'·i·an
in'·fun·dib'·u·lo·pel'·vic
in'·fun·dib'·u·lo·ven·tric'·u·lar
in'·fun·dib'·u·lum *pl.* ·la, *gen. sg.* ·li
in·fuse' ·fused', ·fus'·ing
in·fus'·i·ble
in·fu'·sion
in·fu'·sor
In'·fu·so'·ria
in·gest'
in·ges'·ta
in·ges'·tant
in·ges'·tion
in·ges'·tive
in'·gra·ves'·cent
in'·guen *pl.* in'·gui·nes, *gen. sg.* in'·gui·nis
in'·gui·nal
in'·gui·na'·le *neut. of* inguinalis
in'·gui·na'·lis *pl.* ·les
in'·gui·no·
in'·gui·no·cru'·ral
in'·gui·no·fem'·o·ral
in'·gui·no·la'·bi·al
in'·gui·no·scro'·tal
in·hal'·ant *also* ·ent
in'·ha·la'·tion
in·hale' ·haled', ·hal'·ing
in·hal'·er
in·her'·i·tance
in·hib'·in
in·hib'·it
in'·hi·bi'·tion
in·hib'·i·tive
in·hib'·i·tor *also* ·it·er
in·hib'·i·to'·ry
in'·ho'·mo·ge·ne'·ity
in'·ho'·mo·ge'·ne·ous
in'·i·al
in'·i·en·ceph'·a·ly
in'·i·on
in'·i·op'·a·gus
ini'·ti·a'·tor
in·ject'
in·ject'·a·ble
in·jec'·tion
in·jec'·tor
in'·jure ·jured, ·jur·ing
in'·ju·ry
in'·lay
in'·let
in·nate'
in·na'·tus
in'·ner·vate ·vat'·ed, ·vat'·ing
in'·ner·va'·tion
in·nid'·i·a'·tion
in'·no·cent
in·noc'·u·ous
in·nom'·i·nate
in·nom'·i·na'·tus *fem. sg. & neut. pl.* ·ta, *neut. sg.* ·tum
in·nox'·ious
in'o·
in·oc'·u·la *pl. of* inoculum
in·oc'·u·la·bil'·i·ty
in·oc'·u·la·ble
in·oc'·u·la'·ta
in·oc'·u·late ·lat'·ed, ·lat'·ing
in·oc'·u·la'·tion
in·oc'·u·la·tive
in·oc'·u·la'·tor
in·oc'·u·lum *pl.* ·la
in'·o·cyte
in'o·gen'·e·sis
in·op'·er·a·ble
in'·or·gan'·ic
in·os'·cu·late ·lat'·ed, ·lat'·ing
in·os'·cu·la'·tion
in'·o·se'·mia *Brit.* ·sae'·
in'·o·sine
in'·o·sin'·ic
ino'·si·tol
ino'·si·tu'·ria *also* in'·o·su'·ria
in'·o·tro'·pic [·trop'·ic]
in o'vo
in'·pa·tient
in'·qui·line
in·sal'·i·va'·tion
in'·sa·lu'·bri·ous
in·sane'
in·san'·i·tar'y
in·san'·i·ty

in·scrip′·tio *pl.* in·scrip′·ti·o′·nes
in·scrip′·tion
in′·sect
In·sec′·ta
in·sec′·ti·cide
in·sec′·ti·fuge
In′·sec·tiv′·o·ra
in·sec′·ti·vore
in′·sec·tiv′·o·rous
in·sem′·i·na′·tion
in·sen′·si·ble
in·sen′·si·tiv′·i·ty
in·sert′ *v.*
in′·sert *n.*
in·ser′·tio
in·ser′·tion
in·ser′·tion·al
in·sid′·i·ous
in·sip′·i·dus
in si′·tu
in′·so·la′·tion
in·sol′·u·ble
in·som′·nia
in·som′·ni·ac
in·spec′·tion
in·sper′·sion
in′·spi·ra′·tion
in′·spi·ra′·tor
in·spi′·ra·to′·ry [in′·spi·]
in·spire′ ·spired′, ·spir′·ing
in·spis′·sate [in′·spis·] ·sat·ed, ·sat·ing
in′·spis·sa′·tion
in·spis′·sa·tor [in′·spis·]
in′·sta·bil′·i·ty
in′·step
in′·stil·la′·tion
in′·stinct
in·stinc′·tive
in′·sti·tu′·tion·al·i·za′·tion
in′·sti·tu′·tion·al·ize ·ized, ·iz′·ing
in·struc′·tion

in′·stru·ment
in′·stru·men·tar′·i·um *pl.* ·ia
in′·stru·men·ta′·tion
in·suf·fi′·cien·cy
in′·suf·flate [in·suf′·]
in′·suf·fla′·tion
in′·suf·fla′·tor [in·suf′·fla·tor]
in′·su·la *pl. & gen. sg.* ·lae
in′·su·lar
in′·su·late ·lat′·ed, ·lat′·ing
in′·su·la′·tion
in′·su·la′·tor
in′·su·lin
in′·su·li·no·gen′·ic *also* in′·su·lo·gen′·ic
in′·su·lin·oid′
in′·su·lin·o′·ma *also* in′·su·lo′·ma; *pl.* ·mas *or* ·ma·ta
in′·su·li·no·pe′·nia
in′·su·li·no·priv′·ic
in′·sult
in·sur′·a·ble
in·sur′·ance
in′·take
in′·te·gral [in·teg′·ral]
in′·te·grate ·grat′·ed, ·grat′·ing
in′·te·gra′·tion
in′·teg·ri·ty
in·teg′·u·ment
in·teg′·u·men′·ta·ry
in·teg′·u·men′·tum
in′·tel·lect
in′·tel·lec′·tu·al
in′·tel·lec′·tu·al·i·za′·tion
in·tel′·li·gence
in·ten′·si·fi·ca′·tion
in·ten′·si·fy ·fied, ·fy′·ing
in·ten′·si·ty
in·ten′·sive
in·ten′·tion

in′·ter·
in′·ter·ac·ces′·so·ry
in′·ter·ac′·i·nar *also* ·nous
in′·ter·ac′·tion
in′·ter·al·le′·lic
in′·ter·al·ve′·o·lar
in′·ter·am′·ni·os
in′·ter·an′·gu·lar
in′·ter·an′·nu·lar
in′·ter·ap′·o·phys′·e·al [·apoph′·y·se′·al]
in′·ter·ar·tic′·u·lar
in′·ter·ar·tic′·u·la′·ris
in′·ter·ar′·y·te′·noid *also* ·te·noi′·dal
in′·ter·ar′·y·te·noi′·dea
in′·ter·a′·tri·al
in′·ter·a′·tri·a′·le
in′·ter·au′·ral
in′·ter·au·ric′·u·lar
in′·ter·ax′·o·nal
in′·ter·brain
in·ter′·ca·lar′·y
in·ter′·ca·lat′·ed
in′·ter·can′·thic
in′·ter·cap′·il·lar′·y
in′·ter·cap′·i·tal
in′·ter·ca·pit′·u·lar
in′·ter·ca·pit′·u·la′·ris *pl.* ·res
in′·ter·ca·rot′·i·ca
in′·ter·ca·rot′·id *also* ·ca·rot′·ic
in′·ter·car′·pal
in′·ter·car·pa′·le *neut.* *of* intercarpalis; *pl.* ·lia
in′·ter·car·pa′·lis *pl.* ·les
in′·ter·car′·ti·la·gin′·ea
in′·ter·car′·ti·lag′·i·nous
in′·ter·cav′·er·no′·sus *pl.* ·si
in′·ter·cav′·ern·ous
in′·ter·cel′·lu·lar
in′·ter·cep′·tive
in′·ter·cer′·e·bral

in′·ter·change
in′·ter·chon′·dral
in′·ter·chon·dra′·lis
  pl. ·les
in′·ter·cil′·i·ar′y
in′·ter·cis·tron′·ic
in′·ter·cla·vic′·u·lar
in′·ter·cla·vic′·u·la′·re
in′·ter·cli′·noid   *also*
  ·cli·noi′·dal
in′·ter·col·lic′·u·lar
in′·ter·co·lum′·nar
in′·ter·con′·dy·lar
in′·ter·con′·dy·la′·ris
  neut. ·re
in′·ter·con′·dy·loid
in′·ter·cor′·nu·al
in′·ter·cor′·o·nar′y
in′·ter·cos′·tal
in′·ter·cos·ta′·le   *neut.*
  of intercostalis
in′·ter·cos·ta′·lis   *pl.*
  ·les, *gen. pl.* ·li·um
in′·ter·cos′·to·bra′·chi·al
in′·ter·cos′·to·bra′·chi·a′·lis   *pl.* ·les
in′·ter·course
in′·ter·cris′·tal
in′·ter·cross
in′·ter·cru′·ral
in′·ter·cru·ra′·lis   *pl.*
  ·les
in′·ter·cu·ne′·iform
  [·cu′·ne·]
in′·ter·cu·ne′·ifor′·me
  neut. of intercuneiformis; *pl.* ·mia
in′·ter·cu·ne′·ifor′·mis
  pl. ·mes
in′·ter·cur′·rent
in′·ter·cus′·pal
in′·ter·cus·pa′·tion
in′·ter·def′·er·en′·tial

in′·ter·den′·tal
in′·ter·dig′·i·tal
in′·ter·dig′·i·ta′·lis
in′·ter·dig′·i·tate   ·tat′·ed, ·tat′·ing
in′·ter·dig′·i·ta′·tion
in′·ter·ec·top′·ic
in′·ter·face
in′·ter·fa′·cial
in′·ter·fas′·ci·al
in′·ter·fas·cic′·u·lar
in′·ter·fas·cic′·u·la′·ris
in′·ter·fem′·o·ral
in′·ter·fer′·ence
in′·ter·fer·om′·e·ter
in′·ter·fer·om′·e·try
in′·ter·fer′·on[32]
in′·ter·fi′·bril·lar   *also*
  ·lar′y
in′·ter·fi′·lar
in′·ter·fol·lic′·u·lar
in′·ter·fo·ve′·o·lar
in′·ter·fo·ve′·o·la′·re
in′·ter·fron′·tal
in′·ter·gan′·gli·o·na′·ris
  pl. ·res
in′·ter·gan′·gli·on′·ic
in′·ter·gen′·ic [·ge′·nic]
in′·ter·glob′·u·lar
in′·ter·glob′·u·la′·re
  pl. ·ria
in′·ter·glu′·te·al
in′·ter·grade
in′·ter·gy′·ral
in′·ter·hem′i·spher′·ic
in′·ter·ic′·tal
in·te′·ri·or
in′·ter·ju′·gal
in′·ter·ki·ne′·sis
in′·ter·lam′·i·nar
in′·ter·leu′·kin
in′·ter·lo′·bar
in′·ter·lo·ba′·ris   *pl.*
  ·res

in′·ter·lob′·u·lar
in′·ter·lob′·u·la′·ris
in′·ter·mal·le′·o·lar
in′·ter·mam′·ma·ry
in′·ter·mar′·gin·al
in′·ter·max′·il·la′·ris
in′·ter·max′·il·lar′y
in′·ter·me′·dia   *neut.*
  pl. & fem sg. of
  intermedius; *fem. pl. & gen. sg.* ·di·ae
in′·ter·me′·di·ate
in′·ter·me′·din
in′·ter·me′·dio·lat′·er·a′·lis
in′·ter·me′·dio·lat′·er·al
in′·ter·me′·di·um
  neut. of intermedius;
  pl. ·dia
in′·ter·me′·di·us   *pl. & gen. sg.* ·dii
in′·ter·me·nin′·ge·al
in′·ter·men′·stru·al
in′·ter·mes′·en·ter′·ic
in′·ter·mes′·en·ter′·icus
in′·ter·mes′o·blas′·tic
in′·ter·met′a·car′·pal
in′·ter·met′a·car·pa′·lis
  pl. ·les
in′·ter·met′a·tar′·sal
in′·ter·met′a·tar·sa′·lis
  pl. ·les
in′·ter·mit′   ·mit′·ted, ·mit′·ting
in′·ter·mi·tot′·ic
in′·ter·mit′·tence
in′·ter·mit′·tens
in′·ter·mit′·tent
in′·ter·mo·lec′·u·lar
in′·ter·mus′·cu·lar
in′·ter·mus′·cu·la′·re
  neut. of intermuscularis
in′·ter·mus′·cu·la′·ris
  pl. ·res

---

[32] Greek letters following the word *interferon* are fully spelled out: interferon gamma. Any numbers or letters that follow are joined by a hyphen: interferon gamma-1b.

intern / intervaginal

in′·tern *also* ·terne
in·ter′·na *fem. of* internus; *pl. & gen. sg.* ·nae
in·ter′·nal
in·ter′·nal·i·za′·tion
in′·ter·na′·sal
in′·ter·na·sa′·lis
in′·terne *var. of* intern
in′·ter·neu′·ral
between neural arches: *Cf.* interneuronal
in′·ter·neu′·ron *Brit. also* ·rone
in′·ter·neu·ro′·nal *of interneurons: Cf.* interneural
in·ter′·ni *pl. & gen. sg. of* internus
in·ter′·nist [in′·ter·]
in·ter′·no *ablative of* internus
in′·ter·nod′·al [·no′·dal]
in′·ter·node
in′·tern·ship
in′·ter·nu′·cle·ar
in·ter′·num *neut. of* internus
in′·ter·nun′·ci·al
in·ter′·nus *pl. & gen. sg.* ·ni
in′·ter·oc·clu′·sal
in′·ter·o·cep′·tive
in′·ter·o·cep′·tor
in′·ter·o·fec′·tive
in′·ter·ol′·i·va′·re
in′·ter·ol′·i·var′y
in′·ter·or′·bit·al
in′·ter·os′·sea *fem. sg. & neut. pl. of* interosseus
in′·ter·os′·se·ous
in′·ter·os′·se·um *neut. of* interosseus; *pl.* ·sea, *gen. sg.* ·sei
in′·ter·os′·se·us *pl. & gen. sg.* ·sei

in′·ter·pal′·a·tine
in′·ter·pal′·pe·bral
in′·ter·pap′·il·lar′y
in′·ter·pa·ri′·etal
in′·ter·pa·ri′·eta′·le
in′·ter·par′·ox·ys′·mal
in′·ter·pe·dic′·u·late
in′·ter·pe·dun′·cu·lar
in′·ter·pe·dun′·cu·la′·ris *neut.* ·re
in′·ter·pel′·vi·ab·dom′·i·nal
in′·ter·pha·lan′·gea *gen. pl.* ·pha·lan′·ge·a′rum
in′·ter·pha·lan′·ge·al
in′·ter·pha·lan′·ge·a′lis *pl.* ·a′les, *gen. pl.* ·a′li·um
in′·ter·phase
in′·ter·plant
in′·ter·pleu′·ral
in′·ter·pleu′·ri·cos′·tal
in·ter′·po·late ·lat′·ed, ·lat′·ing
in·ter′·po·la′·tion
in′·ter·pos′·i·tus *pl. & gen. sg.* ·ti
in′·ter·po·si′·tion
in·ter′·pre·ta′·tion
in′·ter·pris·mat′·ic
in′·ter·prox′·i·mal
in′·ter·pu′·bic
in′·ter·pu′·bi·cus
in′·ter·pu′·pil·lar′y
in′·ter·py·ram′·i·dal
in′·ter·ra′·di·al
in′·ter·ra·dic′·u·lar
in′·ter·re′·nal
in′·ter·rupt′·ed
in′·ter·rup′·tus
in′·ter·sa′·cral
in′·ter·scap′·u·lar
in′·ter·scap′·u·lo·tho·rac′·ic
in′·ter·sec′·tio *pl.* ·sec′·ti·o′·nes
in′·ter·sec′·tion

in′·ter·seg·men′·tal
in′·ter·seg′·men·ta′·lis
in′·ter·sep′·tal
in′·ter·sex
in′·ter·sex′·u·al
in′·ter·sex′·u·al′·i·ty
in′·ter·sig′·moid *also* ·sig·moi′·dal
in′·ter·sig·moi′·de·us
in′·ter·space
in′·ter·sphe·noi′·dal
in′·ter·spi′·nal *also* ·nous
in′·ter·spi·na′·le *neut. of* interspinalis; *pl.* ·lia
in′·ter·spi·na′·lis *pl.* ·les
in·ter′·stice *pl.* ·stic·es
in′·ter·sti′·tial
in′·ter·sti′·tio·spi′·nal
in′·ter·sti′·ti·um *pl.* ·sti′·tia
in′·ter·su′·tur·al
in′·ter·tar′·sal
in′·ter·ten′·di·nous
in′·ter·tha·lam′·ic
in′·ter·tho·rac′·i·co·scap′·u·lar
in′·ter·trag′·ic
in′·ter·trag′·i·ca
in′·ter·trans′·ver·sa′·lis *pl.* ·les
in′·ter·trans′·ver·sa′·ri·um *neut. of* intertransversarius; *pl.* ·ria
in′·ter·trans′·ver·sa′·ri·us *pl.* ·rii, *gen. pl.* ·sa′·ri·o′·rum
in′·ter·trans·verse′ [·trans′·verse]
in′·ter·trig′·i·nous
in′·ter·tri′·go
in′·ter·tro′·chan·ter′·ic
in′·ter·tu′·ber·cu·lar
in′·ter·tu′·ber·cu·la′·ris
in′·ter·u′·re·ter′·ic
in′·ter·u′·re·ter′·i·ca
in′·ter·vag′·i·nal

in'·ter·vag'·i·na'·le
  pl. ·lia
in'·ter·val
in'·ter·ve·no'·sum
in'·ter·ve'·nous
in'·ter·ven'·tion
in'·ter·ven·tric'·u·lar
in'·ter·ven·tric'·u·la'·re
  neut. of interventricularis
in'·ter·ven·tric'·u·la'·ris
  pl. ·les
in'·ter·ver'·te·bral
in'·ter·ver'·te·bra'·le
  neut. of intervertebralis; *pl.* ·lia
in'·ter·ver'·te·bra'·lis
  pl. ·les
in'·ter·vil'·lous
in'·ter·zon'·al [·zo'·nal]
in·tes'·ti·nal
in·tes'·ti·na'·lis *pl.*
  ·les
in·tes'·tine
in'·tes·ti'·num *gen.*
  ·ni
in'·ti·ma *pl. & gen.*
  sg. ·mae
in'·ti·mal
in'·ti·mec'·to·my
in'·ti·mi'·tis
in'·toe
in·tol'·er·ance
in·tor'·sion
in·tort'·er
in·tox'·i·cant
in·tox'·i·ca'·tion
in'·tra·
in'·tra-ab·dom'·i·nal
in'·tra-ad'·ven·ti'·tial
in'·tra-al·ve'·o·lar
in'·tra-al'·ve·o·la'·ris
  gen. pl. ·la'·ri·um
in'·tra-aor'·tic
in'·tra-ar·te'·ri·al
in'·tra-ar·tic'·u·lar
in'·tra-ar·tic'·u·la'·re
in'·tra-a'tri·al

in'·tra-au'·ral
in'·tra·bon'·y
in'·tra·bron'·chi·al
in'·tra·bul'·bar
in'·tra·cal'·i·ce'·al
  [·ca'·li·]
in'·tra·can'·a·lic'·u·lar
in'·tra·cap'·su·lar
in'·tra·cap'·su·la'·re
  pl. ·ria
in'·tra·car'·di·ac
in'·tra·car'·ti·lag'·i·
  nous
in'·tra·cav'·i·tar'y
in'·tra·cel'·lu·lar
in'·tra·cer'·e·bral
in'·tra·chi'·as·mat'·ic
in'·tra·chon'·dri·al
in'·tra·chor'·dal
  [·chord'·al]
in'·tra·cho'·ri·on'·ic
in'·tra·chro'·mo·som'·
  al [·so'·mal]
in'·tra·cis·ter'·nal
in'·tra·cis·tron'·ic
in'·tra·cor'·dal
in'·tra·cor'·o·nal [·co·
  ro'·nal]
in'·tra·cor·po'·re·al
  also ·cor'·po·ral
in'·tra·cor·pus'·cu·lar
in'·tra·cor'·ti·cal
in'·tra·cos'·tal
in'·tra·cra'·ni·al
in'·tra·cris'·tal
in·trac'·ta·ble
in'·tra·cu·ta'·ne·ous
in'·tra·cys'·tic
in'·tra·cy'·to·plas'·mic
in'·tra·der'·mal
in'·tra·duc'·tal
in'·tra·du'·ral
in'·tra·em'·bry·on'·ic
in'·tra·ep'·i·der'·mal
in'·tra·ep'·i·the'·li·al
in'·tra·eryth'·ro·cyt'·ic
in'·tra·fis'·sur·al
in'·tra·fol·lic'·u·lar

in'·tra·fu'·sal
in'·tra·gas'·tric
in'·tra·gen'·ic [·ge'·nic]
in'·tra·glan'·du·lar
in'·tra·glu'·te·al
in'·tra·he·pat'·ic
in'·tra·ic'·tal
in'·tra·jug'·u·lar
in'·tra·jug'·u·la'·ris
in'·tra·le'·sion·al
in'·tra·leu'·ko·cyt'·ic
in'·tra·lig'·a·men'·tous
in'·tra·lim'·bi·cus
in'·tra·lin'·gual
in'·tra·lo'·bar
in'·tra·lob'·u·lar
in'·tra·lu'·mi·nal
in'·tra·mam'·ma·ry
in'·tra·max'·il·lar'y
in'·tra·med'·ul·lar'y
in'·tra·mem'·bra·nous
in'·tra·mo·lec'·u·lar
in'·tra·mu·co'·sal
in'·tra·mu'·ral
in'·tra·mus'·cu·lar
in'·tra·na'·sal
in'·tra·neu'·ral
in'·tra·nu'·cle·ar
in'·tra·oc'·u·lar
in'·tra·op'·er·a·tive
in'·tra·op'·tic
in'·tra·o'ral
in'·tra·os'·se·ous
in'·tra·ov'u·lar [·o'·vu·]
in'·tra·pap'·il·la'·ris
  neut. ·re
in'·tra·par'·en·chym'·a·
  tous [·chy'·ma·]
in'·tra·pa·ri'·eta·lis
in'·tra·pa·rot'·i·de'·us
in'·tra·par'·tum
in'·tra·per'·i·car'·di·al
in'·tra·per'i·os'·te·al
in'·tra·per'·i·ne'·al
in'·tra·per'·i·to·ne'·al
in'·tra·pi·tu'·i·tar'y
in'·tra·pleu'·ral
in'·tra·psy'·chic

in'·tra·pul'·mo·nar'y
in'·tra·py·ret'·ic
in'·tra·re'·nal
in'·tra·ret'·i·nal
in'·tra·scle'·ral
in'·tra·seg·men'·tal
in'·tra·seg'·men·ta'·lis
in'·tra·sep'·tal
in'·tra·spi'·nal
in'·tra·sti'·tial
in'·tra·sy·no'·vi·al
[·syn·o'·]
in'·tra·ten·din'·ea
in'·tra·the'·cal
in'·tra·tho·rac'·ic
in'·tra·ton'·sil·lar
in'·tra·tu'·bu·lar
in'·tra·tym·pan'·ic
in'·tra·ure'·thral
in'·tra·u'ter·ine
in'·tra·va·ga'·le
in'·tra·vag'·i·nal
in·trav'·a·sa'·tion
in'·tra·vas'·cu·lar
in'·tra·ve'·nous
in'·tra·ven·tric'·u·lar
in'·tra·ver'·te·bral
in'·tra·ves'·i·cal
in'·tra·vi'·tal
in'·tra vi'·tam
in'·tra·vit'·re·ous
in·trin'·sic
in'·tro·
in'·tro·duc'·er
in'·tro·flex'·ion
in·tro'·itus
in'·tro·jec'·tion
in'·tro·mis'·sion
in'·tro·mit'·tent
in'·tron
in'·tro·pu'·ni·tive
in·tror'·sum
in'·tro·spec'·tion
in'·tro·spec'·tive
in'·tro·ver'·sion
in'·tro·vert
in'·tro·vert'·ed

in'·tu·bate ·bat'·ed,
  ·bat'·ing
in'·tu·ba'·tion
in'·tu·i'·tion
in'·tu·mes'·cence
in'·tu·mes'·cent
in·tu'·mes·cen'·tia pl.
  ·ti·ae
in'·tus·sus·cep'·tion
in'·tus·sus·cep'·tum
in'·tus·sus·cip'·i·ens
in'·u·lase var. of
  inulinase
in'·u·lin
in'·u·lin·ase
in·unc'·tion
in·unc'·tum
in u'tero
in vac'·uo
in·vag'·i·nate ·nat'·ed,
  ·nat'·ing
in·vag'·i·na'·tion
in·vag'·i·na'·tor
in·vag'·i·na'·tus
in'·va·lid
in'·va·lid·is'm
in·va'·sion
in·va'·sive
in·va'·sive·ness
in·ver'·sion
in·ver'·sus
in'·vert adj. & n.
in·vert' v.
in·ver'·tase
in·ver'·te·brate
in·ver'·tin var. of
  invertase
in·ver'·tor
in·vest'
in·vest'·ment
in vi'·tro
in vi'·vo
in'·vo·lu'·crum pl.
  ·cra
in·vol'·un·tar'y
in'·vo·lute ·lut'·ed,
  ·lut'·ing

in'·vo·lu'·tion
in'·vo·lu'·tion·al
Iod' amoe'·ba
  I. beutsch'·lii
i'o·date n. & v. ·dat'·
  ed, ·dat'·ing
i'od-Ba'·se·dow var.
  of Jod-Basedow
iod'·ic
i'o·dide
i'o·dim'·e·try
i'o·di·nate ·nat'·ed,
  ·nat·ing
i'o·di·na'·tion
i'o·dine
iod'·i·nin
i'o·din'·o·phil
i'o·dip'·a·mide
i'o·dis'm
i'o·dize ·dized, ·diz'·
  ing
i'o·do·
i'o·do·acet'·a·mide
  [·ac'et·am'·ide]
i'o·do·ace'·tic
i'o·do·al'·phi·on'·ic
i'o·do·an'·ti·py'·rine
i'o·do·ca'·sein [·ca·
  sein']
i'o·do·chlor'·hy·drox'y·
  quin
i'o·do·de·ox'y·u'ri·dine
i'o·do·der'·ma
io'·do·form
i'o·do·hip'·pur·ate
i'o·do·meth'·a·mate
i'o·do·met'·ric
i'o·dom'·e·try
i'o·do·phil [io'·]
i'o·do·phil'·ia
io'·do·phor
i'o·do·pro'·tein
i'o·dop'·sin
i'o·do·pyr'·a·cet
i'o·do·stick
i'o·do·thi'o·u'ra·cil
i'o·do·thy'·ro·nine

i′o·do·ty′·ro·sine
i′on
ion′·ic
i′on·i·za′·tion
i′on·ize   ·ized, ·iz′·ing
i′on·o·gen′·ic
i′on·om′·e·try
ion′·o·phore
ion′·o·pho·re′·sis
ion′·to·pho·re′·sis
ion′·to·pho·ret′·ic
i′o·phen′·dy·late
i′o·phen·ox′·ic
i′o·py′·dol
i′o·py′·done
i′o·thal′·a·mate
i′o·tha·lam′·ic
i′o·thi′o·u′ra·cil
ip′·e·ca·cu·a′·nha
    also ip′·e·cac
i′po·date
ip′·o·me′a   also ·moe′a
ip′ra·tro′·pi·um
iprin′·dole
i′pro·ni′·a·zid
ip′·si·lat′·er·al
i′ri·dal [ir′i·]   var. of
    iridic
ir′id·aux·e′·sis [i′rid·]
ir′i·dec′·tome
ir′i·dec′·to·my
ir′i·den·clei′·sis
ir′i·de·re′·mia
i′ri·des   pl. of iris
ir″·i·des′·cence
ir″·i·des′·cent
irid′·e·sis [ir′·i·de′·sis]
irid′·i·al
irid′·ic
irid′·i·ca
i′ri·dis   gen. of iris
irid′·i·um
ir′i·di·za′·tion
ir′i·do· [i′ri·do·]
ir′i·do·cap′·su·li′·tis
ir′i·do·cap′·su·lot′·o·my

ir′i·do·cho′·roid·i′·tis
ir′i·do·cil′·i·ar′y
ir′i·do·con·stric′·tor
ir′i·do·cor′·ne·al
ir′i·do·cor′·ne·a′lis
ir′i·do·cor′·neo·scle·
    rec′·to·my
ir′i·do·cy·clec′·to·my
ir′i·do·cy·cli′·tis
ir′i·do·cy′·clo·cho′·
    roid·i′·tis
ir′i·dod′·e·sis [·do·de′·
    sis]
ir′i·do·di·al″·y·sis
ir′i·do·di′·la·tor [·di·
    la′·]
ir′i·do·do·ne′·sis
ir′i·do·ker′·a·ti′·tis
ir′i·do·ki·net′·ic
ir′i·dol′·y·sis
ir′i·do·mes′o·di·al″·y·
    sis
ir′i·don′·cus
ir′i·do·ple′·gia
ir′i·do·rhex′·is
ir′i·dos′·chi·sis
ir′i·do·scle·rot′·o·my
ir′i·dot′·a·sis
irid′·o·tome [ir′i·do·]
ir′i·dot′·o·my
i′ris   pl. i′ri·des, gen.
    sg. i′ri·dis
iri′·tis
ir′i·to·ec′·to·my
irit′·o·my
ir″·i·um
i′ron
ir·ra′·di·ate   ·at′·ed,
    ·at′·ing
ir·ra′·di·a′·tion
ir·ra′·tio·nal
ir″·re·duc′·i·ble
ir·reg′·u·lar
ir·reg′·u·lar′·i·ty
ir″·re·me′·di·a·ble
ir·res″·pi·ra·ble [ir″·re·
    spi′·]

ir″·re·spon′·si·bil″·i·ty
ir″·re·vers′·i·bil″·i·ty
ir″·re·vers′·i·ble
ir″·ri·gant
ir″·ri·gate   ·gat′·ed,
    ·gat′·ing
ir″·ri·ga′·tion
ir″·ri·ga′·tor
ir′·ri·ta·bil″·i·ty
ir″·ri·ta·ble
ir″·ri·tant
ir″·ri·ta′·tion
ir″·ri·ta′·tive
i′sa·tin
is′·aux·e″·sis
is·che″·mia [isch·e′·]
    Brit. ·chae′·
is·che″·mic [isch·e′·]
    Brit. ·chae′·
is″·chia   pl. of ischium
is″·chi·ad′·ic
is″·chi·ad′·i·ca   fem. of
    ischiadicus
is″·chi·ad′·i·cum   neut.
    of ischiadicus
is″·chi·ad′·i·cus   pl. &
    gen. sg. ·i·ci
is″·chi·al
is″·chi·al′·gia
is″·chi·ec′·to·my
is″·chii   gen. of ischium
is″·chio·
is″·chio·ana′·lis
is″·chio·cap′·su·lar
is″·chio·cav′·er·no′·sus
is″·chio·cav′·ern·ous
is″·chio·coc·cyg′·e·us
is″·chio·fem′·o·ral
is″·chio·fem′·o·ra′·lis
    neut. ·le
is″·chi·om″·e·lus
is″·chi·op′·a·gus
is″·chio·pu′·bic
is″·chio·rec′·tal
is″·chio·tho″·ra·cop′·a·
    gus

is′·chi·um *pl.* is′·chia,
  gen. sg. is′·chii
is′·cho·gy′·ria
is′·cho·sper′·mia
is·chu′·ria [isch·u′·ria]
i′sei·ko′·nia *also* ·co′·
  nia
i′sei·kon′·ic *also*
  ·con′·ic
is′·ethi′·o·nate
i′sin·glass
is′·let
i′so·
i′so·ac·cep′·tor
i′so·ag·glu′·ti·na′·tion
i′so·ag·glu′·ti·nin
i′so·al·lele′
i′so·al·lox′·a·zine
i′so·am′·yl
i′so·am′·y·lase
i′so·an·dros′·ter·one
i′so·an′·ti·bod′y
i′so·an′·ti·gen
i′so·bar
i′so·bar′·ic
i′so·bu′·caine
i′so·bu′·tyl
i′so·ca·lo′·ric
i′so·car·box′·a·zid
i′so·cho′·ric
i′so·chro·mat′·ic
i′so·chro′·ma·tid
i′so·chro′·mo·some
i′so·chron′·ic *also*
  isoch′·ro·nous
i′soch′·ro·nis′m
i′so·cit′·rate
i′so·cit′·ric
i′so·com′·ple·ment
i′so·con′·tour
i′so·co′·ria
i′so·cor′·tex
i′so·cy′·a·nate
i′so·cy′·a·nide
i′so·cy′·clic
i′so·cy·to′·sis
i′so·dose

i′so·dy·nam′·ic
i′so·elec′·tric
i′so·elec′·tron′·ic
i′so·en′·zyme
i′so·eth′·a·rine
i′so·gam′·ete [·ga·
  mete′]
i′so·ga·met′·ic
isog′·a·mous
i′sog′·a·my
i′so·ge·ne′·ic
i′so·gen′·ic
isog′·e·nous
i′so·graft
i′so·he·mol′·y·sin [·he′·
  mo·ly′·sin] *Brit.*
  ·hae·
i′so·he·mol′·y·sis
  Brit. ·hae·
i′so·hy′·dric
i′so·ico′·nia *var. of*
  iseikonia
i′so·icon′·ic *var. of*
  iseikonic
i′so·im·mune′
i′so·im′·mu·ni·za′·tion
i′so·in·dic′·i·al
i′so·ion′·ic
i′so·ki·net′·ic
i′so·late *n. & v.* ·lat′·
  ed, ·lat′·ing
i′so·la′·tion
i′so·la′·tor
i′so·lec′·i·thal
i′so·leu′·cine
isol′·o·gous
i′so·mer
isom′·er·ase
i′so·mer′·ic
isom′·er·is′m
isom′·er·i·za′·tion
isom′·er·ous
i′so·meth′·a·done
i′so·me·thep′·tene
i′so·met′·ric *also* ·ri·
  cal
i′so·me·tro′·pia
i′so·morph

i′so·mor′·phism
i′so·mor′·phous *also*
  ·mor′·phic
i′so·ni′·a·zid
i′so·nic′·o·tin′·ic
i′so·nip′·e·caine
i′so-on·cot′·ic
i′so-os·mot′·ic *var. of*
  isosmotic
i′so·pen′·te·nyl
i′so·pep′·tide
i′so·per′·i·stal′·tic
i′so·phan
i′so·phane
i′so·phene
i′so·pho′·ria
i′so·pren′·a·line
i′so·prene
i′so·pro′·pa·mide
i′so·pro′·pa·nol
i′so·pro′·pyl
i′so·pro·ter′·e·nol
isop′·ter
i′so·pyk′·nic *also*
  ·pyc′·
i′so·pyk·no′·sis *also*
  ·pyc·
i′so·pyk·not′·ic *also*
  ·pyc·
i′so·quin′·o·line
i′so·re·sponse′
i′so·rhyth′·mic
i′so·se′·rum
i′so·sex′·u·al
is′·os·mot′·ic
i′so·sor′·bide
Isos′·po·ra
  I. bel′·li
isos′·po·ri′·a·sis *also*
  ·po·ro′·sis
i′so·stere
i′so·sthe·nu′·ria [isos′·
  the·]
i′so·therm
i′so·therm′·ag·no′·sia
i′so·ther′·mal *also*
  ·mic

isothiazine / kakidrosis

i'so·thi'·a·zine
i'so·thi'o·cy'·a·nate
i'so·thi·pen'·dyl
i'so·tone
i'so·ton'·ic
i'so·to·nic'·i·ty
i'so·tope[33]
i'so·top'·ic [·to'·pic]
i'so·trans'·plant
i'so·tret'·i·noin
i'so·tro'·pic [·trop'·ic]
isot'·ro·py
i'so·typ'·ic *also* ·i·cal
i'so·va·ler'·ic
i'so·va·ler'·ic·ac'·id·e'·mia *Brit.* ·ae'·mia
i'so·vol'·u·met'·ric
i'sox·az'·o·lyl
isox'·su·prine
i'so·zyme *var. of* isoenzyme
is'·sue
isth·mec'·to·my
isth'·mi·an
isth'·mus *pl. & gen. sg.* ·mi
isu'·ria
it'·a·con'·ic
itai'-itai'
itch
itch'·ing
i'ter
it'·er·a·tive
ith'·yo·ky·pho'·sis
i'ver·mec'·tin
Ix·o'·des
  I. dam·mi'·ni
  I. per'·sul·ca'·tus
  I. ric'·i·nus
ix'·o·di'·a·sis
ix·od'·id
Ix·od'·i·dae

ix'·o·dis'm
Ix'·o·doi'·dea

J

jack'·screw
jack·so'·ni·an
jac'·ti·ta'·tion *also* jac·ta'·tion
jal'·ap
ja·mais vu'
jan'·i·ceps
ja'·ra·ra'·ca
jar'·gon
jaun'·dice
jaw
jaw'·bone
je·ju'·nal
je'·ju·na'·lis *pl.* ·les
je'·ju·nec'·to·my
je'·ju·ni'·tis
je·ju'·no-
je·ju'·no·ce·cos'·to·my *Brit.* ·cae·cos'·
je·ju'·no·co·los'·to·my
je·ju'·no·gas'·tric
je·ju'·no·il'e·i'tis
je·ju'·no·il'e·os·to·my
je·ju'·no·je'·ju·nos'·to·my
je'·ju·nos'·to·my
je'·ju·not'·o·my
je·ju'·num
jel'·ly
jel'·ly·fish
jen·ne'·ri·an
je·quir'·i·ty
jig'·ger
Jod'-Ba'·se·dow
joint
joule
ju'·ga *pl. of* jugum

ju'·gal
ju'·gate
ju'·glone
ju'·go·max'·il·lar'y
jug'·u·lar
jug'·u·la'·re *neut. of* jugularis
jug'·u·la'·ris *pl.* ·res
jug'·u·lo·di·gas'·tric
jug'·u·lo·di·gas'·tri·cus
jug'·u·lo-o'mo·hy'·oid
jug'·u·lo-o'mo·hy·oi'·de·us
ju'·gu·lum
ju'·gum *pl.* ·ga
juice
junc'·tion
junc'·tion·al
junc·tu'·ra *pl. & gen. sg.* ·rae
jung'·i·an
jus'·to
ju'·ve·nile
jux'·ta-ar·tic'·u·lar
jux'·ta·cor'·ti·cal
jux'·ta·fol·lic'·u·lar
jux'·ta·glo·mer'·u·lar
jux'·tal'·lo·cor'·tex
jux'·ta·med'·ul·lar'y
jux'·ta·pap'·il·lar'y
jux'·ta·po·si'·tion
jux'·ta·py·lo'·ric
jux'·ta·spi'·nal

K

ka·fin'·do
kai'·no· *var. of* caeno-
kak'·es·the'·sia *Brit.* ·aes·the'·; *var. of* cacesthesia
kak'·i·dro'·sis

---

[33] For isotopes of specific elements, no hyphen is used after the fully written out name of the element: carbon 14 (except when used attributively: carbon-14 dating). The isotope number is written as a superscript to the left of the symbol for the element: ^{14}C.

kak′·ke
kak′·o· *var. of* caco-
ka′·la-azar′
ka′·la·fun′·gin
ka′li·o·pe′·nic [kal′i·]
ka′li·ure′·sis [kal′i·]
kal′·li·din
kal′·li·kre′·in
kal′·li·kre′·in·o·gen [·kre·in′·o·]
kal′·ure′·sis
kal′·uret′·ic
ka′′·ma·la [ka·ma′′·la]
kan′·a·my′·cin
ka′·nin·lo′·ma
ka·nyem′·ba
ka′·o·lin
ka′·o·lin·o′·sis
kar′·a·kurt′
ka·ra′·ya
kar′y·ap′·sis
kar′yo·
kar′y·oc′·la·sis
kar′y·o·clas′·tic
kar′y·o·gam′·ic
kar′y·og′·a·my
kar′yo·ki·ne′·sis
kar′yo·ki·net′·ic
kar′yo·lo′·bic
kar′yo·lo′·bism
kar′y·ol′·o·gy
kar′yo·lymph
kar′y·ol′·y·sis
kar′y·o·lyt′·ic
kar′yo·meg′·a·ly
kar′y·o·mere
kar′y·om′·e·try
kar′y·on
kar′y·o·nide
kar′y·o·phage
kar′y·o·plas′m
kar′y·o·plas′′·mic
kar′yo·pyk·no′·sis
kar′yo·pyk·not′·ic
kar′y·or·rhex′·is
kar′y·o·some
kar′y·os′·ta·sis
kar′y·o·the′·ca

kar′y·o·type
kar′y·o·typ′·ic
kar′y·o·typ′·ing
ka·sai′
ka·su′·ga·my′·cin
kat′a· *var. of* cata-
ka·tab′·o·lis′m *var. of* catabolism
ka·tal′ [kat′·al]
kat′a·phy·lax′·is *var. of* cataphylaxis
Ka′·ta·ya′·ma
kath′·a·rom′·e·ter *var. of* catharometer
kath′·i·so·pho′·bia
kat′·ine
kat′·i′on *var. of* cation
ka·tol′·y·sis
kat′o·pho′·ria *var. of* cataphoria
kat′o·tro′·pia *var. of* catatropia
ka′′·va *also* ka′·va-ka′·va
ka′′·va·is′m
ke·da′·ni
keel
ke′·loid
ke·loi′·dal
ke·lot′·o·my
Kel′·vin *temperature scale*
kel′·vin *SI base unit*
ker′·a·sin
ker′·a·tec·ta′·sia
ker′·a·tec′·to·my
ke·rat′·ic
ker′·a·tin
ker′·a·tin·ase′
ker′·a·tin·i·za′·tion
ker′·a·tin·ize ·ized, ·iz′·ing
ke·rat′·i·no·cyte
ke·rat′·i·noid [ker′·a·ti·]
ker′·a·tit′·ic
ker′·a·ti′·tis
ker′·a·to·

ker′·a·to·ac′·an·tho′·ma
ker′·a·to·cele
ker′·a·to·con·junc′·ti·vi′·tis
ker′·a·to·co′·nus
ker′·a·to·cyst
ker′·a·to·cyte
ker′·a·to·der′·ma *also* ·der′·mia
ker′·a·to·gen′·e·sis
ker′·a·to·gen′·ic
ker′·a·tog′·e·nous
ker′·a·to·glo′·bus
ker′·a·to·hy′·a·lin
ker′·a·to·hy′·a·line
ker′·a·toid
ker′·a·to·ir′i·do·cy·cli′·tis
ker′·a·to·irid′·o·scope [·ir′i·do·]
ker′·a·to·leu·ko′·ma
ker′·a·tol′·y·sis
ker′·a·to·lyt′·ic
ker′·a·to′·ma *pl.* ·mas *or* ·ma·ta
ker′·a·to·ma·la′·cia
ker′·a·tom′·e·ter
ker′·a·to·met′·ric
ker′·a·tom′·e·try
ker′·a·to·mi·leu′·sis
ker′·a·to·nyx′·is
ker′·a·top′·a·thy
ker′·a·to·pha′·kia
ker′·a·to·plas′·tic
ker′·a·to·plas′·ty
ker′·a·to·scope
ker′·a·tos′·co·py
ker′·a·to′·sis *pl.* ·ses
ker′·a·to·sul′·fate Brit. ·sul′·phate
ker′·a·to·sul′·fa·tu′·ria Brit. ·sul′·pha·
ker′·a·tot′·ic
ker′·a·tot′·o·my
ke·rec′·ta·sis
ke′·ri·on
ker′·ma

ker·nic′·ter·us
ke′·ta·mine
ke′·ti·mine
ke′·to·
ke′·to·ac′·i·do′·sis
ke′·to·ac′·i·du′·ria
ke′·to·ami′·no·ac′·id·e′·mia *Brit.* ·ae′·mia
ke′·to·de·ox′y·glu′·co·nate
ke′·to·de·ox′y·oc′·to·nate
ke′·to·gen′·e·sis
ke′·to·gen′·ic
ke′·to·glu′·ta·rate
ke′·to·glu·tar′·ic
ke′·tol
ke′·to·lyt′·ic
ke′·tone
ke′·ton·e′·mia [·to·ne·′] *Brit.* ·ae′·mia
ke·ton′·ic
ke′·ton·u′·ria [·to·nu′·]
ke′·tose
ke·to′·sis
ke′·to·ste′·roid
ke·tot′·ic
key′·way
kid′·ney *pl.* kid′·neys
kil′o·
kil′o·bec′·que·rel
ki′lo·cal′·o·rie
kil′o·cu′·rie
kil′o·cy′·cle
kil′o·dal′·ton
kil′o·elec′·tron·volt′
kil′o·gram
kil′o·hertz
kil′·ohm *also* kil′o·ohm
kil′o·joule
kil′o·volt
kil′o·watt
kin′·aes·the′·sia *Brit.* *spel.* *of* kinesthesia
kin′·aes·the′·si·om′·e·ter *Brit.* *spel.* *of* kinesthesiometer

kin·an′·es·the′·sia *Brit.* ·an′·aes·
ki′·nase
kin′·dling
ki′ne· [kin′e·]
ki′ne·mat′·ic
ki′ne·plas′·tic
ki′ne·plas′·ty [kin′e·]
ki′ne·sal′·gia *also* ki·ne′·si·al′·gia
ki·ne′·si· *var.* *of* kinesio-
ki·ne′·sia
ki·ne′·sic
ki·ne′·si·gen′·ic
ki′ne·sim′·e·ter
ki·ne′·sio·
ki·ne′·si·ol′·o·gy
ki·ne′·sis
ki·ne′·si·ther′·a·py *also* ki·ne′·sio· *or* ki·ne′·so·
ki·ne′·so·
kin′e·sod′·ic *also* ki·ne′·si·od′·ic
ki·ne′·so·gen′·ic
kin′·es·the′·sia *Brit.* ·aes·the′·; *also* ·sis
kin′·es·the′·si·om′·e·ter *Brit.* ·aes·the′·
kin′·es·thet′·ic *Brit.* ·aes·thet′·
ki·net′·ic
ki·net′·ics
ki′·ne·tin [ki·ne′·tin]
ki·net′o· [ki·ne′to·]
ki·net′o·car′·di·o·gram
ki·net′o·car′·di·og′·ra·phy
ki·net′o·chore
ki·net′o·gen′·ic
ki·net′o·plas′m
ki·net′o·plast
Ki·net′o·plas′·ti·da
ki′·ne·to′·sis [kin′e·]
ki·net′o·some [·ne′to·]
ki·net′o·ther′·a·py
king′·dom

ki′·nin
ki·nin′·o·gen
ki·nin′·o·gen·ase [ki′·nin·og′·e·nase]
ki′·no·
ki′·no·cil′·i·um *pl.* ·lia
ki′·no·mom′·e·ter
kin′·ship
ki′·o·no· *var.* *of* ciono-
kir′·ro·my′·cin
kit′·a·sa·my′·cin
kit′·ing
Kleb′·si·el′·la
   K. ozae′·nae
   K. pneu·mo′·ni·ae
   K. rhi′·no·scle·ro′·ma·tis
klep′·to·lag′·nia
klep′·to·ma′·nia
klep′·to·ma′·ni·ac
knead′·ing
knee′·cap
knife *pl.* knives
knit ·knit′·ted, knit′·ting
knis′·mo·gen′·ic
knob
knock
knock′-knee
knot
knuck′·le
koch′·er·i·za′·tion
koi′·lo·
koi′·lo·cy·to′·sis
koi′·lo·nych′·ia
koi′·lo·ster′·nia
koi′·no· *var.* *of* coeno-
ko′·jic
kol′·po· *var.* *of* colpo-
ko·nim′·e·ter
ko′·nio·cor′·tex
kop′·ro· *var.* *of* copro-
krait
krau·ro′·sis
kre′o·tox′·in
kryp′·to· *var.* *of* crypto-
kryp′·ton

ku'·ru
kut·tar'·o·some
kwa'·shi·or'·kor [·or·kor']
ky'·a·no· var. of cyano-
ky'·mo·gram
ky'·mo·graph
ky·mog'·ra·phy
kyn'·u·ren'·ic
kyn'·u·ren'·i·nase
kyn·u'·re·nine [·u·ren'·ine]
ky'·pho·ra·chit'·ic
ky'·pho·ra·chi'·tis
ky'·pho·sco'·lio·ra·chit'·ic
ky'·pho·sco'·li·o'·sis
ky·pho'·sis
ky·phot'·ic
kyr'·tor·rhach'·ic

L

la'·bel n. & v. ·bled or ·belled, ·bel·ing or ·bel·ling
la'·bia pl. of labium
la'·bi·al
la'·bi·a'·lis pl. ·les
la'·bi·al·is'm
la'·bii gen. sg. of labium
la'·bile
la·bil'·i·ty
la'·bio·
la'·bio·al·ve'·o·lar
la'·bio·cer'·vi·cal
la'·bi·o·cli·na'·tion
la'·bio·den'·tal
la'·bio·gin'·gi·val
la'·bio·glos'·so·la·ryn'·ge·al
la'·bio·glos'·so·pha·ryn'·ge·al
la'·bio·men'·tal
la'·bio·na'·sal
la'·bi·o·plas'·ty
la'·bio·scro'·tal
la'·bio·te·nac'·u·lum
la'·bi·um pl. ·bia, gen. sg. ·bii, gen. pl. la'·bi·o'·rum
la'·bor Brit. ·bour
lab'·o·ra·to'·ri·an
lab'·o·ra·to'·ry [la·bor'·a·to·ry]
lab'·ro·cyte
la'·brum pl. ·bra
lab'·y·rinth
lab'·y·rin·thec'·to·my
lab'·y·rin'·thi pl. & gen. sg. of labyrinthus
lab'·y·rin'·thic
lab'·y·rin'·thi·cus
lab'·y·rin'·thine
lab'·y·rin·thi'·tis
lab'·y·rin·thot'·o·my
lab'·y·rin'·thus pl. & gen. sg. ·thi
lac gen. lac'·tis
lac'·er·ate ·at'·ed, ·at'·ing
lac'·er·a'·tion
la·cer'·tus pl. ·ti
Lach'·e·sis
la·cin'·i·ate
la·cis'
lac'·ri·ma pl. ·mae
lac'·ri·mal
lac'·ri·ma'·le neut. of lacrimalis
lac'·ri·ma'·lis pl. ·les
lac'·ri·ma'·tion
lac'·ri·ma'·tor
lac'·ri·ma·to'·ry
lac'·ri·mo·con'·chal
lac'·ri·mo·con·cha'·lis
lac'·ri·mo·eth'·moid
lac'·ri·mo·eth·moi'·dal
lac'·ri·mo·max'·il·la'·ris
lac'·ri·mo·max'·il·lar'y
lac'·ri·mo·na'·sal
lac'·ri·mot'·o·my
lact·ac'·i·de'·mia Brit. ·dae'·mia; var. of lacticacidemia
lact·ac'·i·du'·ria
lac'·ta·gogue
lact'·al·bu'·min
lac'·tam
lac'·ta·mase
lac'·tase
lac'·tate n. & v. ·tat·ed, ·tat·ing
lac·ta'·tion
lac·ta'·tion·al
lac'·te·al
lac·tes'·cent
lac'·tic
lac'·tic·ac'·id·e'·mia Brit. ·ae'·mia
lac'·ti·ce'·mia Brit. ·cae'·mia; var. of lacticacidemia
lac·tif'·er·ous
lac·tif'·er·us pl. ·eri
lac'·ti·fuge
lac'·tis gen. of lac
lac'·to·
Lac'·to·ba·cil'·lus
L. ac'·i·doph'·i·lus
L. sal'i·va'·ri·us
lac'·to·ba·cil'·lus pl. ·li
lac'·to·bi'·o·nate
lac'·to·fer'·rin
lac'·to·fla'·vin
lac'·to·gen
lac'·to·gen'·e·sis
lac'·to·gen'·ic
lac'·to·glob'·u·lin
lac·tom'·e·ter
lac'·tone
lac'·to-o'vo·veg'·e·tar'·i·an
lac'·to·per·ox'·i·dase
lac'·to·phe'·nol
lac'·to·phos'·phate
lac'·tor·rhe'a Brit. ·rhoe'a
lac'·tose

lac′·tos·u′·ria [·to·su′·]
lac′·to·veg′·e·tar′·i·an
lac′·tu·lose
la·cu′·na *pl.* ·nae
la·cu′·nar
lac′·u·na′·ris *neut.* ·re
lac′·u·no′·sus *neut.*
  ·sum
la′·cus *pl.* lacus
Lae′·laps
lae′·sa
la′·e·trile
lae′·ve
lae′·vo· *Brit. spel. of*
  levo-
lag *n. & v.* lagged,
  lag′·ging
la·ge′·na *pl.* ·nae
la·ge′·nar
Lag′·o·chi·las′·ca·ris
mi′·nor
lag′·oph·thal′·mic
lag′·oph·thal′·mos
  also ·mus
la grippe′
lake *n.& v.* laked,
  lak′·ing
la′ky
lal·la′·tion
lal′o·
lal′·or·rhe′a *Brit.*
  ·rhoe′a
la·marck′·ism
lamb′·da
lamb′·da·cis′m
lamb′·doid *also* lamb·
  doi′·dal
lamb·doi′·de·us *fem.*
  ·dea
lam′·bert
Lam′·blia
  L. in·tes′·ti·na′·lis
lam·bli′·a·sis *also*
  lam′·bli·o′·sis
la·mel′la *pl.* ·lae
la·mel′·lar
lam′·el·late [la·mel′·
  late] *also* lam′·el·lat·
  ed

la·mel′·li·form
la·mel′·li·po′·di·um
  pl. ·dia
lam′·el·lo′·sum *pl.* ·sa
lam′·i·na *pl. & gen.*
  sg. ·nae
lam′·i·na·graph *var.*
  of laminograph
lam′·i·nag′·ra·phy
  var. of laminography
lam′·i·nar
Lam′·i·nar′·ia
lam′·i·nar′·in
lam′·i·nate *also* ·nat′·
  ed
lam′·i·na′·tion
lam′·i·nec′·to·my
lam′·i·ni′·tis
lam′·i·no·graph
lam′·i·nog′·ra·phy
lam′·i·not′·o·my
lance *n. & v.* lanced,
  lanc′·ing
lan′·ce·o·late
lan′·cet
lan′·ci·nat′·ing
land′·mark
lan′·guage
lan′·o·lin
la·nos′·ter·ol
lan′·tha·nide
lan′·tha·num
lan′·tho·pine
la·nu′·go
la·pac′·tic
lap′·a·rec′·to·my
lap′·a·ro·
lap′·a·ro·cele
lap′·a·ro·co·los′·to·my
lap′·a·ro·cys·tec′·to·my
lap′·a·ro·cys·tot′·o·my
lap′·a·ro·en′·ter·os′·to·
  my
lap′·a·ro·en′·ter·ot′·o·
  my
lap′·a·ro·gas·tros′·co·
  py
lap′·a·ro·gas·trot′·o·my

lap′·a·ro·hep′·a·tot′·o·
  my
lap′·a·ro·il′e·ot′·o·my
lap′·a·ro·my′·o·mec′·
  to·my
lap′·a·ro·my′·o·mot′·o·
  my
lap′·a·ro·ne·phrec′·to·
  my
lap′·a·ror′·rha·phy
lap′·a·ro·scope
lap′·a·ros′·co·py
lap′·a·ro·sple·not′·o·my
lap′·a·rot′·o·my
lap′·a·thin
lap′·is
lap′·pa
lap′·sus *pl.* lapsus
lar·da′·ceous
lar′·i·at
lar′·va *pl. & gen. sg.*
  ·vae
lar·va′·ceous
lar′·val
lar′·vate
lar′·vi·cide
lar·vip′·a·rous
la·ryn′·gea *fem. of*
  ·laryngeus
la·ryn′·ge·al
la·ryn′·ge·a′·lis *pl.*
  ·les
lar′·yn·gec′·to·my
la·ryn′·ge·us *pl. &*
  gen. sg. ·gei, *ablative*
  ·geo
la·ryn′·gis *gen. of*
  larynx
lar′·yn·gis′·mus
lar′·yn·git′·ic
lar′·yn·gi′·tis
la·ryn′·go·
la·ryn′·go·cele
la·ryn′·go·fis′·sure
lar′·yn·gog′·ra·phy
lar′·yn·gol′·o·gist
lar′·yn·gol′·o·gy
la·ryn′·go·ma·la′·cia

laryngopathy / lemmocyte

lar'·yn·gop·a·thy
la·ryn'·go·pha·ryn'·ge·al
la·ryn'·go·pha·ryn'·ge·us *pl. & gen. sg.* ·gei
la·ryn'·go·phar'·yn·gi'·tis
la·ryn'·go·phar'·ynx
la·ryn'·go·plas'·ty
la·ryn'·gor·rhe'a *Brit.* ·rhoe'a
la·ryn'·go·scope
la·ryn'·go·scop'·ic
lar'·yn·gos'·co·py
la·ryn'·go·spas'm
la·ryn'·go·stro'·bo·scope
lar'·yn·got'·o·my
la·ryn'·go·tra'·che·al
la·ryn'·go·tra'·che·i'tis
la·ryn'·go·tra'·cheo·bron·chi'·tis
la·ryn'·go·tra'·cheo·bron'·chi·al
la·ryn'·go·tra'·che·os'·co·py
lar'·ynx *L. pl.* la·ryn'·ges, *gen. sg.* la·ryn'·gis
la'·ser
las'·si·tude
la'·ta *catatonic disorder; also* la'·tah
la'·ta *fem. sg. & neut. pl. of* latus (*broad*); *gen. sg.* ·tae
la'·ten·cy
la'·tent
la·ten'·ti·a'·tion
lat'·er·ad
lat'·er·al
lat'·er·a'·le *neut. of* lateralis; *pl.* ·lia
lat'·er·a'·lis *pl.* ·les, *gen. pl.* ·li·um
lat'·er·al'·i·ty
lat'·er·al·i·za'·tion
lat'·er·is *gen. of* latus (*side*)

lat'·ero·
lat'·ero·ab·dom'·i·nal
lat'·er·o·duc'·tion
lat'·ero·flex'·ion
lat'·ero·pul'·sion
lat'·ero·tor'·sion
lat'·ero·tru'·sion
lat'·ero·ver'·sion
la'·tex
lath'·y·ris'm
lath'·y·rit'·ic
lath'·y·ro·gen
lath'·y·ro·gen'·ic
Lath'·y·rus
la·tis'·si·mus *pl. & gen. sg.* ·mi
lat'·ro·dec'·tism
Lat'·ro·dec'·tus
  L. mac'·tans
lat'·tice
la'·tus *broad; fem.* ·ta, *neut.* ·tum
lat'·us *side; pl.* lat'·era, *gen. sg.* lat'·er·is
laud'·a·ble
lau·dan'·i·dine
lau'·da·nine
lau'·da·num
lau'·reth
lau'·ric
la·vage'
la·va'·tion
law·ren'·ci·um
lax'a
lax·a'·tion
lax'·a·tive
lax'·a·tor
lax'·i·ty
lay'·er
laz'·a·ret'·to
leach *to dissolve out: Cf.* leech
lead
leaf'·let
learn'·ing
lec'·a·no·so'·ma·top'·a·gus
lec'·i·thal

lec'·i·thin
lec'·i·thin·ase
lec'·i·tho·
lec'·tin
leech *bloodsucking worm: Cf.* leach
left'-hand'·ed
Le'·gion·el'·la
  L. pneu·moph'·i·la
le'·gion·el·lo'·sis
le·gume' [leg'·ume]
lei'o·
Lei'o·gnath'·us ba·co'·ti
lei'o·my'o·blas·to'·ma *pl.* ·mas *or* ·ma·ta
lei'o·my·o'·ma *pl.* ·mas *or* ·ma·ta
lei'o·my·o'·ma·to'·sis
lei'o·my'o·sar·co'·ma *pl.* ·mas *or* ·ma·ta
lei'·po·
Leish·man'·ia [·ma'·nia]
  L. ae'·thi·op'·i·ca
  L. bra·sil'·i·en'·sis
  L. cha'·ga·si
  L. don'·o·va'·ni
  L. mex'·i·ca'·na
  L. pi·fa'·noi
  L. trop'·i·ca
leish·man'·ia [·ma'·nia] *pl.* ·i·ae
leish·man'·i·al [·ma'·ni·al]
leish'·man·i'·a·sis *also* ·man·i·o'·sis
leish'·man·i·cid'·al [·ci'·dal]
leish'·man·oid
le'·ma
le·me'·mia
lem'·ma *pl.* ·ma·ta
lem'·mo·blast *also* lem'·no·
lem'·mo·cyte *also* lem'·no·

lem·nis′·cus pl. &
  gen. sg. ·ci, gen. pl.
  lem′·nis·co′·rum
len′·i·tive
lens L. pl. len′·tes,
  gen. sg. len′·tis
lens·om′·e·ter
len·tec′·to·my also
  lens·ec′·to·my
len′·ti·cel
len′·ti·co′·nus
len·tic′·u·la
len·tic′·u·lar
len·tic′·u·la′·ris
len·tic′·u·lo·stri′·ate
len·tic′·u·lo·tha·lam′·ic
len·tic′·u·lus pl. ·li
len′·ti·form
len′·ti·for′·mis pl.
  ·mes
len·tig′·i·no′·sis
len·tig′·i·nous
len′·ti·glo′·bus
len·ti′·go pl. len·tig′·i·
  nes
len′·tis gen. of lens
len·ti′·tis
len′·ti·vi′·rus
le′·on·ti′·a·sis
lep′·er
lep′·i·do·
Lep′·i·dop′·tera
lep′·o·ri·pox′·vi′·rus
lep′·o·thrix
lep′·ra
lep′·re·chaun·is′m
lep′·ro·lin
le·prol′·o·gist
le·prol′·o·gy
le·pro′·ma pl. ·mas or
  ·ma·ta
le·pro′·ma·to′·sis
le·prom′·a·tous [·pro′·
  ma·]

lep′·ro·min
lep′·ro·pho′·bia
lep′·ro·sar′·i·um pl.
  ·ia
lep′·ro·stat′·ic
le·pro′·sum
lep′·ro·sy
le·prot′·ic
lep′·rous
lep′·ta·zol
lep′·to·
lep′·to·ce·phal′·ic
lep′·to·ceph′·a·ly
lep′·to·cyte
lep′·to·cyt′·ic
lep′·to·cy·to′·sis
lep′·to·dac′·ty·ly
lep′·to·me·nin′·ge·al
lep′·to·me·nin′·ges
  sg. ·me′·ninx
lep′·to·me·nin′·gi·o′·ma
lep′·to·men′·in·gi′·tis
lep′·to·men′·in·gop′·a·
  thy
lep·tom′·o·nad [lep′·to·
  mo′·nad]
lep′·to·ne′·ma
lep′·to·pel′·lic
lep′·to·pro·so′·pia
Lep′·to·psyl′·la
lep′·tor·rhine
lep′·to·scope
Lep′·to·spi′·ra
  L. in·ter′·ro·gans
lep′·to·spi′·ral
lep′·to·spire
lep′·to·spi·ro′·sis
lep′·to·tene
lep′·to·tri·cho′·sis
Lep′·to·trom·bid′·i·um
Lep′·tus
les′·bi·an
les′·bi·an·is′m

le′·sion
le·ta′·lis
let′-down
le′·thal
le·thal′·i·ty
le·thar′·gic
le·thar′·gi·ca
leth′·ar·gy
leu·ce′·mia Brit.
  ·cae′·; var. of leukemia
leu′·cine
leu′·ci·no′·sis
leu′·cin·u′·ria [·ci·nu′·]
leu′·co·[34] var. of
  leuko-
leu′·co·ci′·din Brit.
  spel. of leukocidin
leu′·co·cyte Brit. spel.
  of leukocyte
leu′·co·cy·thae′·mia
  Brit. spel. of leukocy-
  themia
leu′·co·cy·to′·sis Brit.
  spel. of leukocytosis
leu′·co·der′·ma Brit.
  spel. of leukoderma
leu′·co·fluo·res′·ce·in
leu·co′·ma Brit. spel.
  of leukoma
Leu′·co·nos′·toc
leuc′·o·nych′·i·a Brit.
  spel. of leukonychia
leu′·co·pe′·nia Brit.
  spel. of leukopenia
leu′·co·pla′·kia Brit.
  spel. of leukoplakia
leu′·co·plast
leu′·co·poi·e′·sis Brit.
  spel. of leukopoiesis
leu′·cor·rhoe′a Brit.
  spel. of leukorrhea
leu′·cor·rhoe′·al Brit.
  spel. of leukorrheal

---

[34] In medical and medical-related terms, the preferred American spelling of this word element is generally with *k*, but *c* is used in most chemical and pharmaceutical terms (e.g., *leucovorin*) and taxonomic names (e.g., *Leuconostoc*). In British spelling, *c* is widely preferred except in *leukaemia* and its derivatives.

leu·cot′·o·my *var. of* leukotomy
leu′·co·vo′·rin
Leu′-en·keph′·a·lin *also* leu′-
leuk′·ag·glu′·ti·nin *var. of* leukoagglutinin
leuk′·apher·e′·sis [·apher′·e·]
leu·ke′·mia *Brit.* ·kae′·
leu·ke′·mic *Brit.* ·kae′·
leu·ke′·mi·cus *also* ·kae·
leu·ke′·mid *Brit.* ·kae′·
leu·ke′·mo·gen *Brit.* ·kae′·
leu·ke′·mo·gen′·e·sis *Brit.* ·kae′·
leu·ke′·mo·gen′·ic *Brit.*·kae′·
leu·ke′·moid *Brit.* ·kae′·
leu′·kin
leu′·ko· *also* ·leuco-
leu′·ko·ag·glu′·ti·nin
leu′·ko·blas·to′·sis
leu′·ko·ci′·din
leu′·ko·co′·ria
leu′·ko·cyte
leu′·ko·cy·the′·mia
leu′·ko·cyt′·ic
leu′·ko·cy′·to·blast
leu′·ko·cy′·to·gen′·e·sis
leu′·ko·cy′·toid [·cyt′·oid]
leu′·ko·cy·tol′·y·sis
leu′·ko·cy′·to·lyt′·ic
leu′·ko·cy·tom′·e·ter
leu′·ko·cy′·to·pe′·nia
leu′·ko·cy′·to·poi·e′·sis
leu′·ko·cy·to′·sis
leu′·ko·cy′·to·tro′·pic [·trop′·ic]
leu′·ko·cy·tu′·ria
leu′·ko·der′·ma *also* ·der′·mia
leu′·ko·der′·ma·tous
leu′·ko·dys·tro′·phia
leu′·ko·dys′·tro·phy
leu′·ko·en·ceph′·a·li′·tis
leu′·ko·en·ceph′·a·lop′·a·thy
leu′·ko·eryth′·ro·blas′·tic
leu′·ko·eryth′·ro·blas·to′·sis
leu′·ko·ker′·a·to′·sis
leu′·ko·ki·net′·ics
leu′·ko·ko′·ria *var. of* leukocoria
leu′·ko·lym′·pho·sar·co′·ma
leu·ko′·ma *pl.* ·mas *or* ·ma·ta
leu·ko′ma·tous [·kom′a·]
leu′·kon
leuk′·o·nych′·ia
leu′·ko·path′·ia
leu·kop′·a·thy
leu′·ko·pe·de′·sis
leu′·ko·pe′·nia
leu′·ko·pe′·nic
leu′·ko·pla′·kia
leu′·ko·pla′·kic
leu′·ko·poi·e′·sis
leu′·ko·poi·et′·ic
leu·kop′·sin
leu′·kor·rhe′a
leu′·kor·rhe′·al
leu′·ko·sar·co′·ma *pl.* ·mas *or* ·ma·ta
leu′·ko·scope
leu·ko′·sis
leu′·ko·tac′·tic
leu′·ko·tax′·ine
leu′·ko·tax′·is
leu′·ko·ther′·a·py
leu·kot′·ic
leu′·ko·tome
leu·kot′·o·my
leu′·ko·tox′·in
leu′·ko·trich′·ia
leu′·ko·tri′·ene
leu′·pro·lide
lev′·al·lor′·phan
lev′·am·fet′·a·mine *also* ·phet′·
le·vam′·i·sole
lev′·an
lev′·ar·ter′·e·nol [lev·ar′·te·re′·nol]
le·va′·tor *pl.* lev′·a·to′·res, *gen. sg.* ·to′·ris
lev′·el
lev′·i·gate ·gat′·ed, ·gat′·ing
le′·vo *Brit.* lae′·vo·
le′·vo·a′trio·car′·di·nal
le′·vo·car′·dia
le′·vo·car′·di·o·gram
le′·vo·con′·dy·lis′m
le′·vo·do′·pa
le′·vo·duc′·tion
le′·vo·nor·def′·rin [·nor′·de·frin]
le′·vo·ro′·ta·to′·ry
lev·or′·pha·nol
le′·vo·thy·rox′·ine
le′·vo·tor′·sion
le′·vo·ver′·sion
le·vox′·a·drol
lev′·u·li·nate
lev′·u·lin′·ic
lev′·u·lose
lev′·u·los·e′·mia [·lo·se′·mia] *Brit.* ·ae′·mia
lew′·is·ite
li′·a·bil′·i·ty
li′·ber *fem.* li′·bera
li·bid′·i·nal
li·bid′·i·nous
li·bi′·do
lice *pl. of* louse

li′·cence[35]
li′·cense ·censed,
 ·cens·ing
li·cen′·ti·ate
li′·chen
li·chen′·i·fi·ca′·tion
li′·chen·i·for′·min
li′·chen·oid
li′·chen·oi′·des
li′·chen·ous
lic″·o·rice *Brit.* liq′·
 uo·rice
li′·do·caine
li′·do·fla′·zine
li″·en *gen.* li·e′nis
li′·enal [li·e′nal]
li′·ena′·lis
li·en′·cu·lus *pl.* ·li
li′·eno· [li·e′no·]
li′·enog′·ra·phy
li′·eno·med′·ul·lar′y
li′·eno·my′·e·lo·ma·la′·
 cia
li′·eno·phren′·ic [li·
 e′no·]
li′·eno·re′·nal
li′·en·ter′·ic
li′·en·ter′y [li·en′·tery]
life *pl.* lives
lig′·a·ment
lig′·a·men′·to·pex′y
lig′·a·men′·tous
lig′·a·men′·tum *pl.*
 ·ta, *gen. sg.* ·ti
lig′·and [li′·gand]
li′·gase
li′·gate ·gat·ed, ·gat·ing
li·ga′·tion
li′·ga·tor
lig′·a·ture
light′-adapt′·ed
light′·en·ing
light′-head′·ed
lig′·nin

lig′·no·caine
lig′·no·cer′·ic
lig′·u·la
Li′·max
limb
lim′·bal
lim′·bic
lim′·bi·cus
lim·bo′·sa
lim′·bus *pl. & gen. sg.*
 ·bi
li′·men *pl.* lim′·i·na
li′·mes *pl.* lim′·i·tes
lim′·i·nal
lim′·i·nom′·e·ter
lim′·it
lim′·i·tans
lim′·o·nene
li′·mo·ther′·a·py
lin′·co·my′·cin
linc′·tus
lin′·dane
lin′·ea *pl. & gen. sg.*
 ·e·ae
lin′·e·age
lin′·e·al
lin′·e·ar
lin′·e·a′·ris
line′·breed·ing
lin′·er
lin′·gua *gen.* ·guae
lin′·gual
lin·gua′·lis *pl.* ·les
Lin·guat′·u·la
lin·guat′·u·li′·a·sis
lin·guat′·u·lid
lin′·gui·form
lin′·gu·la *pl.* ·lae
lin′·gu·lar
lin′·gu·la′·ris
lin′·guo·
lin′·guo·cer′·vi·cal
lin′·guo·cli·na′·tion
lin′·guo·den′·tal

lin′·guo·fa′·cial
lin′·guo·fa′·ci·a′·lis
lin′·guo·gin′·gi·val
 [·gin·gi′·val]
lin′·guo·ver′·sion
lin′·i·ment
li′·nin
lin′·ing
li·ni′·tis
link′·age
lin′·o·le′·ic
lin′·o·len′·ic
li′o· *var. of* leio-
li′o·thy′·ro·nine
lip′·a·ro·cele
li′·pase
li·pec′·to·my
li·pe′·mia *Brit.* ·pae′·
li·pe′·mic *Brit.* ·pae′·
lip′·id
lip′·i·dol″·y·sis [lip′·id·
 ol′·]
lip′·i·do·lyt′·ic
lip′·i·do′·sis
lip′·id·u″·ria [·i·du′·]
lip′o· [li′po·]
lip′o·ad′·e·no′·ma
li′po·am′·ide
lip′o·ar·thri′·tis
lip′o·atro′·phic
 [·atroph′·ic]
lip′o·at′·ro·phy
lip′o·blast
lip′o·blas·to′·ma *pl.*
 ·mas *or* ·ma·ta
lip′o·blas′·to·ma·to′·sis
lip′·o·cele
lip′o·chon′·dro·dys′·
 tro·phy
lip′o·cyte
lip′o·der′·ma·to·scle·
 ro″·sis
lip′o·dys′·tro·phy
lip′o·fi·bro′·ma *pl.*
 ·mas *or* ·ma·ta

---

[35] In British spelling *licence* is used for the noun while the verb is usually *license.* American spelling has *license* regularly for both.

lipofuscin / lobomycosis 156

lip'o·fus'·cin
lip'o·gen'·ic
lip'o·gran'·u·lo'·ma *pl.* ·mas *or* ·ma·ta
lip'o·gran'·u·lo'·ma·to'·sis
li·po'·ic
lip'·oid
li·poi'·dal
lip'·oi·do'·sis
li·pol'·y·sis
lip'o·lyt'·ic
li·po'·ma *pl.* ·mas *or* ·ma·ta
li·po'·ma·to'·des
li·po'·ma·toid
li·po'·ma·to'·sis
li·po'·ma·to'·sus
li·pom'a·tous [·po'ma·]
lip'o·me·lan'·ic
lip'o·me·nin'·go·cele
lip'o·met'·a·bol'·ic
lip'o·me·tab'·o·lis'm
lip'o·mi'·cron
lip'o·myx·o'·ma *pl.* ·mas *or* ·ma·ta
lip'o·myx'o·sar·co'·ma *pl.* ·mas *or* ·ma·ta
Lip'·o·nys·soi'·des
Lip'·o·nys'·sus
lip'o·pe'·nia
lip'o·pe'·nic
lip'o·phage
lip'o·phag'·ic
li·poph'·a·gy
lip'o·phan'·er·o'·sis
lip'o·phil'·ic
lip'o·phore
lip'o·pol'y·sac'·cha·ride
lip'o·pro'·tein
lip'o·pro'·tein·o'·sis
lip'o·sar·co'·ma *pl.* ·mas *or* ·ma·ta
li·po'·sis
lip'o·some
lip'o·tei·cho'·ic

lip'o·tro'·phic [·troph'·ic]
lip'o·tro'·pic [·trop'·ic]
lip'o·tro'·pin
lip'o·tu·ber'·cu·lin
lip'o·vac·cine'
lip·ox'·y·gen·ase
li·pox'·ysm
lip'·ping
li·pu'·ria *var. of* lipiduria
liq'·ue·fa'·cient
liq'·ue·fac'·tion
liq'·ue·fy ·fied, ·fy'·ing
liq'·uid
liq'·uor *L. pl.* li·quo'·res
liq'·uo·rice *Brit. spel. of* licorice
lis'·sen·ce·phal'·ic
lis'·sen·ceph'·a·ly
lis'·sive
Lis·te'·ria mon'·o·cy·tog'·e·nes
lis·te'·ri·o'·sis *also* lis'·ter·el·lo'·sis
lis'·ter·is'm
li'·ter *Brit.* ·tre
lith'·a·gogue
li·than'·gi·u'·ria
li·thec'·ta·sy
li·the'·mia *Brit.* ·thae'·
li·the'·mic *Brit.* ·thae'·
li·thi'·a·sis
lith'·ic
lith'·i·um
lith'o·
lith'·o·cho'·lic
lith'·o·clast
lith'·o·clas'·ty
lith'o·cys·tot'·o·my
lith'o·gen'·e·sis
li·thog'·e·nous
lith'o·kel'·y·pho·pe'·di·on
lith'·o·labe
li·thol'·a·pax'y
li·thol'·o·gy

li·thol'·y·sis
lith'·o·lyte
lith'·o·lyt'·ic
lith'o·ne·phrot'·o·my
lith'o·pe'·di·on *Brit.* ·pae'·
lith'·o·scope
lith'·o·tome
li·thot'·o·my
lith'·o·tre'·sis
lith'·o·trip'·sy
lith'·o·trip'·tic
lith'·o·trip'·tor *also* ·ter
lith'·o·trip'·to·scope
lith'·o·trip·tos'·co·py
lith'·o·trite
li·thot'·ri·ty
lith'·ure'·sis
lith'·ure·ter'·ia
lit'·mus
li'·tre *Brit. spel. of* liter
lit'·ter
lit·tri'·tis
live'-born
li·ve'·do
liv'·er
liv'·id
li·vid'·i·ty
li'·vor
lix·iv'·i·a'·tion
Lo'a
lo'a·i'a·sis *var. of* loiasis
lo'·bar
lo·ba'·ris *pl.* ·res
lo'·bate
lo·ba'·tion
lo·ba'·tum
lobe
lo·bec'·to·my
lo·be'·lia
lo'·be·line
lo'·be·lis'm
lo'·bi *pl. & gen. sg. of* lobus
lo'·bo·my·co'·sis

lo'·bo·po'·di·um *pl.*
  ·dia
lo'·bose
lo·bot'·o·my
lob'·u·lar
lob'·u·lat'·ed
lob'·u·la'·tion
lob'·ule
lob'·u·lose
lob'·u·lus *pl.* ·li
lo'·bus *pl. & gen. sg.*
  ·bi
lo'·cal
lo'·cal·i·za'·tion
lo'·cal·ize ·ized, ·iz'·
  ing
lo'·cal·iz'·er
lo'·chia
lo'·chi·al
lo'·chio·me·tri'·tis
lo'·ci *pl. of* locus
lock'·jaw
lo'·co·mo'·tion
lo'·co·mo'·tive
lo'·co·mo'·tor
lo'·co·mo·to'·ri·al
lo'·co·mo'·to·ry
loc'·u·lar
loc'·u·late *also* ·lat'·ed
loc'·u·la'·tion
loc'·ule
loc'·u·lus *pl.* ·li
lo'·cum ten'·ens *pl.*
  lo'·cum te·nen'·tes
lo'·cus *pl.* ·ci,
  accusative sg. ·cum
loef·fler'·ia
loe·mae'·mia *Brit.*
  spel. of lememia
log·a·dec'·to·my
log'·am·ne'·sia
log'·apha'·sia
log'·a·rith'·mic
log'·it
log'o·
log'·o·clo'·nia
log'o·ma'·nia

log'·o·pe'·dia *Brit.*
  ·pae'·; *var. of*
  logopedics
log'·o·pe'·dics *Brit.*
  ·pae'·
log'·or·rhe'a *Brit.*
  ·rhoe'a
log'o·ther'·a·py
lo·i'a·sis
loin
lo'·li·is'm *also* lo'·lism
lon'·ga *fem. of* longus;
  pl. & gen. sg. ·gae
lon·gev'·i·ty
lon'·gi *pl. & gen. sg.*
  of longus
lon·gis'·si·mus
lon'·gi·tu'·di·nal
lon'·gi·tu'·di·na'·le
  neut. of longitudinalis
lon'·gi·tu'·di·na'·lis
  pl. ·les
long·sight'·ed·ness
lon'·gum *neut. of*
  longus
lon'·gus *pl. & gen. sg.*
  ·gi
loop'·ful
loos'·en·ing
loph'·o·dont
Lo·phoph'·o·ra wil·
  liam'·sii
lo·phoph'·o·rine
lo·phot'·ri·chous
lor·az'·e·pam
lor·bam'·ate
lor'·do·sco'·li·o'·sis
lor·do'·sis
lor·dot'·ic
lo'·tio
lo'·tion
loud'·ness
loupe
loup'·ing-ill'
louse *pl.* lice
lous'·i·cide
lou'·si·ness
lou'·sy ·si·er, ·si·est

lo'·va·stat'·in
low'-spin'
lox'·a·pine
lox'·ia
lox'·oph·thal'·mus
Lox·os'·ce·les
  L. lae'·ta
  L. re·clu'·sa
lox·os'·ce·lis'm
loz'·enge
lubb'-dupp'
lu'·bri·cant
lu·can'·thone
lu'·cent
lu'·cid
lu'·ci·dus *fem.* ·da,
  neut. ·dum
lu·cif'·er·ase
lu·cif'·er·ine
Lu·cil'·ia
  L. cae'·sar
lück'·en·schä'·del
lu'·co·ther'·a·py
lu'·es
lu·et'·ic
lu'·etin
lu·lib'·er·in
lum·ba'·go
lum·ba'·le *neut. of*
  lumbalis; *pl.* ·lia
lum·ba'·lis *pl.* ·les,
  gen. pl. ·li·um
lum'·bar
lum·ba'·ris
lum'·bar·i·za'·tion
lum'·bo·
lum'·bo·cos'·tal
lum'·bo·cos·ta'·lis
  neut. ·le
lum'·bo·cos'·to·ab·
  dom'·i·nal
lum'·bo·dor'·sal
lum'·bo·il'i·ac
lum'·bo·in'·gui·nal
lum·bo'·rum *gen. pl.*
  of lumbus
lum'·bo·sa'·cral

lum'·bo·sa·cra'·lis
lum'·bri·cal
lum'·bri·ca'·lis *pl.* ·les
lum'·bri·coid
lum'·bri·cus *pl.* ·ci
lum'·bus *pl & gen. sg.*
 ·bi, *gen. pl.* lum·bo'·
 rum
lu'·men *pl.* ·mens *or*
 ·mi·na
lu'·mi·chrome
lu'·mi·fla'·vin
lu'·mi·nal
lu'·mi·nes'·cence
lu'·mi·nif'·er·ous
lu'·mi·nous
lu'·mi·rho·dop'·sin
lu'·mi·some
lu·mis'·ter·ol
lump·ec'·to·my
lu'·nar
lu'·nate
lu·na'·to·ma·la'·cia
 [lu'·na·to·]
lu·na'·tus *fem.* ·ta,
  neut. ·tum
lung
lung'·worm
lu'·nu·la *pl.* ·lae
lu'·nule
lu'·pi·form
lu'·pi·nine
lu'·poid
lu·po'·ma
lu'·pous
lu'·pus
lu·so'·ria
lu'·tea *fem. sg. &*
  neut. pl. of luteus
lu'·te·al
lu'·te·ec'·to·my
lu'·te·in
lu'·te·in·i·za'·tion
lu'·te·in·ize ·ized, ·iz'·
 ing
lu'·teo·
lu'·te·o·gen'·ic

lu'·te·o·lin [lu'·te·o'·
 lin]
lu'·te·ol'·y·sis
lu'·te·o'·ma *pl.* ·mas
 or ·ma·ta
lu'·te·o·tro'·phic
 [·troph'·ic] *var. of*
 luteotropic
lu'·te·o·tro'·pic [·trop'·
 ic]
lu'·te·o·tro'·pin *also*
 ·tro'·phin
lu·te'·ti·um
lu'·te·us *fem.* ·tea,
 neut. ·te·um
lut'·ing
lu'·tu·trin
Lutz' o my'·ia
  L. *fla' vi scu' tel·la'·
  ta*
  L. *lon'·gi·pal'·pis*
  L. *pes·so'·ai*
lux'·ans
lux·a'·tio
lux·a'·tion
lux'·us
ly'·ase
ly·can'·thro·py
ly'·co·pene
ly'·co·pen·e'·mia
 Brit. ·ae'·mia
Ly'·co·per'·don
ly'·co·per'·do·no'·sis
ly'·co·po'·di·um
Ly·co'·sa
ly'·ing-in'
Lym·nae'a
lymph
lym'·pha
lym'·pha·den
lym·phad'·e·nec'·to·my
lym·phad'·e·ni'·tis
lym·phad'·e·no·cyst
lym·phad'·e·noid
lym·phad'·e·no'·ma
lym·phad'·e·nom·a'·
 tous [·no'·ma·]
lym·phad'·e·nop'·a·thy

lym·phad'·e·no'·sis
lym·phad'·e·not'·o·my
lym·phad'·e·no·var'·ix
lymph'·a·gogue
lym·phan'·ge·i'·tis
 var. of lymphangitis
lym·phan'·gi·al
lym·phan'·gi·ec'·ta·sis
 also ·ec·ta'·sia
lym·phan'·gi·ec'·to·my
lym'·phan'·gi·i'·tis
 var. of lymphangitis
lym·phan'·gio·
lym·phan'·gio·ad'·e·
 nog'·ra·phy
lym·phan'·gio·en'·do·
 the'·li·al
lym·phan'·gio·en'·do·
 the'·li·o'·ma
lym·phan'·gi·o·gram
lym'·phan'·gi·og'·ra·
 phy
lym·phan'·gio·lei'·o·
 my·o'·ma·to'·sis
lym'·phan'·gi·ol'·o·gy
lym·phan'·gi·o'·ma
  pl. ·mas *or* ·ma·ta
lym·phan'·gi·om·a'·
 tous [·o'·ma·]
lym·phan'·gio·my·o'·
 ma
lym·phan'·gio·phle·bi'·
 tis
lym·phan'·gi·o·plas'·ty
lym·phan'·gio·sar·co'·
 ma *pl.* ·mas *or* ·ma·
 ta
lym·phan'·gi·ot'·o·my
lym'·phan·gi'·tis
lym·phat'·ic
lym·phat'·i·ca *fem.*
 sg. & neut. pl. of
 lymphaticus
lym·phat'·i·co·splen'·ic
lym·phat'·i·cos'·to·my
lym·phat'·i·co·ve'·nous
lym·phat'·i·cum *neut.*
 of lymphaticus

lym·phat′·i·cus *pl. & gen. sg.* ·ci
lym″·pha·tis′m
lym′·pha·tog′·e·nous
lym′·pha·tol′·o·gy
lymph′·ede′·ma Brit. ·oe·de′·ma
lymph′·en′·do·the′·li·o′·ma
lym′·pho·
lym′·pho·blast
lym′·pho·blas′·tic
lym′·pho·blas′·toid
lym′·pho·blas·to′·ma *pl.* ·mas *or* ·ma·ta
lym′·pho·blas·to′·sis
lym′·pho·cele
lym′·pho·cyte
lym′·pho·cyt′·ic
lym′·pho·cy′·to·blast
lym′·pho·cy′·toid [·cyt′·oid]
lym′·pho·cy·to′·ma *pl.* ·mas *or* ·ma·ta
lym′·pho·cy′·to·pe′·nia
lym′·pho·cy′·to·poi·e′·sis
lym′·pho·cy′·to·poi·et′·ic
lym′·pho·cy·to′·sis
lym′·pho·cy·tot′·ic
lym′·pho·cy′·to·tox′·in
lymph′·oe·de′·ma Brit. spel. of lymphedema
lym′·pho·ep′·i·the′·li·al
lym′·pho·ep′·i·the′·li·oid
lym′·pho·ep′·i·the′·li·o′·ma
lym′·pho·gen′·e·sis
lym·phog′·e·nous
lym′·pho·gram
lym′·pho·gran′·u·lo′·ma *pl.* ·mas *or* ·ma·ta
lym′·pho·gran′·u·lo′·ma·to′·sis

lym·phog′·ra·phy
lym′·phoid
lym·phoi′·do·cyte
lym′·pho·ken′·tric
lym′·pho·kine
lym·phol′·o·gy
lym·pho′·ma *pl.* ·mas *or* ·ma·ta
lym·pho′·ma·toid
lym′·pho·ma·to′·sis *pl.* ·ses
lym·pho′·ma·to′·sum
lym·pho′·ma·tous [·phom′·a·]
lym′·pho·no′·dus *pl.* ·di
lym′·pho·pe′·nia
lym′·pho·pe′·nic
lym′·pho·plas′·ty
lym′·pho·poi·e′·sis
lym′·pho·poi·et′·ic
lym′·pho·poi′·e·tin
lym′·pho·pro·lif″·er·a·tive
lym′·pho·re·tic′·u·lar
lym′·pho·re·tic′·u·lo′·sis
lym′·phor·rhage
lym′·phor·rhe′a Brit. ·rhoe′a
lym′·phor·rhoid
lym′·pho·sar·co′·ma *pl.* ·mas *or* ·ma·ta
lym′·pho·sar·co″·ma·tous [·com′·a·]
lym·phos′·ta·sis
lym′·pho·stat′·ic
lym′·pho·tax′·is
lym′·pho·tox′·ic
lym′·pho·tox′·in
lym′·pho·tro′·phic [·troph′·ic]
lym·phot′·ro·phy
lym′·pho·tro′·pic [·trop′·ic]
lymph·u′·ria
lyn·es′·tre·nol
ly′·o·

ly′·on·i·za′·tion
ly′·o·phile
ly′·o·phil′·ic
ly·oph′·i·li·za′·tion
ly·oph′·i·lized
ly′o·pho′·bic
ly′·o·tro′·pic [·trop′·ic]
ly·pres′·sin
ly′·ra
ly′·sate
lyse lysed, lys′·ing
ly·sen′·ko·is′m
ly·ser′·gic
ly′·sin
ly′·sine
ly′·sis
ly′·so·
ly′·so·gen′·ic
ly·sog′·e·ni·za′·tion
ly·sog′·e·ny
ly′·so·ki′·nase
ly′·so·lec′·i·thin
ly′·so·phos′·pha·ti′·dyl·cho′·line
ly′·so·som′·al [·so′·mal]
ly′·so·some
ly′·so·staph′·in
ly′·so·type
ly′·so·zyme
ly′·so·zy·mu′·ria
lys′·sa
Lys′·sa·vi′·rus
ly′·syl
lyt′·ic
Lyt′·ta
lyx′·ose

M

Ma·ca′·ca
  M. mu·lat′·ta
ma·caque′
mac′·er·ate ·at′·ed, ·at′·ing
mac′·er·a′·tion
mac′·er·a′·tive

ma·chine′
ma′·ci·es
Mac′·ra·can′·tho·rhyn′·chus
   M. hi·ru′·di·na′·ce·us
mac′·ro·
mac′·ro·ag′·gre·gate
mac′·ro·am′·y·las·e′· mia Brit. ·ae′·mia
Mac′·ro·bdel′·la
   M. de·co′·ra
mac′·ro·bi′·ote
mac′·ro·bi·ot′·ic
mac′·ro·blast
mac′·ro·bra′·chia
mac′·ro·car′·dia
mac′·ro·car′·di·us
mac′·ro·ceph′·a·lous also ·ce·phal′·ic
mac′·ro·ceph′·a·lus
mac′·ro·ceph′·a·ly
mac′·ro·chei′·lia
mac′·ro·chy′·lo·mi′·cron
mac′·ro·chy′·lo·mi′·cro·ne′·mia [·cron·e′·mia] Brit. ·nae′·
mac′·ro·cra′·nia
mac′·ro·cyst
mac′·ro·cyte
mac′·ro·cyt′·ic
mac′·ro·cy·to′·sis
mac′·ro·dac′·ty·ly
mac′·ro·dont
mac′·ro·don′·tia
mac′·ro·dys·tro′·phia
mac′·ro·en·ceph′·a·ly
mac′·ro·eryth′·ro·blast
mac′·ro·eryth′·ro·cyte
mac′·ro·es·the′·sia Brit. ·aes·the′·
mac′·ro·fol·lic′·u·lar
mac′·ro·gam′·ete
mac′·ro·ga·me′·to·cyte
mac′·ro·gen′·e·sis
mac′·ro·gen′·i·to·so′·mia

mac·rog′·lia
mac·rog′·li·al
mac′·ro·glob′·u·lin
mac′·ro·glob′·u·lin·e′· mia Brit. ·ae′·mia
mac′·ro·glos′·sia
mac′·ro·gna′·thia
mac′·ro·gy′·ria
mac′·ro·lec′·i·thal
mac′·ro·lide
mac′·ro·mas′·tia also ·ma′·zia
mac′·ro·me′·lia
mac′·ro·mere
mac′·ro·meth′·od
mac′·ro·mo·lec′·u·lar
mac′·ro·mol′·e·cule
mac′·ro·mu·ta′·tion
mac′·ro·nod′·u·lar
mac′·ro·nor′·mo·blast
mac′·ro·nu′·cle·us pl. ·clei
mac′·ro·nu′·tri·ent
mac′·ro·nych′·ia
mac′·ro·phage
mac′·ro·phag′·o·cy·to′·sis
mac′·roph·thal′·mia
mac·ro′·pia var. of macropsia
mac′·ro·po′·dia
mac′·ro·pol′y·cyte
mac′·ro·pro·my′·e·lo·cyte
mac′·ro·pro·so′·pia
mac·rop′·sia
mac′·ro·scop′·ic
mac′·ros·mat′·ic
mac′·ro·so′·mia
mac′·ro·spore
mac′·ro·sto′·mia
mac′·ro·struc′·tur·al
mac′·ro·struc′·ture
mac·ro′·tia
mac′·ro·tome
mac′·u·la pl. & gen. sg. ·lae, gen. pl. mac′·u·la′·rum

mac′·u·lar
mac′·u·la′·ris
mac′·u·lar′y
mac′·ule
mac′·u·lo·cer′·e·bral [·ce·re′·]
mac′·u·lo·pap′·u·lar
mac′·u·lo·pap′·ule
mac′·u·lo′·sus
mad′·a·ro′·sis
Mad′·u·rel′·la
mad′·u·ro·my·co′·sis [ma·du′·]
maf′·e·nide
mag′·al·drate
ma′·gen·bla′·se
ma′·gen·stras′·se
ma·gen′·ta
mag′·got
mag′·is·ter′y
mag′·is·tral
mag′·ma
mag′·na fem. of magnus; pl. & gen. sg. ·nae
mag·ne′·sia
mag′·ne·site
mag·ne′·si·um
mag′·net
mag·net′·ic
mag′·net·is′m [ne·tis′m]
mag′·net·i·za′·tion [·ne·ti·]
mag·ne′·to·car′·di·o·gram
mag·ne′·to·car′·di·o·graph
mag·ne′·to·car′·di·og′·ra·phy
mag·ne′·to·en·ceph′·a·lo·graph
mag·ne′·to·graph
mag′·ne·tom′·e·ter
mag′·ne·ton
mag′·ne·tron
mag′·ni·fi·ca′·tion

mag′·ni·fy ·fied, ·fy′·ing
mag′·no·cel′·lu·lar also mag′·ni·
mag′·nus pl. & gen. sg. ·ni
maid′·en·head
maim
main′·te·nance
maize
ma′·jor pl. ma·jo′·res, gen. sg. ma·jo′·ris
ma′·jus neut. of major
mal
ma′·la
mal′·ab·sorp′·tion
ma·la′·cia
ma·la′·cic
mal′·a·co·
mal′·a·co·pla′·kia
mal′·a·cot′·ic
mal′·a·cot′·o·my
ma·lac′·tic
mal′·a·die′
mal′·ad·just′·ment
mal′·a·dy
ma·lag′·ma
ma·laise′
mal′·a·ko·pla′·kia
mal′·align′·ment
ma′·lar
ma·lar′·ia
ma·lar′·i·ae
ma·lar′·i·al
ma·lar′·i·cid′·al [·ci′·dal] also ma·lar′·i·a·
ma·lar·i·ol′·o·gy
ma·lar′·io·ther′·a·py
ma·lar′·i·ous
ma·la′·ris
mal′·ar·tic′·u·la′·tion
Mal′·as·se′·zia
  M. fur′·fur
  M. ova′·le
mal′·as·sim′·i·la′·tion

ma′·late
mal′·a·thi′·on
mal′·ax·ate ·at′·ed, ·at′·ing
mal′·ax·a′·tion
mal′·de·vel′·op·ment
mal′·di·ges′·tion
male
ma′·le·ate
ma·le′·ic
mal′·erup′·tion
mal·eth′·a·mer
ma′·le·yl·ace′·to·ac′·e·tate [·ac′e·to·]
mal′·for·ma′·tion
mal·func′·tion
mal′·ic [ma′·lic]
ma·lig′·nan·cy
ma·lig′·nant
ma·lig′·nus fem. ·na, neut. ·num
ma·lin′·ger
mal′·le·al also mal′·le·ar
mal′·le·a′·ris
mal′·lei gen. of malleus
mal′·leo·in′·cu·dal
ma·le′·o·lar
mal′·le·o·la′·re neut. of malleolaris
mal′·le·o·la′·ris gen. pl. ·ri·um
mal·le′·o·lus pl. & gen. sg. ·li
Mal′·le·o·my′·ces
mal′·le·ot′·o·my
mal′·le·us pl. & gen. sg. ·lei
Mal·loph′·a·ga
mal′·nu·tri′·tion
mal′·oc·clu′·sion
ma′·lo·max′·il·lar′·y
mal′·o·nal
mal′·o·nate

ma·lon′·ic [ma·lo′·nic]
mal′·o·nyl
mal′·o·nyl·ure′a
mal·pi′·ghi·an
mal·posed′
mal′·po·si′·tion
mal·prac′·tice
mal′·pres′·en·ta′·tion
mal′·ro·ta′·tion
malt′·ase
mal·thu′·sian
mal·thu′·sian·is′m
malt′·ose
mal′·um
mal·u′nion
ma·man′·pi·an′
mam′·ba
mam′·e·lon
ma·mil′·la[36] pl. & gen. sg. ·lae
mam′·il·la′·ris neut. ·re
mam′·il·lar′y var. of mammillary
mam′·il·lat′·ed var. of mammillated
mam′·il·la′·tion var. of mammillation
ma·mil′·li·form
ma·mil′·li·plas′·ty
mam′·il·li′·tis
ma·mil′·lo· also mam·mil′·lo·
ma·mil′·lo·in′·fun·dib′·u·lar
ma·mil′·lo·in′·ter·pe·dun′·cu·lar
ma·mil′·lo·pe·dun′·cu·lar
ma·mil′·lo·teg·men′·tal
ma·mil′·lo·tha·lam′·ic
ma·mil′·lo·tha·lam′·i·cus
mam′·ma pl. & gen. sg. ·mae

---

36 See note at *mammilla*.

mam′·mal
Mam·ma′·lia
mam·ma′·li·an
mam·mal′·o·gy
mam′·ma·plas′·ty
　var. of mammoplasty
mam·ma′·ria　fem. of
　mammarius; pl. & gen.
　sg. ·ri·ae
mam·ma′·ri·us　pl. &
　gen. sg. ·rii
mam′·ma·ry
mam·mec′·to·my
mam·mif′·er·ous
mam′·mi·form
mam·mil′·la[37]　var. of
　mamilla
mam′·mil·la′·ris　var.
　of mamillaris
mam′·mil·lar′y
mam′·mil·lat′·ed
mam′·mil·la′·tion
mam·mil′·li·form　var.
　of mamilliform
mam·mil′·li·plas′·ty
　var. of mamilliplasty
mam′·mil·li′·tis　var.
　of mamillitis
mam·mil′·lo-　var. of
　mamillo-
mam·mi′·tis
mam′·mo-
mam′·mo·gen
mam′·mo·gram
mam·mog′·ra·phy
mam·mo·plas′·ty
mam·mose′ [mam′·
　mose]
mam·mot′·o·my
mam·mo·tro′·phic
　[·troph′·ic]
mam′·mo·tro′·pic
　[·trop′·ic]

man′·a·ca
man′·age·ment
man′·de·late
man·del′·ic
man′·di·ble
man·dib′·u·la　pl. &
　gen. sg. ·lae
man·dib′·u·lar
man·dib′·u·la′·ris
　neut. ·re
man·dib′·u·lec′·to·my
man·dib′·u·lo·fa′·cial
man·dib′·u·lo·mar′·gi·
　na′·lis
man·dib′·u·lo·oc′·u·lo·
　fa′·cial
man′·drake
man′·drel　also ·dril
man′·drin
ma·neu′·ver　Brit.
　·noeu′·vre
man′·ga·nese
man·gan′·ic
man′·ga·nis′m
man′·ga·nous
mange
ma′·nia
man′·ic
man′·ic-de·pres′·sive
man′·i·fest
man′·i·fes·ta′·tion
man′·i·kin
man′i·pha′·lanx
man′·i·ple
ma·nip′·u·late　·lat′·
　ed, ·lat′·ing
ma·nip′·u·la′·tion
ma·nip′·u·la′·tive
ma·nip′·u·lus　pl. ·li
man′·ni·tol
man′·nose
man′·no·si·dase [man′·
　no·si′·]

man′·no·side
man′·no·si·do′·sis
man′·no·si′·do·strep′·
　to·my′·cin
ma·noeu′·vre　Brit.
　spel. of maneuver
ma·nom′·e·ter
man′·o·met′·ric
ma·nom′·e·try
man·op′·to·scope
man′·slaugh′·ter
Man′·son·el′·la
　M. oz·zar′·di
　M. per′·stans
　M. strep′·to·cer′·ca
man′·son·el·li′·a·sis
Man·so′·nia
man′·tle
man′·u·al
ma·nu′·bri·al
ma·nu′·brio·ster′·nal
ma·nu′·bri·um　pl.
　·bria, gen. sg. ·brii
man′·u·duc′·tion
man′·us　pl. & gen. sg.
　manus
map′·ping
ma·pro′·ti·line
ma·ran′·tic
ma·ras′·mic
ma·ras′·moid
ma·ras′·mus
mar′·ble·iza′·tion
marc
march
marche′ à pe·tits′ pas′
mar′·gin
mar′·gin·al
mar′·gi·na′·lis　neut.
　·le
mar′·gin·a′·tion
mar′·gi·na′·tum
mar′·gin·o·plas′·ty
　[mar·gin′·o·]

---

[37] Single *m* between the vowels is the preferred spelling for this word and its Latin derivatives such as *mamillaris*. The double-*m* spelling is well established, however, in some
English derivatives such as *mammillary* and *mammillated*.

mar'·go *pl.* mar'·gi·nes, *gen. sg.* mar'·gi·nis
mar'·i·an
mar'·i·jua'·na *also* mar'·i·hua'·na
mar'·i·no·bu'·fa·gin [ma·ri'·no·]
mark'·er
mark'·ing
mar'·mo·rat'·ed
mar'·mo·ra'·tion
mar'·row
mar'·row·brain
mar·su'·pi·al
mar·su'·pi·al·i·za'·tion
mar·su'·pi·um *pl.* ·pia
mas'·cu·la'·ta
mas'·cu·li·na *fem. of* masculinus; *pl. & gen. sg.* ·nae
mas'·cu·line
mas'·cu·lin'·i·ty
mas'·cu·lin·i·za'·tion
mas'·cu·lin·ize ·ized, ·iz'·ing
mas'·cu·lin·o'·vo·blas·to'·ma
mas'·cu·li'·nus
mask'·er
mas'·och·is'm
mas'·och·ist
mass
mas'·sa *pl. & gen. sg.* ·sae
mas·sage' ·saged', ·sag'·ing
mas·se'·ter *gen.* mas'·se·ter'·is *or* mas·se'·ter·is
mas'·se·ter'·ic
mas'·se·ter'·i·cus *fem.* ·ca
mas·seur'
mas·seuse'
mast·ad'·e·no·vi'·rus
mas·tal'·gia
mas·tec'·to·my

mas'·tic
mas'·ti·cate
mas'·ti·ca'·tion
mas'·ti·ca·to'·ri·us
mas'·ti·ca·to'·ry
Mas'·ti·goph'·o·ra
mas'·ti·gote
mas·ti'·tis
mas'·ti·toi'·des
mas'·to·
mast'·oc·cip'·i·tal *var. of* masto-occipital
mas'·to·cyte
mas'·to·cy'·to·gen'·e·sis
mas'·to·cy·to'·ma *pl.* ·mas *or* ·ma·ta
mas'·to·cy·to'·sis
mas'·to·dyn'·ia
mas'·toid
mas·toi'·dal
mas·toi'·dea *fem. of* mastoideus; *pl. & gen. sg.* ·de·ae
mas'·toid·ec'·to·my
mas·toi'·de·um *neut. of* mastoideus
mas·toi'·de·us *pl. & gen. sg.* ·dei
mas'·toid·i'·tis
mas'·to·oc·cip'·i·tal
mas'·to·pa·ri'·etal
mas·top'·a·thy *also* mas'·to·path'·ia
mas'·to·pex'y
mas'·to·plas'·ty
mas·to'·sis
mas'·to·squa'·mous
mas·tos'·to·my
mas·tot'·ic
mas·tot'·o·my
mas'·tur·ba'·tion
match'·ing
ma'·ter *gen.* ma'·tris
ma·te'·ria
ma·te'·ri·es
ma·ter'·nal
ma·ter'·ni·ty

ma·ter'·no·he'·mo·ther'·a·py *Brit.* ·hae'·mo·
mat'·ing
ma'·tri·cal [mat'·ri·] *also* ma·tri'·cial
ma'·tri·cli'·nous [mat'·ri·] *var. of* matroclinous
mat'·ri·lin'·e·al
ma'·tris *gen. of* mater
ma'·trix *pl.* ma'·tri·ces, *gen. sg.* ma'·tri·cis
ma'·tro·cli'·nous [mat'·ro·]
ma'·tro·cli'·ny [mat'·ro·]
ma'·tron
mat'·ter
mat'·tress
mat'·u·rant
mat'·u·rate ·rat'·ed, ·rat'·ing
mat'·u·ra'·tion
ma·ture' *adj. & v.* ·tured, ·tur'·ing
ma·tu'·ri·ty
max'i·cell
max·il'·la *pl. & gen. sg.* ·lae
max·il·la'·re *neut. of* maxillaris
max·il·la'·ris *pl.* ·res
max'·il·lar'y
max'·il·lec'·to·my
max'·il·li'·tis
max·il'·lo·fa'·cial
max·il'·lo·man·dib'·u·lar
max·il'·lo·na'·sal
max'·il·lot'·o·my
max·il'·lo·tur'·bi·nal
max'·i·mal
max'·i·mum *pl.* ·ma *or* ·mums
max'·i·mus *pl. & gen. sg.* ·mi
max'·well

may′·ap′·ple
may′·hem
maze
ma′·zin·dol
ma′·zo·
ma′·zo·dyn′·ia
ma′·zo·pex′y
ma′·zo·pla′·sia
meal
mean
mea′·sles
mea′·sly
mea′·sure [meas′·ure]
mea′·sure·ment [meas′·ure·]
me·a′tal
me′·ati′·tis
me·a′to· [me·at′o·]
me′·atom′·e·ter
me·a′to·plas′·ty [me·at′o·]
me′·ator′·rha·phy
me·at′o·tome *also* me′·atome
me′·atot′·o·my
me·a′tus *L. pl. & gen. sg.* meatus
me·ben′·da·zole
me·bev′·er·ine
me·bu′·ta·mate
mec′·a·mine
mec′·a·myl′·a·mine
me·chan′·i·cal
me·chan′·ics
mech′·a·nis′m
mech′·a·no·
mech′·a·no·re·cep′·tor *also* me·chan′·i·co·
mech′·a·no·ther′·a·py
me′·cism
mec′·li·zine
mec′·lo·cy′·cline
mec′·lo·qua′·lone
me·com′·e·ter
me·con′·ic
me·co′·ni·um
me·cys′·ta·sis
me·daz′·e·pam

me′·dia *pl. of* medium, *fem. of* medius; *pl. & gen. sg.* ·di·ae
me′·di·ad
me′·di·al
me′·di·a′·le *neut. of* medialis
me′·di·a′·lis *pl.* ·les, *gen. pl.* ·li·um
me′·di·an
me′·di·a′·na *fem. of* medianus
me′·di·a′·num *neut. of* medianus
me′·di·a′·nus *pl. & gen. sg.* ·ni
me′·di·as·ti′·na *pl. of* mediastinum
me′·di·as·ti′·nal
me′·di·as′·ti·na′·le *neut. of* me′·di·as′·ti·na′·lis
me′·di·as′·ti·na′·lis *pl.* ·les
me′·di·as′·ti·ni′·tis
me′·di·as·ti′·no·bron′·chi·al
me′·di·as′·ti·nog′·ra·phy
me′·di·as·ti′·no·per′i·car·di′·tis
me′·di·as·ti′·no·scope
me′·di·as′·ti·nos′·co·py
me′·di·as′·ti·not′·o·my
me′·di·as·ti′·num *pl.* ·na
me′·di·ate *adj. & v.* ·at′·ed, ·at′·ing
me′·di·a′·tor
med′·ic
med′·i·ca·ble
med′·i·cal
med′·i·ca·ment [me·dic′·a·ment]
med′·i·ca·men·to′·sus *fem.* ·sa
med′·i·ca·men′·tous

med′·i·cate ·cat′·ed, ·cat′·ing
med′·i·ca′·tion
med′·i·ca′·tor
me′·di·cer′·e·bral [·ce·re′·bral]
me·dic′·i·nal
med′·i·cine
med′·i·co·
med′·i·co·bi′·o·log′·ic
med′·i·co·chi·rur′·gic *also* ·gi·cal
med′·i·co·den′·tal
med′·i·co·le′·gal
med′·i·co·so′·cial
me′·dii *pl. of* medius, *gen. sg. of* medius & medium
me′·dio·
me′·dio·car′·pal
me′·dio·car·pa′·lis
me′·di·oc·cip′·i·tal
me′·dio·fron′·tal
me′·dio·lat′·er·al
me′·dio·ne·cro′·sis
me′·dio·pe·dun′·cle [pe′·dun·cle]
me′·dio·pon′·tine
me′·dio·tar′·sal
me′·dio·tem′·po·ral
me′·dio·tho·rac′·ic
me′·di·o·tru′·sion
me′·di·sect
me′·di·um *neut. of* medius; *pl.* ·dia, *gen. sg.* ·dii
me′·di·us *pl. & gen. sg.* ·dii
med′·pha·lan
me·drox′y·pro·ges′·ter·one
me·dul′·la *pl. & gen. sg.* ·lae
med′·ul·la′·re *neut. of* medullaris
med′·ul·la′·ris *pl.* ·res
med′·ul·lar′y [me·dul′·la·ry]

med′·ul·lat′·ed
med′·ul·la′·tion
med′·ul·lec′·to·my
me·dul′·lo· [med′·ul·lo·]
me·dul′·lo·blast
me·dul′·lo·blas·to′·ma *pl.* ·mas *or* ·ma·ta
me·dul′·lo·ep′·i·the′·li·al
me·dul′·lo·ep′·i·the′·li·o′·ma *pl.* ·mas *or* ·ma·ta
me·dul′·lo·ther′·a·py
me·du′·sa *pl. & gen. sg.* ·sae
mef′·e·nam′·ic
me·fex′·a·mide
mef′·lo·quine
mef′·ru·side
meg′a·
meg′a·car′y·o·blast *var. of* megakaryoblast
meg′a·car′y·o·cyte *var. of* megakaryocyte
meg′a·ce·phal′·ic
meg′a·ceph′·a·ly
meg′a·co′·lon
meg′·a·co′·ni·al
meg′a·cu′·rie
meg′a·cy′·cle
meg′a·cys′·tic
meg′a·dose
meg′a·du′·o·de′·num
meg′a·esoph′·a·gus
meg′a·hertz
meg′a·kar′y·o·blast
meg′a·kar′y·o·cyte
meg′a·kar′y·o·cy′·to·pe′·nia
meg′a·kar′y·o·cy·to′·sis
meg′a·lec′·i·thal
meg′·a·lo·
meg′·a·lo·blast
meg′·a·lo·blas′·tic
meg′·a·lo·blas′·toid
meg′·a·lo·blas·to′·sis
meg′·a·lo·car′·dia
meg′·a·lo·ce·phal′·ic
meg′·a·lo·ceph′·a·ly
meg′·a·lo·cor′·nea
meg′·a·lo·cys′·tis
meg′·a·lo·cyte
meg′·a·lo·cyt′·ic
meg′·a·lo·dac′·ty·ly
meg′·a·lo·dont
meg′·a·lo·en·ceph′·a·ly
meg′·a·lo·en′·ter·on
meg′·a·lo·glos′·sia
meg′·a·lo·kar′y·o·cyte *var. of* megakaryocyte
meg′·a·lo·ma′·nia
meg′·a·loph·thal′·mia
meg′·a·lo·po′·dia
meg′·a·lop′·sia *also* ·lo′·pia
Meg′·a·lop′·y·ge [·lo·py′·ge]
M. oper′·cu·la′·ris
meg′·a·lo·syn·dac′·ty·ly
meg′·a·lo·ure′·ter
meg′·a·lo·ure′·thra
meg′a·nu′·cle·us
meg′a-oe·soph′·a·gus *Brit. spel. of* megaesophagus
meg′a·rec′·tum
Meg′·a·se′·lia
meg′a·sig′·moid
meg′·a·some
meg′·a·so′·mia
meg′a·u′nit
meg′a·volt′
meg′a·volt′·age
me·ges′·trol
meg′·lu·mine
mei·bo′·mi·an
mei·bo′·mi·a·ni′·tis
mei′o·
mei′·o·gen′·ic
mei·o′·sis
mei′o·spore
mei·ot′·ic
me·lae′·na *Brit. spel. of* melena
me·lae′·nic *Brit. spel. of* melenic
mel·al′·gia
mel′·a·mine
mel′·an·cho′·lia
mel′·an·ede′·ma *Brit.* ·oe·de′·
mel′·an·em′·e·sis *var. of* melenemesis
mel′·ane′·mia *Brit.* ·anae′·
Me·la′·nia
me·lan′·ic
mel′·a·nif′·er·ous
mel′·a·nin
mel′·a·nis′m
mel′·a·nis′·tic
mel′·a·no·
mel′·a·no·ac′·an·tho′·ma
mel′·a·no·blast [me·lan′·o·]
mel′·a·no·blas·to′·ma [me·lan′·o·]
mel′·a·no·blas·to′·sis [me·lan′·o·]
mel′·a·no·car′·ci·no′·ma
mel′·a·no·cyte [me·lan′·o·]
mel′·a·no·cyt′·ic [me·lan′·o·]
mel′·a·no·cy·to′·ma [me·lan′·o·]
mel′·a·no·derm [me·lan′·o·]
mel′·a·no·der′·ma
mel′·a·no·der′·mic
mel′·an·oe·de′·ma *Brit. spel. of* melanedema
mel′·a·no·ep′·i·the′·li·o′·ma
me·lan′·o·gen [mel′·a·no·]

melanogenemia / meningocortical

me·lan'·o·gen·e'·mia
[mel'·a·no·] Brit.
 ae'·mia
mel'·a·no·gen'·e·sis
mel'·a·no·gen'·ic
mel'·a·noid
Mel'·a·noi'·des
Mel'·a·no·les'·tes pi'·ci·pes
mel'·a·no'·ma pl.
 ·mas or ·ma·ta
mel'·a·no'·ma·to'·sis
mel'·a·no'ma·tous
 [·nom'a·]
mel'·a·no·nych'·ia
mel'·a·no·phage [me·lan'·o·]
mel'·a·no·phore [me·lan'·o·]
mel'·a·no·phor'·in [me·lan'·o·]
mel'·a·no·pla'·kia [me·lan'·o·]
mel'·a·nop'·ty·sis
mel'·a·nor·rha'·gia
mel'·a·no'·sis
mel'·a·no·some [me·lan'·o·]
mel'·a·not'·ic
mel'·a·no·trich'·ia
mel'·a·no·tro'·pic [me·lan'·o·, ·trop'·ic]
mel'·a·no·tro'·pin [me·lan'·o·]
mel'·a·nu'·ria
mel'·a·nu'·ric
mel·ar'·so·prol
me·las'·ma
mel'·a·to'·nin
me·le'·na Brit. me·lae'·na
mel'·e·nem'·e·sis
me·le'·nic Brit. me·lae'·nic
mel'·i·bi'·ose
mel'·i·ce'·ra
mel'·i·lo·tox'·in

me'·li·oi·do·do'·sis [mel'·i·]
me·lis'·so·ther'·a·py
mel'·i·ten'·sis
mel'·i·tin brucellosis test antigen: Cf.
melittin
me·li'·tis
me·lit'·tin [mel'·it·tin]
 bee venom toxin: Cf.
melitin
mel'·i·tu'·ria also
 mel'·li·
mel'·i·tu'·ric also
 mel'·li·
mel·li'·tus neut. ·tum
mel'o·
mel'o·cer'·vi·co·plas'·ty
mel'·o·me'·lia
mel'·o·plas'·tic
mel'·o·plas'·ty
mel'o·rhe'·os·to'·sis
me·los'·chi·sis
me·lo'·tia
mel'·pha·lan
mem'·ber
mem'·bra pl. of
 membrum
mem·bra'·na pl. & gen. sg. ·nae
mem'·bra·na'·ceous
mem'·bra·na'·ce·us fem. ·cea
mem'·bra·nal
mem'·brane
mem'·bra·nelle
mem·bra'·ni·form
mem'·bra·no·car'·ti·lag'·i·nous
mem'·bra·no·cra'·ni·um
mem'·bra·noid
mem'·bra·no·pro·lif'·er·a·tive
mem'·bra·nous
mem'·broid

mem'·brum pl. ·bra,
 gen. sg. ·bri
mem'·o·ry
men·ac'·me
men'·a·di'·ol
men'·a·di'·one
men'·a·qui·none'
 [·quin'·one]
men'·ar·che
men'·de·le'·vi·um
men·de'·li·an
men'·del·iz'·ing
men'·go·vi'·rus also
 Mengo virus
men'·hi·dro'·sis also
 men'·idro'·sis
me·nin'·gea fem. of
 meningeus; pl. & gen. sg. ·ge·ae
me·nin'·ge·al
me·nin'·ge·or'·rha·phy
me·nin'·ges sg. me'·ninx
me·nin'·ge·us pl. & gen. sg. ·gii, ablative ·geo
me·nin'·gi·o'·ma pl.
 ·mas or ·ma·ta
me·nin'·gi·o'·ma·to'·sis
me·nin'·gism [men'·in·] also men'·in·gis'·mus
men'·in·git'·ic
men'·in·git'·i·form
men'·in·gi'·tis pl.
 ·git'·i·des
me·nin'·go·
me·nin'·go·blast
me·nin'·go·blas·to'·ma
 pl. ·mas or ·ma·ta
me·nin'·go·cele
me·nin'·go·coc'·cal
me·nin'·go·coc·ce'·mia
 Brit. ·cae'·mia
me·nin'·go·coc'·cus
 pl. ·coc'·ci
me·nin'·go·cor'·ti·cal

me·nin'·go·en·ceph'·a·li'·tis
me·nin'·go·en·ceph'·a·lo·cele
me·nin'·go·en·ceph'·a·lo·my'·e·li'·tis
me·nin'·go·en·ceph'·a·lo·my'·e·lop'·a·thy
me·nin'·go·en·ceph'·a·lo·my'·e·lo·ra·dic'·u·lo·neu·ri'·tis
me·nin'·go·en·ceph'·a·lop'·a·thy
me·nin'·go·my'·e·li'·tis
me·nin'·go·my'·e·lo·cele
me·nin'·go·my'·e·lo·en·ceph'·a·li'·tis
me·nin'·go·my'·e·lo·ra·dic'·u·li'·tis
me·nin'·go·os'·teo·phle·bi'·tis
men'·in·gop'·a·thy
me·nin'·go·ra·chid'·i·an
me·nin'·go·ra·dic'·u·lar
me·nin'·go·ra·dic'·u·li'·tis
me·nin'·go·ra·dic'·u·lo·my'·e·li'·tis
me·nin'·gor·rha'·gia
me·nin'·go·the'·li·o'·ma *pl.* ·mas *or* ·ma·ta
me·nin'·go·the'·li·om'a·tous [·o'ma·]
me·nin'·go·vas'·cu·lar
me'·ninx *sg. of* meninges
me·nis'·cal
men'·is·cec'·to·my
me·nis'·ci *pl. of* meniscus
men'·is·ci'·tis
me·nis'·co·cyte
me·nis'·co·fem'·o·ra'·le
me·nis'·co·pex'y
men'·is·cot'·o·my
me·nis'·cus *pl.* ·ci
men'o·

men'o·me'·tror·rha'·gia
men'o·paus'·al [·pau'·sal]
men'o·pause
men'·or·rha'·gia
men'·or·rhe'a *Brit.* ·rhoe'a
me·nos'·che·sis [men'·o·sche'·sis]
me·nos'·ta·sis [men'·o·sta'·sis]
men'·o·tro'·pins
men'·ses
men'·strua *pl. of* menstruum
men'·stru·al
men'·stru·ant
men'·stru·ate ·at'·ed, ·at'·ing
men'·stru·a'·tion
men'·stru·ous
men'·stru·um *pl.* ·strua
men'·tal
men·ta'·le *neut. of* mentalis
men·ta'·lis *pl.* ·les
men·tal'·i·ty
men'·thol
men'·tho·lat'·ed
men'·thyl
men'·ti *gen. of* mentum
men'·to·
men'·to·an·te'·ri·or
men'·to·la'·bi·al
men'·to·la'·bi·a'·lis
men'·to·oc·cip'·i·tal
men'·to·plas'·ty
men'·to·pos·te'·ri·or
men'·to·trans·verse'
men'·tum *gen.* ·ti
mep'·a·crine
me·par'·fy·nol
mep'·a·zine
me·pen'·zo·late
me·per'·i·dine
me·phen'·a·mine

me·phen'·e·sin
meph'·en·ox'·a·lone
me·phen'·ter·mine
me·phen'·y·to'·in
me·phit'·ic
me·phi'·tis
meph'o·bar'·bi·tal
me·piv'·a·caine
me·pred'·ni·sone
mep'·ro·bam'·ate [me·pro'·ba·mate]
mep'·ryl·caine
me·pyr'·a·mine
meq'·ui·dox
mer·al'·ein
me·ral'·gia
mer·al'·lu·ride
mer·bro'·min
mer·cap'·tan
mer·cap'·tide
mer·cap'·to·
mer·cap'·to·eth'·a·nol
mer·cap'·to·ethyl'·amine [eth'·yl·amine']
mer·cap'·to·im'·id·az'·ole
mer'·cap·tom'·er·in [mer·cap'·to·mer'·in]
mer·cap'·to·pu'·rine
mer'·cap·tu'·ric
mer·cu'·ri·al
mer·cu'·ri·a·len'·tis
mer·cu'·ri·al·is'm
mer·cu'·ri·ben'·zo·ate
mer·cu'·ric
mer'·cu·ro·phyl'·line
mer·cu'·rous
mer'·cu·ry
mer'·ethox'·yl·line
me·rid'·i·an
me·rid'·i·a'·nus *pl. & gen. sg.* ·ni
me·rid'·i·o·nal
me·rid'·i·o·na'·lis *pl.* ·les
me·ris'·tic
mer'o· *part, partial*

mero- / mesophile

me′·ro· *thigh, femoral*
mer′o·an′·en·ceph′·a·ly
mer′·o·blas′·tic
me′·ro·cele
mer′·o·crine
mer′o·en·ceph′·a·ly
mer′·o·gon′·ic
me·rog′·o·ny
mer′·o·me′·lia
mer′o·mi′·cro·so′·mia
mer′o·my′·o·sin
mer′o·ra·chis′·chi·sis
  also mer′·or·rha·
me·rot′·o·my
mer′·o·zo′·ite
mer′o·zy′·gote
mer′·pha·lan
mer·sal′·yl [mer′·sal·yl]
me′·sad *var. of* mesiad
me′·sal *var. of* mesial
mes·an′·gi·al
mes·an′·gio·cap′·il·lar′y
mes·an′·gi·ol′·y·sis
mes·an′·gi·um *pl.* ·gia
mes′·a·or·ti′·tis
mes′·ar′·ter·i′·tis
me·sat′i·ce·phal′·ic
me·sat′·i·pel′·lic
mes·ax′·on
mes·cal′
mes′·ca·line
mes·ec′·to·derm
mes′·en·ce·phal′·ic
mes′·en·ce·phal′·i·cus
  fem. ·ca
mes′·en·ceph′·a·li′·tis
mes′·en·ceph′·a·lon
  gen. ·li
mes′·en·ceph′·a·lot′·o·my
mes·en′·chy·mal [mes′·en·chym′·mal]
mes′·en·chy′·ma·tous [chym′a·]
mes′·en·chyme *also*
  mes·en′·chy·ma
mes′·en·chy·mo′·ma

mes′·en·ter′·ic
mes′·en·ter′·i·ca *fem.*
  of mesentericus
mes′·en·ter′·i·co·pa·ri′·etal
mes′·en·ter′·i·cum
  neut. of mesentericus
mes′·en·ter′·i·cus *pl.*
  & gen. sg. ·ci
mes′·en·ter′·ii *gen. of*
  mesenterium
mes·en′·ter·i′·o·lum
mes′·en·ter′·i·o·pex′y
mes′·en·ter′·i·or′·rha·phy
mes′·en·ter′i·pli·ca′·tion
mes′·en·ter·i′·tis
mes′·en·ter′·i·um
  gen. ·ter′·ii
mes·en′·ter·on
mes′·en·ter′y
mes′·en·tor′·rha·phy
mes·eth′·moid
mesh′·work
me′·si·ad
me′·si·al
me′·sio·
me′·sio·clu′·sion *var.*
  of mesio-occlusion
me′·sio·dens *pl.* me′·sio·den′·tes
me′·sio·dis′·tal
me′·sio·lin′·gual
me′·sio-oc·clu′·sal
me′·sio-oc·clu′·sion
me′·sio-oc·clu′·so·dis′·tal
me′·sio·ver′·sion
mes′o· [me′so·]
mes′o·a·or·ti′·tis
mes′o·ap·pen′·di·ci′·tis
mes′o·ap·pen′·dix
mes′o·a′tri·al
mes′o·blast
mes′o·blas·te′·ma
mes′o·blas′·tic
mes′o·car′·dia

mes′o·car′·di·um *pl.*
  ·dia
mes′o·car′·pal
mes′o·ca′·val
mes′o·ce·phal′·ic
mes′o·ceph′·a·ly
mes′o·chon′·dri·um
mes′o·co′·lic
mes′o·co′·li·ca *fem.*
  of mesocolicus
mes′o·co′·li·cus *pl.*
  ·ci
mes′o·co′·lon
mes′o·co′·lo·pex′y
mes′o·co′·lo·pli·ca′·tion
mes′o·cor′·tex
mes′o·derm
mes′o·der′·mal *also*
  ·mic
mes′o·du′·o·de′·nal
mes′o·du′·o·de′·num
mes′o·esoph′·a·gus
mes′o·gas′·tric
mes′o·gas′·tri·um
mes′o·gnath′·ic
mes′o·gna′·thi·on
mes′o·il′e·um
mes′o·je·ju′·num
mes′o·lat′·er·al
mes′o·lec′·i·thal
mes′o·me′·lia
mes′o·mel′·ic [·me′·lic]
mes′o·mere
mes′o·me′·tri·um
mes′o·morph
mes′o·mor′·phic
mes′o·mor′·phy
mes′·on [me′·son]
mes′o·neph′·ric
mes′o·ne·phro′·ma
mes′o·neph′·ros *pl.*
  ·roi
mes′o-oe·soph′·a·gus
  Brit. spel. of meso-esophagus
mes′o·pex′y
mes′o·phile

mes′o·phil′·ic
me·so′·pic
mes′o·pneu′·mon
mes′o·por′·phy·rin
mes′o·pro·so′·pic
mes′o·pul·mo′·non
   also ·mo′·num
me·sor′·chi·um
mes′o·rec′·tum
mes′·o·rid′·a·zine
mes·or′·rha·phy
mes′o·sal′·pinx
mes′o·sig′·moid
mes′o·sig·moi′·do·
   pex′y
mes′o·some
mes′o·tar′·sal
mes′o·ten·din′·e·um
   pl. ·din′·ea
mes′o·ten′·don
mes′o·the′·li·al
mes′o·the′·li·o′·ma
   pl. ·mas *or* ·ma·ta
mes′o·the′·li·um *pl.*
   ·lia
mes′o·tron
mes′·ovar′·i·an *also*
   ·i·al
mes′·ovar′·i·cus
mes′·ovar′·i·um
mes·ox′·a·lyl·ure′a
mes′·sen·ger
mes′·tra·nol
mes′·u·prine
mes′·y·late
met′a·
met′a·bi·o′·sis
met′a·bi·sul′·fite
met′·a·bol′·ic
me·tab′·o·lim′·e·ter
me·tab′·o·lis′m
me·tab′·o·lite
me·tab′·o·liz′·a·ble
me·tab′·o·lize ·lized,
   ·liz′·ing
met′a·but·eth′·a·mine
met′a·car′·pal

met′a·car·pa′·le *neut.*
   of metacarpalis; *pl.* ·lia
met′a·car·pa′·lis *pl.*
   ·les, *gen. pl.* ·li·um
met′a·car·pec′·to·my
met′a·car′·pe·um
met′a·car′·pi *pl. &*
   gen. sg. of metacarpus
met′a·car′·po·car′·pal
met′a·car′·po·hy′·po·
   the′·nar
met′a·car′·po·pha·lan′·
   gea *gen. pl.* ·pha·
   lan′·ge·a′·rum
met′a·car′·po·pha·lan′·
   ge·al
met′a·car′·po·pha·lan′·
   ge·a′·lis *pl.* ·les,
   gen. pl. ·li·um
met′a·car′·po·the′·nar
met′a·car′·pus *pl. &*
   gen. sg. ·pi
met′a·cen′·tric
met′a·cer·car′·ia *pl.*
   ·i·ae
met′a·chro·ma′·sia
met′a·chro·mat′·ic
met′a·chro′·ma·tin
met′a·chro′·ma·tis′m
met′a·chro′·mo·phil
   also ·phile
met′·a·coele
met′a·cone
met′a·co′·nid
met′a·cor·tan′·dra·cin
met′a·cor·tan′·dra·lone
met′a·cryp′·to·zo′·ite
met′a·cy′·clic
met′a·fe′·male
met′a·glob′·u·lin
met′·a·gon′·i·mi′·a·sis
Met′·a·gon′·i·mus
   M. yo′·ko·ga′·wai
met′a·gran′·u·lo·cyte
met′a·hy′·po·phys′·i·al
met′a·in·fec′·tive
met′·a·ken′·trin
met′·al

me·tal′·lic
me·tal′·lo·en′·zyme
me·tal′·lo·fla′·vo·de′·
   hy·drog′·e·nase [·de·
   hy′·dro·gen·ase]
me·tal′·lo·fla′·vo·pro′·
   tein
me·tal′·lo·phil
me·tal′·lo·phil′·ic
me·tal′·lo·pro′·tein
me·tal′·lo·thi′·o·ne′·in
met′a·male
met′·a·mer *type of*
   isomer: Cf. metamere
met′·a·mere
   embryonic segment: Cf.
   metamer
met′·a·mer′·ic
me·tam′·er·is′m
met′·a·mor′·phic
met′·a·mor·phop′·sia
met′·a·mor′·pho·sis
   pl. ·ses
met′a·my′·e·lo·cyte
met′a·myx′o·vi′·rus
met′a·neph′·ric
met′a·neph′·ro·gen′·ic
met′a·neph′·ros *pl.*
   ·roi
met′a·phase
met′a·phos′·phate
met′·a·phys′·e·al [me·
   taph′·y·se′·al] *var.*
   of metaphysial
met′·a·phys′·i·al
me·taph′·y·sis *pl.* ·ses
me·taph′·y·si′·tis
met′·a·pla′·sia
   abnormal growth: Cf.
   metaplasis
me·tap′·la·sis
   completed growth: Cf.
   metaplasia
met′·a·plas′·tic
met′a·pneu·mon′·ic
met′·apoph′·y·sis
met′a·pro′·tein
met′a·pro·ter′·e·nol

met′·a·py′·rone
met′·a·ram′·i·nol
met′·a·rho·dop′·sin
met′·ar·te′·ri·ole
met′a·sta′·ble [met′a·sta′·ble]
me·tas′·ta·sec′·to·my
me·tas′·ta·sis   *pl.*   ·ses
me·tas′·ta·size   ·sized, ·siz′·ing
met′·a·stat′·ic
met′a·syn·ap′·sis
met′a·syn′·de·sis [·syn·de′·sis]
met′a·syph′·i·lit′·ic
met′a·tar′·sal
met′a·tar·sa′·le   *neut. of* metatarsalis; *pl.* ·lia
met′a·tar·sal′·gia
met′a·tar·sa′·lis   *pl.* ·les, *gen. pl.* ·li·um
met′a·tar·sec′·to·my
met′a·tar′·so·pha·lan′·gea   *gen. pl.* ·pha·lan′·ge·a′·rum
met′a·tar′·so·pha·lan′·ge·al
met′a·tar′·so·pha·lan′·ge·a′·lis   *pl.* ·les, *gen. pl.* ·li·um
met′a·tar′·sus   *pl. & gen. sg.* ·si
met′a·thal′·a·mus   *pl. & gen. sg.* ·mi
me·tath′·e·sis
met′·a·troph
met′·a·tro′·phic [·troph′·ic]
met′a·typ′·i·cal
me·tax′·a·lone
Met′·a·zo′a
met′·a·zo′·an
met′a·zo′·o·no′·sis
me·te′·cious   *also* me·toe′·cious

met′·en′·ce·phal′·ic
met′·en·ceph′·a·lon
Met′-en·keph′·a·lin   *also* met′-
me′·te·o·ris′m
me′·te·o·ro·pa·thol′·o·gy
me′·te·o·ro·tro′·pic [·trop′·ic]
me′·te·o·ro·tro′·pism
me′·ter[38]   *Brit.* me′·tre
met·es′·trus
met·for′·min
meth·ac′·e·tin [meth′·acet′·in]
meth′a·cho′·line
meth·ac′·ry·late
meth′·acryl′·ic
meth′a·cy′·cline
meth′·a·done
met′·haem′·al·bu′·min   *Brit. spel. of* methemalbumin
met·hae′·mo·glo′·bin   *Brit. spel. of* methemoglobin
meth′·al′le·nes′·tril
meth′·am·phet′·a·mine
meth·an′·dri·ol
meth·an′·dro·sten′·o·lone
meth′·ane
meth′·ane·sul′·fo·nate
Meth′·a·no·bac·te′·ri·a′·ce·ae
meth·an′·o·gen [meth′·a·no·gen]
me·than′·o·gen′·ic [meth′·a·no·gen′·ic]
meth′·a·nol
meth·an′·the·line
meth′·a·pyr′·i·lene
meth·aq′·ua·lone
meth·ar′·bi·tal

meth′·a·zol′·a·mide
meth·dil′·a·zine
met′·hem′·al·bu′·min   *Brit.* ·haem′·
met′·heme   *Brit.* ·haem
met·he′·mo·glo′·bin   *Brit.* ·hae′·mo·glo′·
met′·he′·mo·glo′·bin·e′·mia   *Brit.* ·hae′·, ·ae′·mia
met′·he′·mo·glo′·bin·e′·mic   *Brit.* ·hae′·, ·ae′·mic
met′·he′·mo·glo′·bin·u′·ria   *Brit.* ·hae′·
me·the′·na·mine
me·the′·to·in
meth′·i·cil′·lin
meth·im′·a·zole
meth·i′·o·dal
meth·i′·o·dide
me·thi′·o·nine
me·thix′·ene
meth′·o·car′·ba·mol
meth′o·chlo′·ride
meth′·od
meth′·od·ol·o′·o·gy
meth′·o·hex′·i·tal
meth′·o·trex′·ate
meth′·o·tri·mep′·ra·zine
me·thox′·a·mine
me·thox′·sa·len
me·thox′y
me·thox′y·chlor
me·thox′y·in′·dole
me·thox′·yl
me·thox′y·phen′·a·mine
me·thox′y·pro′·ma·zine
me·thox′y·pso′·ra·len
meth′·sco·pol′·a·mine
meth·sux′·i·mide
meth′·y·clo·thi′·a·zide

---

[38] The British spelling *metre* is used only for the measurement, not for a type of instrument.

methyl / microbody

meth′·yl
meth′·yl·al
meth′·yl·amine′ [·am′·ine]
meth′·yl·as·par′·tate
meth′·yl·at′·ed
meth′·yl·a′·tion
meth′·yl·benz′·e·tho′·ni·um
meth′·yl·bro′·mide
meth′·yl·cat′·e·chol
meth′·yl·cel′·lu·lose
meth′·yl·cho·lan′·threne
meth′·yl·do′·pa
meth′·yl·ene
meth′·yl·ene·tet′·ra·hy′·dro·fo′·late
meth′·yl·er′·go·no′·vine
meth′·yl·glu′·ca·mine
meth′·yl·gua′·no·sine
meth′·yl·hex·ane′·amine
meth′·yl·ma·lon′·ic
meth′·yl·ma·lon′·ic·ac′·id·u′·ria
meth′·yl·mal′·o·nyl
meth′·yl·phen′·i·date
meth′·yl·pred·nis′·o·lone
meth′·yl·pu′·rine
meth′·yl·sul′·fate
meth′·yl·tes·tos′·ter·one
meth′·yl·thi′o·u′ra·cil
meth′·yl·trans′·fer·ase
meth′·y·ser′·gide
met·my′o·glo′·bin
met′·o·cu′·rine
me·toe′·cious *var. of* metecious
met·oes′·trus *Brit. spel. of* metestrus
me·ton′·y·my
me·top′·a·gus
me·top′·ic
me·top′·i·ca

me·to′·pi·on
met′·o·pis′m
met′·o·pon
me·tox′·e·nous
me·tox′·e·ny
me′·tra
me·tral′·gia
me′·tra·to′·nia
me′·tra·tro′·phia
me′·tre *Brit. spel. of* meter
me′·trec·ta′·sia
me′·treu·ryn′·ter
me·treu′·ry·sis
me′·tri·al
met′·ric
met′·ri·fo′·nate
me·trit′·ic
me·tri′·tis
me·triz′·a·mide
met′·ri·zo′·ate
met′·ri·zo′·ic
me′·tro· *denoting the uterus*
met′·ro· *denoting measurement*
me·trog′·e·nous
met′·ro·log′·i·cal
me·trol′·o·gy
me′·tro·ma·la′·cia
met′·ro·ni′·da·zole
me·tron′·o·scope
me′·tro·path′·ia
me′·tro·path′·ic
me·trop′·a·thy
me′·tro·per′·i·to·ne′·al
me′·tro·pex′·y
me′·tro·phle·bi′·tis
me′·tro·plas′·ty
me′·tro·pto′·sis
me′·tror·rha′·gia
me′·tro·sal′·pinx *pl.* ·sal·pin′·ges
me′·tro·scope
me′·tro·ste·no′·sis
me·trot′·o·my
me·tyr′·a·pone
me·val′·o·nate

mev′·a·lon′·ic
me·ze′·re·um *also* ·re·on
mi′·ca
mi·ca′·tion
mi·celle′
mi·con′·a·zole
mi′·cra *pl. of* micron
mi′·cra·cous′·tic
mi′·cren·ceph′·a·ly
mi′·cro·
mi′·cro·ab′·scess
mi′·cro·ad′·e·no′·ma *pl.* ·mas *or* ·ma·ta
mi′·cro·aer′·o·phil
mi′·cro·al·bu′·min·u′·ria [·mi·nu′·]
mi′·cro·am′·pere
mi′·cro·anal′·y·sis *pl.* ·ses
mi′·cro·anat′·o·mist
mi′·cro·anat′·o·my
mi′·cro·an′·eu·rys′m
mi′·cro·an′·gi·og′·ra·phy
mi′·cro·an′·gi·o·path′·ic
mi′·cro·an′·gi·op′·a·thy
mi′·cro·an′·gi·os′·co·py
mi′·cro·bal′·ance
mi′·crobe
mi·cro′·bi·al *also* ·bic
mi·cro′·bi·cid′·al [·ci′·dal]
mi·cro′·bi·cide
mi′·cro·bi′o·as′·say [·as·say′]
mi′·cro·bi′·o·log′·ic *also* ·i·cal
mi′·cro·bi·ol′·o·gist
mi′·cro·bi·ol′·o·gy
mi′·cro·bi·o′·ta
mi′·cro·bi·ot′·ic
mi′·cro·bis′m [mi′·crob·is′m]
mi′·cro·blast
mi′·cro·bleph′·a·ry
mi′·cro·bod′y

mi'·cro·bra'·chia
mi'·cro·bren'·ner
mi'·cro·bu·ret'
mi'·cro·cal'·cu·lus   *pl.*
   ·li
mi'·cro·cal'·o·rie
mi'·cro·cal'·o·rim'·e·try
mi'·cro·cap'·sule
mi'·cro·car'·dia
mi'·cro·car'·ri·er
mi'·cro·cav'·i·ta'·tion
mi'·cro·ce·phal'·ic
mi'·cro·ceph'·a·ly
mi'·cro·chem'·is·try
mi'·cro·cir'·cu·la'·tion
mi'·cro·cir'·cu·la·tory
Mi'·cro·coc·ca'·ce·ae
mi'·cro·coc'·cal
mi'·cro·coc'·cin
Mi'·cro·coc'·cus
mi'·cro·coc'·cus   *pl.*
   ·ci
mi'·cro·col'·o·ny
mi'·cro·co·nid'·i·um   *pl.* ·nid'·ia
mi'·cro·co'·ria
mi'·cro·cor'·nea
mi'·cro·cra'·nia
mi'·cro·crys'·tal·line
mi'·cro·cu'·rie
mi'·cro·cyst
mi'·cro·cys'·tic
mi'·cro·cys·tom'·e·ter
mi'·cro·cyte
mi'·cro·cy·the'·mia   *Brit.* ·thae'·
mi'·cro·cyt'·ic
mi'·cro·cy·to'·sis
mi'·cro·dis·sec'·tion
mi'·cro·dont
mi'·cro·don'·tia
mi'·cro·don'·tism
mi'·cro·elec'·trode
mi'·cro·elec'·tro·pho·re'·sis
mi'·cro·em'·bo·lus   *pl.* ·li

mi'·cro·en·ceph'·a·ly   *var. of* micrencephaly
mi'·cro·far'·ad
mi'·cro·fi'·bril
mi'·cro·fil'·a·ment
mi'·cro·fil'·a·re'·mia   *Brit.* ·rae'·
mi'·cro·fi·lar'·ia   *pl.* ·i·ae
mi'·cro·fi·lar'·i·al
mi'·cro·fil'·a·ri'·a·sis
mi'·cro·fol·lic'·u·lar
mi'·cro·frac'·ture
mi'·cro·gam'·ete   [·ga·mete']
mi'·cro·ga·me'·to·cyte
mi'·cro·gas'·tria
mi'·cro·ge'·nia
mi'·cro·gen'·i·tal·is'm
mi·crog'·lia
mi·crog'·li·al
mi·crog'·li·o'·ma
mi·crog'·li·o'·ma·to'·sis
mi'·cro·glob'·u·lin
mi'·cro·glos'·sia
mi'·cro·gna'·thia
mi'·cro·gram
mi'·cro·graph
mi'·cro·graph'·ia
mi·crog'·ra·phy
mi'·cro·gray
mi'·cro·gy'·ria
mi'·cro·hem'·ag·glu'·ti·na'·tion   *Brit.* ·haem'·
mi'·cro·he·mat'·o·crit   [he'·ma·to·]   *Brit.* ·hae·mat'·
mi'·cro·he·pat'·ia
mi'·cro·het'·er·o·ge·ne'·ity
mi'·cro·in·cin'·er·a'·tion
mi'·cro·in'·farct
mi'·cro·in·jec'·tion
mi'·cro·in·va'·sion
mi'·cro·ka·tal'   [·kat'·al]

mi'·cro·lar'·yn·gos'·co·py
mi'·cro·lec'·i·thal
mi'·cro·li'·ter   *Brit.* ·li'·tre
mi'·cro·lith
mi'·cro·li·thi'·a·sis
mi'·cro·ma·nip'·u·la'·tion
mi'·cro·ma·nip'·u·la'·tor
mi'·cro·ma·nom'·e·ter
mi'·cro·mas'·tia
mi'·cro·me'·lia
mi'·cro·mel'·ic   [·me'·lic]
mi'·cro·mere
mi'·cro·me·tas'·ta·sis   *pl.* ·ses
mi'·cro·me'·ter   *unit of length; Brit.* ·me'·tre
mi·crom'·e·ter   *instrument*
mi'·cro·meth'·od
mi·crom'·e·try
mi'·cro·mole
Mi'·cro·mo·nos'·po·ra
mi'·cro·mo'·tor
mi'·cro·my·e'·lia
mi'·cro·my'·e·lo·blast
mi'·cro·my'·e·lo·blas'·tic
mi'·cron
mi'·cro·nee'·dle
mi'·cro·neme
mi'·cron·ize   ·ized,   ·iz'·ing
mi'·cro·nod'·u·lar
mi'·cro·nor'·mo·blast
mi'·cro·nu'·cle·us   *pl.* ·clei
mi'·cro·nu'·tri·ent
mi'·cro·nych'·ia
mi'·cro-or·chid'·ia   *var. of* microrchidia
mi'·cro·or'·gan·is'm
mi'·cro·par'·a·site
mi'·cro·pe'·nis

mi'·cro·per·fu"·sion
mi'·cro·phage
mi'·cro·pha'·kia
mi'·cro·phal'·lus
mi'·cro·phon'·ics
mi'·cro·pho'·no·graph
mi'·cro·pho'·to·graph
mi'·croph·thal'·mia
mi'·croph·thal'·mic
mi'·croph·thal'·mos
   also ·mus
mi·cro'·pia *var. of*
   micropsia
mi'·cro·pi'·no·cy·tot'·ic
mi'·cro·pi·pet' *also*
   ·pi·pette'
mi'·cro·pla"·sia
mi'·cro·pli'·ca *pl.* ·cae
mi'·cro·pore
mi'·cro·probe
mi·crop'·sia
mi·crop'·tic
mi'·cro·punc'·ture
mi'·cro·pyk·nom'·e·ter
mi'·cro·pyle
mi'·cro·ra'·di·o·graph
   also ·gram
mi'·cro·ra'·di·og'·ra·phy
mi'·cror·chid'·ia
mi'·cro·re'·frac·tom'·e·ter
mi'·cro·res'·pi·rom'·e·ter
mi'·cro·roent'·gen
mi'·cro·scope
mi'·cro·scop'·ic *also*
   ·i·cal
mi·cros'·co·pist
mi·cros'·co·py
mi'·cro·sec'·ond
mi'·cro·sec'·tion
mi'·cro·som'·al [·so'·mal]
mi'·cro·some
mi'·cro·so'·mia
mi'·cro·spec·trog'·ra·phy

mi'·cro·spec'·tro·pho·tom'·e·ter
mi'·cro·spec'·tro·pho·tom'·e·try
mi'·cro·spec'·tro·scope
mi'·cro·sphere
mi'·cro·sphe"·ro·cy·to"·sis [·spher'·o·]
mi'·cro·spher'·ule
mi'·cro·splanch"·nic
mi'·cro·sple"·nia
Mi·cros'·po·ra [·cro·spo'·]
mi·cros'·po·rid [·cro·spo'·]
Mi'·cro·spo·rid'·ia
mi'·cro·spo·rid'·i·an
mi'·cro·spo·ro"·sis
Mi·cros'·po·rum [·cro·spo'·]
mi'·cro·steth'·o·phone
mi'·cro·sto'·mia
mi'·cro·struc'·ture
mi'·cro·sur'·gery
mi'·cro·su'·ture
mi'·cro·throm'·bus
   pl. ·bi
mi·cro'·tia
mi'·cro·ti'·ter *Brit.*
   ·ti'·tre
mi'·cro·tome
mi'cro·to·mog'·ra·phy
mi·crot'·o·my
mi'·cro·to·nom'·e·ter
Mi'·cro·trom·bid'·i·um
mi'·cro·tu'·bule
mi'·cro·vas'·cu·lar
mi'·cro·vas'·cu·la·ture
mi'·cro·vil'·lus *pl.* ·li
mi'·cro·volt
mi'·cro·vol·tom'·e·ter
mi'·cro·wave
mi'·cro·zo"·on *pl.* ·zo'a
mi'·crur·gy
Mi'·cru·roi"·des
Mi·cru'·rus
mic'·tion

mic'·tu·rate ·rat'·ed, ·rat'·ing
mic'·tu·ri'·tion
mid·az'·o·lam
mid'·body
mid'·brain
mid·car'·pal
mid'·cla·vic'·u·lar
mid'·dle·piece
mid·ep'i·gas"·tric
mid·fa"·cial
mid·for'·ceps
mid·fron'·tal
midge
midg'·et
mid'·gut
mid'·line
mid'·pha·lan'·ge·al
mid'·piece
mid'·plane
mid'·riff
mid·sag'·it·tal
mid'·sec·tion
mid·tar'·sal
mid·ven'·tral
mid'·wife
mid·wif"e·ry [mid'·wife·ry]
mi'·graine
mi"·grain·oid
mi"·grain·ous
mi"·grans
mi'·grate ·grat·ed, ·grat·ing
mi·gra'·tion
mi'·gra·to'·ry
mil
mil'·dew
mil'·i·ar'·ia
mil'·i·a'·ris
mil'·i·ar'y
mi·lieu' *pl.* ·lieux'
mil'·i·um *pl.* mil'·ia
milk'·pox
milk'y   milk'·i·er, milk'·i·est
mil'·li·
mil'·li·am'·me·ter

mil′·li·am′·pere
mil′·li·bar
mil′·li·cu′·rie
mil′·li·equiv′·a·lent
mil′·li·gram
mil′·li·gray
mil′·li·li′·ter Brit. ·li′·tre
mil′·li·me′·ter Brit. ·me′·tre
mil′·li·mi′·cro·
mil′·li·mi′·cron
mil′·li·mole
mil′·li·os′·mole
mil′·li·rad
mil′·li·rem
mil′·li·roent′·gen
mil′·li·sec′·ond
mil′·li·volt
milz′·brand
mi·me′·sis
mi·met′·ic
mim′·ic mim′·icked, mim′·ick·ing
mim′·ic·ry
Mi′·na·ma′·ta
min′·er·al
min′·er·al·i·za′·tion
min′·er·alo·cor′·ti·coid
min′i·cell
min′·im
min′·i·ma fem. of minimus; pl. & gen. sg. ·mae, gen. pl. ·ma′·rum
min′·i·mal
min′·i·mum pl. ·ma or ·mums
min′·i·mus pl. & gen. sg. ·mi
min′i·pill
min′i·pol′y·my′o·clo′·nus [·my·oc′·lo·nus]
min′·o·cy′·cline
mi·nom′·e·ter
mi′·nor pl. mi·no′·res, gen. sg. ·ris
mi′·nus neut. of minor; pl. mi·no′·ra

min′·ute unit of time
mi·nute′ extremely small
mi′o·
mi′·o·car′·dia
mi′o·did′·y·mus
mi′o·lec′·i·thal
mi·o′·sis
mi·ot′·ic
mi·ra′·bi·le
mi′·ra·cid′·i·um pl. ·cid′·ia
mir′·ror
mis·car′·riage
mis·car′·ry ·ried, ·ry·ing
mis′·ce·ge·na′·tion
mis′·ci·ble
mis′·di′·ag·nose′ [di′·ag·nose] ·nosed′, ·nos′·ing
mis′·di′·ag·no′·sis pl. ·ses
mis′·match
mi·sog′·y·ny
mi·sog′·y·nous
mis′·sense
mis·tu′·ra pl. & gen. sg. ·rae
mith′·ra·my′·cin
mith′·ri·da′·tism [mith·rid′·a·]
mi′·ti·cid′·al [·ci′·dal]
mi′·ti·cide
mit′·i·gate ·gat′·ed, ·gat′·ing
mi′·tis neut. ·te
mi′·to·
mi′·to·chon′·dri·al
mi′·to·chon′·dri·on pl. ·dria
mi′·to·cro′·min
mi′·to·gen
mi′·to·gen′·e·sis also ·ge·ne′·sia
mi′·to·gen′·ic also ·ge·net′·ic
mi′·to·mal′·cin

mi′·to·my′·cin
mi·to′·sis pl. ·ses
mi′·to·some
mi·tot′·ic
mi′·tral
mi′·tral·i·za′·tion
mi′·troid
mit′·tel·schmerz
mix′·er
mix′·ing
mix′·o·sco′·pia also mix·os′·co·py
mix′·o·tro′·phic
mix′·ture
Mi′·ya·ga′·wa·nel′·la
mne·mon′·ic
mo′·bile
mo′·bi·lis neut. ·le
mo·bil′·i·ty
mo′·bi·li·za′·tion
mo′·bi·lize ·lized, ·liz′·ing
mo′·bi·liz′·er
moc′·ca·sin
mo·dal′·i·ty
mode
mod′·el n. & v.
mod′·eled or mod′·elled, mod′·el·ing or mod′·el·ling
mod′·er·ate adj. & v. ·at′·ed, ·at′·ing
mod′·i·cum
mod′·i·fi·ca′·tion
mod′·i·fy ·fied, ·fy′·ing
mo·di′·o·lus pl. & gen. sg. ·li
mod′·u·lar
mod′·u·la′·tion
mod′·u·la′·tor
mod′·u·lus pl. ·li
mog′i·
mog′·i·ar′·thria
mog′·i·graph′·ia
mog′·i·la′·lia
moi′·ety
mol′·al [mo′·lal]
mo·lal′·i·ty

mo′·lar
mo·la′·ris pl. ·res
mo·lar′·i·ty
mold Brit. mould
mole
mo·lec′·u·lar
mo·lec′·u·la′·re
mol′·e·cule
mo·li′·men pl. mo·lim′·i·na
mol′·le neut. of mollis
Mol′·li·cu′·tes
mol′·lis pl. ·les
mol·li′·ti·es
Mol·lus′·ca
mol·lus′·cous
mol·lus′·cum
mol′·lusk also ·lusc
mo·lyb′·date
mo·lyb′·de·num
mo·men′·tum
mo′·nad
mon′·ar·tic′·u·lar var. of monoarticular
mon·as′·ter
mon′·atom′·ic
mon·auch′·e·nos
mon·au′·ral
mon·ax′·i·al
mon′·es·thet′·ic Brit. ·aes·
mon·es′·trous Brit. ·oes′·
mon′·gol·is′m
mon′·gol·oid also Mongoloid
mo·nil′·e·thrix
Mo·nil′·ia
Mo·nil′·i·a′·ce·ae
mo·nil′·i·al
mo′·ni·li′·a·sis
mo·nil′·i·form
mo·nil′·i·id
mon′·i·tor
mon′·o·
mon′·o·am′·ine
mon′·o·am′·ni·ot′·ic
mon′·o·ar·tic′·u·lar

mon′·o·bac·te′·ri·al
mon′·o·bal′·lism
mon′·o·ba′·sic
mon′·o·ben′·zone
mon′·o·blast
mon′·o·bloc [mo′no·]
mon′·o·car·box·yl′·ic
mon′·o·cel′·lu·lar
mon′·o·cen′·tric
mon′·o·chlo′·ride
mon′·o·chord
mon′·o·cho′·ri·al
mon′·o·cho′·ri·on′·ic
mon′·o·chro′·ic
mon′·o·chro′·ma·sy
mon′·o·chro′·mat
mon′·o·chro·mat′·ic
mon′·o·chro′·ma·tis′m
mon′·o·chro·mat′o·phil [·chro′·ma·to·]
mon′·o·chro·mat′o·phil′·ic also ·chro′·mo·
mon′·o·chro′·ma·tor
mon′·o·chro′·mic
mon′·o·clon′·al [·clo′·nal]
mon′·o·con·tam′·i·nat′·ed
mon′·o·con·tam′·i·na′·tion
mon′·o·cra′·ni·us
mon′·o·crot′·ic
mo·noc′·ro·tis′m
mon·oc′·u·lar
mon·oc′·u·lus
mon′·o·cy′clic
mon′·o·cyte
mon′·o·cyt′·ic
mon′·o·cy′·toid
mon′·o·cy′·to·pe′·nia
mon′·o·cy′·to·poi·e′·sis
mon′·o·cy·to′·sis
mon·o′·dal
mon′·o·der′·mal
mon′·o·did′·y·mus
mon′·o·dis·perse′
mon′·o·es′·ter·ase

mon·oes′·trous Brit. spel. of monestrous
mon′·o·fac·to′·ri·al
mon′·o·fil′·a·ment
mo·nog′·a·mous
mo·nog′·a·my
mon′·o·gen′·e·sis
mon′·o·ge·net′·ic
mon′·o·gen′·ic
mo·nog′·e·nous
mon′·o·glyc′·er·ide
mon′·o·graph
mon′·o·hy′·brid
mon′·o·hy′·drate
mon′·o·hy′·dric
mon′·o·in·fec′·tion
mon′·o·i′odo·ty′·ro·sine
mon′·o·lay′·er
mon′·o·lep′·tic
mon′·o·lob′·u·lar
mon′·o·loc′·u·lar
mon′·o·ma′·nia
mon′·o·mas′·ti·gote
mon′·o·mel′·ic [·me′·lic]
mon′·o·mer
mon′·o·mer′·ic
mon′·o·meth′·yl·mor′·phine
mon′·o·mo·lec′·u·lar
mon′·o·mor′·phic
mon′·o·mor′·phism
mon′·o·mor′·phous
mon·om′·pha·lus
mon′·o·neu·ri′·tis
mon′·o·neu·rop′·a·thy
mon′·o·ni′·trate
mon′·o·nu′·cle·ar
mon′·o·nu′·cle·ate
mon′·o·nu′·cle·o′·sis
mon′·o·nu′·cle·o·tide
mon′·o·nu′·cle·o·tide
mon′·o-os′·te·it′·ic
mon′·o·ox′·y·gen·ase
mon′·o·pha′·sic
mon′·o·phe′·nol
mon′·o·pho′·bia
mon′·o·phos′·phate

mon′·o·phy·let′·ic
mon′o·phy′·le·tis′m
mon′·o·plas′·tic
mon′·o·ple′·gia
mon′·o·ploid
mon′·o·po′·dia
mon′o·po′·lar
mon′·o·pus
mon·or′·chia
mon·or′·chi·dis′m
    also ·or′·chism
mon′o·rhyth′·mic
mon′o·sac′·cha·ride
mon′o·sex′·u·al
mon′o·so′·di·um
mon′·o·some
mon′·o·so′·mic
mon′·o·so′·my
mon′·o·sper′·my
Mon′·o·spo′·ri·um
mon′·os·tot′·ic
mon′o·stra′·tal
mon′o·strat′·i·fied
mon′o·sul′·fo·nate
mon′o·sym′·me·tros
mon′o·symp′·tom
mon′o·symp′·to·mat′·ic
mon′o·syn·ap′·tic
mon′o·ter′·pene
mon′o·ther′·a·py
mon·o′tic
mo·not′·ri·chous
mon′o·typ′·ic
mon′o·un·sat′·u·rat′·ed
mon′o·va′·lent
mon·ov′u·lar [·o′vu·]
mon·ov′u·la·to′·ry
    [·o′vu·]
mon′o·xen′·ic
mo·nox′·e·nous
mo·nox′·e·ny
mon·ox′·ide
mon′o·zy·gos′·i·ty
mon′o·zy·got′·ic
mons
mon′·stro·cel′·lu·lar
mon·tage′
mon·tic′·u·lus

Mor′·ax·el′·la lac′·u·na′·ta
mor′·bi gen. of morbus
mor′·bid
mor·bid′·i·ty
mor·bif′·ic
mor·bil′·li
mor·bil′·li·form
Mor·bil′·li·vi′·rus
mor′·bus gen. ·bi
mor·cel′ ·celled′, ·cel′·ing
mor′·cel·la′·tion
mor′·celle·ment′
mor′·dant
Mo·re′·ra·stron′·gy·lus
mor·ga′·gni·an
mor′·gan
morgue
mo′·ria
mor′·i·bund
mo′·ron
mor·phe′a Brit. ·phoe′a; type of scleroderma: Cf. morphia
mor·phe′·ic
mor′·phia var. of morphine: Cf. morphea
mor′·phine
mor·phin′·ic
mor′·phin·is′m
mor′·phin·i·za′·tion
mor′·phi·om′·e·try
mor′·pho·
mor′·pho·dif′·fer·en′·ti·a′·tion
mor·phoe′a Brit. spel. of morphea
mor′·pho·gen′·e·sis
mor′·pho·ge·net′·ic
mor′·pho·gen′·ic
mor′·pho·log′·ic also ·i·cal
mor·phol′·o·gy
mor′·pho·met′·ric
mor·phom′·e·try
mor′·pho·plas′m

mor′·pho·syn′·the·sis
mor′·rhu·ate
mor·rhu′·ic
mors gen. mor′·tis, accusative mor′·tem
mor′·sal
mor′·sel·ize ·ized, ·iz′·ing
mor′·tal
mor·tal′·i·ty
mor′·tar
mor′·tem accusative of mors
mor′·ti·fi·ca′·tion
mor′·ti·na·tal′·i·ty
mor′·tis gen. of mors
mor′·tise
mor′·tu·ar′y
mor′·tu·us
mor′·u·la pl. ·lae or ·las
mor′·u·la′·tion
mor′·u·lus pl. ·li
mo′·rus
mo·sa′·ic
mo·sa′·i·cis′m
mos·qui′·ti·cid′·al [·ci′·dal] also ·qui′·to·
mos·qui′·ti·cide also ·qui′·to·
mos·qui′·to pl. ·toes or ·tos
mo′·tile
mo·til′·in
mo·til′·i·ty
mo′·tion
mo′·ti·va′·tion
mo′·tive
mo′·to·fa′·cient
mo′·to·neu′·ron Brit. ·rone
mo′·to·neu′·ro·ni′·tis [·ron·i′·]
mo′·tor
mo·to′·ri·al
mo·to′·ri·um
mo·to′·ri·us fem. ·ria

mo'·to·ro·ger'·mi·na·tive
mot'·tle mot'·tled, mot'·tling
mou·lage'
mould Brit. spel. of mold
mound
mount
moun'·tant [mount'·ant]
mount'·ing
mouse pl. mice
mouse'·pox
mouth'-to-mouth'
mouth'·wash
move'·ment
mov'·er
mox'·a·lac'·tam
mox'·i·bus'·tion
mo'·ya·mo'·ya
mu'·cate
mu'·ci·car'·mine
mu·cif'·er·ous
mu'·ci·fi·ca'·tion
mu'·ci·form
mu·cig'·e·nous
mu'·ci·hem'·a·te'·in Brit. ·haem'·
mu'·ci·lage
mu'·ci·lag'·i·nous
mu'·ci·la'·go
mu'·cil·loid
mu'·cin
mu'·cin·ase
mu'·cin·e'·mia Brit. ·ae'·mia
mu·cin'·o·blast
mu·cin'·o·gen
mu'·ci·no·lyt'·ic
mu'·ci·no'·sis
mu'·ci·nous
mu'·cin·u'·ria
mu·cip'·a·rous
mu·civ'·o·rous
mu'·co
mu'·co·al·bu'·mi·nous
mu'·co·buc'·cal

mu'·co·cele
mu'·co·cel'·lu·la'·re
mu·coc'·la·sis
mu'·co·col'·pos
mu'·co·cu·ta'·ne·ous
mu'·co·ep'·i·der'·moid
mu'·co·gin'·gi·val
mu'·coid
mu'·co·la'·bi·al
mu'·co·lip'·i·do'·sis
mu'·co·lyt'·ic
mu'·co·mem'·bra·nous
mu'·co·pep'·tide
mu'·co·per'·i·os'·te·al
mu'·co·per'·i·os'·te·um
mu'·co·poi·e'·sis
mu'·co·pol'·y·sac'·cha·ride
mu'·co·pol'·y·sac'·cha·ri·do'·sis pl. ·ses
mu'·co·pro'·tein
mu'·co·pu'·ru·lent
mu'·co·pus
Mu'·cor
Mu'·co·ra'·ce·ae
mu'·co·ra'·ceous
mu'·cor·my·co'·sis
mu·co'·sa fem. of mucosus; pl. & gen. sg. ·sae
mu·co'·sal
mu'·co·sal'·pinx
mu'·co·san·guin'·e·ous
mu'·co·se'·rous
mu·co'·sin
mu'·co·stat'·ic
mu·co'·sus fem. ·sa, neut. ·sum
mu'·co·tome
mu'·cous
mu'·co·vis'·ci·do'·sis
mu'·cro pl. mu·cro'·nes
mu'·cro·nate
mu'·cus
mu'·li·eb'·ris neut. pl. ·ria
mull

mul·tan'·gu·lar [mult·an'·] also mul'·ti·an'·gu·lar
mul'·ti·
mul'·ti·al·le'·lic
mul'·ti·cel'·lu·lar
mul'·ti·cen'·tric
Mul'·ti·ceps
mul'·ti·cip'·i·tal
mul'·ti·clon'·al [·clo'·nal]
mul'·ti·core
mul'·ti·cus'·pid
mul'·ti·cus'·pi·date
mul'·ti·den'·tate
mul'·ti·de·ter'·mi·na'·tion
mul'·ti·fac·to'·ri·al
mul'·ti·fe·ta'·tion Brit. also ·foe·
mul'·ti·fid
mul·tif'·i·dus pl. ·di
mul'·ti·flag'·el·late
mul'·ti·fo'·cal
mul'·ti·form
mul'·ti·for'·me
mul'·ti·gan'·gli·on'·ic
mul'·ti·gem'·i·ni
mul'·ti·glan'·du·lar
mul'·ti·grav'·i·da pl. ·dae or ·das
mul'·ti·lo'·bar
mul'·ti·lob'·u·lar
mul'·ti·loc'·u·lar
mul'·ti·nod'·u·lar
mul'·ti·nu'·cle·ar
mul'·ti·nu'·cle·ate also ·at'·ed
mul·tip'·a·ra pl. ·rae or ·ras
mul·tip'·ar·i·ty
mul·tip'·a·rous
mul'·ti·par'·tial
mul'·ti·par'·tite
mul'·ti·pen'·nate also ·pen'·ni·form
mul'·ti·pha'·sic
mul'·ti·ple

mul′·ti·plex
mul′·ti·pli·ca′·tive
mul′·ti·plic′·i·tas
mul′·ti·po′·lar
mul·tip′·o·tent
mul′·ti·stage
mul′·ti·syn·ap′·tic
mul′·ti·sys′·tem
mul′·ti·va′·lent
mul′·ti·var′·i·ate
mul′·ti·ve·sic′·u·lar
mul′·ti·vi′·ta·min
mum′·mi·fi·ca′·tion
mum′·mi·fy ·fied, ·fy′·ing
mumps
mu′·ni·ty
mu′·ral
mu·ram′·ic
mu·ram′·i·dase
mu′·rein
mu·rex′·ide
mu′·ri·ate
mu′·ri·at′·ic
Mu′·ri·dae
mu′·rine
mur′·mur
Mus
Mus′·ca
  M. do·mes′·ti·ca
mus′·ca pl. ·cae
mus′·ca·rine
mus′·ca·rin′·ic
mus′·ca·rin·is′m
mus′·ci·cide
Mus′·ci·dae
mus′·cle
mus′·coid
mus′·cu·lar
mus·cu·la′·re neut.
  of muscularis
mus′·cu·la′·ris pl. ·res
mus′·cu·lar′·i·ty
mus′·cu·la·ture
mus′·cu·li pl. & gen.
  sg. of musculus
mus′·cu·lo·

mus′·cu·lo·ap′·o·neu·rot′·ic
mus′·cu·lo·cu·ta′·ne·ous
mus′·cu·lo·cu·ta′·ne·us pl. & gen. sg. ·nei
mus′·cu·lo·elas′·tic
mus′·cu·lo·fas′·cial
mus′·cu·lo·fi′·brous
mus′·cu·lo·mem′·bra·nous
mus′·cu·lo·phren′·ic
mus′·cu·lo·phren′·i·ca pl. & gen. sg. ·cae
mus′·cu·lo·ra·chid′·i·an
mus′·cu·lo′·rum gen. pl. of musculus
mus′·cu·lo·skel′·e·tal
mus′·cu·lo·spi′·ral
mus′·cu·lo·ten′·di·nous
mus′·cu·lo·tro′·pic [·trop′·ic]
mus′·cu·lo·tu′·bal
mus′·cu·lo·tu·ba′·ri·us pl. & gen. sg. ·rii
mus′·cu·lus pl. & gen. sg. ·li, gen. pl. mus′·cu·lo′·rum
mu′·si·co·gen′·ic
mus′·si·ta′·tion
mu′·ta·ble
mu′·ta·fa′·cient
mu′·ta·gen
mu′·ta·gen′·e·sis
mu′·ta·gen′·ic
mu′·ta·ge·nic′·i·ty
mu′·ta·gen·ize ·ized, ·iz′·ing
mu′·tant
mu′·tase
mu′·tate ·tat′·ed, ·tat′·ing
mu·ta′·tion
mu·ta′·tion·al
mu′·ta·tor
mute
mu′·ti·late ·lat′·ed, ·lat′·ing

mu′·ti·la′·tion
mut′·ism
mu′·ton
mu″·tu·al·is′m
my·al′·gia
my·al′·gic
my′·as·the′·nia
my′·as·then′·ic
  showing abnormal
  muscle fatigue: Cf.
  myosthenic
my′·a·to′·nia
  reduction in muscle
  tone: Cf. myotonia;
  also my·at′·o·ny
my·at′·ro·phy
my′·au·ton′·o·my
my·ce′·li·al
my·ce′·li·oid
my·ce′·li·um pl. ·lia
my′·ce·the′·mia Brit.
  ·thae′·
my′·ce·tis′·mus also
  my′·ce·tis′m
my′·ce·to· [my·ce′·to·]
my′·ce·toid
my′·ce·to′·ma pl.
  ·mas or ·ma·ta
my′·co·
my′·co·bac·te′·ri·o′·sis
My′·co·bac·te′·ri·um
  M. bo′·vis
  M. che·lo′·nei
  M. lep′·rae
  M. par′a·tu·ber′·cu·lo′·sis
  M. scrof·u·la′·ce·um
  M. tu·ber′·cu·lo′·sis
  M. ul′·cer·ans
my′·co·bac·te′·ri·um
  pl. ·ria
my′·co·bac′·tin
my′·coid
my·col′·o·gist
my·col′·o·gy
my′·co·path′·o·gen
my′·co·pa·thol′·o·gy
my′·co·phage

my′·co·phe·no′·lic
My′·co·plas′·ma
M. hom′·i·nis
M. ora′·le
M. pneu·mo′·ni·ae
my′·co·plas′·ma
my·co′·sis *pl.* ·ses
my′·co·stat
my′·co·stat′·ic
my·cot′·ic
my·cot′·i·ca
my′·co·tox′·i·col′·o·gy
my′·co·tox′·i·co′·sis
my′·co·tox′·in
my·dri′·a·sis
myd′·ri·at′·ic
my·ec′·to·my
my·ec′·to·py *also*
  my′·ec·to′·pia
my′·el·en·ceph′·a·li′·tis
my′·el·en·ceph′·a·lon
my·el′·ic
my′·e·lin
my′·e·lin·at′·ed
my′·e·lin·a′·tion *also*
  ·i·za′·tion
my′·e·lin′·ic
my′·e·li·no·gen′·e·sis
my′·e·li·no·ge·net′·ic
my′·e·li·nol′·y·sis
my′·e·li·nop′·a·thy
my′·e·li·no′·sis
my′·e·lit′·ic
my′·e·li′·tis
my′·e·lo·
my′·e·lo·ar′·chi·tec′·ture
my′·e·lo·blast
my′·e·lo·blas·te′·mia
  Brit. ·tae′·
my′·e·lo·blas′·tic
my′·e·lo·blas·to′·ma
my′·e·lo·blas·to′·sis
my′·e·lo·cele *neural tube defect: Cf.* myelocoele
my′·e·lo·clast

my′·e·lo·coele
  embryonic spinal canal: Cf. myelocele
my′·e·lo·cyst
my′·e·lo·cys·tog′·ra·phy
my′·e·lo·cyte
my′·e·lo·cy·the′·mia
  Brit. ·thae′·
my′·e·lo·cyt′·ic
my′·e·lo·cy·to′·sis
my′·e·lo·di·as′·ta·sis
my′·e·lo·dys·pla′·sia
my′·e·lo·en′·ce·phal′·ic
my′·e·lo·fi·bro′·sis
my′·e·lo·gen′·e·sis
my′·e·log′·e·nous
  also my′·e·lo·gen′·ic
my′·e·lo·gram
my′·e·log′·ra·phy
my′·e·loid
my′·e·lo·ken′·tric
my′·e·lo·li·po′·ma
my′·e·lol′·y·sis
my′·e·lo·lyt′·ic
my′·e·lo′·ma *pl.* ·mas *or* ·ma·ta
my′·e·lo·ma·la′·cia
my′·e·lo′ma·toid
  [·lom′a·]
my′·e·lo′·ma·to′·sis
my′·e·lo′ma·tous
my′·e·lo·me·nin′·go·cele
my′·e·lo·mon′·o·cyte
my′·e·lo·mon′·o·cyt′·ic
my′·e·lo·neu·ri′·tis
my′·e·lo-op′·ti·co·neu·rop′·a·thy
my′·e·lo·path′·ic
my·e·lop′·a·thy
my′·e·lo·per·ox′·i·dase
my′·e·lo·phthis′·ic
my′·e·lo·phthi′·sis
  [·loph′·thi·]
my′·e·lo·plas′m
my′·e·lo·poi·e′·sis

my′·e·lo·pro·lif′·er·a·tive
my′·el·op′·ti·co·neu·rop′·a·thy *var. of*
  myelo-opticoneuropathy
my′·e·lo·ra·dic′·u·li′·tis
my′·e·lo·ra·dic′·u·lo·dys·pla′·sia
my′·e·lo·ra·dic′·u·lop′·a·thy
my′·e·lor·rha′·gia
my′·e·los′·chi·sis
my′·e·lo·scle·ro′·sis
my′·e·lo·scle·rot′·ic
my′·e·lo′·sis
my′·e·lo·spas′m
my′·e·lo·spon′·gi·um
  pl. ·gia
my′·e·lo·syr′·in·go′·sis
my′·e·lot′·o·my
my′·e·lo·tox′·ic
my′·e·lo·tox·ic′·i·ty
my′·e·lo·tox′·in
my′·e·lo·tro′·pic
  [·trop′·ic]
my′·en·ter′·ic
my′·en·ter′·i·cus
my·en′·ter·on
my′·es·the′·sia *Brit.*
  ·aes·
my·i′·a·sis *pl.* ·ses
my·i′tis
my′·lo·hy′·oid
my′·lo·hy·oi′·de·an
my′·lo·hy·oi′·de·us
my′·lo·pha·ryn′·gea
my′·lo·pha·ryn′·ge·al
my′o·
my′·o·blast
my′·o·blas′·tic
my′o·blas·to′·ma *pl.*
  ·mas *or* ·ma·ta
my′·o·car′·di·al
my′·o·car′·di·o·graph
my′·o·car′·di·op′·a·thy
my′·o·car′·di·or′·rha·phy

my'·o·car·di'·tis
my'·o·car'·di·um
my'·o·car·do'·sis
my'·o·cele *muscle
hernia: Cf.* myocoele
my'·o·cep'·tor
my'·o·clo'·nia
my'·o·clon'·ic
my'·o·clon'·i·ca
my'·o·clo'·nus [my·oc'·
  lo·nus]
my'·o·coele *also
  ·coel; myotome cavity:
  Cf.* myocele
my'·o·col·pi'·tis
my·oc'·u·la'·tor
my'·o·cu·ta'·ne·ous
my'·o·cyte
my'·o·cy·tol'·y·sis
my'·o·di·as'·ta·sis *pl.*
  ·ses
my'·o·di·op'·ter *Brit.*
  ·tre
my'·o·dy·nam'·ics
my'·o·dy'·na·mom'·e·
  ter
my'·o·dys·pla'·sia
my'·o·dys·to'·nia
my'·o·dys·tro'·phia
  also ·dys'·tro·phy
my'·o·ede'·ma *var. of*
  myoidema
my'·o·elas'·tic
my'·o·elec'·tric
my'·o·ep'·i·the'·li·al
my'·o·ep'·i·the·li·o'·ma
my'·o·ep'·i·the'·li·um
  pl. ·lia
my'·o·fas'·ci·al
my'·o·fas·ci'·tis
my'·o·fi'·bril
my'·o·fi·bril'·la *pl.*
  ·lae; *var. of* myofibril
my'·o·fi'·bril·lar
my'·o·fi'·bro·blast
my'·o·fi·bro'·ma *pl.*
  ·mas *or* ·ma·ta
my'·o·fi·bro'·sis

my'·o·fi'·bro·si'·tis
my'·o·fil'·a·ment
my'·o·func'·tion·al
my'·o·gen'·e·sis
my'·o·gen'·ic *also*
  my·og'·e·nous
my·og'·lia
my'·o·glo'·bin
my'·o·glo'·bin·u'·ria
  [·bi·nu'·]
my·og'·na·thus
my'·o·graph
my'·o·graph'·ic
my·og'·ra·phy
my'·o·he'·mo·glo'·bin
  Brit. ·hae'·mo·glo'·
my'·o·hy·per·tro'·phia
my'·oid
my'·oi·de'·ma *also*
  myoedema
my'·o·in'·ti·mal
my'·o·ki'·nase
my'·o·kin'e·sim'·e·ter
  [·ki'·ne·]
my'·o·ki·ne'·si·og'·ra·
  phy
my'·o·ki·net'·ic
my'·o·ky'·mia
my'·o·lo'·gia
my'·o·log'·ic
my·ol'·o·gy
my·ol'·y·sis
my·o'·ma *pl.* ·ma *or*
  ·ma·ta
my'·o·ma·la'·cia
my·om'·a·tous [·o'·ma·]
my'·o·mec'·to·my
my'·o·mere
my'·o·me'·tri·al
my'·o·me·tri'·tis
my'·o·me'·tri·um
my'·on
my'·o·ne·cro'·sis
my'·o·neph'·ro·path'·ic
my'·o·neph'·ro·pex'y
my'·o·neu'·ral
my'·o·neu·ro'·ma *pl.*
  ·mas *or* ·ma·ta

my'·o·path'·ia
my'·o·path'·ic
my·op'·a·thy
my'·ope
my'·o·per'i·car·di'·tis
my'·o·phos·pho'·ry·lase
my·o'·pia
my·op'·ic [·o'·pic]
my'·o·plas'm
my'·o·plas'·tic
my'·o·plas'·ty
my·or'·rha·phy
my'·or·rhyth'·mia
my'·o·sal'·pinx
my'·o·sar·co'·ma
my'·o·scle·ro'·sis
my'·o·sep'·tum *pl.* ·ta
my'·o·sin
my·o'·sis
my'·o·sit'·ic
my'·o·si'·tis
my'·o·spas'm
my'·o·stat'·ic
my'·o·sthen'·ic
  *relating to muscle
  strength: Cf.*
  myasthenic
my'·o·tac'·tic
my·ot'·a·sis
my'·o·tat'·ic
my'·o·ten'·di·nous
my'·o·te·not'·o·my
my·ot'·ic *var. of*
  miotic
my'·o·tome
my·ot'·o·my
my'·o·to'·nia *muscle
  contraction disorder:
  Cf.* myatonia; *also* my·
  ot'·o·ny
my'·o·ton'·ic
my'·o·ton'·i·ca
my·ot'·o·nus
my'·o·tro'·phic
  [·troph'·ic]
my'·o·tro'·pic [·trop'·
  ic]
my'·o·tube

my′o·tu′·bu·lar
my′o·vas′·cu·lar
myr′·i·cin
my·rin′·ga
myr′·in·gi′·tis
my·rin′·go·
my·rin′·go·plas′·ty
my·rin′·go·sta·pe′·di·o·pex′y
my·rin′·go·tome
myr′·in·got′·o·my
myr′·inx [my′·rinx]
my·ris′·tate
my·ris′·ti·cin
myrrh
myr′·ti·form
myr′·ti·for′·mis *pl.*
·mes
my′·so·phil′·ia
my′·so·pho′·bia
myth′o·ma′·nia
myx′·ad′·e·ni′·tis
myx′·ede′·ma *Brit.*
·oe·de′·
myx′·edem′·a·tous [·ede′·ma·] *Brit.*
·oe·dem′·
myx·e′·mia *Brit.* ·ae′·mia
myx′o·
myx′o·blas·to′·ma
myx′o·cys·ti′·tis
myx′o·cys·to′·ma
myx′·o·cyte
myx′o·fi·bro′·ma *pl.*
·mas *or* ·ma·ta
myx′o·fi′·bro·sar·co′·ma
myx′·oid
myx′o·lip′o·fi′·bro·sar·co′·ma [·li′po·]
myx′o·li·po′·ma *pl.*
·mas *or* ·ma·ta
myx·o′·ma *pl.* ·mas *or* ·ma·ta
myx·o′·ma·to′·des
myx′·o′·ma·to′·sis

myx·o′·ma·tous [·om′a·]
Myx′·o·my·ce′·tes
myx′o·pap′·il·lar′y
myx′o·poi·e′·sis
myx′o·sar·co′·ma *pl.*
·mas *or* ·ma·ta
myx′o·vi′·rus

N

na·bo′·thi·an
Nae·gle′·ria
N. fow′·leri
nae′·void *Brit. spel. of*
nevoid
nae′·vous *Brit. spel. of* nevous
nae′·vus *Brit. spel. of*
nevus; *pl.* ·vi
naf·cil′·lin
na·ga′·na
Na′·ja
na′·ked
nal′·i·dix′·ic
nal·or′·phine
nal·ox′·one
nal·trex′·one
nan′·dro·lone
na′·nism [nan′·ism]
nan′o· [na′no·]
 denoting dwarf
nan′o· [na′no·]
 denoting 1 billionth
nan′o·ce·phal′·ic
nan′o·ceph′·a·ly
nan′o·cu′·rie
nan′o·gram
nan′o·li′·ter *Brit.* ·li′·tre
nan′o·me′·lia
nan′o·me′·ter *Brit.* ·me′·tre
Na′·no·phy·e′·tus
nan′o·so′·mia *also*
·so′·ma

na′·nu·ka′·ya·mi [·ka·ya′·mi]
na·phaz′·o·line
naph′·tha
naph′·tha·lene
naph′·tha·len′·ic
naph′·thol
naph′·thol·is′m
naph′·tho·qui·none′ [·quin′·one]
naph′·thyl
naph·thyl′·amine
na·prox′·en
nar′·ce·ine
nar′·cis·sis′m *also*
nar′·cism
nar′·cis·sis′·tic
nar′·co·
nar′·co·anal′·y·sis
nar′·co·hyp′·nia
nar′·co·lep′·sy
nar′·co·lep′·tic
nar′·co·lo′·cal
nar·co′·sis *pl.* ·ses
nar′·co·stim′·u·lant
nar′·co·syn′·the·sis
nar′·co·ther′·a·py
nar·cot′·ic
nar′·co·tine
nar′·co·tize ·tized,
·tiz′·ing
na′·res *sg.* ·ris
na′·sal
na·sa′·le *neut. of*
nasalis
na·sa′·lis *pl.* ·les
na·sal′·i·ty
na′·scent
na′·si *gen. of* nasus
na′·si·on
na′·so·
na′·so·al·ve′·o·lar
na′·so·bron′·chi·al
na′·so·buc′·co·pha·ryn′·ge·al
na′·so·cil′·i·a′·ris
na′·so·cil′·i·ar′y
na′·so·en′·do·scope

na′·so·en·dos′·co·py
na′·so·fa′·cial
na′·so·fron′·tal
na′·so·fron·ta′·lis
na′·so·gas′·tric
na′·so·la′·bi·al
na′·so·la′·bi·a′·lis
na′·so·lac′·ri·mal
na′·so·lac′·ri·ma′·lis
na′·so·max′·il·la′·ris
na′·so·max′·il·lar′y
na′·so·men′·tal
na′·so-oc′·u·lar
na′·so-op′·tic
na′·so-o′ral
na′·so·pal′·a·tine
na′·so·pal′·a·ti′·nus
na′·so·pha·ryn′·ge·al
na′·so·pha·ryn′·ge·us
na′·so·phar′·yn·gi′·tis
na′·so·pha·ryn′·go·scope
na′·so·phar′·yn·gos′·co·py
na′·so·phar′·ynx
na′·so·pul′·mo·nar′y
na′·so·ros′·tral
na′·so·scope
na′·so·sep′·tal
na′·so·tra′·che·al
na′·so·tur′·bi·nal
na′·sus *gen.* ·si
na′·tal
na·tal′·i·ty
na′·tes *sg.* ·tis
na′·ti·form
na′·ti·mor·tal′·i·ty
na′·tive
na′·tiv·is′m
na′·tri·ure′·sis *also* na′·tru·re′·sis
na′·tri·uret′·ic *also* na′·tru·ret′·ic
nat′·u·ral
na′·tur·o·path
na′·tur·o·path′·ic
na′·tur·op′·a·thy
nau′·sea

nau′·se·ant
nau′·se·ate ·at′·ed, ·at·ing
nau′·seous
nau′·ti·lus
na′·vel
na·vic′·u·lar
na·vic′·u·la′·ris *neut.* ·re
na·vic′·u·lo·cu′·boid
near′·sight′·ed
near′·sight′·ed·ness
ne′·ar·thro′·sis *var. of* neoarthrosis; *pl.* ·ses
ne′·ben·kern′
neb′·ra·my′·cin
neb′·u·la *pl.* ·lae *or* ·las
neb′·u·lize ·lized, ·liz′·ing
neb′·u·liz′·er
Ne·ca′·tor
N. amer′·i·ca′·nus
ne·ca′·to·ri′·a·sis
ne·ces′·si·tas *gen.* ne·ces′·si·ta′·tis
ne·crec′·to·my *var. of* necronectomy
nec′·ro·
nec′·ro·bac′·il·lo′·sis
nec′·ro·bi·o′·sis
nec′·ro·bi·ot′·ic
nec′·ro·cy′·to·tox′·in
nec′·ro·gen′·ic *also* ne·crog′·e·nous
nec′·ro·gran′·u·lom′a·tous [·lo′ma·]
nec′·ro·log′·ic *also* ·i·cal
ne·crol′·o·gy
ne·crol′·y·sis
nec′·ro·nec′·to·my
nec′·ro·phil′·ia
nec′·ro·phil′·ic
ne·croph′·i·lous
nec′·ro·pho′·bia
nec′·rop·sy

ne·crose′ [nec′·rose] ·crosed′, ·cros′·ing
ne·cro′·sis *pl.* ·ses
nec′·ro·sper′·mia
ne·cros′·te·o′·sis
ne·crot′·ic
ne·crot′·i·ca
ne·crot′·i·cans
nec′·ro·tize ·tized, ·tiz′·ing
ne·crot′·o·my
nec′·ro·zo′·o·sper′·mia
Nec·tu′·rus
nee′·dle *n. & v.* ·dled, ·dling
ne′·en·ceph′·a·lon
ne·ga′·tion
neg′·a·tive
neg′·a·tiv·is′m
neg′·a·tol
neg′·a·tron
ne·glect′
ne·glec′·ta
neg′·li·gence
ne′·groid *also* Negroid
neigh′·bor·wise *Brit.* ·bour·
Neis·se′·ria
N. gon′·or·rhoe′·ae
N. men′·in·git′·i·dis
neis·se′·ria *pl.* ·ri·ae
neis·se′·ri·ol′·o·gy
nek′·ro· *var. of* necro-
nel′·a·vane
nem′·a·line
nem′·a·thel′·minth
Nem′·a·thel·min′·thes
nem′·a·ti·cide [ne·mat′·i·] *var. of* nematocide
nem′·a·to·
Nem′·a·toc′·era
nem′·a·to·cide [ne·mat′·o·]
nem′·a·to·cyst [ne·mat′·o·]
Nem′·a·to′·da
nem′·a·tode

nem'·a·to·di'·a·sis
Nem'·a·to·di'·rus
nem'·a·to·do'·sis
nem'·a·toid
nem'·a·tol'·o·gist
nem'·a·tol'·o·gy
nem'·a·to'·sis
nem'·a·to·sper'·mia
ne'o·
ne'o·an'·ti·gen
ne'o·ars·phen'·a·mine
ne'o·ar·thro'·sis
ne'·o·blas'·tic
ne'o·cer'·e·bel'·lar
ne'o·cer'·e·bel'·lum
ne'o·cor'·tex
ne'o·cor'·ti·cal
ne'o·cys·tos'·to·my
ne'·o·cyte
ne'·o·cy·to'·sis
ne'o·dar'·win·is'm
ne'o·den·ta'·tum
ne'·o·dym'·i·um
ne'o·fe'·tus
ne'o·for·ma'·tion
ne'o·for'·ma·tive
ne'o·gen'·e·sis
ne'o·glot'·tis
ne'o·ki·net'·ic
ne·ol'·o·gis'm
ne'·o·morph
ne'·o·my'·cin
ne'·on
ne'o·na'·tal
ne'·o·nate
ne'·o·na·tol'·o·gy
ne'·o·na'·tus gen. pl.
 ne'·o·na·to'·rum
ne'o-ol'·ive
ne'o·pal'·li·um
ne'o·pho'·bia
ne'·o·pla'·sia
ne'·o·plas'm
ne'·o·plas'·tic
Ne'o·rick·ett'·sia hel'·
 min·thoe'·ca
ne'·o·stig'·mine
ne·os'·to·my

ne'o·stri·a'·tal
ne'o·stri·a'·tum
ne'o·stro·phin'·gic
ne·ot'·e·ny
ne'o·thal'·a·mus
ne'o·u'·ni·tar'·i·an
ne'o·vas'·cu·lar
ne'o·vas'·cu·lar·i·za'·
 tion
ne·pen'·thic
neph'·e·lom'·e·ter
neph'·e·lom'·e·try
ne·phral'·gia
neph'·rec·ta'·sia
ne·phrec'·to·mize
 ·mized, ·miz'·ing
ne·phrec'·to·my
neph'·ric
ne·phrit'·ic
ne·phri'·tis pl. ne·
 phrit'·i·des
neph'·ri·to·gen'·ic
neph'·ro·
neph'·ro·blas·to'·ma
 pl. ·mas or ·ma·ta
neph'·ro·cal'·ci·no'·sis
neph'·ro·cap'·su·lec'·
 to·my also ·cap·
 sec'·to·my
neph'·ro·cap'·su·lot'·o·
 my
neph'·ro·cele
 herniated kidney: Cf.
 nephrocoele
neph'·ro·coele also
 ·coel; cavity containing
 nephrotome: Cf.
 nephrocele
neph'·ro·co'·lic
neph'·ro·co'·lo·pex'y
neph'·ro·gen'·e·sis
neph'·ro·gen'·ic
ne·phrog'·e·nous
neph'·ro·gram
neph'·ro·graph'·ic
ne·phrog'·ra·phy
neph'·roid
neph'·ro·lith

neph'·ro·li·thi'·a·sis
neph'·ro·li·thot'·o·my
neph'·ro·log'·ic also
 ·i·cal
ne·phrol'·o·gist
ne·phrol'·o·gy
neph'·ro·lum'·bar
ne·phrol'·y·sis
ne·phro'·ma pl. ·mas
 or ·ma·ta
neph'·ro·meg'·a·ly
neph'·ro·mere
neph'·ron
ne·phron'·ic
neph'·ro·noph'·thi·sis
neph'·ro·path'·ic
ne·phrop'·a·thy also
 neph'·ro·path'·ia
neph'·ro·pex'y
neph'·rop·to'·sis
neph'·ro·py'·e·lo·li·
 thot'·o·my
neph'·ro·py'·e·lo·plas'·
 ty
ne·phror'·rha·phy
neph'·ro·scle·ro'·sis
neph'·ro·scle·rot'·ic
ne·phro'·sis pl. ·ses
neph'·ro'·so·ne·phri'·tis
ne·phros'·to·gram
ne·phros'·to·li·thot'·o·
 my
ne·phros'·to·my
ne·phrot'·ic
neph'·ro·tome
neph'·ro·to·mog'·ra·
 phy
ne·phrot'·o·my
neph'·ro·tox'·ic
neph'·ro·tox·ic'·i·ty
neph'·ro·tox'·in
neph'·ro·tre'·sis
neph'·ro·tro'·phic
 [·troph'·ic]
neph'·ro·tro'·pic
 [·trop'·ic]
neph'·ro·ure'·ter·ec'·
 to·my

neph'·ro·ure'·tero·cys·tec'·to·my
nep·tu'·ni·um
nerve
ner'·vi *pl. & gen. sg.* of nervus
ner'·vone
ner·von'·ic
ner·vo'·sa *fem. sg. & neut. pl.* of nervosus
ner·vo'·sum *neut. sg.* of nervosus
ner·vo'·sus
ner'·vous
ner'·vus *pl. & gen. sg.* ·vi, *ablative* ·vo, *gen. pl.* ner·vo'·rum
ne·sid'·i·ec'·to·my
ne·sid'·i·o·blast
ne·sid'·i·o·blas·to'·ma
ne·sid'·i·o·blas·to'·sis
ness·ler·i·za'·tion
nes'·te·os'·to·my
net'·work
neu'·ral
neu·ral'·gia
neu·ral'·gic
neu·ral'·gi·form
neur'·amin'·ic
neur'·amin'·i·dase
neur'·apoph'·y·sis *pl.* ·ses
neur'·aprax'·ia
neur'·ar·throp'·a·thy
neur'·as·the'·nia
neur'·as·then'·ic
neur·ax'·i·al
neur·ax'·is
neur·ax'·on
neur·ec'·to·derm
neu·rec'·to·my
neur·ec'·to·py
neur'·en·ter'·ic
neur'·ep'·i·the'·li·al
neur'·ep'·i·the'·li·um
neur'·ex·er'·e·sis
neu·ric'·i·ty
neu'·ri·lem'·ma

neu'·ri·lem'·mal
neu'·ri·lem·mi'·tis
neu'·ri·lem·mo'·ma *pl.* ·mas *or* ·ma·ta
neu'·ri·lem'·mo·sar·co'·ma *pl.* ·mas *or* ·ma·ta
neu·ril'·i·ty
neu'·ri·mo·til'·i·ty
neu'·ri·mo'·tor
neu'·ri·no'·ma
neu'·rite
neu·rit'·ic
neu·ri'·tis *pl.* ·rit'·i·des
neu'·ro·
neu'·ro·anas'·to·mo'·sis
neu'·ro·anat'·o·my
neu'·ro·ar·throp'·a·thy
neu'·ro·as'·tro·cy·to'·ma
neu'·ro·avi'·ta·min·o'·sis
neu'·ro·ax'·o·nal
neu'·ro·bi·ol'·o·gy
neu'·ro·bi'·o·tax'·is
neu'·ro·blast
neu'·ro·blas·to'·ma *pl.* ·mas *or* ·ma·ta
neu'·ro·car'·di·ac
neu'·ro·cen'·trum *pl.* ·tra
neu'·ro·cep'·tor
neu'·ro·cer'·a·tin *var.* of neurokeratin
neu'·ro·chem'·is·try
neu'·ro·chron·ax'·ic
neu'·ro·cir'·cu·la·to'·ry
neu·roc'·la·dis'·m
neu'·ro·coele
neu'·ro·cra'·ni·al
neu'·ro·cra'·ni·um
neu'·ro·crine
neu'·ro·cu·ta'·ne·ous
neu'·ro·cyte
neu'·ro·cy·tol'·o·gy
neu'·ro·cy·tol'·y·sin

neu'·ro·cy·to'·ma *pl.* ·mas *or* ·ma·ta
neu'·ro·de·gen'·er·a·tive
neu'·ro·den'·drite
neu'·ro·den'·dron
neu'·ro·derm
neu'·ro·der'·mal
neu'·ro·der'·ma·ti'·tis
neu'·ro·der'·ma·to·my'·o·si'·tis
neu'·ro·di'·ag·no'·sis *pl.* ·ses
neu'·ro·ec'·to·derm
neu'·ro·elec·tric'·i·ty
neu'·ro·en'·do·crine
neu'·ro·en'·do·cri·nol'·o·gy
neu'·ro·en·ter'·ic
neu'·ro·ep'·i·der'·mal
neu'·ro·ep'·i·the'·li·al
neu'·ro·ep'·i·the'·li·a'·lis *neut.* ·le
neu'·ro·ep'·i·the'·li·o'·ma *pl.* ·mas *or* ·ma·ta
neu'·ro·ep'·i·the'·li·um *pl.* ·lia
neu'·ro·fi'·bril
neu'·ro·fi·bril'·la *pl.* ·lae
neu'·ro·fi'·bril·lar
neu'·ro·fi·bro'·ma *pl.* ·mas *or* ·ma·ta
neu'·ro·fi·bro'·ma·to'·sis
neu'·ro·fi'·bro·sar·co'·ma *pl.* ·mas *or* ·ma·ta
neu'·ro·fil'·a·ment
neu'·ro·gan'·gli·o'·ma *pl.* ·mas *or* ·ma·ta
neu'·ro·gan'·gli·on
neu'·ro·gan'·gli·on·i'·tis
neu'·ro·gan·gli'·tis
neu'·ro·gas'·tric
neu'·ro·gen
neu'·ro·gen'·e·sis

neu'·ro·ge·net'·ics
neu'·ro·gen'·ic *also*
   neu·rog'·e·nous
neu·rog'·lia [neu'·ro·gli'a]
neu·rog'·li·al [neu'·ro·gli'·al
neu·rog'·li·o·cy·to'·ma *pl.* ·mas *or* ·ma·ta
neu'·ro·gli·o'·ma *pl.* ·mas *or* ·ma·ta
neu'·ro·gli·o'·sis
neu'·ro·he'·mal *Brit.* ·hae'·
neu'·ro·his·tol'·o·gy
neu'·ro·hor·mo'·nal [·hor'·mon·al]
neu'·ro·hor'·mone
neu'·ro·hu'·mor *Brit.* ·mour
neu'·ro·hu'·mor·al
neu'·ro·hu'·mor·al·is'm
neu'·ro·hy'·po·phys'·e·al [·hy·poph'·y·se'·al] *var. of* neurohypophysial
neu'·ro·hy·poph'·y·sec'·to·my
neu'·ro·hy'·po·phys'·i·al
neu'·ro·hy·poph'·y·sis
neu'·roid
neu'·ro·ker'·a·tin
neu'·ro·lem'·ma *var. of* neurilemma
neu'·ro·lem·mo'·ma *var. of* neurilemmoma
neu'·ro·lept
neu'·ro·lept'·an·al·ge'·sia
neu'·ro·lept'·an·al·ge'·sic
neu'·ro·lept'·an·es·the'·sia *Brit.* ·aes·the'·
neu'·ro·lept'·an·es·thet'·ic *Brit.* ·aes·thet'·
neu'·ro·lep'·tic
neu'·ro·li·po'·ma·to'·sis

neu'·ro·log'·ic *also* ·i·cal
neu·rol'·o·gist
neu·rol'·o·gy
neu'·ro·lym'·pho·ma·to'·sis
neu·rol'·y·sis
neu'·ro·lyt'·ic
neu·ro'·ma *pl.* ·mas *or* ·ma·ta
neu'·ro·ma·la'·cia
neu·ro'·ma·to'·sa
neu·ro'·ma·tous [·rom'a·]
neu'·ro·mech'·an·is'm
neu'·ro·mere
neu'·ro·mod'·u·la'·tor
neu'·ro·mus'·cu·lar
neu'·ro·my'·al
neu'·ro·my'·e·li'·tis
neu'·ro·my'o·ar·te'·ri·al
neu'·ro·my'·o·car'·di·um
neu'·ro·my·op'·a·thy
neu'·ro·my'·o·si'·tis
neu'·ro·my'·o·to'·nia
neu'·ron *Brit. also* ·rone
neu·ro'·nal [neu'·ro·nal]
neu'·ro·ne'·vus *Brit.* ·nae'·vus
neu'·ro·ni'·tis [·ron·i'·]
neu'·ro·nog'·ra·phy
neu·ron'·o·phage
neu'·ro·no·pha'·gia *also* ·noph'·a·gy
neu·ro'·no·tro'·pic [·trop'·ic]
neu'·ro·oph'·thal·mol'·o·gy
neu'·ro·op'·tic
neu'·ro·otol'·o·gy
neu'·ro·pap'·il·li'·tis
neu'·ro·par'·a·lyt'·ic
neu'·ro·path'·ic
neu'·ro·path'·o·gen'·ic

neu'·ro·path'·o·ge·nic'·i·ty
neu'·ro·pa·thol'·o·gy
neu·rop'·a·thy
neu'·ro·phar'·ma·col'·o·gy
neu'·ro·phil'·ic
neu'·ro·phy'·sin
neu'·ro·phys'·i·ol'·o·gy
neu'·ro·pil *also* ·pile
neu'·ro·plas'm
neu'·ro·ple'·gic
neu'·ro·po'·di·um *pl.* ·dia
neu'·ro·pore
neu'·ro·po'·ric
neu'·ro·pro·ba'·sia
neu'·ro·pros·the'·sis *pl.* ·ses
neu'·ro·psy·chi'·a·try
neu'·ro·psy·chol'·o·gy
neu'·ro·psy·chop'·a·thy
neu'·ro·psy'·cho·phar'·ma·col'·o·gy
neu'·ro·ra'·di·ol'·o·gy
neu'·ro·ret'·i·ni'·tis
neu'·ro·ret'·i·nop'·a·thy
neuror'·rha·phy
neu'·ro·sci'·ence
neu'·ro·se·cre'·tion
neu'·ro·se·cre'·to·ry
neu'·ro·sen'·so·ry
neu·ro'·sis *pl.* ·ses
neu'·ro·so·mat'·ic
neu'·ro·splanch'·nic
neu'·ro·spon'·gi·um
Neu·ros'·po·ra
neu'·ro·stim'·u·la'·tor
neu'·ro·sur'·geon
neu'·ro·sur'·gery
neu'·ro·syph'·i·lis
neu'·ro·ten'·di·nous
neu'·ro·the'·le [neur'·ro·thele]
neu·rot'·ic
neu·rot'·i·cis'm
neu'·ro·ti·za'·tion

neurotmesis / noctambulation 186

neu′·rot·me′·sis
neu·rot′·o·gen′·ic
neu′·ro·tome
neu·rot′·o·my
neu′·ro·tox′·ic
neu′·ro·tox·ic′·i·ty
neu′·ro·tox′·in
neu′·ro·trans·mit′·ter
neu′·ro·trau′·ma
neu′·ro·tro′·phic
[·troph′·ic]
neu·ro′·tro·phy
neu′·ro·tro′·pic [·trop′·ic]
neu·rot′·ro·pis′m
neu′·ro·tu′·bule
neu′·ro·vas′·cu·lar
neu′·ro·veg′·e·ta′·tive
neu′·ro·vir′·u·lence
neu′·ro·vir′·u·lent
neu′·ro·vi′·rus
neu′·ro·vis′·cer·al
neu′·ru·la pl. ·lae or ·las
neu′·ru·la′·tion
neu′·tral
neu·tral′·i·ty
neu′·tral·i·za′·tion
neu′·tral·ize ·ized, ·iz′·ing
neu·tri′·no
neu′·tro·clu′·sion
neu′·tro·cyte
neu′·tron
neu′·tro·pe′·nia
neu′·tro·phil
neu′·tro·phil′·ia
neu′·tro·phil′·ic
neu′·tro·tax′·is
ne′·vi pl. of nevus
ne′·vo·cyt′·ic
ne′·void
ne′·vo·li·po′·ma
ne′·vous also ·vose
ne′·vus Brit. nae′·; pl. ·vi
new′·born
new′·ton

nex′·us
n'ga′·na var. of nagana
ni′·a·cin
ni′·a·cin′·a·mide
ni·al′·a·mide
niche
nick′·el
nick′·ing
nick′·krampf
ni·clo′·sa·mide
nic′·o·tin′·a·mide
nic′·o·tine
nic′·o·tin′·ic
nic′·o·tin·is′m
nic′·o·tin′·o·lyt′·ic
nic′·o·tin′o·mi·met′·ic
nic′·o·tin·u′·ric [·ti·nu′·]
nic·ta′·tio
nic·ta′·tion
nic′·ti·tans
nic′·ti·tate ·tat′·ed, ·tat′·ing
nic′·ti·ta′·tion
ni′·dal
ni·da′·tion
ni′·dus pl. ·di
ni′·ger fem. ni′·gra
night′·mare
night′·shade
ni′·gra fem. of niger
ni′·gral
ni′·gri·cans
ni′·gro·ru′·bral
ni′·gro·sine also ·sin
ni′·gro·stri·a′·tal
ni′·hil·is′m
nik·eth′·a·mide
nim′·a·zone
nin·hy′·drin
ni·o′·bi·um
niph′·a·blep′·sia
nip′·pers
nip′·ple
Nip′·po·stron′·gy·lus
ni′·sin
ni′·sus pl. nisus

ni′·trate
ni·traz′·e·pam
ni·tre′·mia Brit. ·trae′·
ni′·tric
ni′·tride
ni′·tri·fi·ca′·tion
ni′·trile
ni′·tri·lo·
ni′·trite
ni′·tri·toid
ni′·tro·
ni′·tro·ben′·zene [·ben·zene′]
ni′·tro·ben·zo′·ic
ni′·tro·fu′·ran
ni′·tro·fu·ran′·to·in
ni′·tro·fu′·ra·zone
ni′·tro·gen
ni·trog′·e·nous
ni′·tro·glyc′·er·in
ni′·tro·mer′·sol
ni·trom′·e·ter
ni′·tro·phe′·nol
ni′·tro·phen′·yl
ni′·tro·prus′·side
ni·tro′·sa·mine [·tros′·a·]
ni·tro′·so·
ni′·tro·sul′·fa·thi′·a·zole Brit. ·sul′·pha·
ni·tro′·syl [ni′·tro·]
ni′·trous
njo·ver′a
no·bel′·i·um
No·car′·dia
N. as′·ter·oi′·des
N. bra·sil′·i·en′·sis
no·car′·di·al
no·car′·din
no·car′·di·o′·sis
no′·ci·
no′·ci·cep′·tion
no′·ci·cep′·tive
no′·ci·cep′·tor
no′·ci·fen′·sor
no′·ci·per·cep′·tion
noct·am′·bu·la′·tion [noc·tam′·]

noc·tu′·ria
noc·tur′·na
noc·tur′·nal
noc′·u·ous
nod′·al [no′·dal]
node
no′·di *pl. & gen. sg. of*
    nodus
no′·dose
no·dos′·i·ty
no·do′·sus *fem.* ·sa,
    neut. ·sum
nod′·u·lar
nod′·u·lat′·ed
nod′·u·la′·tion
nod′·ule
nod′·u·lo·ul′·cer·a·tive
nod′·u·lus *pl. & gen.*
    sg. ·li
no′·dus *pl. & gen. sg.*
    ·di
no·gal′·a·my′·cin [no′·
    ga·la·]
noise
no′·ma
no′·men *pl.* no′·mi·na
no′·men·cla′·ture
No′·mi·na An′·a·tom′·
    i·ca
nom′·i·nal
nom′o· [no′mo·]
nom′·o·gram *also*
    ·graph
nom′·o·thet′·ic
nom′·o·top′·ic
no′·na·
non′·ab·sorb′·a·ble
non·ac′·cess
no′·nan
non·bac′·il·lar′y
non′·bac·te′·ri·al
non′·cal·car′·e·ous
non·chro′·maf·fin
non·com′·i·tance
non·com′·i·tant
non′·com·mu′·ni·cat′·
    ing
non′ com′·pos men′·tis

non′·con·duc′·tor
non′·de·po′·lar·iz′·er
non′·di·rec′·tive
non′·dis·junc′·tion
non′·elec′·tro·lyte
non′·en·cap′·su·lat′·ed
non′·es·ter′·i·fied
non·fil′·a·ment·ed
non′·gon′o·coc′·cal
non′·gran′·u·lom′a·
    tous [·lo′ma·]
non·grav′·id
non′·he′·mo·lyt′·ic
    Brit. ·hae′·
non′·ho·mol′·o·gous
non·hom′·o·logue
    [·ho′·mo·]
non′·in·fec′·tious
non′·in·flam′·ma·to′·ry
non′·in·va′·sive
non′·ion′·ic
non′·ke·tot′·ic
non′·la·mel′·lar
non·lam′·el·lat′·ed
non·lin′·e·ar
non·mo′·tile
non′·mo′·to·fa′·cient
non·my′·e·lin·at′·ed
non-nu′·cle·at′·ed
non·nu′·tri·tive
non′·ob·struc′·tive
non′·oc·clu′·sion
non′·ol′·i·gu′·ric
non′·on′·co·gen′·ic
non′·opaque′
non′·or·gan′·ic
non·os′·si·fy′·ing
non·ov′u·la·to′·ry
    [·o′vu·]
no·nox′·y·nol
non′·par′·a·lyt′·ic
non′·par′·a·met′·ric
non·par′·ous
non′·path′·o·gen′·ic
non′·pe·dun′·cu·lat′·ed
non′·pen′·e·trant
non·pen′·e·trat′·ing
non·pha′·sic

non·pig′·ment·ed
non·po′·lar
non′·pro·pri′·etar′y
non′·ro·ta′·tion
non′·se·cre′·tor
non′·self
non′·spe·cif′·ic
non′·sphe′·ro·cyt′·ic
non′·ste·roi′·dal
non·stri′·at·ed
non·sur′·gi·cal
non·tast′·er
non′·throm′·bo·cy′·to·
    pe′·nic
non·u′nion
non′·ve·ne′·re·al
non·vi′·a·ble
non·vi′·tal
no′·o·tro′·pic [·trop′·ic]
nor′·adren′·a·line
nor′·ep′·i·neph′·rine
nor′·eth·an′·dro·lone
nor·eth′·in·drone
nor′·e·thy′·no·drel
nor·flox′·a·cin
nor·leu′·cine
norm
nor′·ma
nor′·mal
nor′·mal·cy
nor·mal′·i·ty
nor′·mal·ize ·ized,
    ·iz′·ing
nor·mer′·gic
nor·met′a·neph′·rine
nor′·mo·
nor′·mo·blast
nor′·mo·blas′·tic
nor′·mo·blas·to′·sis
nor′·mo·cal·ce′·mia
    Brit. ·cae′·
nor′·mo·cal·ce′·mic
    Brit. ·cae′·
nor′·mo·cap′·nia
nor′·mo·cap′·nic
nor′·mo·cho·les′·ter·e′·
    mic *Brit.* ·ae′·mic;

var. of normocholester-
olemic
nor'·mo·cho·les'·ter·ol
  e'·mia *Brit.* ·ae'·mia
nor'·mo·cho·les'·ter·ol
  e'·mic *Brit.* ·ae'·mic
nor'·mo·chro·mat'·ic
nor'·mo·chro'·mia
nor'·mo·chro'·mic
nor'·mo·cyte
nor'·mo·cyt'·ic
nor'·mo·cy·to'·sis
nor'·mo·eryth'·ro·cyte
nor'·mo·gly·ce'·mia
  Brit. ·cae'·
nor'·mo·gly·ce'·mic
  Brit. ·cae'·
nor'·mo·ka·le'·mia
  Brit. ·lae'·
nor'·mo·ka·le'·mic
  Brit. ·lae'·
nor'·mo·re·flex'·ia
nor'·mo·sper'·ma·to·
  gen'·ic
nor'·mo·sthen·u'·ria
nor'·mo·ten'·sion
nor'·mo·ten'·sive
nor'·mo·ther'·mia
nor'·mo·ther'·mic
nor'·mo·thet'·ic
nor'·mo·to'·nia
nor'·mo·ton'·ic
nor'·mo·tro'·phic
  [·troph'·ic]
nor'·mo·vol·e'·mia
  [·vo·le'·] *Brit.* ·ae'·
  mia
nor'·mo·vol·e'·mic
  [·vo·le'·] *Brit.* ·ae'·
  mic
nor'·oph·thal'·mic
nor'·pseu'·do·ephed'·
  rine
nor·trip'ty·line
nos'·ca·pine
nose'·bleed
nose'·gay
nose'·piece

nos'o·
nos'·o·co'·mi·al
nos'·o·graph'·ic
no·sog'·ra·phy
nos'·o·log'·ic *also* ·i·
  cal
no·sol'·o·gy
nos'o·my·co'·sis
nos'o·par'·a·site
nos'o·pho'·bia
Nos'·o·psyl'·lus
  N. fas'·ci·a'·tus
nos'o·ther'·a·py
nos'o·tox'·i·co'·sis
nos'o·tox'·in
nos'·o·tro'·pic [·trop'·
  ic]
nos'·tras
nos'·tril
nos'·trum
no'·tal
no·tal'·gia
notch
No·te'·chis
not'·en·ceph'·a·lo·cele
no'·ti·fi'·a·ble
no'·ti·fi·ca'·tion
no'·to·
no'·to·chord
no'·to·chor·do'·ma
no'·to·gen'·e·sis
no'·to·ge·net'·ic
nour'·ish·ment
nov'·ar'·se·no·ben'·
  zene *also* ·zol
nov'·au·ran'·tia
no'·vo·bi'·o·cin
no'·vum
nox'a *pl.* nox'·ae
nox'·ious
noy
nu·bil'·i·ty
nu'·cha *gen.* ·chae
nu'·chal
nu'·cle·ar
nu'·cle·a'·re
nu'·cle·ase

nu'·cle·at'·ed *also*
  ·ate
nu'·cle·a'·tion
nu'·clei *pl. & gen. sg.*
  of nucleus
nu·cle'·ic
nu·cle'·iform
nu'·cle·in
nu'·cleo·
nu'·cleo·cap'·sid
nu'·cleo·cy'·to·plas'·
  mic
nu'·cle·og'·ra·phy
nu'·cleo·his'·tone
nu'·cle·oid
nu·cle'·o·lar
nu'·cle·ol'·i·form
nu·cle'·o·lo·ne'·ma
nu·cle'·o·lus *pl.* ·li
nu'·cleo·lymph
nu'·cleo·mi'·cro·some
nu'·cle·on
nu'·cle·on'·ic
nu'·cle·o·phile
nu'·cle·o·phil'·ic
nu'·cle·o·plas'm
nu'·cle·o·plas'·mic
nu'·cleo·pro'·tein
nu'·cle·or·rhex'·is
nu'·cle·o·si'·dase
  [·sid'·ase]
nu'·cle·o·side
nu'·cle·o·side·di·phos'·
  pha·tase
nu'·cle·o·side·mon'o·
  phos'·phate
nu'·cle·o·sin
nu'·cle·o·some
nu'·cleo·spin'·dle
nu'·cle·o·ti'·dase [·tid'·
  ase]
nu'·cle·o·tide
nu'·cle·o·ti'·dyl
nu'·cle·o·ti'·dyl·trans'·
  fer·ase
nu'·cle·o·tro'·pic
  [·trop'·ic]

nu′·cle·us *pl. & gen.
  sg.* ·clei
nu′·clide
nul′·li·grav′·id
nul′·li·grav′·i·da *pl.*
  ·das *or* ·dae
nul·lip′·a·ra *pl.* ·ras *or*
  ·rae
nul′·li·par′·i·ty
nul·lip′·a·rous
nul′·li·so′·mic
numb
numb′·ness
nu·mer′·ic *also* ·i·cal
num′·mi·form
num′·mu·lar
nun·na′·tion
nup·tial′·i·ty
nurse *n. & v.* nursed,
  nurs′·ing
nurs′·ery
nu′·tans
nu·ta′·tion
nu′·ta·to′·ry
nu·tri′·cia *fem. of*
  nutricius; *pl.* ·ci·ae
nu·tri′·ci·us *fem.* ·cia,
  neut. ·ci·um
nu′·tri·ent
nu′·tri·lite
nu′·tri·ment
nu·tri′·tion
nu·tri′·tion·al
nu·tri′·tion·ist
nu·tri′·tious
nu′·tri·tive
nu′·tri·ture
nux′ vom′·i·ca
nych·the′·mer·al *also*
  nyc′·ter·o·he′·mer·al
nyc′·ta·lope
nyc′·ta·lo′·pia
nyc′·to·
nyc′·to·pho′·bia
nyc·tu′·ria
nymph
nym′·pha *pl.* ·phae
nym′·phal

nym·phec′·to·my
nym′·pho·
nym′·pho·ma′·nia
nym·phot′·o·my
Nys′·so·rhyn′·chus
nys·tag′·mic
nys·tag′·mo·graph
nys′·tag·mog′·ra·phy
nys·tag′·moid
nys·tag′·mus
nys′·ta·tin

O

oar′·io·
oast′·house
oath
obe′·di·ence
obe′·li·on
obese′
obe′·si·ty
o′bex
ob′·ject
ob·jec′·tive
ob′·li·gate
ob·li′·qua *fem. of*
  obliquus; *pl. & gen. sg.*
  ·quae
ob·lique′
ob·li′·quum *neut. of*
  obliquus
ob·li′·quus *pl. & gen.
  sg.* ·qui
ob·lit′·er·ans
ob·lit′·er·ate ·at′·ed,
  ·at′·ing
ob·lit′·er·a′·tion
ob·lit′·er·a·tive
ob·lon′·ga
ob′·lon·ga′·ta *gen.*
  ·tae
ob·nu′·bi·la′·tion
ob·scu′·ra
ob·ses′·sion
ob·ses′·sive
ob′·so·les′·cence
ob′·sol·ete′

ob·stet′·ric *also* ·ri·cal
ob·stet′·ri·ca
ob′·ste·tri′·cian
ob·stet′·rics
ob·stet′·rist
ob′·sti·pa′·tion
ob·struct′·ed
ob·struc′·tion
ob·struc′·tive
ob′·stru·ent
ob·tund′
ob′·tun·da′·tion
ob·tun′·dent
ob·tun′·di·ty
ob′·tu·ra′·tion
ob′·tu·ra′·tor *gen.*
  ob′·tu·ra·to′·ris
ob′·tu·ra·to′·ria *fem.
  of* obturatorius; *pl. &
  gen. sg.* ·ri·ae
ob′·tu·ra·to′·ri·um
  neut. of obturatorius
ob′·tu·ra·to′·ri·us *pl.
  & gen. sg.* ·rii
ob′·tu·ra′·tum
ob·tu′·sion
oc·cip′·i·tal
oc·cip′·i·ta′·le *neut.
  of* occipitalis
oc·cip′·i·ta′·lis *pl.* ·les
oc·cip′·i·tal·i·za′·tion
oc·cip′·i·to·
oc·cip′·i·to·an·te′·ri·or
oc·cip′·i·to·at·lan′·tal
oc·cip′·i·to·ax′·i·al
oc·cip′·i·to·bas′·i·lar
oc·cip′·i·to·cal′·ca·rine
oc·cip′·i·to·cer′·vi·cal
oc·cip′·i·to·fron′·tal
oc·cip′·i·to·fron·ta′·lis
  pl. ·les
oc·cip′·i·to·mas′·toid
oc·cip′·i·to·mas·toi′·
  dea
oc·cip′·i·to·men′·tal
oc·cip′·i·to·odon′·toid
oc·cip′·i·to·pa·ri′·etal

oc·cip′·i·to·pon′·tine
  also ·tile
oc·cip′·i·to·pon·ti′·nus
oc·cip′·i·to·pos·te′·ri·or
oc·cip′·i·to·sa′·cral
oc·cip′·i·to·sphe·noi′·dal
oc·cip′·i·to·tem′·po·ral
oc·cip′·i·to·tem′·po·ra′·lis
oc·cip′·i·to·tha·lam′·ic
oc·cip′·i·to·trans·verse′
oc′·ci·put gen. oc·cip′·i·tis
oc·clude′ ·clud′·ed, ·clud′·ing
oc·clu′·dens
oc·clud′·er
oc·clu′·sal
oc·clu′·sion
oc·clu′·sive
oc′·clu·som′·e·ter
oc·cult′ [oc′·cult]
oc·cul′·tus fem. ·ta, neut. ·tum
oc′·cu·pan·cy
oc′·cu·pa′·tion·al
ocel′·lus pl. ·li
o′chre also o″cher
O′chro·gas′·ter con·trar′·ia
o′chro·no′·sis also ·sus
o′chro·not′·ic
oc′·ta·
oc′·ta·he′·dral
oc′·ta·he′·dron
oc′·tan
oc′·ta·no′·ic
oc·tar′·i·us
oc′·ti· var. of octa-
oc′·to· var. of octa-
oc′·tose
oc′·tyl
oc′·u·lar
oc′·u·len′·tum
oc′·u·li pl. & gen. sg. of oculus

oc′·u·list
oc′·u·lo·
oc′·u·lo·au′·di·to′·ry
oc′·u·lo·au·ric′·u·lar
oc′·u·lo·au·ric′·u·lo·ver′·te·bral
oc′·u·lo·buc′·co·gen′·i·tal
oc′·u·lo·car′·di·ac
oc′·u·lo·ce·phal′·ic
oc′·u·lo·ceph′·a·lo·gy′·ric
oc′·u·lo·cer′·e·bro·re′·nal
oc′·u·lo·cu·ta′·ne·ous
oc′·u·lo·den′·to·dig′·i·tal
oc′·u·lo·den′·to-os′·se·ous
oc′·u·lo·en′·ce·phal′·ic
oc′·u·lo·fa′·cial
oc′·u·lo·fron′·tal
oc′·u·lo·gas′·tric
oc′·u·lo·glan′·du·lar
oc′·u·lo·gy′·ria
oc′·u·lo·gy′·ric
oc′·u·lo·met′·ro·scope
oc′·u·lo·mo′·tor
oc′·u·lo·mo·to′·ria fem. of oculomotorius
oc′·u·lo·mo·to′·ri·us pl. & gen. sg. ·rii
oc′·u·lo·my·co′·sis
oc′·u·lop′·a·thy
oc′·u·lo·pha·ryn′·ge·al
oc′·u·lo·pleth′·ys·mog′·ra·phy
oc′·u·lo·pneu′·mo·pleth′·ys·mog′·ra·phy
oc′·u·lo·pu′·pil·lar′y
oc′·u·lo·sen′·so·ry
oc′·u·lo·va′·gal
oc′·u·lo·ver′·te·bral
oc′·u·lo·ves·tib′·u·lar
oc′·u·lo·ves·tib′·u·lo·au′·di·to′·ry

oc′·u·lus pl. & gen. sg. ·li
o′cy·o·din′·ic
o′dax·et′·ic
odif′·er·ous var. of odoriferous
od′o·gen′·e·sis
o′don·tal′·gia
o′don·tex′·e·sis
odon′·tic
odon′·to·
odon′·to·am′·e·lo·blas·to′·ma
odon′·to·at·lan′·tal
odon′·to·blast
odon′·to·blas′·tic
odon′·to·blas·to′·ma pl. ·mas or ·ma·ta
odon′·to·cele
odon′·to·clast
odon′·to·dys·pla′·sia
odon′·to·gen′·e·sis
  also o′don·tog′·e·ny
odon′·to·gen′·ic
odon′·toid
odon·toi′·de·um
odon′·to·log′·i·cal
o′don·tol′·o·gy
o′don·tol′·y·sis
o′don·to′·ma pl. ·mas or ·ma·ta; also odon′·tome
o′don·top′·a·thy
odon′·to·per′i·os′·te·um
odon′·to·plas′·ty
odon′·to·sar·co′·ma pl. ·mas or ·ma·ta
odon′·to·sei′·sis
odon′·to·the′·ca
o′don·tot′·o·my
o′dor Brit. o′dour
o′dor·ant
o′dor·if′·er·ous
o′dor·im′·e·try
o′dor·o·gram
o′dor·ous

o′dyn·acu′·sis *also*
 ·acou′·sis
odyn′·o· [o′dy·no·]
o′dy·nom′·e·ter
odyn′·o·pha′·gia
o′dy·nu′·ria
oe- *See also words beginning e-*
oe′·co·site *var. of* ecosite
oe·de′·ma *Brit. spel. of* edema
oe′·di·pal [oed′·i·pal]
Oe′·di·pus [Oed′·i·pus]
oe·soph′·a·go· *Brit. spel. of* esophago-
Oe·soph·a·gos′·to·mum
oe·soph′·a·gus *var. of* esophagus; *gen.* ·gi
oes′·tra·di′·ol *Brit. spel. of* estradiol
oes·tri′·a·sis
oes′·trid
Oes′·tri·dae
oes′·trin *Brit. spel. of* estrin
oes′·trin·i·sa′·tion *Brit. spel. of* estrinization
oes′·tro·gen *Brit. spel. of* estrogen
oes′·trous *Brit. spel. of* estrous
oes′·trus *Brit. spel. of* estrus
Oes′·trus o′vis
of′·fice
of′·fi·cer
of·fi′·cial
of·fic′·i·nal [of′·fi·ci′·nal]
ohm
ohm′·me·ter
oid′·io·my·co′·sis
Oid′·i·um
oi′·ko· *var. of* eco-
oi′·ko·site *var. of* ecosite

oint′·ment
o′le·ag′·i·nous
o′le·an′·do·my′·cin
o′le·an′·drin
o′le·ate
olec′·ra·nal
olec′·ra·nar·throc′·a·ce
olec′·ra·nar·throp′·a·thy
olec′·ra·non *gen.* ·ni
o′le·fin
ole′·ic
o′le·in
o′leo·
o′leo·ar·thro′·sis
o′leo·chrys′o·ther′·a·py
o′leo·in·fu′·sion
o′le·om′·e·ter
o′leo·res′·in
o′le·um
ol·fac′·tion
ol·fac′·tism
ol·fac′·tive
ol·fac′·to·ha·ben′·u·lar
ol·fac′·to·hy′·po·tha·lam′·ic
ol′·fac·tol′·o·gy
ol′·fac·tom′·e·ter
ol′·fac·tom′·e·try
ol′·fac·to′·ria *fem. of* olfactorius; *pl. & gen. sg.* ·ri·ae
ol′·fac·to′·ri·um *neut. of* olfactorius
ol′·fac·to′·ri·us *pl. & gen. sg.* ·rii
ol·fac′·to·ry
ol·fac′·tus *gen.* olfactus
ol′·i·ge′·mia *Brit.* ·gae′·
ol′·i·ge′·mic *Brit.* ·gae′·
ol′·i·go·
ol′·i·go·as′·tro·cy·to′·ma
ol′·i·go·blast
Ol′·i·go·chae′·ta

ol′·i·go·chro·ma′·sia
ol′·i·go·clon′·al [·clo′·nal]
ol′·i·go·cy·the′·mia *Brit.* ·thae′·
ol′·i·go·dac′·ty·ly *also* ·dac·tyl′·ia
ol′·i·go·den′·dro·blast
ol′·i·go·den′·dro·cyte
ol′·i·go·den·drog′·lia
ol′·i·go·den·drog′·li·al
ol′·i·go·den′·dro·gli·o′·ma
ol′·i·go·dip′·sia
ol′·i·go·don′·tia [olig′·odon′·tia]
ol′·i·go·ga·lac′·tia
ol′·i·gog′·lia
ol′·i·go·hi·dro′·sis
ol′·i·go·hy·dram′·ni·os
ol′·i·go·hy′·per·men′·or·rhe′a *Brit.* ·rhoe′a
ol′·i·go·hy′·po·men′·or·rhe′a *Brit.* ·rhoe′a
ol′·i·go·lec′·i·thal
ol′·i·go·leu′·ko·cy·the′·mia *Brit.* ·thae′·
ol′·i·go·leu′·ko·cy·to′·sis
ol′·i·go·men′·or·rhe′a *Brit.* ·rhoe′a
olig′·o·mer
olig′·o·mer′·ic [ol′·i·go·]
ol′·i·go·my′·cin
ol′·i·go·ne·phron′·ic
ol′·i·go·nu′·cle·o·tide
ol′·i·go·ov′u·la′·tion [-o′vu·]
ol′·i·go·pep′·tide
ol′·i·go·phre′·nia
ol′·i·go·phren′·ic
ol′·i·go·plas′·mia
ol′·i·go·plas′·tic
ol′·i·go·pne′a [·gop′·nea] *Brit.* ·pnoe′a

ol'·i·go·py'·rene *also*
·py'·rous
ol'·i·go·sac'·cha·ride
ol'·i·go·sper·mat'·ic
ol'·i·go·sper'·mia *also*
·sper'·ma·tis'm
ol'·i·go·ste'·ato'·sis
ol'·i·go·symp'·to·mat'·ic
ol'·i·go·syn·ap'·tic
ol'·i·go·zo'·o·sper'·mia
ol'·i·gu'·ria
olis'·thero·chro'·ma·tin
oli'·va *pl. & gen. sg.*
·vae, *gen. pl.* ol'·i·va'·rum
ol'·i·va'·ris *neut.* ·re
ol'·i·var'y
ol'·ive
ol'·i·vif'·u·gal
ol'·i·vip'·e·tal
ol'·i·vo·cer'·e·bel'·lar
ol'·i·vo·cer'·e·bel·la'·ris
ol'·i·vo·coch'·le·ar
ol'·i·vo·cor'·ti·cal
ol'·i·vo·nu'·cle·ar
ol'·i·vo·pon'·to·cer'·e·bel'·lar
ol'·i·vo·spi'·nal
ol'·i·vo·spi·na'·lis
ol·sal'·a·zine
ol'·ti·praz
oma'·sum
ome'·ga
omen'·ta *pl. of*
omentum
omen'·tal
o'men·ta'·le *neut. of*
omentalis
o'men·ta'·lis *pl.* ·les
o'men·tec'·to·my
o'men·ti'·tis
omen'·to·pex'y
omen'·to·plas'·ty
omen'·to·por·tog'·ra·phy
o'men·tor'·rha·phy

omen'·to·sple'·no·pex'y [·splen'·o·]
o'men·tot'·o·my
omen'·to·vol'·vu·lus
omen'·tum *pl.* ·ta
omen'·tum·ec'·to·my *var. of* omentectomy
ome'·pra·zole
om·nip'·o·tence
om·niv'·o·rous
o'mo·
o'mo·ceph'·a·lus
o'mo·cer'·vi·ca'·lis
o'mo·cla·vic'·u·lar
o'mo·cla·vic'·u·la'·re
o'mo·hy'·oid
o'mo·hy·oi'·de·us *pl. & gen. sg.* ·dei
o'mo·pha'·gia
o'mo·ster'·num
o'mo·thy'·roid
om'·pha·lec'·to·my
om·phal'·ic
om'·pha·li'·tis
om'·pha·lo·
om'·pha·lo·cele [om·phal'·o·]
om'·pha·lo·did'·y·mus
om'·pha·lo'·ma
om'·pha·lo·mes'·en·ter'·ic
om'·pha·lop'·a·gus
om'·pha·lo·phle·bi'·tis
om'·pha·los *also* ·lus
om'·pha·lo·site
om'·pha·lo·spi'·nous
om'·u·no'·no
o'nan·is'm
on'·cho·
On'·cho·cer'·ca
on'·cho·cer'·cal
on'·cho·cer·ci'·a·sis
on'·cho·cer'·cid
On'·cho·cer'·ci·dae
on'·cho·cer·co'·ma
on'·cho·cer·co'·sis
on'·cho·der'·ma·ti'·tis
On·cic'·o·la

on'·co·
On'·co·cer'·ca *var. of* Onchocerca
on'·co·cer·ci'·a·sis *var. of* onchocerciasis
on'·co·cyte
on'·co·cyt'·ic
on'·co·cy·to'·ma *pl.* ·mas *or* ·ma·ta
on'·co·cy·to'·sis
on'·co·gene
on'·co·gen'·e·sis
on'·co·ge·net'·ic
on'·co·gen'·ic
on'·co·ge·nic'·i·ty
on'·co·graph
on'·co·log'·ic *also* ·i·cal
on·col'·o·gist
on·col'·o·gy
on·col'·y·sis
on'·co·lyt'·ic
On'·co·me·la'·nia
on·com'·e·ter
On·cor'·na·vi'·ri·nae
on·cor'·na·vi'·rus
on'·co·sphere
on·cot'·ic
on·cot'·o·my
on'·co·tro'·pic [·trop'·ic]
on'·co·vi'·rus
onei'·ric *also* oni'·
onei'·rism
onei'·ro *also* oni'·ro·
onei'·ro·phre'·nia
on·kin'·o·cele
on'·lay
on'·o·mat'o·ma'·nia
on'·o·mat'o·poi·e'·sis
on'·set
on'·to·ge·net'·ic
on·tog'·e·ny *also* on'·to·gen'·e·sis
on'y·al'·ai [o'ny·]
on'·ych·a·tro'·phia
on'·y·chec'·to·my [·ych·ec'·]

onych′·ia
on′·y·chi′·tis
on′·y·cho·
on′·y·cho·dys′·tro·phy
on′·y·chog′·ra·phy
on′·y·cho·gry·po′·sis
on′·y·chol′·o·gy
on′·y·chol′·y·sis
on′·y·cho·ma·de′·sis
on′·y·cho·my·co′·sis
on′·y·cho-os′·teo·dys·pla′·sia
on′·y·chop′·a·thy
on′·y·cho·pha′·gia
 also on′·y·choph′·a·gy
on′·y·chor·rhex′·is
on′·y·cho·schiz′·ia
on′·y·chot′·o·my
onyx′·is
o′·o·
o′·o·ci′·nete *var. of* ookinete
o′·o·cy·e′·sis
o′·o·cyst
o′·o·cyte
oog′·a·mous
oog′·a·my
o′·o·gen′·e·sis
o′·o·ge·net′·ic
o′·o·gen′·ic *also* oog′·e·nous
o′·o·go′·ni·um *pl.* ·nia
o′·o·ki·ne′·sis
o′·o·ki′·nete
o′·o·pho·ral′·gia [ooph′·o·]
o′·o·pho·rec′·to·mize [ooph′·o·] ·mized, ·miz′·ing
o′·o·pho·rec′·to·my [ooph′·o·]
o′·o·pho·ri′·tis [ooph′·o·]
ooph′·o·ro· [o′·o·pho·ro·]
ooph′·o·ro·cys·tec′·to·my

ooph′·o·ro·hys′·ter·ec′·to·my
ooph′·o·rop′·a·thy
ooph′·o·ro·pex′y
ooph′·o·ro·plas′·ty
ooph′·o·ro·sal′·pin·gec′·to·my
ooph′·o·ro·sal′·pin·gi′·tis
ooph′·o·ros′·to·my
ooph′·o·rot′·o·my
ooph′·o·rus
o′·o·plas′m
o′·o·some
o′·o·the′·ca
o′·o·the′·co·
o′·o·the′·co·cy·e′·sis
o′·o·tid
oot′·o·my
o′·o·type
opac′·i·fi·ca′·tion
opac′·i·fy ·fied, ·fy′·ing
opac′·i·ty
o′·pal·es′·cent
opaque′
o′pen
o′pen·ing
op′·er·a·bil′·i·ty
op′·er·a·ble
op′·er·ant
op′·er·ate ·at′·ed, ·at′·ing
op′·er·a′·tion
op′·er·a·tive
op′·er·a′·tor
oper′·cu·lat′·ed *also* ·late
oper′·cu·lec′·to·my
oper′·cu·lum *pl.* ·la, *gen. sg.* ·li
op′·er·on
oper′·tus *pl.* ·ti
o′phi·as′·ic
ophi′·a·sis
o′phi·di′·a·sis
o′phi·dis′m
o′phio·

O′phi·oph′·a·gus han′·nah
oph′·ry·on
oph·thal′·ma·cro′·sis
oph·thal′·ma·tro′·phia
oph′·thal·mec′·to·my
oph·thal′·mia
oph·thal′·mic
oph·thal′·mi·ca *fem. of* ophthalmicus; *pl. & gen. sg.* ·cae
oph·thal′·mi·cus *pl. & gen. sg.* ·ci
oph′·thal·mit′·ic
oph′·thal·mi′·tis
oph·thal′·mo·
oph·thal′·mo·di·a·phan′·o·scope [·di·aph′·a·no·]
oph·thal′·mo·do·ne′·sis
oph·thal′·mo·dy′·na·mom′·e·ter
oph·thal′·mo·dy′·na·mom′·e·try
oph·thal′·mo·graph
oph′·thal·mog′·ra·phy
oph·thal′·mo·gy′·ric
oph·thal′·mo·log′·ic *also* ·i·cal
oph′·thal·mol′·o·gist
oph′·thal·mol′·o·gy
oph·thal′·mo·ma·la′·cia
oph′·thal·mom′·e·ter
oph′·thal·mom′·e·try
oph·thal′·mo·my·i′·a·sis
oph·thal′·mo·my·ot′·o·my
oph·thal′·mo·neu·ri′·tis
oph·thal′·mo·neu′·ro·my′·e·li′·tis
oph′·thal·mop′·a·thy
oph·thal′·mo·pha·com′·e·ter
oph′·thal·moph′·thi·sis
oph·thal′·mo·plas′·tic
oph·thal′·mo·plas′·ty
oph·thal′·mo·ple′·gia
oph·thal′·mo·ple′·gic

oph·thal·mop·to′·sis
oph·thal′·mo·re·ac′·
  tion
oph·thal′·mo·scope
oph·thal′·mo·scop′·ic
oph′·thal·mos′·co·py
oph·thal′·mo·stat
oph·thal′·mo·sta·tom′·
  e·ter
oph·thal′·mo·ste·re′·sis
oph·thal′·mo·tox′·in
oph·thal′·mo·trope
oph·thal′·mo·tro·pom′·
  e·ter
oph·thal′·mo·vas′·cu·
  lar
o′pi·an
o′pi·a·nine
o′pi·ate
opin′·ion
o′pi·oid
opis′·the·nar
opis′·then·ceph′·a·lon
opis′·thio·ba′·si·al
opis′·thi·on
opis′·thio·na′·si·al
opis′·tho·
opis′·tho·cra′·ni·on
opis′·tho·glyph′·ic
o′pis·thog′·na·this′m
  [op′is·]
o′pis·thog′·na·thous
  [op′is·]
opis′·thor·chi′·a·sis
  [op′is·]
o′pis·thor′·chid [op′is·]
O′pis·thor′·chis [Op′is·]
o′pis·thot′·ic [op′is·]
opis′·tho·ton′·ic
o′pis·thot′·o·nos
  [op′is·] *also* ·nus
o′pi·um
o′po·ceph′·a·lus
o′po·did′·y·mus *also*
  opod′·y·mus
op′·plo·ten′·tes
op·po′·nens *pl.* op′·
  po·nen′·tes

op′·por·tu′·nist
op′·por·tu·nis′·tic
op′·sin
op′·si·om′·e·ter
op′·so·clo′·nus *also*
  ·nia
op·son′·ic
op·son′·i·fi·ca′·tion
op′·so·nin
op′·so·ni·za′·tion
op′·so·nize ·nized,
  ·niz′·ing
op′·so·no·cy′·to·phag′·
  ic
op′·tic
op′·ti·ca *fem. sg. &*
  neut. pl. of opticus
op′·ti·cal
op′·ti·ci *pl. & gen. sg.*
  of opticus
op·ti′·cian
op·ti′·cian·ry
op′·ti·co·
op′·ti·co·ag·no′·sia
op′·ti·co·fa′·cial
op′·ti·co·ki·net′·ic
op′·ti·co·pal′·pe·bral
op′·ti·co·pu′·pil·lar′y
op′·ti·co·py·ram′·i·dal
op′·ti·co·stri′·ate
op′·tics
op′·ti·cum *neut. of*
  opticus; *pl.* ·ca
op′·ti·cus *pl. & gen.*
  sg. ·ci
op′·ti·mal
op′·ti·mi·za′·tion
op′·ti·mum *pl.* ·ma
op′·to·
op′·to·acous′·tic
op′·to·gram
op′·to·ki·net′·ic
op·tom′·e·ter
op·tom′·e·trist
op·tom′·e·try
op′·to·my·om′·e·ter
op′·to·phone
op′·to·type

o′ra *edge; pl. & gen.*
  sg. o′rae
o′ra *pl. of* os (*mouth*)
o′rad
o′ral
ora′·lis *neut.* ·le
oral′·i·ty
or′·ange
orb
or·bic′·u·lar
or·bic′·u·la′·ris *neut.*
  ·re
or·bic′·u·lo·an′·tero·
  cap′·su·lar
or·bic′·u·lo·cil′·i·ar′y
or·bic′·u·lo·pos′·tero·
  cap′·su·lar
or·bic′·u·lo·pu′·pil·lar′y
or·bic′·u·lus
or′·bit
or′·bi·ta *pl. & gen. sg.*
  ·tae
or′·bi·tal
or′·bi·ta′·le *neut. of*
  orbitalis
or′·bi·ta′·lis *pl.* ·les
or′·bi·to·nom′·e·ter
or′·bi·to·nom′·e·try
or′·bi·top′·a·gus
or′·bi·to·sphe′·noid
  also ·sphe·noi′·dal
or′·bi·tot′·o·my
or′·bi·vi′·rus
or′·ce·in
or′·chi· *var. of* orchio-
or′·chi·al′·gia *also*
  ·chi·dal′·
or′·chi·dec′·to·my
  var. of orchiectomy
or·chid′·ic
or′·chi·do· *var. of*
  orchio-
or′·chi·do·ep′·i·did′·y·
  mec′·to·my
or′·chi·dom′·e·ter
or′·chi·do·pex′y *var.*
  of orchiopexy

or'·chi·do·plas'·ty
  var. of orchioplasty
or'·chi·dop·to'·sis
or'·chi·dot'·o·my   var.
  of orchiotomy
or'·chi·ec'·to·my
or'·chi·ep'·i·did'·y·mi'·
  tis
or'·chil
or'·chio·
or'·chi·o·cele
or'·chi·o·dyn'·ia
or'·chi·op'·a·thy
or'·chi·o·pex'y
or'·chi·o·plas'·ty
or'·chi·ot'·o·my
or·chit'·ic
or·chi'·tis
or'·cin·ol
or'·der·ly
orec'·tic
orex'·ia
orex'·i·gen'·ic
orex'·i·ma'·nia
orex'·is
orf
or'·gan
or'·ga·na   pl. of
  organum
or'·gan·elle'
or·gan'·ic
or·gan'·i·cis'm
or·gan'·i·fi·ca'·tion
or'·gan·is'm
or'·gan·i·za'·tion
or'·gan·ize   ·ized, ·iz'·
  ing
or'·gan·iz'·er
or'·ga·no·
or'·ga·no·gen'·e·sis
or'·gan·oid
or'·ga·no·lep'·tic
or·ga·nol'·o·gy
or'·ga·no·me·tal'·lic
or·ga·no·ther'·a·py
or·gan'·o·trope
or'·ga·no·tro'·phic
  [·troph'·ic]

or'·ga·no·tro'·pic
  [·trop'·ic]
or'·ga·no·tro'·pism
or'·ga·num   pl. ·na,
  gen. sg. ·ni
or'·gasm
or·gas'·mic
or·gas'·mo·lep'·sy
or·gas'·tic
o'ri·ens
o'ri·ent
o'ri·en·ta'·tion
or'·i·fice
or'·i·fi'·cial
o'ri·fi'·ci·um   pl. ·cia
or'·i·form
or'·i·gin
o'ris   gen. of os
  (mouth)
or·met'·o·prim
or'·ni·thine
or'·ni·thin·e'·mia [·thi·
  ne'·]   Brit. ·ae'·mia
Or'·ni·thod'·o·ros
  O. mou·ba'·ta
  O. ru'·dis
  O. ta·la'·je
  O. tho'·lo·za'·ni
Or'·ni·tho·nys'·sus
or'·ni·tho'·sis
o'ro·
o'ro·an'·tral
o'ro·dig'·i·to·fa'·cial
o'ro·fa'·cial
o'ro·fa'·cio·dig'·i·tal
o'ro·gen'·i·tal
o'ro·na'·sal
o'ro·pha·ryn'·ge·al
o'ro·phar'·ynx
O'ro·psyl'·la
  O. i'·da·ho·en'·sis
  O. si·lan'·tiew'i
or'·o·so·mu'·coid
or'·o·tate
orot'·ic
orot'·ic·ac'·id·u'·ria
orot'·i·dine
orot'·i·dyl'·ic

o'ro·tra'·che·al
or·phen'·a·drine
or'·ris
or·the'·sis   var. of
  orthosis; pl. ·ses
or·thet'·ic   var. of
  orthotic
or'·tho·
or'·tho·car'·di·ac
or'·tho·ce·phal'·ic
  also ·ceph'·a·lous
or'·tho·chro·mat'·ic
or'·tho·chro'·mia
or'·tho·chro'·mic
or'·tho·dac'·ty·lous
or'·tho·den'·tin
or'·tho·di'·a·graph
or'·tho·di·ag'·ra·phy
or'·tho·di'·a·scope
or'·tho·di·as'·co·py
or'·tho·don'·tia
or'·tho·don'·tic
or'·tho·don'·tics
or'·tho·don'·tist
or'·tho·don·tol'·o·gy
or'·tho·drom'·ic [·dro'·
  mic]
or'·tho·gly·ce'·mic
  Brit. ·cae'·
or'·thog·nath'·ic   also
  or·thog'·na·thous
or·thog'·na·this'm
or·thog'·o·nal
or'·tho·grade
or'·tho·ki·net'·ics
or'·tho·mel'·ic [·me'·
  lic]
or·thom'·e·ter
or'·tho·mo·lec'·u·lar
Or'·tho·myx'o·vi'·ri·
  dae
or'·tho·myx'o·vi'·rus
or'·tho·pe'·dic   also
  ·pae'·
or'·tho·pe'·dics   also
  ·pae'·
or'·tho·pe'·dist   also
  ·pae'·

or′·tho·pe′·dist *also*
  ·pae′·
or′·tho·pho′·ria
or′·tho·pho′·ric
or′·tho·phos′·phate
or′·tho·phos·pho′·ric
or′·tho·plast
or′·tho·pne′a *Brit.*
  ·pnoe′a
or′·tho·pne′·ic *Brit.*
  ·pnoe′·ic
or′·tho·pox′·vi′·rus
or′·tho·prax′y
or′·tho·psy·chi′·a·try
or·thop′·tic
or·thop′·tist
or′·tho·ra′·di·os′·co·py
or′·tho·roent′·gen·og′·
  ra·phy
or′·tho·scope
or′·tho·scop′·ic
or·tho′·sis *pl.* ·ses
or′·tho·stat′·ic
or′·tho·stat′·ism
or′·tho·ste′·re·o·scope
  [·ster′·e·]
or′·tho·ther′·a·py
or·thot′·ic
or′·tho·tist
or′·tho·tol·u′·i·dine
or·thot′·o·nos *also*
  ·nus
or′·tho·top′·ic
or′·tho·volt′·age
or·thu′·ria
os *mouth; pl.* o′ra,
  gen. sg. o′ris
os *bone; pl.* os′·sa,
  gen. sg. os′·sis, *gen.*
  pl. os′·si·um
o′sa·zone
os′·che·al
os′·che·i′tis *also* os·
  chi′·tis
os′·cheo·
os′·che·o·cele
os′·che·o·lith
os′·che·o·plas′·ty

os′·cil·lat′·ing
os′·cil·la′·tion
os′·cil·la′·tor
os·cil′·lo·gram
os·cil′·lo·graph
os′·cil·lom′·e·ter
os′·cil·lo·met′·ric
os′·cil·lom′·e·try
os′·cil·lop′·sia
os·cil′·lo·scope
os′·ci·ta′·tion
os′·cu·lum
os′·la·din
os·mat′·ic
os′·mes·the′·sia *Brit.*
  ·maes·
os′·mic
os′·mics
os′·mi·o·phil′·ic
os′·mi·um
os′·mo·
os′·mo·cep′·tor *var.*
  of osmoreceptor
os′·mol
os·mo′·lal
os′·mo·lal′·i·ty
os·mo′·lar
os′·mo·lar′·i·ty
os′·mole
os·mom′·e·ter
os·mom′·e·try
os′·mo·phil′·ic
os′·mo·phore
os′·mo·re·cep′·tor
os′·mo·reg′·u·la′·tor
os′·mose ·mosed,
  ·mos·ing
os·mo′·sis
os′·mo·ther′·a·py
os·mot′·ic
os·phre′·si·o·lag′·nia
os·phre′·si·ol′·o·gy
os′·phyo·my′·e·li′·tis
os′·phy·ot′·o·my
os′·sa *pl. of* os (*bone*)
os′·sa·ture
os′·sea *neut. pl. &*
  fem. sg. of osseus; *fem.*
  pl. & gen. sg. ·se·ae

os′·se·in
os′·seo·
os′·seo·car·ti·lag′·i·
  nous
os′·seo·fi′·brous
os′·seo·mu′·cin
os′·seo·mu′·coid
os′·seo·so·nom′·e·ter
os′·seo·so·nom′·e·try
os′·se·ous
os′·se·um *neut. of*
  osseus; *pl.* ·sea
os′·se·us *pl. & gen.*
  sg. ·sei
os′·si·cle
os·sic′·u·la *pl. of*
  ossiculum
os·sic′·u·lar
os′·si·cu·lec′·to·my
os·sic′·u·lo·plas′·ty
os′·si·cu·lot′·o·my
os·sic′·u·lum *pl.* ·la,
  gen. sg. ·li, *gen. pl.* os·
  sic′·u·lo′·rum
os·sif′·er·ous
os·sif′·ic
os·sif′·i·cans
os′·si·fi·ca′·tion
os′·si·fy ·fied, ·fy′·ing
os′·sis *gen. sg. of* os
  (*bone*)
os′·si·um *gen. pl. of*
  os (*bone*)
os′·te·al
os′·te·al′·gia *also* os·
  tal′·gia
os′·te·ar·thri′·tis *var.*
  of osteoarthritis
os·tec′·to·my *also*
  os′·te·ec′·to·my
os′·te·in
os′·te·ite
os′·te·it′·ic
os′·te·i′tis
ost·em′·py·e′·sis
os′·teo·
os′·teo·an′a·gen′·e·sis
os′·teo·ar·thri′·tis

os′·te·o·ar·throp′·a·thy
os′·te·o·ar·throt′·o·my
os′·te·o·ar·tic′·u·lar
os′·te·o·blast
os′·te·o·blas′·tic
os′·te·o·blas·to′·ma
os′·te·o·car′·ti·lag′·i·nous
os′·te·o·cele
os′·te·o·chon′·dral
os′·te·o·chon·dri′·tis
os′·te·o·chon′·dro·dys·pla′·sia
os′·te·o·chon′·dro·dys′·tro·phy *also* ·dys·tro′·phia
os′·te·o·chon′·dro·gen′·ic
os′·te·o·chon·dro′·ma *pl.* ·mas *or* ·ma·ta
os′·te·o·chon·dro′·ma·to′·sis
os′·te·o·chon·drop′·a·thy *also* ·chon′·dro·path′·ia
os′·te·o·chon′·dro·phyte
os′·te·o·chon·dro′·sis
os′·te·o·chon′·drous
os′·te·o·cla′·sia
os′·te·oc′·la·sis
os′·te·o·clast
os′·te·o·clas′·tic
os′·te·o·clas·to′·ma *pl.* ·mas *or* ·ma·ta
os′·te·o·clas′·ty
os′·te·o·col·lag′·e·nous
os′·te·o·cra′·ni·um
os′·te·o·cyte
os′·te·o·den′·tal
os′·te·o·den′·tin
os′·te·o·der′·mia
os′·te·o·des·mo′·sis
os′·te·o·di·as′·ta·sis
os′·te·o·dyn′·ia
os′·te·o·dys·pla′·sia
os′·te·o·dys·plas′·tic
os′·te·o·dys·plas′·ti·ca
os′·te·o·dys′·plas·ty

os′·te·o·dys′·tro·phy *also* ·dys·tro′·phia
os′·teo·fi·bro′·ma *pl.* ·mas *or* ·ma·ta
os′·teo·fi·bro′·ma·to′·sis
os′·teo·fi·bro′·sis
os′·teo·fluo·ro′·sis
os′·teo·gen′·e·sis *also* os′·te·og′·e·ny
os′·teo·ge·net′·ic
os′·te·o·gen′·ic
os′·teo·ge·net′·i·cum
os′·te·o·gen′·ic
os′·teo·hy′·da·ti·do′·sis
os′·teo·hy′·per·tro′·phic [·troph′·ic]
os′·te·oid
os′·te·o·lith
os′·te·o·lo′·gia
os′·te·ol′·o·gist
os′·te·ol′·o·gy
os′·te·ol′·y·sis
os′·te·o·lyt′·ic
os′·te·o′·ma *pl.* ·mas *or* ·ma·ta
os′·teo·ma·la′·cia
os′·teo·ma·la′·cic
os′·te·o′·ma·toid
os′·te·o′·ma·to′·sis
os′·te·o·mere
os′·te·o·met′·ric
os′·te·om′·e·try
os′·teo·mu′·coid *var. of* osseomucoid
os′·teo·my′·e·lit′·ic
os′·teo·my′·e·li′·tis
os′·teo·my′·e·lo·dys·pla′·sia
os′·teo·my′·e·lo·fi·brot′·ic
os′·teo·my′·e·lo·scle·ro′·sis
os′·te·on *gen.* os′·te·o′·ni
os′·te·one *var. of* osteon
os′·teo·ne·cro′·sis

os′·teo·neu·ral′·gia
os′·te·o·path
os′·te·o·path′·ia
os′·te·o·path′·ic
os′·te·op′·a·thy
os′·te·o·pe′·nia
os′·teo·per′i·os·ti′·tis
os′·teo·pe·tro′·sis
os′·teo·pe·trot′·ic
os′·te·o·pha′·gia
os′·teo·phle·bi′·tis
os′·te·o·phyte
os′·te·o·phyt′·ic
os′·te·o·phy·to′·sis
os′·te·o·pla′·sia
os′·te·o·plas′·tic
os′·te·o·plas′·ty
os′·teo·poi′·ki·lo′·sis
os′·teo·po·ro′·sis
os′·teo·ra′·dio·ne·cro′·sis
os′·teo·sar·co′·ma *pl.* ·mas *or* ·ma·ta
os′·teo·sar·co′ma·tous [·com′a·]
os′·teo·scle·ro′·sis
os′·teo·scle·rot′·ic
os′·te·o′·sis
os′·teo·syn′·the·sis
os′·teo·throm′·bo·phle·bi′·tis
os′·teo·throm·bo′·sis
os′·te·o·tome
os′·te·ot′·o·my
os′·teo·tym·pan′·ic
os′·ti·al
os·ti′·tis
os′·ti·um *pl.* ·tia, *gen. sg.* ·tii
os′·to·mate
os′·to·my
os·to′·sis
os·tra′·cea
os·tra′·ceous
os′·treo·tox′·ism
otal′·gia
otal′·gic
o′tic

o′ti·cum *neut. of*
  oticus; *gen.* ·ci
o′ti·cus *pl. & gen. sg.*
  ·ci
otit′·ic
oti′·tis
o′to·
o′to·acous′·tic
o′to·ce·phal′·ic
o′to·ceph′·a·ly
o′to·co′·nia *sg.* ·ni·um
o′to·cra′·ni·al
o′to·cra′·ni·um
o′to·cyst
o′to·en·ceph′·a·li′·tis
otog′·e·nous *also*
  o′to·gen′·ic
o′to·lar′·yn·gol′·o·gist
o′to·lar′·yn·gol′·o·gy
o′to·lite
o′to·lith
o′to·lith′·ic
o′to·log′·ic *also* ·i·cal
otol′·o·gist
otol′·o·gy
o′to·man·dib′·u·lar
o′to·my·co′·sis
o′to·my·i′a·sis
o′to·neu·rol′·o·gy
o′to·pal′·a·to·dig′·i·tal
o′to·plas′·ty
o′to·rhi′·no·lar′·yn·gol′·o·gist
o′to·rhi′·no·lar′·yn·gol′·o·gy
o′tor·rhe′a *Brit.*
  ·rhoe′a
o′to·scle·ro′·sis
o′to·scle·rot′·ic
o′to·scope
otos′·co·py
o′to·spon′·gi·o′·sis
otos′·te·on
o′to·tox′·ic
o′to·tox·ic′·i·ty
oua·ba′·in
ou·li′·tis *var. of* ulitis
ou′·lo· *var. of* ulo-

out′·break
out′·breed·ing
out′·cross
out′·flow
out′·frac·ture
out′·let
out′·li·er
out′·pa′·tient
out′·pock′·et·ing
out′·pouch′·ing
o′va *pl. of* ovum
o′val
ov′·al·bu′·min
ova′·lis *neut.* ·le
oval′·o·cyte
oval′·o·cy·to′·sis
ovar′·i·al′·gia
ovar′·i·an
ovar′·i·ca *fem. of*
  ovaricus; *pl. & gen. sg.*
  ·cae
ova′·ri·cus *pl. & gen.*
  sg. ·ci
ovar′·i·ec′·to·my
ova′·rii *gen. of*
  ovarium
ovar′·io·
ovar′·i·o·cele
ovar′·io·cen·te′·sis
ovar′·io·cy·e′·sis
ovar′·io·hys′·ter·ec′·to·my
ovar′·i·o·pex′y
ovar′·io·sal′·pin·gec′·to·my
ovar′·i·ot′·o·my
o′va·ri′·tis
ova′·ri·um *pl.* ·ria,
  gen. sg. ·rii
o′va·ry
o′ver·achiev′·er
o′ver·bite
o′ver·breath′·ing
o′ver·clo′·sure
o′ver·com′·pen·sate
  ·sat′·ed, ·sat′·ing
o′ver·com′·pen·sa′·tion
o′ver·cor·rec′·tion

o′ver·den′·ture
o′ver·de·ter′·mi·na′·tion
o′ver·dom′·i·nance
o′ver·dose *n.*
o′ver·dose′ *v.*
  ·dosed′, ·dos′·ing
o′ver·erup′·tion
o′ver·graft *n.*
o′ver·graft′ *v.*
o′ver·growth
o′ver·jet
o′ver·lap *n.*
o′ver·lap′ *v.* ·lapped′,
  ·lap′·ping
o′ver·lay
o′ver·lie′ ·lay′, ·lain′,
  ·ly′·ing
o′ver·load
o′ver·nu·tri′·tion
o′ver·ride′ ·rode′,
  ·rid′·den, ·rid′·ing
o′ver·stain
o′ver·stim′·u·la′·tion
o′ver·sup·pres′·sion
overt′
o′ver·toe
o′ver·tone
o′ver·weight′
o′vi *gen. of* ovum
o′vi·
o′vi·cid′·al [·ci′·dal]
o′vi·cide
o′vi·duct
o′vi·duc′·tal *also*
  ·du′·cal
ovif′·er·ous
o′vi·form
o′vi·gen′·ic
o′vine
ovip′·a·rous
o′vi·pos′·it
o′vi·po·si′·tion
o′vi·pos′·i·tor
o′vo *ablative of* ovum
o′vo·
o′vo·cyte
o′void

o′vo·lar·vip′·a·rous
o′vo·mu′·coid
o′vo·plas′m
o′vo·tes·tic′·u·lar
o′vo·tes′·tis *pl.* ·tes′·
  tes
o′vo·trans·fer′·rin
o′vo·vi·tel′·lin
o′vo·vi·vip′·a·rous
ov′u·la [o′vu·] *pl. of*
  ovulum
ov′u·lar [o′vu·]
ov′u·late [o′vu·] ·lat′·
  ed, ·lat′·ing
ov′u·la′·tion [o′vu·]
ov′u·la·to′ry [o′vu·]
ov′ule [o′vule]
ov′u·lo· [o′vu·lo·]
ov′u·lo·cy′·clic [o′vu·]
ov′u·lum [o′vu·] *pl.*
  ·la
o′vum *pl.* o″va, *gen.*
  sg. o″vi, *ablative* o″vo
ox′·a·cil′·lin
ox′·a·late
ox′·a·lat′·ed
ox′·a·le′·mia *Brit.*
  ·lae′·
ox·al′·ic
ox′·a·lis′m
ox′·a·lo·ac′·e·tate
ox′·a·lo·ace′·tic
ox′·a·lo′·sis
ox′·a·lo·suc′·ci·nate
ox′·a·lo·suc·cin′·ic
ox′·a·lu′·ria
ox·am′·ni·quine
ox·an′·a·mide
ox·an′·dro·lone
ox·az′·e·pam
ox′·a·zo′·li·dine [·zol′·
  i·]
ox·eth′·a·zaine
ox′·gall
ox′·i·dant
ox′·i·dase
ox′·i·da′·tion
ox′·i·da′·tive

ox′·ide
ox′·i·diz′·a·ble
ox′·i·dize ·dized,
  ·diz′·ing
ox′·i·do·cy′·clase
ox′·i·do·re·duc′·tase
ox′·i·do·re·duc′·tion
ox′·ime
ox·im′·e·ter
ox·im′·e·try
ox′o·
ox′o·ac′·id
ox′o·ac′·yl
ox′·o·ges′·tone
ox′o·glu′·ta·rate
ox′o·glu·tar′·ic
ox′·o·lin′·ic
ox·o′·ni·um
ox′o·phen·ar′·sine
ox′·tri·phyl′·line
  [·triph′·yl·]
ox′y·
ox′y·ben·zo′·ic
ox′y·bu·tyr′·ic·ac′·id·
  e′·mia *Brit.* ·ae′·mia
ox′y·cal′·o·rim′·e·ter
ox′y·ce·phal′·ic
ox′y·ceph′·a·ly
ox′y·chlo′·ride
ox′y·chro·mat′·ic
ox′y·chro′·ma·tin
ox′y·cy′·a·nide
ox′·y·gen
ox′·y·gen·ase
ox′·y·gen·ate ·at′·ed,
  ·at′·ing
ox′·y·gen·a′·tion
ox′·y·gen·a′·tor
ox′y·geu′·sia
ox′y·he′·ma·tin *Brit.*
  ·hae′·
ox′y·he′·mo·cy′·a·nin
  Brit. ·hae′·
ox′y·he′·mo·glo′·bin
  Brit. ·hae′·mo·glo′·
ox′y·hy′·dro·ceph′·a·
  lus
ox′y·la′·lia

ox′y·me·taz′·o·line
ox′y·meth′·o·lone
ox′y·mor′·phone
ox′y·my′o·glo′·bin
ox·yn′·tic
ox′y·op′·ter
ox′y·os′·mia
ox′y·per′·tine
ox′y·phen·bu′·ta·zone
ox′y·phen·cy′·cli·mine
ox′y·phil
ox′y·phil′·ic *also* ox·
  yph′·i·lous
ox′y·plas′m
ox′y·quin′·o·line
ox′y·sa·lic′·y·late
ox′y·spore
ox·yt′·a·lan
ox′y·tet′·ra·cy′·cline
ox′y·to′·cic
ox′y·to′·cin
ox′y·to′·cin·ase
ox′y·u′·ria
ox′y·u·ri′·a·sis *also*
  ·u·ro′·sis
ox′y·u′·ri·cide
ox′y·u′·rid
Ox′y·u′·ri·dae
Ox′y·u′·ris
oze′·na *Brit.* ozae′·
oze′·nous *Brit.* ozae′·
o′zone
o′zon·ide
o′zon·ize ·ized, ·iz′·
  ing
o′zon·iz′·er

P

pab′·u·lar
pab′·u·lin
pab′·u·lum
pac′·chi·o′·ni·an
pace′·mak′·er
pach′y·
pach′y·ceph′·a·ly
  also ·ce·pha′·lia

pach′y·der′·ma·to·cele
 [·der·mat′·o·]
pach′y·der′·ma·tous
 also ·der′·mic
pach′y·der′·mia also
 ·der′·ma
pach′y·der′·mo·per′i·
 os·to′·sis
pach′y·gy′·ria
pach′y·lep′·to·men′·in·
 gi′·tis
pach′y·men′·in·gi′·tis
pach′y·me′·ninx
pach′y·ne′·ma
pach′y·onych′·ia
pach′y·pel′·vi·per′·i·to·
 ni′·tis
pach′y·per′·i·to·ni′·tis
pach′y·pleu·ri′·tis
pach′y·sal′·pin·gi′·tis
pach′y·sal·pin′·go·o′va·
 ri′·tis
pach′y·tene
pac′·i·fi′·er
pa·cin′·i·an
pac′·i·ni′·tis
pad′·i·mate
Pae′·ci·lo·my′·ces
 P. li′·la·ci′·num
 P. var′·i·o′·tii
paed- *See also words*
 beginning ped-
pae′·der·as′·ty *Brit.*
 spel. of pederasty
pae′·di·at′·ric *var. of*
 pediatric
pae′·di·a·tri′·cian *var.*
 of pediatrician
pae′·di·at′·rics *var. of*
 pediatrics
pae′·do· *var. of* pedo-
 (*child*)
pae′·do·gen′·e·sis
 var. of pedogenesis
pae′·do·mor′·pho·sis
 var. of pedomorphosis
pae′·do·phil′·ia *var.*
 of pedophilia

pag′·et·oid
pain′·kill′·er
pa′·ja·ro·el′·lo
pal′·aeo· *Brit. spel. of*
 paleo-
pal′·a·tal
pal′·ate
pa·la′·ti *gen. of*
 palatum
pal′·a·ti′·na *fem. of*
 palatinus; *pl. & gen.*
 sg. ·nae
pal′·a·tine
pal′·a·ti′·num *neut. of*
 palatinus; *gen.* ·ni
pal′·a·ti′·nus *pl. &*
 gen. sg. ·ni
pal′·a·to·
pal′·a·to·eth·moi′·dal
pal′·a·to·eth′·moi·da′·
 lis
pal′·a·to·glos′·sal
pal′·a·to·glos′·sus
pal′·a·tog′·na·thous
pal′·a·to·graph
pal′·a·tog′·ra·phy
pal′·a·to·max′·il·la′·ris
pal′·a·to·max′·il·lar′y
pal′·a·to·my′·o·graph
pal′·a·to·pha·ryn′·ge·al
pal′·a·to·pha·ryn′·ge·us
pal′·a·to·pha·ryn′·go·la·
 ryn′·ge·al
pal′·a·to·pha·ryn′·go·
 plas′·ty
pal′·a·to·plas′·ty
pal′·a·to·ple′·gia
pal′·a·tor′·rha·phy
pal′·a·tos′·chi·sis
pal′·a·to·vag′·i·nal
pal′·a·to·vag′·i·na′·lis
pa·la′·tum *gen.* ·ti
pa′·leo· *Brit.* pal′·aeo·
pa′·leo·cer′·e·bel′·lar
pa′·leo·cer′·e·bel′·lum
pa′·leo·cor′·tex
pa′·leo·gen′·e·sis
pa′·leo·ol′·ive

pa′·leo·pal′·li·um
pa′·leo·pa·thol′·o·gy
pa′·leo·ru′·brum
pa′·leo·stri·a′·tum
pa′·leo·thal′·a·mus
pal′i·
pal′·i·graph′·ia
pal′i·ki·ne′·sia
pal′·i·la′·lia
pal′·in·drome
pal′·in·dro′·mia
pal′·in·drom′·ic [·dro′·
 mic]
pal′·in·gen′·e·sis
pal′·in·graph′·ia
pal′·in·mne′·sis
pal′·i·phra′·sia
pal′·i·sade′
pal·la′·di·um
pal′·lan′·es·the′·sia
 Brit. ·aes·the′·
pal′·les·the′·sia *Brit.*
 ·laes·
pal′·les·thet′·ic *Brit.*
 ·laes·
pal′·li·al
pal′·li·ate ·at′·ed, ·at′·
 ing
pal′·li·a·tive
pal′·li·dal
pal′·li·dec′·to·my
pal′·li·do·
pal′li·dof′·u·gal [·do·
 fu′·gal]
pal′·li·do·hy′·po·tha·
 lam′·ic
pal′·li·do·re·tic′·u·lar
pal′·li·do·sub′·tha·lam′·
 ic
pal′·li·do·teg·men′·tal
pal′·li·do·tha·lam′·ic
pal′·li·dot′·o·my
pal′·li·dus *fem.* ·da,
 neut. ·dum
pal′·lio·pon′·tine
pal′·li·um
pal′·lor
palm

pal'·ma *pl. & gen. sg.*
 ·mae
pal'·mar
pal·ma'·re *neut. of*
 palmaris; *pl.* ·ria
pal·ma'·ris *pl.* ·res,
 gen. pl. ·ri·um
pal·ma'·ta *pl.* ·tae
pal'·mate
pal'·ma·ture
pal'·mes·thet'·ic *Brit.*
 ·maes·
pal'·mi·tate
pal·mit'·ic
pal'·mi·to·le'·ic
pal'·mi·to'·yl *also*
 pal'·mi·tyl
pal·mod'·ic
pal'·mo·men'·tal
pal'·mo·plan'·tar
palm'·print
pal'·mus
pal'·pa·ble
pal'·pate ·pat·ed, ·pat·
 ing
pal·pa'·tion
pal'·pa·tom'·e·try
pal'·pa·to·per·cus'·sion
pal'·pa·to'·ry
pal'·pe·bra *pl. & gen.*
 sg. ·brae, *gen. pl.* pal'·
 pe·bra'·rum
pal'·pe·bral
pal'·pe·bra'·lis *pl.* ·les
pal'·pe·bro·na'·sal
pal'·pe·bro·na·sa'·lis
pal'·pi·tate ·tat'·ed,
 ·tat'·ing
pal'·pi·ta'·tion
pal'·sy
pa·lu'·dal [pal'·u·]
pal'·u·dis'm
pam'·a·brom
pam'·a·quine
pam'·o·ate
pam·pin'·i·form
pam·pin'·i·for'·mis
pam·ple'·gia

pan'·a·ce'a
pan·ac'·i·nar
pan'·ag·glu'·ti·na·ble
pan'·ag·glu'·ti·na'·tion
pan'·ag·glu'·ti·nin
pan'·anx·i'·ety
pan'·a·ris
pan'·a·ri'·ti·um
pan'·ar'·ter·i'·tis
pan'·ar·thri'·tis
pan·at'·ro·phy
pan'·car·di'·tis
pan'·cav'·er·no·si'·tis
pan'·chro·mat'·ic
pan'·co·lec'·to·my
pan'·cre·as *L. pl.* pan·
 cre'·a·ta, *gen. sg.* pan·
 cre'·a·tis
pan'·cre·a·tec'·to·my
pan'·cre·at'·ic
pan'·cre·at'·i·ca *fem.*
 of pancreaticus; *pl. &*
 gen. sg. ·cae
pan'·cre·at'·i·ci *pl. &*
 gen. sg. of pancreaticus
pan'·cre·at'·i·co· *var.*
 of pancreato-
pan'·cre·at'·i·co·du'·o·
 de'·nal
pan'·cre·at'·i·co·du'·o·
 de·na'·lis *pl.* ·les
pan'·cre·at'·i·co·du'·o·
 de·nec'·to·my
pan'·cre·at'·i·co·du'·o·
 de·nos'·to·my
pan'·cre·at'·i·co·en'·
 ter·os'·to·my
pan'·cre·at'·i·co·gas'·
 tric
pan'·cre·at'·i·co·gas·
 tros'·to·my
pan'·cre·at'·i·co·je'·ju·
 nos'·to·my
pan'·cre·at'·i·co·li'·enal
pan'·cre·at'·i·co·li·ena'·
 lis *pl.* ·les
pan'·cre·at'·i·co·splen'·
 ic

pan'·cre·at'·i·cus *pl.*
 & gen. sg. ·ci
pan·cre'·a·tin [pan'·
 cre·]
pan·cre'·a·tis *gen. of*
 pancreas
pan'·cre·a·ti'·tis
pan'·cre·a·to· [pan·
 cre'·a·to·]
pan'·cre·a·to·du'·o·de·
 nec'·to·my
pan'·cre·a·to·du'·o·de·
 nos'·to·my
pan'·cre·a·to·en'·ter·
 os'·to·my
pan'·cre·a·tog'·e·nous
 also ·to·gen'·ic
pan'·cre·a·tog'·ra·phy
pan'·cre·a·to·li'·pase
pan'·cre·at'·o·lith
pan'·cre·a·to·li·thec'·
 to·my
pan'·cre·a·to·li·thi'·a·
 sis
pan'·cre·a·to·li·thot'·o·
 my
pan'·cre·a·tol'·y·sis
 var. of pancreolysis
pan'·cre·a·to·lyt'·ic
 var. of pancreolytic
pan'·cre·a·to·meg'·a·ly
pan'·cre·a·tot'·o·my
 also pan'·cre·at'·o·my
pan'·cre·a·to·tro'·pic
 [·trop'·ic]
pan'·cre·ec'·to·my
 var. of pancreatectomy
pan'·cre·li'·pase
pan'·cre·o·li·thot'·o·my
 var. of pancreatoli-
 thotomy
pan'·cre·ol'·y·sis
pan'·cre·o·lyt'·ic
pan'·cre·o·tro'·pic
 [·trop'·ic] *var. of*
 pancreatotropic
pan'·cre·o·zy'·min

pan'·cu·ro'·ni·um
pan'·cy·tol'·y·sis
pan'·cy'·to·pe'·nia
pan'·cy·to'·sis
pan·dem'·ic
pan·dic'·u·la'·tion
pan'·el
pan'·elec'·tro·scope
pan'·en·ceph'·a·li'·tis
pan·en'·do·scope
pan'·en·dos'·co·py
pan'·es·the'·sia Brit.
  ·aes·the'·
pan·fa'·cial
pan·gen'·e·sis
pan'·hi·dro'·sis
pan'·hy·per·e'·mia
  Brit. ·ae'·mia
pan'·hy'·po·pan'·cre·a·tis'm
pan'·hy'·po·pi·tu'·i·tar·is'm
pan'·hy'·po·pi·tu'·i·tar'y
pan'·hys'·ter·ec'·to·my
pan'·ic n. & v. pan'·icked, pan'·ick·ing
pa·nic'·u·lus
pan'·i·dro'·sis var. of
  panhidrosis
pan·lob'·u·lar
pan·mic'·tic
pan·mix'·ia
pan·mu'·ral
pan·my'·e·loid
pan'·my'·e·lop'·a·thy
pan·my'·e·lo·phthi'·sis
  [·loph'·thi·sis]
pan'·my'·e·lo'·sis
pan'·neu·ri'·tis
pan·nic'·u·li'·tis
pan·nic'·u·lus var. of
  paniculus

pan'·nus pl. ·ni
pan·od'·ic var. of
  panthodic
pan'o·pho'·bia var. of
  panphobia
pan'·oph'·thal·mi'·tis
pan·op'·tic
pan'·os'·te·i'tis also
  pan'·os·ti'·tis
pan·pho'·bia
pan'·proc'·to·co·lec'·to·my
pan'·si'·nus·i'·tis
Pan·stron'·gy·lus
  P. ge·nic'·u·la'·tus
  P. me·gis'·tus
pan'·sys·tol'·ic
pant'·ach'·ro·mat'·ic
pant'·an'·en·ceph'·a·ly
pan'·te·the'·ine
pan·thod'·ic
pan'·to·
pan'·to·graph
pan'·to·graph'·ic
pan·to'·ic
pan'·to·mim'·ic
pan'·to·mog'·ra·phy
pan'·to·mor'·phic
pan'·to·pho'·bia var.
  of panphobia
pan'·to·scop'·ic
pan'·to·then'·ate
pan'·to·then'·ic
pan·tro'·pic [·trop'·ic]
pan·tur'·bi·nate
pan'·u've·i'tis
pan'·zer·herz'
pa·pa'·in
pa·pav'·er·ine
pa·pa'·ya
pa·pil'·la pl. & gen.
  sg. ·lae
pap'·il·la'·re neut. of
  papillaris; pl. ·ria

pap'·il·la'·ris pl. ·res
pap'·il·lar'y
pap'·il·late
pap'·il·lec'·to·my
pap'·il·le·de'·ma Brit.
  ·loe·
pap'·il·lif'·er·ous
pap'·il·lif'·er·us
pa·pil'·li·form
pap'·il·li'·tis
pap'·il·lo· [pa·pil'·lo·]
pap'·il·loe·de'·ma
  Brit. spel. of
  papilledema
pap'·il·lo'·ma pl. ·mas
  or ·ma·ta
pap'·il·lo'·ma·to'·sa
pap'·il·lo'·ma·to'·sis
pap'·il·lom'a·tous
  [·lo'·ma·]
pap'·il·lo'·ma·vi'·rus
pap'·il·lop'·a·thy
pap'·il·lose
pap'·il·lo·sphinc'·ter·ot'·o·my
Pa·po'·va·vi'·ri·dae
pa·po'·va·vi'·rus
pap'·pa·ta'·ci
pap'·u·lar
pap'·ule
pap'·u·lo·ero'·sive
pap'·u·lo·er'·y·the'·ma·tous [·them'a·]
pap'·u·lo·ne·crot'·ic
pap'·u·lo·pus'·tu·lar
pap'·u·lo'·sis
pap'·u·lo·squa'·mous
pap'·u·lo'·sus fem.
  ·sa, neut. ·sum
pap'·u·lo·ve·sic'·u·lar
par'a[39]
par'a·
par'a-am'·y·loid

---

[39] This term is derived from the ending of terms like *primipara* and *secundipara*. It is followed by a numeral (usually Roman) indicating the number of times a woman has given birth: para I (primipara), para II (secundipara).

par′a·aor′·tic
par′a·aor′·ti·cum pl.
 ·ca
par′a·ba′·sal
par′·ab·du′·cent
par′a·bi·gem′·i·nal
par′a·bi·o′·sis
par′a·bi·ot′·ic
par′a·blast
par′·a·bu′·lia
par′a·car′·di·ac
par′a·cen·te′·sis pl.
 ·ses
par′a·cen′·tral
par′a·cen·tra′·lis
par′a·cer′·e·bel′·lar
par′·ac′·et·al′·de·hyde
par′a·chlo′·ro·met′a·
 xy′·le·nol
par′a·chlo′·ro·phe′·nol
par′a·chol′·era
par′a·chor′·dal
 [·chord′·al]
par′a·clo′·nus
Par′a·coc·cid′·i·oi′·des
par′a·coc·cid′·i·oi′·do·
 my·co′·sis
par′a·co′·lic
par′a·co′·li·cus pl. ·ci
par′a·col·pi′·tis
par′·a·col′·pi·um
par′a·cone
par′a·co′·nid
par′a·cox·al′·gia
par′·a·cu′·sia also
 ·cou′·sia
par′·a·cu′·sis also
 ·cou′·sis
par′a·cy′·clic
par′a·cys′·tic
par′a·cys·ti′·tis
par′·a·cys′·ti·um
par′·a·den′·tal
par′·a·den·ti′·tis
par′·a·den′·ti·um
par′·a·derm
par′a·did′·u·mis

par′a·di·meth′·yl·ami′·
 no·benz·al′·de·hyde
par′·a·don·to′·sis
par′·a·dox
par′·a·dox′·i·cal
par′a·dox′·us fem.
 ·dox′a
par′a·du′·o·de·na′·lis
par′a·dys′·en·ter′y
par′a·en′·do·crine
par′a·en·ter′·ic var.
 of parenteric
par′a·ep′·i·lep′·sy
par′a·esoph′·a·ge′·al
 Brit. ·oe·soph′·
par′·aes·the′·sia Brit.
 spel. of paresthesia; pl.
 ·si·as or ·si·ae
par′·aes·thet′·i·ca
par′a·fas·cic′·u·lar
par′·af·fin
par′·af·fin·o′·ma [·fi-
 no′·ma]
par′a·flag′·el·late
par′a·floc′·cu·lar
par′a·floc′·cu·lus pl.
 ·li
par′a·fol·lic′·u·lar
par′a·for·mal′·de·hyde
Par′a·fos·sar′·u·lus
par′a·fo′·ve·al
par′a·fre′·nal
par′a·gam′·ma·cis′m
par′a·gan′·gli·o′·ma
 pl. ·mas or ·ma·ta
par′a·gan′·gli·on pl.
 ·glia
par′a·gen′·e·sis
par′a·ge·net′·ic
par′a·gen′·i·ta′·lis pl.
 ·les
par′·a·geu′·sia
par′·ag·glu′·ti·na′·tion
par′a·gle·noi′·dal
pa·rag′·na·thus [·par′·
 ag·nath′·us]
par′·ag·no′·sis
par′a·gom·pho′·sis

par′·a·gon′·i·mi′·a·sis
 also ·mo′·sis
Par′·a·gon′·i·mus
 P. kel′·li·cot′·ti
 P. wes′·ter·man′i
par′a·gram′·ma·tis′m
par′a·gran′·u·lo′·ma
par′·a·graph′·ia
par′a·he′·mo·phil′·ia
 Brit. ·hae′·mo·
par′a·hep′·a·ti′·tis
par′a·he·red′·i·ty
par′a·hex′·yl
par′a·hi·a′·tal
par′a·hip′·po·cam′·pal
par′a·hip′·po·cam·pa′·
 lis
par′a·hor′·mone
par′a·hy·poph′·y·sis
par′a·in′·flu·en′·za
par′a·in′·flu·en′·zal
par′a·ker′·a·to′·sis
par′a·ki·ne′·sia
par′a·ki·net′·ic
par′·a·la′·lia
par′a·lamb′·da·cis′m
par·al′·de·hyde
par·al′·de·hyd·is′m
par′·a·lex′·ia
par′·a·lex′·ic
par′·al·ge′·sia
par′·al·ge′·sic
par′·al·lac′·tic
par′·al·lax
par′·al·lel·is′m
par′·al·lel·om′·e·ter
par′·a·lo′·gia
par′a·lu′·te·al
par′a·lu′·te·in
pa·ral′·y·sis pl. ·ses
par′a·lys′·sa
par′·a·lyt′·ic
par′·a·lyz′·ant [pa·ral′·
 y·zant] Brit. ·lys′·
 ant
par′·a·lyze ·lyzed,
 ·lyz′·ing; Brit. ·lyse,
 ·lysed, ·lys′·ing

par′·a·mag·net′·ic
par′·a·mag′·net·is′m
  [·ne·tis′m]
par′·a·mal′·ta
par′·a·mas′·ti·gote
par′·a·mas·ti′·tis
par′·a·mas′·toid
par′·a·mas·toi′·de·us
par′·a·me′·cin
Par′·a·me′·ci·um
par′·a·me′·ci·um pl.
  ·cia
par′·a·me′·di·al
par′·a·me′·di·an
par′·a·med′·ic
par′·a·med′·i·cal
par′·a·me′·nia
par′·a·me′·si·al
par′·a·mes′o·neph′·ric
pa·ram′·e·ter
par′·a·meth′·a·di′·one
par′·a·meth′·a·sone
par′·a·me′·tri·al
par′·a·me′·tric
  adjacent to uterus
par′·a·met′·ric
  relating to a parameter
par′·a·me·tris′·mus
par′·a·me·tri′·tis
par′·a·me′·tri·um
par′·a·me·trop′·a·thy
par′·am·ne′·sia
par′·am·ne′·sic
par′·a·mo′·lar
par′·a·morph
par′·a·mor′·phia
par′·a·mor′·phine
par′·a·mu′·sia
par′·a·mu′·ta·ble
par′·a·mu′·ta·gen′·ic
par′·a·mu·ta′·tion
par′·a·my′o·clo′·nus
  [·my·oc′·lo·nus]
par′·a·my′·o·to′·nia
Par′·a·myx′o·vi′·ri·dae
par′·a·myx′o·vi′·rus
par′·a·na′·sal

par′·a·na·sa′·lis pl.
  ·les
par′·a·ne′·o·pla′·sia
par′·a·ne′·o·plas′·tic
par′·a·neph′·ric
par′·a·neu′·ral
par′·a·noi′a
par′·a·noi′·ac
par′·a·noid
par′·a·no′·mia
par′a·nor′·mal
par′·a·no′·sic
par′·a·no′·sis
par′·a·nu·cle′·o·lus pl.
  ·li
par′·a·nu′·cle·us pl.
  ·clei
par′·a·op′·er·a·tive
par′·a·o′ral
par′·aor′·tic var. of
  para-aortic
par′·a·pa·re′·sis
par′·a·pa·ret′·ic
par′·a·per′·i·to·ne′·al
par′·a·per·tus′·sis
par′·a·pha·ryn′·ge·al
par′·a·pha′·sia
par′·a·pha′·sic
par′·a·phe′·mia
pa·raph′·ia [pa·ra′·
  phia]
par′·a·phil′·ia
par′·a·phil′·i·ac
par′·a·phi·mo′·sis
par′·a·phra′·sia
par′·a·phre′·nia
par′·a·phys′·e·al [pa·
  raph′·y·se′·al]
pa·raph′·y·sis pl. ·ses
par′·a·plec′·tic
par′·a·ple′·gia
par′·a·ple′·gic
par′a·pox′·vi′·rus
par′·a·prax′·ia
par′·a·proc′·ti·um
par′·a·pro·fes′·sion·al
par′·a·pros′·ta·ti′·tis
par′·a·pro′·tein

par′·a·pro′·tein·e′·mia
  Brit. ·ae′·mia
par′·a·pso·ri′·a·sis
par′·a·psy·chol′·o·gy
par′·a·py′·e·lit′·ic
par′·a·py·ram′·i·dal
par′·a·quat
par′·a·rec′·tal
par′·a·rec·ta′·lis pl.
  ·les
par′·a·re′·nal
par′·a·ros·an′·i·line
par′·ar·rhyth′·mia
par′·a·sa′·cral
par′·a·sag′·it·tal
par′·a·sal·pin′·ge·al
par′·a·sal′·pin·gi′·tis
par′·a·scar′·la·ti′·na
par′·a·sel′·lar
par′·a·sep′·tal
par′·a·sex′·u·al
par′·a·sex′·u·al′·i·ty
par′·a·si·noi′·dal
par′·a·site
par′·a·sit·e′·mia Brit.
  ·ae′·mia
par′·a·sit′·ic
par′·a·sit′·i·cid′·al [·ci′·
  dal]
par′·a·sit′·i·cide
par′·a·sit′·i·cus
par′·a·sit·is′m
par′·a·sit·i·za′·tion
par′·a·sit·ize ·ized,
  ·iz′·ing
par′·a·si′·to·gen′·e·sis
par′·a·si′·toid
par′·a·si′·toid·is′m
par′·a·si·tol′·o·gist
par′·a·si·tol′·o·gy
par′·a·si′·to·tro′·pic
  [·trop′·ic]
par′·a·small′·pox
par′·a·som′·nia
par′·a·spa′·di·as
par′·a·spe·cif′·ic
par′·a·sple′·ni·al
par′·a·splen′·ic

par′a·ster′·nal
par′a·ster·na′·lis *pl.*
  ·les
par′a·stri′·ate
par′a·sym′·pa·thet′·ic
par′a·sym·pa·thet′·i·
  cus *fem.* ·ca, *neut.*
  ·cum
par′a·sym·path′·i·co·
  to′·nia
par′·a·sym·pa·thet′·i·
  cus *fem.* ·ca, *neut.*
  ·cum
par′a·sym′·pa·tho·lyt′·
  ic
par′a·sym′·pa·tho·mi·
  met′·ic
par′a·sym′·pa·tho·to′·
  nia
par′a·syph′·i·lis
par′a·sys′·to·le
par′a·sys·tol′·ic
par′·a·tax′·ic
par′·a·te·ne′·sis
par′·a·ten′·ic
par′a·ten′·on
par′a·ter′·mi·nal
par′a·ter′·mi·na′·lis
par′·a·thi′·on
par′·a·thor′·mone
par′·a·thy′·mia
par′·a·thy′·rin
par′a·thy′·roid
par′a·thy·roi′·dal
par′a·thy·roi′·dea *pl.*
  ·de·ae
par′a·thy′·roid·ec′·to·
  my
par′a·thy′·ro·pri′·val
  also ·priv′·ic
par′a·thy′·ro·pri′·via
par′a·thy′·ro·tro′·pic
  [·trop′·ic]
par′·a·to′·nia
par′·a·ton′·ic
par′a·ton′·sil·lar
par′·a·tope
par′·a·tose
par′a·tra′·che·al
par′a·tra′·che·a′·lis
  pl. ·les
par′a·tra·cho′·ma
par′a·tri·gem′·i·nal
par′·a·tro′·phic
  [·troph′·ic]
par′a·tub′·al [·tu′·bal]
par′a·tu·ber′·cu·lo′·sis
par′a·tu·ber′·cu·lous
par′a·ty′·phoid
par′a·typ′·i·cal *also*
  ·typ′·ic
par′a·um·bil′·i·cal
par′a·um·bil′·i·ca′·lis
  pl. ·les
par′a·un′·du·lant
par′a·un′·gual
par′a·u′re·ter′·ic
par′a·ure′·thra
par′a·ure′·thral
par′a·u′re·thra′·lis *pl.*
  ·les
par′a·u′re·thri′·tis
par′a·u′ter·ine
par′a·vac·cin′·ia
par′a·vag′·i·nal
par′a·vag′·i·ni′·tis
par′a·val′·vu·lar
par′a·ve′·nous
par′a·ven·tric′·u·lar
par′a·ven·tric′·u·lo·hy′·
  po·phys′·i·a′·lis
par′a·ver′·te·bral
par′a·ves′·i·cal
par′a·ves′·i·ca′·lis
par·ax′·i·al
par′a·zone
par′·a·zo′·on *pl.* ·zo′a
par′·e·gor′·ic
pa·rei′·ra
par′·en·ceph′·a·li′·tis
par′·en·ceph′·a·lo·cele
pa·ren′·chy·ma
pa·ren′·chy·mal [par′·
  en·chy′·mal]
par′·en·chy′·ma·tous
  [·chym′·a·]
par′·ent
pa·ren′·tal
par·en′ter·al
par′·en·ter′·ic
par′·ent·ing
par′·ep′·i·did′·y·mal
par′·ep′·i·did′·y·mis
pa·re′·sis [par′·e·sis]
par′·e·so·an′·al·ge′·sia
  [pa·re′·so′·]
par′·es·the′·sia *Brit.*
  ·aes·the′·; *pl.* ·si·as *or*
  ·si·ae
par′·es·thet′·ic *Brit.*
  ·aes·thet′·
par′·es·thet′·i·ca *also*
  ·aes·
pa·ret′·ic
par·eu′·nia
par·fo′·cal
par′·gy·line
par′·i·es *pl.* pa·ri′·
  etes, *gen. sg.* pa·ri′·etis
pa·ri′·etal
pa·ri′·eta′·le *neut. of*
  parietalis
pa·ri′·eta′·lis *pl.* ·les
pa·ri′·eto·
pa·ri′·eto·fron′·tal
pa·ri′·etog′·ra·phy
pa·ri′·eto·mas′·toid
pa·ri′·eto·mas·toi′·dea
pa·ri′·eto-oc·cip′·i·tal
pa·ri′·eto-oc·cip′·i·ta′·
  lis
pa·ri′·eto·per′·i·to·ne′·
  al
pa·ri′·eto·pon′·tine
pa·ri′·eto·pon·ti′·nus
pa·ri′·eto·tem′·po·ral
par′i pas′·su
par′·i·ty
par′·kin·so′·ni·an
par′·kin·son·is′m
par′·o·don′·tal
par′·o·don·ti′·tis
par′·o·don′·ti·um
par′·o·don·top′·a·thy

pa·role′
par′·ol′·fac·to′·ri·us
par′·ol·fac′·to·ry
par·ol′·i·var′y
par′·o·mo·my′·cin
par·om′·pha·lo·cele
par′·o·nych′·ia
par′·o·nych′·i·al
par·on′·y·cho·my·co′·sis
par·o′o·pho′·ric
par·o′o·pho·ri′·tis
par′oöph′·o·ron *also* ·ooph′·
par·or′·chis
par′·orex′·ia
par·os′·mia
par·os′·te·al
par·os′·te·i′tis *also* par′·os·ti′·tis
par·os′·te·o′sis *also* par′·os·to′·sis
pa·rot′·ic
pa·rot′·id
par′·o·tid′·ea *fem. of* parotideus; *pl.* ·de·ae
pa·rot′·i·dec′·to·my
par′·o·tid′·eo·mas′·se·ter′·ic
par′·o·tid′·e·us *pl. & gen. sg.* ·tid′·ei
pa·rot′·i·do·au·ric′·u·la′·ris
pa·ro′·tis *pl.* ·ro′·ti·des, *gen. sg.* ·ro′·ti·dis
par′·o·tit′·ic
par′·o·ti′·tis
par′·ous
par′·ovar′·i·an
par′·ovar′·i·um
par·ox′·ia
par′·ox·ys′m
par′·ox·ys′·mal
pars *pl.* par′·tes, *gen. sg.* par′·tis, *gen. pl.* par′·ti·um
par′·tal
par′·the·no·gen′·e·sis
par′·tial
par′·tial·is′m
par′·ti·cle
par·tic′·u·late
par′·tis *gen. of* pars
par·ti′·tion
par′·tum *accusative of* partus
par·tu′·ri·en·cy
par·tu′·ri·ent
par′·tu·ri·fa′·cient
par′·tu·ri·om′·e·ter
par′·tu·ri′·tion
par′·tus *pl. & gen. sg.* partus, *accusative* ·tum
pa·ru′·lis *pl.* ·li·des
par′·um·bil′·i·cal
par′·va *fem. of* parvus
par′·vi·cel′·lu·lar
par′·vi·col′·lis
par′·vi·loc′·u·lar
Par′·vo·vi′·ri·dae
par′·vo·vi′·rus
par′·vule
par′·vus *fem.* ·va, *neut.* ·vum
pas′·cal
pas′·sage
pas′·sive
pas′·siv·is′m
pas·siv′·i·ty
pas′·ter
Pas′·teu·rel′·la
  P. mul·to′·ci·da
  P. pneu′·mo·tro′·pi·ca
pas′·teur·is′m
pas′·teur·i·za′·tion
pas′·teur·ize ·ized, ·iz′·ing
pas·tille′ *also* pas′·til
past′-point′·ing
patch′·ing
pat′·e·fac′·tion
pa·tel′·la *pl. & gen. sg.* ·lae
pa·tel′·lar
pat′·el·la′·ris
pat′·el·lec′·to·my
pa·tel′·lo·ad·duc′·tor
pa·tel′·lo·fem′·o·ral
pa′·ten·cy
pa′·tent *unobstructed*
pat′·ent *proprietary*
pa·ter′·ni·ty
path′·er·ga′·sia
pa·thet′·ic
path′o·
path′o·bi·ol′·o·gy
path′·o·clis′·is
path′o·cure
path′·o·gen
path′o·gen′·e·sis
path′o·ge·net′·ic
path′·o·gen′·ic
path′·o·ge·nic′·i·ty
path′·og·no·mon′·ic
pa·thog′·no·my
path′·og·nos′·tic
path′·o·log′·ic *also* ·i·cal
pa·thol′·o·gist
pa·thol′·o·gy
path′o·mi·me′·sis
path′o·mim′·i·cry
path′o·mor·phol′·o·gy
path′o·neu·ro′·sis
path′o·phys·i·ol′·ogy
path′·way
pa′·tient
pat′·ri·lin′·e·al
pat′·ro·cli′·nous
pat′·ro·cli′·ny
pat′·ro·gen′·e·sis
pat′·ten
pat′·tern
pat′·tern·ing
pat′·u·lous
pa′·vex
pa·vil′·ion
pav·lov′·i·an
pa′·vor [pav′·or]
peak
pearl
peau
pec′·a·zine

pec′·cant
pec′·tate
pec′·ten
pec′·ten·o′·sis
pec′·ten·ot′·o·my
pec′·tic
pec′·tin
pec′·ti·na′·ta *fem. of* pectinatus
pec′·ti·nate
pec′·ti·na′·tus *pl.* ·ti
pec·tin′·e·al
pec·tin′·e·a′·lis *neut.* ·le
pec·tin′·e·us
pec·tin′·i·form
pec′·to·ral
pec′·to·ra′·lis *pl.* ·les
pec′·to·ril′·o·quous
pec′·to·ril′·o·quy
pec′·to·ris *gen. of* pectus
pec′·to·ro·dor·sa′·lis
pec′·tus *gen.* pec′·to·ris
ped′·al
ped′·er·ast *Brit.* pae′·der·
ped′·er·as′·ty *Brit.* pae′·der·
ped′·es [pe′·des] *pl. of* pes
pe′·di *var. of* pedo- (*child*)
ped′·i· *var. of* pedo- (*foot*)
ped·i·al′·gia
pe′·di·at′·ric *also* pae′·
pe′·di·a·tri′·cian *also* pae′·
pe′·di·at′·rics *also* pae′·
pe′·di·at′·rist *also* pae′·
ped′·i·cel
pe·dic′·el·late *also* ·lat′·ed

ped′·i·cle
ped′·i·cled
pe·dic′·u·lar
pe·dic′·u·lat′·ed *also* ·late
pe·dic′·u·la′·tion
pe·dic′·u·li *pl. of* pediculus
pe·dic′·u·li·cide
Pe·dic′·u·loi′·des
pe·dic′·u·lo′·sis
pe·dic′·u·lous
Pe·dic′·u·lus
  P. hu·ma′·nus cap′·i·tis
pe·dic′·u·lus *pl.* ·li
ped′·i·cure
ped′·i·gree
pe′·di·o·don′·tia *var. of* pedodontia; *also* ·pae′·
pe′·di·on *also* pae′·
ped′i·pha′·lanx
ped′·is *gen. of* pes
pe′·do *child; also* pae′·do·
ped′o· *foot*
pe′·do·bar′o·ma·crom′·e·ter *also* pae′·
pe′·do·ba·rom′·e·ter *also* pae′·
pe′·do·don′·tia *also* pae′·
pe′·do·don′·tics *also* pae′·
pe′·do·don′·tist *also* pae′·
ped′o·dy′·na·mom′·e·ter
pe′·do·gen′·e·sis *also* pae′·
pe′·do·log′·ic *also* pae′·
pe·dol′·o·gist *also* pae·
pe·dol′·o·gy *also* pae·
pe·dom′·e·ter

pe′·do·mor′·phic *also* pae′·
pe′·do·mor′·phism *also* pae′·
pe′·do·mor′·pho·sis *also* pae′·
pe′·do·phile *also* pae′·
pe′·do·phil′·ia *also* pae′·
pe′·do·phil′·ic *also* pae′·
pe·dun′·cle [pe′·dun·cle]
pe·dun′·cu·lar
pe·dun′·cu·la′·ris
pe·dun′·cu·lat′·ed *also* ·late
pe·dun′·cu·lot′·o·my
pe·dun′·cu·lus *pl. & gen. sg.* ·li, *gen. pl.* pe·dun′·cu·lo′·rum
peel′·ing
pee′·nash
pel′·age
pel′·i·di′·si
pel′·i·o′·sis [pe′·li·]
pel·la′·gra
pel·la′·gra·gen′·ic
pel·la′·grin
pel·la′·groid
pel·la′·grous *also* ·grose
pel′·lant
pel′·let
pel′·li·cle
pel·lic′·u·lar
pel·lu′·ci·da *fem. of* pellucidus
pel·lu′·ci·dum *neut. of* pellucidus; *gen.* ·di
pel·lu′·ci·dus *pl. & gen. sg.* ·di
pel·mat′·ic
pe′·lo·
pe′·loid [pel′·oid]
pe′·lo·ther′·a·py
pel′·ta

pel·ta′·tin
pel′·ves *pl. of* pelvis
pel′·vi·
pel′·vic
pel′·vi·ca *fem. of* pelvicus
pel′·vi·ceph′·a·lom′·e·try
pel′·vi·cus *pl.* ·ci
pel′·vi·fem′·o·ral
pel′·vi·fix·a′·tion
pel′·vi·li·thot′·o·my
pel·vim′·e·ter
pel·vim′·e·try
pel·vi′·na *fem. sg. & neut. pl. of* pelvinus
pel·vi′·nus *pl.* ·ni
pel′·vio· *var. of* pelvi-
pel′·vio·il′·eo·ne′o·cys·tos′·to·my
pel′·vio·li·thot′·o·my *var. of* pelvilithotomy
pel′·vio·ne′o·cys·tos′·to·my
pel′·vi·o·plas′·ty
pel′·vi·os′·co·py
pel′·vi·os′·to·my
pel′·vi·ot′·o·my
pel′·vi·rec′·tal
pel′·vis *pl.* ·ves
pel′·vi·scope
pel′·vi·ver′·te·bral
pel′·vo·
pel′·vo·cru′·ral
pel′·vo·spon′·dy·li′·tis
pel′·y·co·
pel′·y·col′·o·gy
pem′·o·line
pem′·phi·goid
pem′·phi·gus
pen′·del·luft
pen′·du·lar
pen′·du·lous
pe·nec′·to·my
pen′·e·trance
pen′·e·trant
pen′·e·trat′·ing
pen′·e·tra′·tion

pen′·e·trom′·e·ter
pen·flu′·ri·dol
pe′·ni·al
pen′·i·cil′·la·mine
pen′·i·cil′·lar *also* ·la·ry
pen′·i·cil′·li *pl. of* penicillus
pen′·i·cil′·lic
pen′·i·cil′·lin
pen′·i·cil′·lin·ase
pen′·i·cil·lin′·ic
Pen′·i·cil′·li·um
pen′·i·cil·lo′·ic
pen′·i·cil′·lus *pl.* ·li
pe′·nile
pe′·nis *pl.* ·nes *or* ·nis·es
pe·nis′·chi·sis
pe·ni′·tis
pen′·nate
pen′·ni·form
pe′·no·pu′·bic
pe′·no·scro′·tal
pen′·ta·
pen′·ta·chlo′·ro·phe′·nol
pen′·ta·chro′·mic
pen′·ta·dac′·tyl
pen′·ta·eryth′·ri·tol
pen′·ta·gas′·trin
pen·tal′·o·gy
pen′·ta·mer
pen′·ta·meth′·a·zene
pent·am′·i·dine
pen′·tane
pen′·ta·ploid
pen′·ta·stome
pen′·ta·sto·mi′·a·sis
pen′·ta·sto′·mid [pen·tas′·to·mid]
Pen′·ta·stom′·i·da
Pen′·ta·trich′·o·mo′·nas [*·tri·chom′·o·nas*]
P. hom′·i·nis
pen′·ta·va′·lent
pen·taz′·o·cine

pen·thi′·e·nate
pen′·ti·lam′·i·nar
pen′·to·bar′·bi·tal
 also ·bi·tone
pen′·ton
pen′·tose
pen′·to·side
pen′·tos·u′·ria
pen′·to·syl
pent·ox′·ide
pen′·tox·if′·yl·line
pen′·tyl
pen′·tyl·ene·tet′·ra·zole
pe·ot′·o·my
pep′·lo·mer
pep′·los
pep′·sic
pep′·si·gogue
pep′·sin
pep′·sin·if′·er·ous
pep·sin′·o·gen
pep′·sin·og′·e·nous
pep′·sin·u′·ria
pep′·tic
pep′·ti·dase
pep′·tide
pep′·ti·do·gly′·can
pep′·ti·dyl
pep′·ti·dyl·trans′·fer·ase
Pep′·to·coc′·cus
pep′·to·gen′·ic *also* pep·tog′·e·nous
pep′·tone
pep·ton′·ic
pep′·to·nize ·nized, ·niz′·ing
pep′·ton·u′·ria [·to·nu′·]
Pep′·to·strep′·to·coc′·cus
pep′·to·tox′·in
per′·aceph′·a·lus
per′·ace′·tic
per·ac′·id
per′·acute′
per a′num
per′·ar·tic′·u·la′·tion

per·ax′·il·lar′y
per·bo′·rate
per·bo′·rax
perc
per·cen′·tile
per′·cept
per·cep′·tion
per·cep′·tive
per·cep′·tu·al
per·cep′·tuo·mo′·tor
per·cer′·vi·cal
per·chlo′·rate
per·chlo′·ric
per·chlo′·ro·eth′·yl·ene
per′·co·late ·lat′·ed, ·lat′·ing
per′·co·la′·tion
per′·co·la′·tor
per con·tig′·u·um
per con·tin′·u·um
per·cuss′
per·cuss′·i·ble
per·cus′·sion
per·cus′·sor
per′·cu·ta′·ne·ous
per cu′·tem
per′·cu·teur′
per′·en·ceph′·a·ly
per·en′·ni·al
per′·fo·rans *pl.* per′·fo·ran′·tes
per′·fo·ra′·ta
per′·fo·rate
per′·fo·ra′·tion
per′·fo·ra′·tor
per·for′·ma·ti′·va
per′·fri·ca′·tion
per·frig′·er·a′·tion
per·frin′·gens
per·fu′·sate
per·fuse′ ·fused′, ·fus′·ing
per·fu′·sion
per′·i
per′i·ac′·i·nal *also* ·nar *or* ·nous
per′i·ad′·e·ni′·tis
per′i·amyg′·da·loid

per′i·a′nal
per′i·an′·gi·i′tis
per′i·an′·gi·o′·ma
per′i·aor′·tic
per′i·a′pex
per′i·ap′i·cal [·a′pi·]
per′i·ap·pen′·di·ce′al
per′i·aq′·ue·duc′·tal
per′i·ar·te′·ri·al
per′i·ar·te′·ri·a′·lis
per′i·ar·te′·ri·o′·lar
per′i·ar′·ter·i′·tis
per′i·ar·thri′·tis
per′i·ar·tic′·u·lar
per′i·ax′·i·al
per′·i·blast
per′i·bron′·chi·al
per′i·bron·chi′·o·lar [·bron′·chi·o′·lar]
per′i·bron·chi′·tis
per′i·bul′·bar
per′i·cal′·i·ce′·al [·ca′·li·]
per′i·cal·lo′·sal
per′i·can′·a·lic′·u·lar
per′i·cap′·il·lar′y
per′·i·car·di′·a·ca *fem. of* pericardiacus; *pl.* ·cae
per′·i·car′·di·a·co·phren′·ic *also* ·car′·dio·
per′·i·car·di′·a·co·phren′·i·ca
per′·i·car·di′·a·cus *pl. & gen. sg.* ·ci
per′·i·car′·di·al *also* ·ac
per′·i·car′·di·a′·lis
per′·i·car′·di·ec′·to·my *also* ·dec′·to·my
per′·i·car′·dii *gen. of* pericardium
per′·i·car′·dio·cen·te′·sis *also* ·car′·di·cen·; *pl.* ·ses
per′·i·car′·di·ol′·y·sis

per′·i·car′·dio·me′·di·as′·ti·ni′·tis
per′·i·car′·dio·per′·i·to·ne′·al
per′·i·car′·dio·pleu′·ral
per′·i·car′·di·os′·to·my
per′·i·car′·di·ot′·o·my
per′·i·car′·dio·ver′·te·bral
per′·i·car·di′·tis
per′·i·car′·di·um *pl.* ·dia, *gen. sg.* ·dii
per′i·car′y·on *var. of* perikaryon
per′i·ce′·cal *Brit.* ·cae′·
per′i·cel′·lu·lar
per′i·ce·men′·tal
per′i·ce′·men·ti′·tis
per′i·ce·men′·tum
per′i·cen′·tric
per′i·cen′·tri·o′·lar
per′i·cho·lan′·gi·o·lit′·ic
per′i·cho′·lan·gi′·tis *also* ·dri·al
per′i·cho′·le·cys·ti′·tis
per′·i·chon′·dral
per′·i·chon·dri′·tis
per′·i·chon′·dri·um
per′·i·chord
per′i·cho·roi′·dal *also* ·ri·oi′·dal
per′i·cho·roi′·de·a′·le
per′i·ci′·sion
per′i·claus′·tral
per′i·co′·lic
per′i·co·li′·tis *also* ·co′·lon·i′·tis
per′i·col·pi′·tis
per′i·con′·chal
per′i·cor′·ne·al
per′i·cor′·o·nal [·co·ro′·]
per′i·cor′·o·ni′·tis
per′i·cor·pus′·cu·lar
per′i·cra′·ni·al
per′i·cra′·ni·um

pericruciate / periostitis

per'i·cru'·ci·ate
per'i·cys'·tic
per'i·cys·ti'·tis
per'·i·cyte
per'·i·cy·to'·ma
per'·i·dec'·to·my
per'i·def'·er·en·ti'·tis
per'i·den·drit'·ic
per'i·dens'
per'i·den'·tal
per'·i·den·ti'·tis
per'·i·den'·ti·um
per'·i·derm
per'i·did'·y·mis
per'i·did'·y·mi'·tis
per'i·di'·ver·tic'·u·li'·tis
per'i·duc'·tal
per'i·du'·o·de·ni'·tis
per'i·du'·ral
per'i·du'·ro·gram
per'i·du·rog'·ra·phy
per'i·en·ceph'·a·log'·ra·phy
per'i·en·ter'·ic
per'i·ep·en'·dy·mal
per'i·esoph'·a·ge'·al
per'i·esoph'·a·gi'·tis
per'i·fo'·cal
per'i·fol·lic'·u·lar
per'i·fol·lic'·u·li'·tis
per'i·gan'·gli·i'·tis
per'i·gan'·gli·on'·ic
per'i·gas·tri'·tis
per'i·he·pat'·ic
per'i·hep'·a·ti'·tis
per'i·hi'·lar
per'i·hy'·po·glos'·sal
per'i·hy'·po·phys'·i·al
per'i-im·plan'·to·cla'·sia
per'i·in'·su·lar
per'i·kar'y·on
per'·i·ky'·ma·ta
per'i·lab'·y·rinth
per'i·lab'·y·rin·thi'·tis
per'i·len·tic'·u·lar
per'i·lig'·a·men'·tous
per'i·lim'·bal

per'i·lu'·nate
per'i·lymph
per'i·lym'·pha
per'i·lym·phad'·e·ni'·tis
per'i·lym·phan'·gi·al
  also ·ge·al
per'i·lym'·phan·gi'·tis
per'i·lym·phat'·ic
per'i·lym·phat'·i·cus
  fem. ·ca, *neut.* ·cum
per'i·mac'·u·lar
pe·rim'·e·ter
per'·i·met'·ric
per'·i·me·tri'·tis
per'·i·me'·tri·um
pe·rim'·e·try
per'i·my'o·car·di'·tis
per'i·my'·o·si'·tis
per'·i·mys'·i·al
per'·i·mys'·i·um *pl.*
  ·sia
per'i·na'·tal
per'i·na·tol'·o·gy
per'·i·ne'·al
per'·i·ne·a'·lis *pl.* ·les
per'·i·ne'i *gen. of*
  perineum
per'·i·ne'o·
per'·i·ne'·o·cele
per'·i·ne·om'·e·ter
per'·i·ne'·o·plas'·ty
per'·i·ne·or'·rha·phy
per'·i·ne·ot'·o·my
per'·i·ne'o·vag'·i·nal
per'·i·ne'o·vul'·var
per'i·neph'·ric
per'i·ne·phri'·tis
per'i·neph'·ri·um
per'·i·ne'·um *gen.*
  ·ne'i
per'i·neu'·ral
per'·i·neu'·ri·al
per'·i·neu·rit'·ic
per'·i·neu·ri'·tis
per'·i·neu'·ri·um
per'i·neu·ro'·nal [·neu'·ro·]
per'i·nod'·al

per'i·nu'·cle·ar
per'i·oc'·u·lar
pe'·ri·od
per'·i·o·date
pe'·ri·od'·ic
pe'·ri·o·dic'·i·ty
per'i·o·dont'·al
per'i·o·don'·tia
per'i·o·don'·tics
per'i·o·don'·tist
per'i·o'·don·ti'·tis
per'i·o·don'·ti·um
per'i·o·don'·to·cla'·sia
per'i·o'·don·tol'·o·gy
per'i·o'·don·to'·sis
per'i·oe·soph'·a·ge'·al
  Brit. spel. of periesoph-
  ageal
per'i·oe·soph'·a·gi'·tis
  Brit. spel. of peri-
  esophagitis
per'i·om·phal'·ic
per'i·o·nych'·ia
per'i·o·nych'·i·al
per'i·o·nych'·i·um
per'i·on'·yx
per'i·o'o·pho·ri'·tis
per'i·op'·tic
per'i·o'ral
per'i·or'·bi·ta
per'i·or'·bit·al
per'i·or·chi'·tis
per'i·os'·te·al
per'i·os'·tei *gen. of*
  periosteum
per'i·os'·te·i'tis *var.*
  of periostitis
per'i·os'·teo·my'·e·li'·tis
per'i·os'·te·o·phyte
per'i·os'·te·o·plas'·tic
per'i·os'·teo·ra'·di·al
per'i·os'·te·or'·rha·phy
per'i·os'·te·o·tome
per'i·os'·te·ot'·o·my
per'i·os'·te·um *gen.*
  ·tei
per'i·os·ti'·tis

per'i·o'tic
per'i·ov'u·lar [·o'vu·]
per'i·pha·ryn'·ge·al
per'i·pha·ryn'·ge·um
pe·riph'·er·ad
pe·riph'·er·al
per'·i·pher'·i·cum
pe·riph'·ery
per'i·phle·bit'·ic
per'i·phle·bi'·tis
Per'·i·pla·ne'·ta
  P. amer'·i·ca'·na
  P. aus'·tra·la'·si·ae
per'·i·plas'm
per'·i·plas'·mic
pe·rip'·lo·cin
per'·i·po·le'·sis
per'·i·po·ri'·tis
per'i·por'·tal
per'i·proc'·tal   *also* ·tic
per'i·proc·ti'·tis
per'i·pros'·ta·ti'·tis
per'i·py'·e·li'·tis
per'i·py'·le·phle·bi'·tis
per'i·py'·lic
per'i·rec'·tal
per'i·re'·nal
per'i·sal·pin'·gi·an
per'i·sal'·pin·gi'·tis
per'i·sal·pin'·go-o'o·pho·ri'·tis
per'·i·scop'·ic
per'i·si·nu·soi'·dal
per'i·sper'·ma·ti'·tis
per'i·sple·ni'·tis
per'i·spon·dyl'·ic
per'i·spon'·dy·li'·tis
per'·i·stal'·sis
per'·i·stal'·tic
per'i·sto'·mal
per'·i·stome
per'i·stri'·ate
per'i·syn'·o·vi'·tis
per'i·tar'·sal
per'·i·tec'·to·my
per'i·ten·din'·e·um
  pl. ·din'·ea

per'i·ten'·di·ni'·tis
per'i·ten'·di·nous
per'i·ten'·on
per'·i·the'·li·al
per'·i·the'·li·o'·ma
per'·i·the'·li·um
pe·rit'·o·my
per'·i·to·nae'·um   *var. of* peritoneum
per'·i·to·ne'·al
per'·i·to·ne·a'·lis
per'·i·to·ne'·al·ize   ·ized, iz'·ing
per'·i·to·ne'i   *gen. of* peritoneum
per'·i·to·ne'o·cen·te'·sis
per'·i·to'·ne·oc'·ly·sis [·to·ne'·o·cly'·sis]
per'·i·to·ne'o·cu·ta'·ne·ous
per'·i·to'·ne·og'·ra·phy
per'·i·to·ne'o·in·tes'·ti·nal
per'·i·to·ne'·o·pex'y
per'·i·to·ne'·o·plas'·ty
per'·i·to·ne'·o·scope
per'·i·to'·ne·os'·co·py
per'·i·to·ne'o·sub'·arach'·noid
per'·i·to·ne'o·the'·cal
per'·i·to·ne'·o·tome
per'·i·to·ne'o·vag'·i·nal
per'·i·to·ne'o·ve'·nous
per'·i·to·ne'·um   *gen.* ·ne'i
per'·i·to·nis'm
per'·i·to·ni'·tis
per'·i·to·ni·za'·tion
per'·i·to·nize   ·nized, ·niz'·ing
per'i·ton'·sil·lar
per'i·tra'·che·al
pe·rit'·ri·chous   *also* per'·i·trich'·ic
per'i·tro'·chan·ter'·ic
per'i·tu'·bu·lar
per'i·typh'·lic

per'i·typh·li'·tis
per'i·um·bil'·i·cal
per'i·un'·gual
per'i·ure'·ter·al   *also* ·u're·ter'·ic
per'i·ure'·ter·i'·tis
per'i·ure'·thral
per'i·u're·thri'·tis
per'i·vag'·i·ni'·tis
per'i·vas'·cu·lar
per'i·vas'·cu·la'·ris
per'i·vas'·cu·li'·tis
per'i·ve'·nous
per'i·ven·tric'·u·lar
per'i·ven·tric'·u·la'·ris   *pl.* ·res
per'i·ves'·i·cal
per'i·ve·sic'·u·li'·tis
per'i·vis'·cer·al
per'i·vi·tel'·line
per·lèche'
perl'·sucht
per·man'·ga·nate
per'·man·gan'·ic
per'·me·abil'·i·ty
per'·me·able
per'·me·ant
per'·me·ase
per'·me·a'tion
per·mis'·sive
per·na'·sal
per·nei'·ras
per·ni'·ci·o'·si·form
per·ni'·cious
per'·ni·o'·sis
per'o·
per'o·bra'·chi·us
per'o·ceph'·a·ly
per'o·dac'·ty·ly
per'·o·me'·lia
per'·o·ne'·al
per·o·ne'o·cu·boi'·de·us
per'·o·ne'·us   *pl.* & *gen. sg.* ·ne'i, *gen. pl.* ·ne·o'·rum
per·o'·ral
per os'

per·ox′·i·dase
per·ox′·i·dat′·ic
per·ox′·ide
per·ox′·i·some
per·ox′y·ac′·yl·ni′·trate
per′·pen·dic′·u·lar
per′·pen·dic′·u·la′·ris
per·phen′·a·zine
per pri′·mam in·ten′·ti·o′·nem
per rec′·tum
per se·cun′·dam in·ten′·ti·o′·nem
per·sev′·er·ate ·at′·ed, ·at′·ing
per·sev′·er·a′·tion
per·sis′·tence [·sist′·ence]
per·sis′·tent [·sist′·ent]
per·sist′·er
per·so′·na
per′·son·al′·i·ty
per′·spi·ra′·tion
per·spi′·ra·to′·ry
per·spire′ ·spired′, ·spir′·ing
per′·stans
per·tech′·ne·tate
per′·tro′·chan·ter′·ic
per tu′·bam
per′·tu·ba′·tion
per′·tur·ba′·tion
per·tus′·sal
per·tus′·sis
per va·gi′·nam
per·ve′·nous
per·ver′·sion
per·vert′ v.
per′·vert n.
per vi′·as na·tu·ra′·les
per′·vi·ous
pes pl. ped′·es, gen. sg. ped′·is
pes′·sa·ry
pes′·ti·ce′·mia Brit. ·cae′·
pes′·ti·cid′·al [·ci′·dal]
pes′·ti·cide

pes·tif′·er·ous
pes′·ti·len′·tial
pes′·tis gen. pestis
pes′·ti·vi′·rus
pes′·tle
pe·te′·chi·ae sg. ·chia
pe·te′·chi·al
pe·te′·chi·om′·e·ter
peth′·i·dine
pet′·i·ole
pe·ti′·o·lus
pe·tit′ mal′
pe·tits′ maux′
pe′·tri also Pe′·tri
pet′·ri·fac′·tion
pé′tris·sage′
pet′·ro·bas′·i·lar
pet′·ro·la′·tum
pe·tro′·le·um
pet′·ro·mas′·toid
pet′·ro·oc·cip′·i·tal
pet′·ro·oc·cip′·i·ta′·lis
pe·tro′·sa fem. of petrosus; pl. & gen. sg. ·sae
pe·tro′·sal
pet′·ro·sec′·to·my
pe·tro′·si pl. & gen. sg. of petrosus
pet′·ro·si′·tis
pet′·ro·sphe′·noid also ·sphe·noi′·dal
pet′·ro·squa·mo′·sus
pet′·ro·squa′·mous also ·squa·mo′·sal
pe·tro′·sum neut. of petrosus
pe·tro′·sus pl. & gen. sg. ·si
pet′·ro·tym·pan′·ic
pet′·ro·tym·pan′·i·ca
pet′·rous
Peu·ce′·tia
P. vir′·i·dans
pex′·in
pex′·is
pe·yo′·te

pha·ci′·tis var. of phakitis
phac′·o·
phac′·o·an′a·phy·lac′·tic
phac′·o·cys·tec′·to·my
phac′·o·cys·ti′·tis
phac′·o·emul′·si·fi·ca′·tion
phac′·o·er′·y·sis
phac′·oid
pha·col′·y·sis
phac′·o·lyt′·ic
pha·co′·ma also phakoma
phac′·o·ma·la′·cia
pha·co′·ma·to′·sis also phakomatosis
pha·com′·e·ter
phac′·o·scope
pha·cos′·co·py
Phae·ni′·cia
P. se′·ri·ca′·ta
phae′·o· var. of pheo·
phae′·o·chro′·mo·cy·to′·ma var. of pheochromocytoma
phae′·o·my·cot′·ic
phage
phag′·e·de′·na Brit. ·dae′·na
phag′·e·de′·nic Brit. ·dae′·nic
phage′-typ′·ing
phag′o·
phag′·o·car′y·o′·sis var. of phagokaryosis
phag′·o·cyte
phag′·o·cyt′·ic
phag′·o·cy·tize ·tized, ·tiz′·ing
phag′·o·cy·tol′·y·sis
phag′·o·cy·tose ·tosed, ·tos′·ing
phag′·o·cy·to′·sis
phag′·o·kar′y·o′·sis
pha·gol′·y·sis
phag′o·ly′·so·some
phag′o·ma′·nia

phag'o·py·ro'·sis
phag'·o·some
pha'·kic
pha·ki'·tis
phak'o·   var. of phaco-
phak'o·lyt'·ic
pha·ko'·ma   var. of
   phacoma
pha·ko'·ma·to'·sis
   var. of phacomatosis
pha·lan'·ge·al
pha'·lan·gec'·to·my
   [phal'·an·]
pha·lan'·ge·us
phal'·an·gi'·tis [pha'·
   lan·]
phal'·an·gi·za'·tion
   [pha'·lan·]
pha'·lanx   pl. pha·lan'·
   ges, gen. sg. pha·lan'·
   gis
phal'·la·nas'·tro·phe
phal·lec'·to·my
phal'·lic
phal'·li·form
phal'·lin
phal·li'·tis
phal'·lo·   also phal'·li·
phal'·lo·camp'·sis
phal'·lo·cryp'·sis
phal'·lo·dyn'·ia
phal'·loid
phal·loi'·din
phal'·lo·plas'·ty
phal'·lor·rha'·gia
phal·lor·rhe'a   Brit.
   ·rhoe'a
phal·lot'·o·my
phal'·lus   pl. ·li or ·lus·
   es
phan'·ero·
phan'·er·o·gen'·ic
   also ·ero·ge·net'·ic
phan'·ero·ma'·nia
phan'·er·o'·sis
phan·ta'·sia
phan'·tasm

phan'·ta·sy   var. of
   fantasy
phan'·tom
phar'·a·on'·ic
phar'·ma·ceu'·ti·cal
   also ·ceu'·tic
phar'·ma·ceu'·tics
phar'·ma·cist
phar'·ma·co·
phar'·ma·co·chem'·is·
   try
phar'·ma·co·di'·ag·no'·
   sis
phar'·ma·co·dy·nam'·
   ics
phar'·ma·co·ep'·i·de'·
   mi·ol'·o·gy
phar'·ma·co·ge·net'·ics
phar'·ma·cog'·no·sist
phar'·ma·cog'·no·sy
   also ·cog·nos'·tics
phar'·ma·co·ki·net'·ics
phar'·ma·co·log'·ic
   also ·i·cal
phar'·ma·col'·o·gist
phar'·ma·col'·o·gy
phar'·ma·co·met'·rics
phar'·ma·co·pe'·dia
   Brit. ·pae'·dia
phar'·ma·co·pe'·ia
   Brit. ·poe'·ia
phar'·ma·co·pe'·ial
   Brit. ·poe'·ial
phar'·ma·co·phore
phar'·ma·co·ther'·a·
   peu'·tics
phar'·ma·co·ther'·a·py
phar'·ma·cy
pha·ryn'·gea   fem. of
   pharyngeus; pl. ·ge·ae
pha·ryn'·ge·al
pha·ryn'·ge·a'·lis   pl.
   ·les
phar'·yn·gec'·to·my
pha·ryn'·ge·um   neut.
   of pharyngeus
pha·ryn'·ge·us   pl. &
   gen. sg. ·gei

pha·ryn'·gi·   var. of
   pharyngo-
pha·ryn'·gis   gen. of
   pharynx
phar'·yn·gi'·tis
pha·ryn'·go·
pha·ryn'·go·bas'·i·lar
pha·ryn'·go·bas'·i·la'·
   ris
pha·ryn'·go·bran'·chi·al
pha·ryn'·go·cele
pha·ryn'·go·con'·junc·
   ti'·val
pha·ryn'·go·con·junc'·
   ti·vi'·tis
pha·ryn'·go·ep'·i·glot'·
   tic
pha·ryn'·go·ep'·i·glot'·
   ti·cus
pha·ryn'·go·esoph'·a·
   ge'·al   Brit. ·go-oe·
   soph'·
pha·ryn'·go·esoph'·a·
   go·plas'·ty   Brit. ·go-
   oe·soph'·
pha·ryn'·go·esoph'·a·
   gus   Brit. ·go-oe·
   soph'·
pha·ryn'·go·la·ryn'·ge·
   al
pha·ryn'·go·lar'·yn·
   gec'·to·my
pha·ryn'·go·lar'·yn·gi'·
   tis
pha·ryn'·go·max'·il·
   lar'y
pha·ryn'·go·na'·sal
pha·ryn'·go-o'·ral
pha·ryn'·go·pal'·a·tine
pha·ryn'·go·pal'·a·ti'·
   nus
pha·ryn'·go·pa·ral'·y·
   sis
phar'·yn·gop'·a·thy
pha·ryn'·go·plas'·ty
pha·ryn'·go·ple'·gia
pha·ryn'·go·rhi·ni'·tis
pha·ryn'·go·scope

phar′·yn·gos′·co·py
pha·ryn′·go·ste·no′·sis
pha·ryn′·go·sto′·ma
  also pha·ryn′·go·stome
phar′·yn·gos′·to·my
phar′·yn·got′·o·my
pha·ryn′·go·tra′·che·al
pha·ryn′·go·tym·pan′·ic
pha·ryn′·go·ty′·phoid
phar′·ynx L. pl. pha·ryn′·ges, gen. sg. pha·ryn′·gis
phase
pha′·sic
phas′·mid
phe′·na·caine [phen′·a·]
phe·nac′·e·mide
phe·nac′·e·tin
phe·nan′·threne [phen·an′·]
phe·naz′·o·cine [phen·az′·]
phe·naz′·o·pyr′·i·dine
phen′·ben·i·cil′·lin
phen·benz′·a·mine
phen·cy′·cli·dine
phen′·di·met′·ra·zine
phene
phen′·el·zine
phe·neth′·i·cil′·lin
phen·eth′·yl
phe·net′·i·dine also ·din
phen·for′·min
phe·nin′·da·mine
phen′·in·di′·one
phen·ir′·a·mine
phen·met′·ra·zine
phe′·no·bar′·bi·tal
  also ·tone
phe′·no·cop′y
phe′·no·ge·net′·ics
phe′·nol
phe′·no·late [phen′·o·]
phe′·nol·e′·mia Brit.
  ·ae′·mia
phe·no′·lic

phe′·nol·phtha′·lein [·phthal′·ein]
phe′·nol·sul·fon′·ic
phe′·nol·sul′·fon·phtha′·lein [·phthal′·ein]
phe·nom′·e·nol′·o·gy
phe·nom′·e·non pl. ·na
phe′·no·thi′·a·zine
phe′·no·type
phe′·no·typ′·ic also ·i·cal
phe·nox′·ide
phe·nox′y· [phen·ox′y·]
phe·nox′y·ben′·za·mine
phe·nox′y·meth′·yl
phe·nox′y·meth′·yl·pen′·i·cil′·lin
phe′·no·
phen′·pro·cou′·mon
phen·pro′·pi·o·nate
phen·sux′·i·mide
phen′·ter·mine
phen·tol′·a·mine
phen′·yl
phen′·yl·ac′·e·tate
phen′·yl·al′·a·nine
phen′·yl·al′·a·nin·e′·mia Brit. ·ae′·mia
phen′·yl·bu′·ta·zone
phen′·yl·ene
phen′·yl·eph′·rine
phen′·yl·hy′·dra·zine
phen′·yl·ke′·ton·u′·ria [·to·nu′·]
phen′·yl·mer·cu′·ric
phen′·yl·pro′·pa·nol′·a·mine
phen′·yl·py′·ru·vate
phen′·yl·py·ru′·vic
phen′·yl·quin′·o·line
phen′·yl·thi′o·car′·ba·mide
phen′·yl·thi′o·hy·dan′·to·in
phen′·yl·thi′o·ure′a

phen′·y·to′·in [phe·nyt′·o·in]
phe′o Brit. phaeo-
phe″o·chrome
phe′o·chro′·mo·blast
phe′o·chro′·mo·cyte
phe′o·chro′·mo·cy·to′·ma
phe·re′·sis var. of apheresis
pher′·o·mone
phi
phi′·al
Phi·a·loph′·o·ra
phil′·trum
phi·mo′·si·ec′·to·my
phi·mo′·sis
phi·mot′·ic
phleb′·ec·ta′·sia
phle·bec′·to·my
phle·bit′·ic
phle·bi′·tis
phleb′o·
phle·boc′·ly·sis [phleb′o·cly′·sis]
phleb′o·dy′·na·mom′·e·try
phleb′·o·gram
phle·bog′·ra·phy
phleb′·o·lith
phleb′o·li·thi′·a·sis
phle·bol′·o·gy
phleb′o·ma·nom′·e·ter
phleb′o·me·tri′·tis
phleb′o·phle·bos′·to·my
phleb′·o·plas′·ty
phleb′o·rhe·og′·ra·phy
phle·bor′·rha·phy
phleb′o·scle·ro′·sis
phleb′o·ste·no′·sis
phleb′o·throm·bo′·sis
phle·bot′·o·mist
Phle·bot′·o·mus
  P. ar·gen′·ti·pes
  P. pap′·a·ta′·sii
  P. ser·gen′·ti
phle·bot′·o·mus

phle·bot′·o·my
phlegm
phleg·ma′·sia
phleg·mat′·ic
phleg′·mon *also* ·mo·na
phleg′·mo·nous
phlo·gis′·tic
phlo′·go· [phlog′o·]
phlo′·go·gen
phlo′·go·gen′·ic *also*
  phlo·gog′·e·nous
phlo′·rhid·zin [phlo·rhid′·zin] *also* ·rid·zin *or* ·ri·zin *or* phlor′·rhi·zin
phlo′·rhid·zin·ize
  ·ized, ·iz′·ing
phlo′·ro·glu′·ci·nol
phlox′·ine
phlyc·ten′·u·la *pl.*
  ·lae; *also* ·ten′·ule
phlyc·ten′·u·lar
phlyc·ten′·u·lo′·sis
pho′·bia
pho′·bic
pho′·co·me′·lia
pho′·co·mel′·ic [·me′·lic]
pho·com′·e·lus
phol′·co·dine
phon
pho′·nal
phon′·an′·gi·og′·ra·phy
phon′·as·the′·nia
pho·na′·tion
pho′·na·to′·ry
pho′·neme
pho·ne′·mic
pho·net′·ic
Pho·neu′·tria
pho′·ni·at′·rics
phon′·ic [pho′·nic]
pho′·nism
pho′·no·
pho′·no·car′·di·o·gram
pho′·no·car′·di·o·graph
pho′·no·car′·di·o·graph′·ic
pho′·no·car′·di·og′·ra·phy
pho′·no·cath′·e·ter
pho·nol′·o·gy
pho′·no·my′o·clo′·nus [·my·oc′·lo·nus]
pho′·no·my·og′·ra·phy
pho·nop′·a·thy
pho·nop′·sia
pho′·no·re·cep′·tor
pho·nos′·co·py
phor′·bin
pho·re′·sis
pho′·ria
Phor′·mia
P. re·gi′·na
pho′·ro·
pho′·ro·blast
pho′·ro·cyte
pho·rol′·o·gy
pho·rom′·e·ter
pho·rom′·e·try
pho′·ro-op·tom′·e·ter
pho′·ro·zo′·on *pl.*
  ·zo′a
phose
pho′·sis
phos′·pha·gen
phos′·pha·tase
phos′·phate
phos′·pha·te′·mia
  Brit. ·tae′·
phos′·pha·ti′·date
phos′·pha·tide
phos′·pha·tid′·ic
phos′·pha·ti′·dyl
phos′·pha·ti′·dyl·cho′·line
phos′·pha·ti′·dyl·eth′·a·nol′·a·mine
phos′·pha·ti′·dyl·glyc′·er·ol
phos′·pha·ti′·dyl·ino′·si·tol
phos′·pha·ti′·dyl·ser′·ine [·se′·rine]
phos′·pha·ti′·dyl·trans′·fer·ase
phos′·pha·tu′·ria
phos′·phene
phos′·phide
phos′·phine
phos′·phite
phos′·pho·
phos′·pho·ar′·gi·nine
phos′·pho·cre′·atine
phos′·pho·di·es′·ter
phos′·pho·di·es′·ter·ase
phos′·pho·dis·mu′·tase [·dis′·mu·]
phos′·pho·e′nol·py′·ru·vate [·py·ru′·vate]
phos′·pho·e′nol·py·ru′·vic
phos′·pho·fruct·al′·do·lase
phos′·pho·fruc′·to·ki′·nase
phos′·pho·fruc′·to·mu′·tase
phos′·pho·ga·lac′·to·isom′·er·ase
phos′·pho·glu′·co·ki′·nase
phos′·pho·glu′·co·mu′·tase
phos′·pho·glu′·co·nate
phos′·pho·glu·con′·ic
phos′·pho·glyc′·er·ac′·e·tal
phos′·pho·glyc′·er·al′·de·hyde
phos′·pho·glyc′·er·ate
phos′·pho·gly·cer′·ic
phos′·pho·glyc′·er·ide
phos′·pho·glyc′·ero·mu′·tase
phos′·pho·hex′o·isom′·er·ase
phos′·pho·ino′·si·tide
phos′·pho·ke′·to·lase [·tol·ase]
phos′·pho·li′·pase
phos′·pho·lip′·id

phosphomevalonate / photosynthetic

phos′·pho·me·val″·o·nate
phos′·pho·mo·lyb″·dic
phos′·pho·mon′o·es″·ter·ase
phos′·pho·mu′·tase
phos′·pho·ne·cro″·sis
phos·phon′·ic
phos·pho′·ni·um
phos′·pho·pan′·te·the′·ine
phos′·pho·pro′·tein
phos′·pho·py·ru″·vic
phos′·phor
phos′·pho·res′·cence
phos′·pho·ri′·bo·ki′·nase
phos′·pho·ri′·bose
phos′·pho·ri′·bo·syl·trans′·fer·ase
phos′·pho·ri′·bu·lo·ki′·nase
phos′·pho·ri′·bu·lose
phos·pho′·ric
phos′·pho·rol″·y·sis
phos″·pho·rous [phos·pho′·]
phos′·pho·rus
phos′·pho·ryl
phos·pho′·ry·lase
phos′·pho·ryl·a″·tion [phos·pho′·ry·la′·tion]
phos′·pho·ser″·ine
phos′·pho·thre″·o·nine
phos′·pho·trans′·fer·ase
phos′·pho·tung′·stic
phos′·sy
phos·vi′·tin
phot
pho′·tic
pho′·tism
pho′·to·
pho′·to·ac·tin″·ic
pho′·to·al″·ler·gen
pho′·to·al·ler′·gic
pho′·to·al″·ler·gy

pho″·to·au″·to·troph
pho″·to·au″·to·tro″·phic
pho″·to·bi·ot″·ic
pho″·to·cath″·ode
pho″·to·cau″·ter·i·za′·tion
pho″·to·cau′·tery
pho″·to·cep′·tor
pho″·to·chem″·i·cal
pho″·to·chem″·is·try
pho″·to·chro′·mic
pho″·to·chro″·mo·gen
pho″·to·chro″·mo·gen′·ic
pho″·to·co·ag″·u·la′·tion
pho″·to·co·ag″·u·la′·tor
pho″·to·con″·duc·tiv′·i·ty
pho″·to·cu·ta′·ne·ous
pho″·to·den″·si·tom″·e·ter
pho″·to·der′·ma·ti′·tis
pho″·to·der′·ma·to′·sis
pho″·to·di′·ode
pho″·to·dy·nam″·ic
pho″·to·elec′·tric
pho″·to·elec′·tron
pho″·to·emis′·sion
pho″·to·flu′o·ro·gram
pho″·to·fluo·rog″·ra·phy
pho″·to·flu′o·ro·scope
pho″·to·fluo·ros″·co·py
pho″·to·gen″·ic
pho″·to·hap′·ten
pho″·to·het″·er·o·troph
pho″·to·ki·ne′·sis
pho″·to·la′·bile
pho″·to·lu″·mi·nes′·cence
pho·tol′·y·sis
pho″·to·lyt′·ic
pho·tom″·e·ter
pho·tom″·e·try
pho″·to·mi″·cro·graph
pho″·to·mi·crog″·ra·phy
pho″·to·mi″·cro·scope
pho″·to·mo′·tor

pho′·to·mul″·ti·pli″·er
pho′·to·my′o·clo″·nus [·my·oc″·lo·nus]
pho′·ton
pho·ton′·ics
pho′·to·nu″·cle·ar
pho′·to-oph·thal″·mia
pho′to-ox″·i·da′·tion
pho′·to·pe″·ri·o·dic″·i·ty
pho′·to·pe″·ri·od·is′m
pho′·to·phil′·ic
pho′·to·pho″·bia
pho′·to·pho″·bic
pho′·to·phos″·pho·ryl·a″·tion
phot′·oph·thal″·mia
var. of photo-ophthalmia
pho·to′·pia
pho·to′·pic [·top″·ic]
pho′·to·pig″·ment
pho′·to·ple·thys″·mo·graph
pho′·to·pro″·ton
pho·top″·sia
pho·top″·sin
phot″·op·tom″·e·ter
pho′·to·re·ac″·ti·va′·tion
pho′·to·re·cep″·tion
pho′·to·re·cep″·tive
pho′·to·re·cep″·tor
pho′·to·res″·pi·ra′·tion
pho′·to·ret″·i·nop′·a·thy
pho′·to·scan
pho′·to·scan′·ner
pho′·to·scin″·ti·gram
pho′·to·sen″·si·tive
pho′·to·sen″·si·tiv′·i·ty
pho′·to·sen″·si·ti·za′·tion
pho′·to·sen″·si·tize
·tized, ·tiz′·ing
pho′·to·sta″·ble
pho′·to·syn″·the·sis
pho′·to·syn·thet″·ic

pho′·to·tac′·tic
pho′·to·tax′·is
pho′·to·ther′·a·py
pho′·to·ther′·mal
pho′·to·ther′·my
pho′·to·to′·pia
pho′·to·tox′·ic
pho′·to·tox·ic′·i·ty
pho′·to·tox′·is
pho′·to·tro′·phic
[·troph′·ic] *utilizing light in nutrition: Cf.* phototropic
pho′·to·tro′·pic [·trop′·ic] *responding to light in orientation: Cf.* phototrophic
pho′·to·tro′·pism [pho·tot′·ro·pis′m]
pho·tox′·y·lin
phren
phre·nec′·to·my
phren′·em·phrax′·is
phren′·i· *var. of* phreno-
phren′·ic
phren′·i·ca *fem. of* phrenicus; *pl. & gen. sg.* ·cae
phren′·i·cec′·to·my
phren′·i·ci *pl. & gen. sg. of* phrenicus
phren′·i·cla′·sia
phren′·i·co· *var. of* phreno-
phren′·i·co·ab·dom′·i·nal
phren′·i·co·ab·dom′·i·na′·lis *pl.* ·les
phren′·i·co·co′·li·cum
phren′·i·co·cos′·tal
phren′·i·co·ex·er′·e·sis
phren′·i·co·li′·enal
phren′·i·co·me′·di·as′·ti·na′·lis

phren′·i·co·per′·i·car′·di·al
phren′·i·co·pleu·ra′·lis
phren′·i·co·splen′·ic *var. of* phrenosplenic
phren′·i·cot′·o·my
phren′·i·cus *pl. & gen. sg.* ·ci
phren′·o·
phren′·o·co′·lic
phren′·o·co′·lo·pex′y
phren′·o·cos′·tal
phren′·o·graph
phre·nol′·o·gist
phre·nol′·o·gy
phren′·o·per′·i·car′·di·al
phren′·op·to′·sis
phren′·o·sin
phren′·o·spas′m
phren′·o·splen′·ic
phryn′·o·der′·ma *also* ·der′·mia
phthal′·ate
phthal′·ein [phtha′·lein]
phthal′·ic
phthal′·o·cy′·a·nine
phthal′·yl·sul′·fa·cet′·a·mide
phthal′·yl·sul′·fa·thi′·a·zole
phthi′·noid
phthi·ri′·a·sis
Phthi′·rus[40] *var. of Pthirus*
phthis′·ic
phthis′·i·cal
phthis′·i·cus *fem.* ·ca
phthi′·sis [phthis′·is]
phy′·co·
phy′·co·bi′·lin
phy′·co·cy′·a·nin
phy′·co·er′·y·thrin
phy′·co·my′·cete
phy′·co·my·co′·sis *also* ·my′·ce·to′·sis

phy′·co·my·cot′·ic
phy′·la *pl. of* phylum
phy·lac′·tic
phy·lac′·to·trans·fu′·sion
phy·lax′·is
phy·let′·ic
phyl′·lo·
phyl′·lode
phyl·lo′·des
phyl′·loid
phyl′·lo·qui·none′ [·quin′·one]
phy′·lo·ge·net′·ic
phy·log′·e·ny *also* phy′·lo·gen′·e·sis
phy′·lum *pl.* ·la
Phy·sa′·lia
phy′·sa·lif′·e·rous *also* ·liph′·o·rous
phy·sal′·i·form
phys′·i·a·tri′·cian
phys′·i·at′·rics
phys′·i·at′·rist [phy·si′·a·trist]
phy·si′·a·try
phys′·ic
phys′·i·cal
phy·si′·cian
phys′·i·cist
phys′·i·co·chem′·i·cal
phys′·i·co·gen′·ic
phys′·ics
phys′·i·no′·sis
phys′·io·
phys′·io·chem′·i·cal
phys′·i·og′·no·my
phys′·i·o·log′·ic *also* ·i·cal
phys′·i·ol′·o·gist
phys′·i·ol′·o·gy
phys′·io·neu·ro′·sis
phys′·io·pa·thol′·o·gy
phys′·io·ther′·a·peu′·tic
phys′·io·ther′·a·pist

---
40 See note at *Pthirus*.

phys'·io·ther'·a·py
phy·sique'
phy'·so·
phy'·so·he'·ma·to·me'·tra *Brit.* ·hae'·
phy'·so·hy'·dro·me'·tra
phy'·so·me'·tra
Phy·sop'·sis
phy'·so·py'o·sal'·pinx
phy'·so·stig'·mine
phy·tan'·ic
phy'·tase
phy'·tate
phy'·tic
phy'·tid
phy'·tin
phy'·to·
phy'·to·be'·zoar
phy'·to·hem'·ag·glu'·ti·nin *Brit.* ·haem'·
phy'·tol
phy'·to·men'·a·di'·one
phy'·to·mi'·to·gen
phy'·to·na·di'·one
phy'·to·no'·sis *pl.* ·ses
phy'·to·pa·thol'·o·gy
phy·toph'·a·gous
phy'·to·pho'·to·der'·ma·ti'·tis
phy'·to·ther'·a·py
phy'·to·tox'·ic
phy'·to·tox·ic'·i·ty
phy'·to·tox'·in
phy'·to·trich'o·be'·zoar
pi'a
pi'a-ar'·ach·ni'·tis
pi'a-arach'·noid
pi'a-gli'a
pi'·al
pi'a ma'·ter
pi'a·ma'·tral
pi'·an [pi·an']
pi'·arach·ni'·tis *var. of* pia-arachnitis
pi'·arach'·noid *var. of* pia-arachnoid
pi·blok'·to

pi'·ca
pick·wick'·i·an
pi'·co·
pi'·co·am'·pere
pi'·co·cu'·rie
pi'·co·far'·ad
pi'·co·gram
pi'·co·lin'·ic
pi'·co·li'·ter *Brit.* ·li'·tre
pi'·co·mole
Pi·cor'·na·vi'·ri·dae
pi·cor'·na·vi'·rus
pic·ram'·ic
pic'·ric
pic'·ro·
pic'·ro·car'·mine
pic'·ro·lon'·ic
pic'·ro·tox'·in
pic'·ro·tox'·in·is'm
pie'·bald
pie'·bald·is'm
pi·e'·dra
pi·es'·es·the'·sia *also* pi·ez'·, *Brit.* ·aes·the'·
pi'·esim'·e·ter *var. of* piezometer
pi·e'·zo·elec'·tric
pi·e'·zo·elec·tric'·i·ty
pi·e'·zo·gen'·ic
pi'·ezom'·e·ter
pig'·bel
pig'·ment
pig'·men·tar'·y
pig'·men·ta'·tion
pig'·ment·ed
pig'·men·to'·sus *fem.* ·sa, *neut.* ·sum
pig'·my *var. of* pygmy
pi·i'·tis
pi'·lar *also* pi'·la·ry
pi·las'·ter
pi·la'·tion
pile
pi'·le·us
pi'·li *pl. & gen. sg. of* pilus
pi'·li·a'·tion

pi·lif'·er·ous
pi'·li·form [pil'·i·]
pi'·li·mic'·tion
pi'·lin
pil'·lar
pil'·let
pil'·lion
pill'·roll'·ing
pi'·lo·
pi'·lo·be'·zoar
pi'·lo·car'·pine
pi'·lo·cys'·tic
pi'·lo·cyt'·ic
pi'·lo·erec'·tion
pi'·lo·jec'·tion
pi'·lo·ma'·trix·o'·ma *also* ·tri·co'·ma
pi'·lo·mo'·tor
pi'·lo·ni'·dal
pi·lo'·rum *gen. pl. of* pilus
pi'·lose *also* ·lous
pi'·lo·se·ba'·ceous
pi·lo'·sus
pil'·u·la *pl.* ·lae
pil'·u·lar
pil'·ule
pi'·lus *pl. & gen. sg.* ·li, *gen. pl.* pi·lo'·rum
pi·mel'·ic
pim'·e·lo·
pim'·e·lo'·ma *pl.* ·mas *or* ·ma·ta
pim'·e·lo·pte·ryg'·i·um
pi·men'·ta
pim'·e·tine
pim'·o·zide
pim'·ple
pin'·cers
pinch
pin'·do·lol
pin'·e·al [pi'·ne·al]
pin'·e·al·ec'·to·my [pi'·ne·]
pi'·ne·a'·lis [pin'·e·]
neut. ·le
pi·ne'·alo·blas·to'·ma *var. of* pineoblastoma

pi·ne′·al·o·cyte
pi·ne′·al·o·cy·to′·ma
  var. of pineocytoma
pin′·e·al·o′·ma
pin′·eo·
pin′·e·o·blas·to′·ma
  pl. ·mas *or* ·ma·ta
pin′·e·o·cy·to′·ma   *pl.*
  ·mas *or* ·ma·ta
pin·guec′·u·la *also*
  ·guic′·
pink′·eye
pin′·lay
pin′·na *pl.* ·nae
pin′·nal
pi′·no·cy·to′·sis
pi′·no·cy·tot′·ic
pin′·sel·haa′·re
pin′·ta *also* pin′·to
pin′·tid
pi′·nus
pin′·worm
Pi·oph′·i·la
  P. ca′·sei
pi·pam′·a·zine
pi·pam′·per·one
pi·paz′·e·thate
pi·pen′·zo·late
pi′·per·acet′·a·zine
pi′·per·a·zine
pi·per′·i·dine
pi′·per·id′′·o·late
pip′·er·ine
pi·per′·o·caine
pi′·per·ox′·an
pipe′·stem
pi·pette′ *also* pi·pet′
pi′·po·bro′·man
pi′·po·sul′·fan
pi·pox′·o·lan
pi′·pra·drol
pip′·to·nych′·ia
pi·qûre′
pir·ac′·e·tam
pir′·i·form
pir′·i·for′·mis
pi′·ro·men

Pir′·o·plas′·ma [*Pi′·ro·*]
pir′·o·plas·mo′·sis
pis′·ci·cide
pi′·si·an′·nu·la′·ris
pi′·si·form
pi′·si·for′·mis *neut.*
  ·me
pi′·si·met′a·car′·pus
pi′·so·cu·ne′·iform
pi′·so·ha′·mate
pi′·so·ha·ma′·tum
pi′·so·met′a·car′·pal
pi′·so·met′a·car′·pe·um
pi′·so·tri·que′·tral
pis′·ton
pitch
pitch′·blende
Pith′·e·can′·thro·pus
pith′·e·coid
pith′·ing
pit′·ting
pi·tu′·i·cyte
pi·tu′·i·ta′·ri·us *fem.*
  ·ria, *neut.* ·ri·um
pi·tu′·i·tar′y
pit′·y·ri·as′·ic [·ri′·a·sic]
pit′·y·ri′·a·sis
pit′·y·roid
Pit′·y·ros′·po·rum
  also ·po·ron
piv′·a·late
piv·am′·pi·cil′·lin
pix′·el
pi·zo′·ty·line
pla·ce′·bo *pl.* ·bos *or*
  ·boes
pla·cen′·ta *L. pl. &*
  gen. sg. ·tae
pla·cen′·tal
pla·cen′·ta·scan
plac′·en·ta′·tion
plac′·en·ti′·tis
plac′·en·tog′·ra·phy
plac′·en·tol′·o·gy
plac′·en·to′·ma *pl.*
  ·mas *or* ·ma·ta

plac′·en·top′·a·thy
plac′·ode
pla′·gio·ce·phal′·ic
pla′·gio·ceph′·a·ly
plague
pla′·na *fem. sg. &*
  neut. pl. of planus
plan′·chet
pla′·ni·form [plan′·i·]
pla·nig′·ra·phy
pla·nim′·e·ter
plan′i·tho′·rax [pla′·ni·]
pla′·no
pla′·no· *flat, plane*
plan′o· *wandering, motile*
pla′·no·cel′·lu·lar
pla′·no·con′·cave
pla′·no·con′·vex
plan′·o·cyte
pla·nog′·ra·phy *var. of* planigraphy
pla·nor′·bid
Pla·nor′·bi·dae
Pla·nor′·bis
pla′·no·val′·gus
plan′·ta *pl. & gen. sg.*
  ·tae
plan·ta′·go *gen.* plan·tag′·i·nis
plan′·tar
plan·ta′·re *neut. of*
  plantaris; *pl.* ·ria
plan·ta′·ris *pl.* ·res
plan′·ti·flex′·ion
plan′·ti·grade
pla′·num *neut. of*
  planus; *pl.* ·na
plan·u′·ria
pla′·nus *fem.* ·na, *neut.* ·num
plaque
plas′m
plas′·ma
plas′·ma·
plas′·ma·blast
plas′·ma·crit
plas′·ma·cyte

plas'·ma·cyt'·ic
plas'·ma·cy'·toid
plas'·ma·cy·to'·ma
plas'·ma·cy·to'·sis
plas'·ma·gel
plas'·ma·gene
plas'·ma·lem'·ma
plas·mal'·o·gen
plas'·ma·pher·e'·sis
 [·pher'·e·]
plas'·ma·sol
plas·mat'·ic
plas'·ma·to· *var. of*
 plasmo-
plas'·ma·tog'·a·my
 var. of plasmogamy
plas'·ma·tor·rhex'·is
 var. of plasmorrhexis
plas'·mic
plas'·mid
plas'·min
plas·min'·o·gen
plas'·mo·
plas'·mo·crine
plas'·mo·cy·to'·ma
plas·mo'·dia *pl. of*
 plasmodium
plas·mo'·di·al
plas'·mo·di·cid'·al
plas·mo'·di·cide
Plas'·mo·di'·idae
Plas·mo'·di·um
 P. fal·cip'·a·rum
 P. ma·lar'·i·ae
 P. ova'·le
 P. vi'·vax
plas·mo'·di·um *pl.*
 ·dia
plas·mog'·a·my
plas·mol'·y·sis
plas'·mo·lyt'·ic
plas'·mon
plas·mop'·ty·sis
plas'·mor·rhex'·is
plas'·ter
plas'·tic
plas·tic'·i·ty
plas'·ti·ciz'·er

plas'·tid
plas'·ti·na'·tion
plas'·tron
plate *n. & v.* plat'·ed,
 plat'·ing
pla·teau'
plate'·let
plate'·let·pher·e'·sis
plat'·i·nec'·to·my
plat'·i·num
plat'·ode
plat'·y·
plat'·y·ba''·sia
plat'·y·ce·phal'·ic *also*
 ·ceph'·a·lous
plat'·y·ceph'·a·ly
plat'·y·cne'·mia
plat'·y·cne'·mic
plat'·y·cra'·nia
plat'·y·glos'·sal
plat'·y·hel'·minth
Plat'·y·hel·min'·thes
plat'·y·hel·min'·thic
plat'·y·hi·er'·ic
plat'·y·kne'·mia *var.*
 of platycnemia
plat'·y·mor'·phia
plat'·y·mor'·phic
plat'·y·onych'·ia
plat'·y·o'pia
plat'·y·o'pic
plat'·y·pel'·lic
plat'·y·pne'a *Brit.*
 ·pnoe'a
plat'·yr·rhine
pla·tys'·ma
pla·tys'·mal
plat'·y·spon·dyl'·ia
plat'·y·staph'·y·line
plat'·y·trope
pleas'·ure [plea'·sure]
plec'·to·ne'·mic
pled'·get
pleg'·a·pho'·nia
ple'·gia
plei'·o·tro'·pic [·trop'·
 ic]

plei'·o·tro'·pism *also*
 ·tro'·pia
ple'o· *also* plei'o·
ple'·o·chro'·ism
ple'o·chro'·mo·cy·to'·
 ma
ple'·o·co'·ni·al
ple'·o·cy·to'·sis
ple'·o·mor'·phic *also*
 ·phous
ple'·o·mor'·phism
ple'·o·nas'm
ple'·on·os'·te·o'·sis
ple·op'·tics
ple·op'·to·phor
ple'·ro·cer'·coid
ple'·si·o·gnath'·us
Ple'·si·o·mo'·nas
ple'·si·o'·pia
ples·sim'·e·ter
ples'·sor
pleth'·o·ra
ple·tho'·ric
ple·thys'·mo·gram
ple·thys'·mo·graph
pleth'·ys·mog'·ra·phy
pleth'·ys·mom'·e·ter
pleu'·ra *pl. & gen. sg.*
 ·rae
pleu'·ra·cen·te'·sis
 var. of pleurocentesis
pleu'·ral
pleu·ral'·gia
pleu·ra'·lis *pl.* ·les
pleu·rec'·to·my
pleu'·ri·sy
pleu·rit'·ic
pleu·ri'·tis
pleu'·ro·
pleu'·ro·bron'·chi·al
pleu'·ro·cen·te'·sis
pleu'·ro·cu·ta'·ne·ous
pleu·rod'·e·sis
pleu'·ro·dyn'·ia
pleu'·ro·esoph'·a·ge'·al
 Brit. pleu'·ro·oe·soph'·
pleu'·ro·esoph'·a·ge''·us
 also pleu'·ro·oe·soph'·

pleu′·ro·hep′·a·ti′·tis
pleu·rol′·y·sis
pleu′·ro·me′·lus [pleu·rom′·e·lus]
pleu′·ro·pa·ri′·eto·pex′y
pleu′·ro·per′·i·car′·di·al
pleu′·ro·per′·i·car′·di·a′·le
pleu′·ro·per′·i·car·di′·tis
pleu′·ro·per′·i·to·ne′·al
pleu′·ro·per′·i·to·ne′·um
pleu′·ro·pneu·mo′·nia
pleu′·ro·pneu′·mo·nol′·y·sis
pleu′·ro·pul′·mo·nar′y
pleu′·ror·rhe′a *Brit.* ·rhoe′a
pleu·ros′·co·py
pleu′·ro·so′·ma
pleu′·ro·thot′·o·nos *also* ·nus
pleu′·ro·tome
pleu·rot′·o·my
plex·ec′·to·my
plex′·i·form
plex′·i·for′·me
plex·im′·e·ter *also* ·om′·e·ter
plex·i′·tis
plex′·or
plex′·us *L. pl. & gen. sg.* plexus, *gen. pl.* plex′·u·um
pli′·a·ble
pli′·ca *pl. & gen. sg.* ·cae
pli′·cate ·cat·ed, ·cat·ing
pli·ca′·tion
plinth *also* plint
ploi′·dy
plom·bage′
plo′·sive
plo′·to·tox′·in

plug plugged, plug′·ging
plug′·ger
plum′·bism
plump′·er
plu′·ri·
plu′·ri·caus′·al
plu′·ri·cys′·tic
plu′·ri·de·fi′·cien·cy
plu′·ri·de·fi′·cient
plu′·ri·fo′·cal
plu′·ri·glan′·du·lar
plu′·ri·grav′·i·da *pl.* ·das *or* ·dae
plu′·ri·o′ri·fi′·ci·a′·lis
plu·rip′·a·ra *pl.* ·ras *or* ·rae
plu′·ri·par′·i·ty
plu·rip′·o·tent
plu′·ri·po·ten′·tial
plu′·ri·po·ten′·ti·al′·i·ty
plu′·ri·re·sis′·tant [·sist′·ant]
plu′·ri·seg·men′·tal
plu′·to·nis′m
plu·to′·ni·um
pne′o·
pne′·o·gram
pne·om′·e·ter
pneum′·ar·throg′·ra·phy *var. of* pneumoarthrography
pneum′·ar·thro′·sis
pneu·ma·the′·mia *Brit.* ·thae′·
pneu·mat′·ic
pneu·mat′·i·ca *fem. of* pneumaticus; *pl.* ·cae
pneu·mat′·i·cus *fem.* ·ca, *neut.* ·cum
pneu′·ma·ti·nu′·ria *var. of* pneumaturia
pneu′·ma·ti·za′·tion
pneu′·ma·tized
pneu′·ma·to·ratio [pneu·mat′o·]
pneu′·ma·to·car′·dia
pneu·mat′·o·cele

pneu′·ma·to·ceph′·a·lus
pneu′·ma·to·en·ter′·ic
pneu·mat′·o·gram
pneu·mat′·o·graph
pneu′·ma·tom′·e·ter
pneu′·ma·tom′·e·try
pneu′·ma·to′·sis
pneu′·ma·tu′·ria
pneu′·mec′·to·my
pneum′·en·ceph′·a·log′·ra·phy
pneu′·mo·
pneu′·mo·ar·throg′·ra·phy
pneu′·mo·blas·to′·ma
pneu′·mo·bul′·bar
pneu′·mo·car′·di·og′·ra·phy
pneu′·mo·cele
pneu′·mo·cen·te′·sis *var. of* pneumonocentesis
pneu′·mo·ceph′·a·lus
pneu′·mo·cho′·le·cys·ti′·tis
pneu′·mo·coc′·cal *also* ·cic
pneu′·mo·coc·ce′·mia *Brit.* ·cae′·mia
pneu′·mo·coc·cid′·al [·ci′·dal]
pneu′·mo·coc′·co·cid′·al [·ci′·dal] *var. of* pneumococcidal
pneu′·mo·coc·co′·sis
pneu′·mo·coc′·cus *pl.* ·coc′·ci
pneu′·mo·co′·lon
pneu′·mo·co′·ni·o′·sis
pneu′·mo·cys′·tic
Pneu′·mo·cys′·tis
  P. *ca·ri′·nii*
pneu′·mo·cys′·tis
pneu′·mo·cys′·to·gram
pneu′·mo·cys·tog′·ra·phy
pneu′·mo·cys·to′·sis
pneu′·mo·cyte

pneu'·mo·en·ceph'·a·lo·cele
pneu'·mo·en·ceph'·a·log'·ra·phy
pneu'·mo·en'·ter·i'·tis
pneu'·mo·er'·y·sip'·e·las
pneu'·mo·gas'·tric
pneu'·mo·gas·trog'·ra·phy
pneu'·mo·gas·tros'·co·py
pneu'·mo·gen'·ic
pneu'·mo·graph
pneu·mog'·ra·phy
pneu'·mo·he'·mo·tho'·rax Brit. ·hae'·mo·
pneu'·mo·hy'·dro·me'·tra
pneu'·mo·hy'·dro·tho'·rax
pneu'·mo·lith
pneu'·mo·li·thi'·a·sis
pneu·mol'·o·gy
pneu·mol'·y·sin
pneu·mol'·y·sis
pneu'·mo·me'·di·as'·ti·nog'·ra·phy
pneu'·mo·me'·di·as·ti'·num
pneu'·mo·my'·e·log'·ra·phy
pneu'·mo·nec'·to·my
pneu'·mo·nere
pneu·mo'·nia
pneu·mon'·ic
pneu'·mo·ni'·tis
pneu'·mo·no· var. of pneumon-
pneu·mon'·o·cele [pneu'·mo·no·]
pneu'·mo·no·cen·te'·sis
pneu'·mo·no·co'·ni·o'·sis var. of pneumoconiosis
pneu'·mo·no·cyte [pneu·mon'·o·] var. of pneumocyte
pneu'·mo·nol'·y·sis
pneu'·mo·no·pex'y
pneu'·mo·no·pleu·ri'·tis
pneu'·mo·no·re·sec'·tion
pneu'·mo·nor'·rha·phy
pneu'·mo·not'·o·my
pneu'·mo·or'·bi·tog'·ra·phy
pneu'·mo·per'·i·car·di'·tis
pneu'·mo·per'·i·car'·di·um
pneu'·mo·per'·i·to·ne'·um
pneu'·mo·per'·i·to·ni'·tis
pneu'·mo·pex'y var. of pneumonopexy
pneu'·mo·pha'·gia
pneu'·mo·pleth'·ys·mog'·ra·phy
pneu'·mo·pleu·ri'·tis var. of pneumonopleuritis
pneu'·mo·pleu'·ro·pa·ri'·eto·pex'y
pneu'·mo·py'·e·log'·ra·phy
pneu'·mo·py'o·per'·i·car'·di·um
pneu'·mo·py'o·tho'·rax
pneu'·mo·ra'·chi·cen·te'·sis
pneu'·mo·ra'·chis
pneu'·mo·ra'·di·og'·ra·phy
pneu'·mo·re·sec'·tion
pneu'·mo·roent'·gen·og'·ra·phy
pneu'·mo·scle·ro'·sis
pneu'·mo·sil'·i·co'·sis
pneu'·mo·tach'·o·graph
pneu'·mo·tax'·ic
pneu'·mo·ther'·mo·mas·sage'
pneu'·mo·tho'·rax pl. ·rax·es or ·ra·ces
pneu·mot'·o·my var. of pneumonotomy
pneu'·mo·tro'·pic [·trop'·ic]
pneu'·mo·ty'·phoid
pneu'·mo·u'ria
pneu'·mo·ven'·tri·cle
pneu'·mo·ven·tric'·u·log'·ra·phy
pneu'·mo·vi'·rus
pock'·et
pock'·mark
poc'·u·li·form
poc'·u·lum
po·dag'·ra
po·dal'·gia
po·dal'·ic
pod'·ar·thri'·tis
pod'·en·ceph'·a·lus
po·di'·a·trist
po·di'·a·try
po·di'·tis
po'·di·um pl. ·ia
pod'o·
pod'·o·cyte
pod'o·dy'·na·mom'·e·ter
pod'·o·dyn'·ia
pod'·o·gram
po·dog'·ra·phy
po·dol'·o·gist
po·dol'·o·gy
po·dom'·e·ter var. of pedometer
pod'·o·phyl'·lin
pod'·o·phyl'·lo·tox'·in
pod'·o·phyl'·lum
pod'o·spas'm also pod'o·spas'·mus
po·go'·ni·on
Po·go'·no·myr'·mex
poi'·ki·lo·
poi'·ki·lo·cyte
poi'·ki·lo·cy·the'·mia Brit. ·thae'·
poi'·ki·lo·cy·to'·sis
poi'·ki·lo·der'·ma

poi′·ki·lo·der′·ma·to·my′·o·si′·tis
poi′·kil·os·mo″·sis
poi′·kil·os·mot′·ic
poi′·ki·lo·therm
poi′·ki·lo·ther′·mic
poi′·ki·lo·ther′·my
point′·er
poi′·son
poi′·son·ing
poi′·son·ous
poke″·weed
po′·lar
po′·lar·im′·e·ter
po·lar′·i·scope
po·lar′·i·ty
po′·lar·i·za′·tion
po′·lar·ize ·ized, ·iz′·ing
po′·lar·iz′·er
po′·lar·og′·ra·phy
pol′·dine
po′·li pl. & gen. sg. of polus
pol′i·clin′·ic
po′·li·en·ceph′·a·li′·tis var. of polioencephalitis
po′·lio
po′·lio·
po′·li·o·clas′·tic
po′·lio·dys′·tro·phy also ·dys·tro′·phia
po′·lio·en·ceph·a·li′·tis
po′·lio·en·ceph′·a·lo·my′·e·li′·tis
po′·lio·en·ceph′·a·lo·my′·e·lop′·a·thy
po′·lio·en·ceph′·a·lop′·a·thy
po′·lio·my′·e·lit′·ic
po′·lio·my′·e·li′·tis
po′·li·o′·sis
po′·lio·vi′·rus
pol′·it·zer·i·za′·tion
pol′·la·ki·dip′·sia
pol′·la·ki·u′ria
pol′·len·o′·sis var. of pollinosis

pol′·lex pl. pol′·li·ces, gen. sg. pol′·li·cis
pol′·li·ci·za′·tion
pol′·li·co·men′·tal
pol·lin′·ic
pol′·li·no′·sis
pol·lod′·ic
pol·lu′·tant
pol·lu′·tion
po·lo′·ni·um
po′·lus pl. & gen. sg. po′·li
pol′y·
pol′y·ac′·id
pol′y·acryl′·a·mide
pol′y·ad′·e·ni′·tis
pol′y·ad′·e·nop′·a·thy
pol′y·aden′·y·late
pol′y·aden′·y·la′·tion
pol′y·ag·glu′·ti·na·bil′·i·ty
pol′y·am′·ide
pol′y·am′·ine
pol′y·an′·gi·i′tis
pol′y·ar′·ter·i′·tis
pol′y·ar′·thric
pol′y·ar·thri′·tis
pol′y·ar·throp′·a·thy
pol′y·ar·thro′·sis
pol′y·ar·tic′·u·lar
pol′y·aux′·o·troph
pol′y·avi′·ta·min·o′·sis
pol′y·ax′·i·al
pol′y·ax′·on
pol′y·ax·on′·ic
pol′y·ba′·sic
pol′y·blast
pol′y·cen′·tric
pol′y·che′·mo·ther′·a·py
pol′y·chlo′·ri·nat′·ed
pol′y·chon·dri′·tis
pol′y·chon·drop′·a·thy
pol′y·chrest
pol′y·chro·ma′·sia
pol′y·chro·mat′·ic
pol′y·chro·mat′·o·cyte

pol′y·chro·mat′·o·cy·to″·sis [·chro′·ma·to′·]
pol′y·chro·mat′·o·phil
pol′y·chro·mat′·o·phil′·ia [·chro′·ma·to′·]
pol′y·chro·mat′·o·phil′·ic [·chro′·ma·to′·]
pol′y·chro′·ma·to″·sis
pol′y·chrome
pol′y·chro′·mia
pol′y·chro′·mo·cy·to″·sis
pol′y·chro′·mo·phil var. of polychromatophil
pol′y·cis·tron′·ic
pol′y·clin′·ic
pol′y·clon′·al [·clo′·nal]
pol′y·co′·ria
pol′y·crot′·ic
pol′y·cy′·clic
pol′y·cys′·tic
pol′y·cyte
pol′y·cy·the″·mia Brit. ·thae′·
pol′y·dac′·ty·lous
pol′y·dac′·ty·ly
pol′y·de·fi′·cient
pol′y·dip′·sia
pol′y·don′·tia also ·den′·tia
pol′y·dys·pla′·sia
pol′y·dys·plas′·tic
pol′y·dys·spon′·dy·lis′m
pol′y·dys·tro′·phic
pol′y·dys′·tro·phy
pol′y·elec′·tro·lyte
pol′y·em′·bry·o·ny
pol′y·e′mia Brit. ae′·mia
pol′y·en′·do·crine
pol′y·ene
pol′y·es′·ter
pol′y·ga·lac′·tia
pol′y·ga·lac·tu′·ro·nase
po·lyg′·a·lin

po·lyg′·a·my
pol′y·gan′·gli·on′·ic
pol′y·gene
pol′y·gen′·ic [·ge′·nic]
pol′y·glan′·du·lar
pol′y·glob′·u·lis′m
pol′y·graph
po·lyg′·y·ny
pol′y·gy′·ria
pol′y·he′·dral
pol′y·het′·er·ox′·e·nous
pol′y·hi·dro′·sis
pol′y·hy′·brid
pol′y·hy·dram′·ni·os
pol′y·hy′·dric
pol′y·hy·drox′y
pol′y·hy·dru′·ria
pol′y·in·fec′·tion
pol′y·kar′y·o·cyte
pol′y·ke′·tide
pol′y·lec′·i·thal
pol′y·lep′·tic
pol′y·lob′·u·lar
pol′y·ly′·sine
pol′y·mas′·tia *also* ·ma′·zia
pol′y·mas′·ti·gote
pol′y·me′·lia
pol′y·me′·nia
pol′y·men′·or·rhe′a *Brit.* ·rhoe′a
pol′y·mer
pol′y·mer·ase [po·lym′·er·ase]
pol′y·mer′·ic
pol′y·mer·i·za′·tion [po·lym′·er·]
pol′y·mer·ize [po·lym′·er·ize] ·ized, ·iz′·ing
pol′y·met′a·car′·pia
pol′y·met′a·tar′·sia
pol′y·mi′·cro·li·po′·ma·to′·sis
pol′y·morph
pol′y·mor′·phic
pol′y·mor′·phism
pol′y·mor′·pho·cel′·lu·lar

pol′y·mor′·pho·cyte
pol′y·mor′·pho·cyt′·ic
pol′y·mor′·pho·nu′·cle·ar
pol′y·mor′·phous
pol′y·my·al′·gia
pol′y·my′·o·clo′·nia
var. of polymyoclonus
pol′y·my′o·clo′·nus [·my·oc′·lo·nus]
pol′y·my·op′·a·thy
pol′y·my′·o·si′·tis
pol′y·myx′·in
pol′y·neme
pol′y·neu′·ral *also* ·ric
pol′y·neu·ral′·gia
pol′y·neu·rit′·ic
pol′y·neu·ri′·tis
pol′y·neu′·ro·my′·o·si′·tis
pol′y·neu·ro′·nal [·neu′·ro·]
pol′y·neu′·ron·i′·tis
pol′y·neu·rop′·a·thy
pol′y·neu′·ro·ra·dic′·u·li′·tis
pol′y·nu′·cle·ar
pol′y·nu·cle′·o·lar
pol′y·nu′·cle·o′·sis
pol′y·nu′·cle·o·tide
pol′y·o′·ma
pol′y·o′·ma·vi′·rus
pol′y·onych′·ia *also* pol′y·nych′·ia
pol′y·o′·pia *also* ·op′·sia
pol′y·or′·chi·dis′m *also* ·or′·chism
pol′y·orex′·ia
pol′y·os·tot′·ic
pol′y·o′·tia
pol′y·ov′u·lar [·o′vu·]
pol′y·ov′u·la·to′·ry [·o′vu·]
pol′·yp
pol′y·pap′·il·lo′·ma
pol′·yp·ec′·to·my

pol′y·pep′·tide
pol′y·per′i·os·ti′·tis
pol′y·pha′·gia
pol′y·pha·lan′·gia *also* ·lan′·gism
pol′y·phar′·ma·ceu′·tic
pol′y·phar′·ma·cy
pol′y·pha′·sic
pol′y·phe′·nic
pol′y·phe′·ny
pol′y·phos′·phate
pol′y·phy·let′·ic
pol′y·phy′·le·tis′m
pol′y·phy′·o·dont
pol′·y·pi *pl. of* polypus
pol′·yp·if′·er·ous
pol′y·plas′·tic
pol′y·pleu′·ro·di′·a·phrag·mot′·o·my
pol′y·ploid
pol′y·ploi′·dy
pol′·y·pne′a *Brit.* ·pnoe′a
pol′·y·pne′·ic *Brit.* ·pnoe′·ic
pol′y·po′·dia
pol′·yp·oid
pol′y·po′·rous
pol′·yp·o′·sa
pol′·yp·o′·sis
pol′·yp·ous
pol′y·prag′·ma·sy
pol′·y·pus *pl.* ·pi
pol′y·ra·dic′·u·li′·tis
pol′y·ra·dic′·u·lo·neu·ri′·tis
pol′y·ra·dic′·u·lo·neu·rop′·a·thy
pol′y·rhyth′·mic
pol′y·ri′·bo·nu′·cle·o·tide
pol′y·ri′·bo·some
pol′y·sac′cha·ri·dase′
pol′y·sac′·cha·ride
pol′y·sce′·lia
pol′y·se′·ro·si′·tis
pol′y·so′·ma·ty

pol'y·some
pol'y·so'·mia
pol'y·so'·mic
pol'y·som'·no·graph
pol'y·som'·no·graph'·ic
pol'y·som·nog'·ra·phy
pol'y·so'·my
pol'y·sper'·my *also* pol'y·sper'·mia
pol'y·spike' [pol'y·spike]
pol'y·sple'·nia
pol'y·sty'·rene
pol'y·syn·ap'·tic
pol'y·syn·dac'·ty·ly
pol'y·ten'·di·ni'·tis
pol'y·tene
pol'y·te·ni·za'·tion
pol'y·te'·ny
pol'y·the'·lia
po·lyt'·o·cous *also* ·kous
pol'y·top'·ic [·to'·pic]
pol'y·typ'·ic
pol'y·un·sat'·u·rat'·ed
pol'y·u'·ria
pol'y·u'·ri·dyl'·ic
pol'y·va'·lent
pol'y·vi'·nyl
pol'y·vi'·nyl·pyr·rol'·i·done
Po·mat'·i·op'·sis
pom'·pho·lyx
pom'·phus
pon·ceau'
po·ne'·si·at'·rics
Pon'·gi·dae
pons *pl.* pon'·tes, *gen. sg.* pon'·tis
pon'·ti·bra'·chi·um
pon'·tic
pon·tic'·u·lus
pon'·tine *also* ·tile
pon'·tis *gen. of* pons
pon'·to·bul'·bar
pon'·to·bul·ba'·re
pon'·to·cer'·e·bel'·lar
pon'·to·med'·ul·lar'·y

pon'·to·pe·dun'·cu·lar
pop'·les *pl.* pop'·li·tes, *gen. sg.* pop'·li·tis
pop·lit'·e·al [pop'·li·te'·al]
pop·lit'·e·a'·lis *pl.* ·les
pop'·li·te'·us *fem.* ·te'a, *neut.* ·te'·um
pop'·u·la'·tion
por'·ad·e·ni'·tis
por'·ce·lain
por'·cine
pore
por'·en·ce·phal'·ic
por'·en·ceph'·a·ly
po'·ri *pl. & gen. sg. of* porus
po'·rin
po'·ri·on
po'·ro·
po'·ro·cele
po'·ro·ceph'·a·li'·a·sis
Po'·ro·ce·phal'·i·dae
Po'·ro·ceph'·a·lus
po'·ro·ker'·a·to'·sis
po'·ro·ker'·a·tot'·ic
po·ro'·ma *pl.* ·mas *or* ·ma·ta
po'·ro·plas'·tic
po·ro'·sis
po·ros'·i·ty
po·rot'·ic
po·rot'·o·my
po'·rous
por'·phin
por'·pho·bi'·lin
por'·pho·bi·lin'·o·gen
por·phyr'·ia
por'·phy·rin
por'·phy·rin'·o·gen
por'·phy·rin·u'·ria [·ri·nu'·] *also* por'·phy·ru'·ria
por'·ta *pl. & gen. sg.* ·tae
por'·ta·ca'·val
por'·tal
por·ta'·lis

por'·ta·re'·nal
por'·ta·sys·tem'·ic *var. of* portosystemic
porte'·ai·guille'
por'·tio *pl.* por'·ti·o'·nes, *gen. sg.* por'·ti·o'·nis
por'·ti·plex'·us
por'·to·az'·y·gos
por'·to·ca'·val *var. of* portacaval
por'·to·gram
por·tog'·ra·phy
por'·to·sys·tem'·ic
por'·to·ve·nog'·ra·phy
po'·rus *pl. & gen. sg.* po'·ri
po·si'·tion
po·si'·tion·al
po·si'·tion·er
pos'·i·tive
pos'·i·tron
po'·so·log'·ic
po·sol'·o·gy
post'·abor'·tal
post'·ac'·i·dot'·ic
post·a'nal
post·an'·es·thet'·ic *Brit.* ·an'·aes·
post'·anox'·ic
post'·aor'·ti·cus *pl.* ·ci
post·ap'·o·plec'·tic
post·au'·di·to'·ry
post'·au·ric'·u·lar
post·ax'·i·al
post·bra'·chi·al
post·bul'·bar
post·cal'·ca·rine
post·cap'·il·lar'·y
post·car'·di·ac
post·car'·di·nal
post'·car'·di·ot'·o·my
post·ca'·va
post·ca'·val
post'·ca·va'·lis *pl.* ·les

post·ce'·cal　*Brit.*
　·cae'·
post·cen'·tral
post'·cen·tra'·lis
post·chi'·as·mat'·ic
post·cho'·le·cys·tec'·
　to·my
post·chrom'·ing
post·ci'·bal
post'·ci'·bum [cib'·um]
post'·cis·ter'·na
post·cli'·val
post·co'·ital
post'·co'·itum
post'·col·lic'·u·lar
post'·com·mis'·su·ral
post'·com·mis'·su·rot'·
　o·my
post'·com·mu'·ni·cal
post'·com·mu'·ni·ca'·
　lis
post'·con·cep'·tu·al
post'·con·cus'·sion·al
post'·con'·dy·la'·re
post'·con·vul'·sive
post·cor'·nu
post·cos'·tal
post·cra'·ni·al
post·cri'·coid
post·crit'·i·cal
post·dam'·ming
post'·di'·as·tol'·ic
post'·di·crot'·ic
post'·diph'·the·rit'·ic
　also ·diph·the'·ric
post·dor'·mi·tal
post·duc'·tal
post'·em'·bry·on'·ic
　also ·o'·nal
post'·en·ceph'·a·lit'·ic
post'·ep'·i·lep'·tic
pos·te'·ri·ad
pos·te'·ri·or　*pl.* pos·
　te'·ri·o'·res, *gen. sg.*
　·ris, *gen. pl* ·rum
pos·te'·ri·us　*neut. of*
　posterior; *pl.* pos·te'·ri·
　o'·ra

pos'·tero·
pos'·tero·an·te'·ri·or
pos'·tero·clu'·sion
pos'·tero·in·fe'·ri·or
pos'·tero·lat'·er·al
pos'·tero·lat'·er·a'·lis
pos'·tero·mar'·gin·al
pos'·tero·me'·dial
pos'·tero·me'·di·a'·lis
pos'·tero·me'·di·an
pos'·tero·me'·di·a'·na
pos'·tero·su·pe'·ri·or
pos'·tero·tem'·po·ral
pos'·tero·trans·verse'
pos'·tero·ve·sic'·u·lar
post'·erup'·tive
post'·evac'·u·a'·tion
post'·ex·an'·the·mat'·ic
post'·ex'·an·them'·a·
　tous [·the'·ma·]
post'·ex·po'·sure
post'·ex'·tra·sys·tol'·ic
post·fe'·brile [·feb'·rile]
post·fi'·bri·nous
post'·gan'·gli·on'·ic
post'·gas·trec'·to·my
post·gle'·noid
post'·glo·mer'·u·lar
post'·hem'·i·ple'·gic
post·hem'·or·rhage
　Brit. ·haem'·
post'·hem'·or·rhag'·ic
　Brit. ·haem'·
post'·he·pat'·ic
post'·hep'·a·tit'·ic
post'·her·pet'·ic
pos'·thi·o·plas'·ty
pos·thi'·tis
pos'·tho·lith
post'·hu·mous
post'·hy·oi'·de·an
post'·hyp·not'·ic
post'·hy'·po·gly·ce'·
　mic　*Brit.* ·cae'·
post'·hy·pox'·ic
post·ic'·tal
pos·ti'·cus　*fem.* ·ca,
　neut. ·cum

post·im'·mu·ni·za'·tion
post'·in·farc'·tion
post'·in·fec'·tious
post'·in·fec'·tive
post'·in'·flu·en'·zal
post'·in'·fun·dib'·u·lar
post'·inoc'·u·la'·tion
post'·ir·ra'·di·a'·tion
post·lu'·nate
post'·ma·lar'·i·al
post'·mas·tec'·to·my
post'·ma·ture'
post'·ma·tu'·ri·ty
post·max'·il·lar'·y
post'·me·a'tal
post'·me'·di·as·ti'·nal
post'·mei·ot'·ic
post'·men'·in·git'·ic
post'·men'o·paus'·al
　[·pau'·sal]
post·men'·stru·al
post'·mil'·i·ar'·i·al
post·min'·i·mus
post'·mi·tot'·ic
post'·mor'·tem　*adv.*
post·mor'·tem　*adj.*
post·na'·sal
post·na'·tal
post'·ne·crot'·ic
post'·ne'o·na'·tal
post'·neu·rit'·ic
post·nod'·u·lar
post·oc'·u·lar
post·ol'·i·var'y
post·op'·er·a·tive
post·o'ral
post·or'·bi·tal
post·ov'u·la·to'·ry
　[·o'·vu·]
post'·par'·a·lyt'·ic
post'·par'·tum　*adv.*
post·par'·tum　*adj.*
post'·per·fu'·sion
post'·per'·i·car'·di·ot'·
　o·my
post'·pha·ryn'·ge·al
post'·phle·bit'·ic
post'·pi·tu'·i·tar'y

post'·pneu·mon'·ic
post·pon'·tile
post·pran'·di·al
post·pri'·ma·ry
post'·py·ram'·i·dal
post'·ra'·di·a'·tion
post'·re'·nal
post'·re·sec'·tion
post'·ro·lan'·dic
post'·ro·ta'·tion·al
post·sphe'·noid
post'·sphe·noi'·dal
post·sphyg'·mic
post·spi'·nal
post'·sple·nec'·to·my
post'·ste·not'·ic
post·syl'·vi·an
post'·syn·ap'·tic
post'·sys·tol'·ic
post-term'
post'-te·tan'·ic
post'-throm·bot'·ic
post'-trau·mat'·ic
post'-tre·mat'·ic
post-tus'·sis
post-tus'·sive
pos'·tu·late
pos'·tur·al
pos'·ture
post·vac'·ci·nal
  following vaccination:
  Cf. postvaccinial
post'·vac·cin'·i·al
  following a vaccinia
  infection: Cf. postvac-
  cinal
post'·val'·vu·lot'·o·my
post·vi'·tal
post·zos'·ter
po'·ta·ble
pot'·ash
pot'·as·se'·mia   Brit.
  ·sae'·
po·tas'·si·um
po'·ten·cy

po'·tent
po·ten'·tial
po·ten'·ti·a'·tion
po·ten'·ti·a'·tor
po·ten'·ti·om'·e·ter
po·ten'·ti·o·met'·ric
po'·ten·tize ·tized,
  ·tiz'·ing
po'·tion
po'·to·ma'·nia
po'·tus   pl. potus
pouch
pou·drage'
poul'·tice
po'·vi·done
pow'·der
pow'·er
pox
Pox·vi'·ri·dae
pox'·vi'·rus
prac'·tice n. & v.
 ·ticed, ·tic·ing
prac'·tise[41] ·tised, ·tis·
  ing
prac·ti'·tion·er
prae'·cox
prae·pu'·ti·a'·lis   var.
  of preputialis
prae·pu'·tium   var. of
  preputium
prae'·sens
prae'·via   var. of
  previa
prag'·mat·ag·no'·sia
prag'·mat·am·ne'·sia
pra·mox'·ine
pran'·di·al
pra'·se·o·dym'·i·um
pra·tique'
prax'·is
pra'·zi·quan'·tel
pra'·zo·sin
pre'·ad·mis'·sion
pre·ag'·o·nal
pre'·al·bu'·min

pre'·am·biv'·a·lent
pre·a'nal
pre·an'·es·the'·sia
  Brit. ·an'·aes·
pre·an'·es·thet'·ic
  Brit. ·an'·aes·
pre'·aor'·tic
pre'·aor'·ti·cus   pl. ·ci
pre'·au·ric'·u·lar
pre'·au·ric'·u·la'·ris
  pl. ·res
pre·ax'·i·al
pre'·be'·ta·lip'o·pro'·
  tein·e'·mia   Brit.
  ·ae'·mia
pre·bra'·chial
pre·bul'·bar
pre·can'·cer·ous
pre·cap'·il·lar'y
pre'·car·cin'·o·gen
pre·car'·di·nal
pre·car'·di·na'·lis
pre·car'·ti·lage
pre·ca'·va
pre·ca'·val
pre'·ca·va'·lis   pl. ·les
pre'·ce·ca'·lis   also
  ·cae·ca'·; pl. ·les
pre·cen'·tral
pre'·cen·tra'·lis
pre·cep'·tor
pre'·chi'·as·mat'·i·cus
pre·chor'·dal [·chord'·
  al]
pre·cip'·i·ta·ble
pre·cip'·i·tant
pre·cip'·i·tate   adj. &
  v. ·tat'·ed, ·tat'·ing
pre·cip'·i·ta'·tion
pre·cip'·i·tin
pre·cip'·i·tin'·o·gen
  also pre·cip'·i·to·gen
pre·ci'·sion
pre·clin'·i·cal
pre·cli'·val

---

[41] In British usage, the noun is spelled *practice* and the verb is spelled *practise*.

pre·co′·cious
pre·coc′·i·ty
pre′·cog·ni′·tion
pre·co′·ital
pre′·col·lag′·e·nous
pre·co′·ma
pre′·com·mis′·su·ral
pre·con′·scious
pre′·con·vul′·sive
pre·cor′·di·al
pre·cor′·di·um also ·dia
pre·cor′·ne·al
pre·cri′·coid
pre·crit′·i·cal
pre·cu′·ne·al
pre·cu′·ne·us
pre·cur′·sor
pre·cur′·so·ry
pre′·de·cid′·u·ous
pre′·de·liv′·ery
pre·den′·tin
pre′·di′·a·be′·tes
pre′·di′·a·bet′·ic
pre·di′·a·stol′·ic
pre·dic′·tor
pre′·di·ges′·ted
pre′·di·ges′·tion
pre′·dis·pose′ ·posed′, ·pos′·ing
pre′·dis·po·si′·tion
pred·nis′·o·lone
pred′·ni·sone
pre·dor′·mi·tal
pre·dor′·sal
pre·duc′·tal
pre′·eclamp′·sia
pre′·eclamp′·tic
pre·emp′·tive
pre′·erup′·tive
pre′·eryth′·ro·cyt′·ic
pre·ex′·ci·ta′·tion
pre′·ex·po′·sure
pre′·fi·brot′·ic
pre′·for·ma′·tion
pre·fron′·tal
pre·func′·tion·al
pre′·gan′·gli·on′·ic

pre·gen′·i·tal
pre·gle′·noid
pre′·glo·mer′·u·lar
preg′·nan·cy
preg′·nane
preg′·nane·di′·ol
preg′·nane·tri′·ol
preg′·nant
preg′·nene
preg′·nen·in′·o·lone
preg·nen′·o·lone
pre·gran′·u·lo′·sa
pre·hal′·lux
pre′·hem′·i·ple′·gic
pre·hen′·sile
pre·hen′·sion
pre·hen′·so·ry
pre′·he·pat′·ic
pre·hor′·mone
pre·hy′·oid
pre·ic′·tal
pre′·in·duc′·tion
pre′·in·farc′·tion
pre·in′·su·la
pre·in′·su·lar
pre·in′·ter·pa·ri′·etal
pre′·in·va′·sive
pre′·kal′·li·kre′·in
pre·lac′·te·al
pre′·la·ryn′·geal
pre′·la·ryn′·ge·a′·lis pl. ·les
pre·lep′·to·tene
pre′·leu·ke′·mia Brit. ·kae′·
pre′·leu·ke′·mic Brit. ·kae′·
pre′·lo′·cal·i·za′·tion
pre·lu′·nate
pre′·ma·lig′·nant
pre·mam′·il·lar′y
pre′·mam′·ma·ry
pre′·ma·ture′
pre′·ma·tu′·ri·ty
pre·max·il′·la
pre′·max′·il·lar′y
pre·med′
pre·med′·i·cal

pre·med′·i·cant
pre·med′·i·cate ·cat′·ed, ·cat′·ing
pre′·med′·i·ca′·tion
pre′·mei·ot′·ic
pre·men′·ar·che
pre′·men′o·paus′·al [·pau′·sal]
pre·men′·stru·al
pre·men′·stru·um pl. ·strua
pre′·mi·tot′·ic
pre·mo′·lar
pre′·mo·la′·ris pl. ·res
pre·mon′·i·to′·ry
pre·mon′·o·cyte var. of promonocyte
pre·mor′·bid
pre·mor′·tal
pre·mo′·tor
pre′·mu·ni′·tion
pre·mu′·ni·tive
pre′·my·cot′·ic
pre·my′·e·lo·cyte var. of promyelocyte
pre·na′·res sg. ·ris
pre·na′·sal
pre·na′·tal
pre′·ne′·o·plas′·tic
pre·nod′·u·lar
pren′·yl
pre′·oc·cip′·i·tal
pre′·oc·cip′·i·ta′·lis
pre·oe′·di·pal [·oed′·i·]
pre·ol′·i·var′y
pre′·op′·er·a′·tion·al
pre·op′·er·a·tive
pre′·oper′·cu·lum
pre·op′·tic
pre·o′ral
pre·ov′u·la·to′·ry [·o′vu·]
pre′·par′·a·lyt′·ic
prep′·a·ra′·tion
pre′·pa·ret′·ic
pre·par′·tal
pre′·pa·tel′·lar

pre·pa′·ten·cy *also*
 pa′·tence
pre·pa′·tent
pre′·per·i·car′·di·ac
pre′·per′·i·car′·di·a′·lis
 pl. ·les
pre′·per′·i·to·ne′·al
pre·pir′·i·form
pre′·pla·cen′·tal
pre·pol′·lex
pre·pon′·der·ance
pre′·po·ten′·tial
pre·pran′·di·al
pre′·pro·hor′·mone
pre′·pro·in′·su·lin
pre′·pro·par′a·thy′·roid
pre·pu′·ber·tal
pre·pu′·ber·ty
pre′·pu·bes′·cence
pre′·pu·bes′·cent
pre′·puce
pre·pu′·tial
pre·pu′·ti·a′·lis *pl.*
 ·les
pre·pu′·tio·la′·bi·al
pre·pu′·ti·ot′·o·my
 also pre′·pu·cot′·o·my
pre·pu′·ti·um *gen.* ·tii
pre′·py·lo′·ric
pre′·py·lo′·ri·ca
pre·rec′·tal
pre′·re·duc′·tion
pre·re′·nal
pre·ren′·nin
pre·ret′·i·nal
pre′·ro·lan′·dic
pre·ru′·bral
pre·sa′·cral
pres′·by *also* pres′·byo·
pres′·by·at′·rics
pres′·by·cu′·sis *also*
 ·acu′·sia *or* ·acu′·sis
pres′·by·ope
pres′·by·o·phre′·nia
pres′·by·o′·pia
pres′·by·o′·pic
pre·scap′·u·la

pre·scribe′ ·scribed′,
 ·scrib′·ing
pre·scrip′·tion
pre′·se·cre′·to·ry
pre·sec′·tion
pre′·seg·ment′·er
pre·se′·nile
pre·sent′ *v.*
pres′·en·ta′·tion
pre·ser′·va·tive
pre·so′·mite
pre·sper′·ma·tid
pre·sphe′·noid
pre′·sphe·noi′·dal
pre·sphyg′·mic
pre′·spon′·dy·lo·lis·
 the′·sis
pres′·sor
pres′·so·re·cep′·tive
pres′·so·re·cep′·tor
pres′·so·sen′·si·tive
pres′·sure
pre·ster′·nal
pre·stri′·ate
pre′·su·bic′·u·lum
pre·sump′·tive
pre·sup′·pu·ra′·tive
pre·syl′·vi·an
pre·symp′·tom
pre′·symp′·to·mat′·ic
pre′·syn·ap′·tic
pre·sys′·to·le
pre′·sys·tol′·ic
pre·tar′·sal
pre·tec′·tal
pre·tec′·tum
pre·term′
pre·ter′·mi·nal
pre′·test *n.*
pre·test′ *v.*
pre·tib′·i·al
pre·tra′·che·al
pre′·tra′·che·a′·lis *pl.*
 ·les
pre′·tre·mat′·ic
pre′·tu·ber′·cu·lous
pre′·ure′·thral
prev′·a·lence

pre·vent′·a·ble *also*
 ·i·ble
pre·ven′·tion
pre·ven′·tive *also* ·ta·
 tive
pre′·ven·to′·ri·um
pre′·ven·tric′·u·lo′·sis
pre′·ven·tric′·u·lus
pre·ver′·te·bral
pre·ves′·i·cal
pre·vi′·a·ble
pre·vil′·lous
pre·vi′·ta·min var. of
 provitamin
pre′·vi·us *fem.* ·via,
 neut. ·vi·um
pre′·zone *var. of*
 prozone
pre·zo′·nu·lar [·zon′·
 u·]
pri′·a·pis′m
pri′·a·pi′·tis
prick′·le
prick′·ly
pril′·o·caine
pri′·ma·cy
pri′·mal
prim′·a·quine [pri′·
 ma·]
pri·ma′·ri·us
pri′·ma·ry
pri′·mate
Pri·ma′·tes
pri′·ma·tol′·o·gy
prime primed, prim′·
 ing
pri′·mer
pri′·mi *gen. of* primus
 & primum
pri′·mi·done
pri′·mi·grav′·id
pri′·mi·grav′·i·da *pl.*
 ·das *or* ·dae
pri·mip′·a·ra *pl.* ·ras
 or rae
pri′·mi·par′·i·ty
pri·mip′·a·rous
pri·mi′·ti·ae

prim'·i·ti·va'·tion
 also ·tiv·i·za'·tion
prim'·i·tive
pri·mor'·di·al
pri·mor'·di·a'·lis
pri·mor'·di·um pl.
 ·dia
pri'·mum neut. of
 primus; gen. ·mi
pri'·mus gen. ·mi
prin'·ceps
prin'·ci·pal most
 important: Cf. principle
prin'·ci·pa'·lis
prin'·ci·ple rule: Cf.
 principal
pri'·on
Pri'·o·nu'·rus
pris'm
pris'·ma pl. ·ma·ta
pris·mat'·ic
pris'·moid
pris'·mop·tom'·e·ter
 also pris'·op·
priv'·i·lege
pro'·ac·cel'·er·in
pro'·ac'·ro·som'·al
 [·so'·mal]
pro'·ac·tin'·i·um var.
 of protactinium
pro·ac'·ti·va'·tor
pro·ac'·tive
pro·an'·gi·o·ten'·sin
pro'·ar·rhyth'·mia
pro·at'·las
prob'·a·bil'·i·ty
pro'·bac·te'·ri·o·phage
pro'·band
pro'·bang
pro·bar'·bi·tal
probe n. & v. probed,
 prob'·ing
pro·ben'·e·cid
pro'·bit
pro·bos'·cis pl. ·ci·des
pro'·bu·col
pro·cain'·a·mide
pro'·caine

pro·cal'·lus
pro·car'·ba·zine
pro'·car·cin'·o·gen
 [·car'·ci·no·gen']
pro·car'y·ote var. of
 prokaryote
pro·car'y·ot'·ic var.
 of prokaryotic
pro'·ca·tarc'·tic
pro'·ca·tarx'·is
pro·ce'·dure
pro·ce'·lia var. of
 procoelia
pro·cen'·tri·ole
pro·cer'·coid
pro·ce'·rus
pro'·cess [proc'·ess]
pro·ces'·sus pl. &
 gen. sg. processus
pro·chei'·lon
pro'·chlor·per'·a·zine
pro·chon'·dral
pro·chor'·dal [·chord'·
 al] var. of pre-
 chordal
pro'·ci·den'·tia
proc'·li·na'·tion
pro'·co·ag'·u·lant
pro·coe'·lia
pro·col'·la·gen
pro'·con·cep'·tive
pro'·con·ver'·tin
pro'·cre·a'·tion
pro'·cre·a'·tive
proc·tal'·gia
proct'·ec·ta'·sia
proc·tec'·to·my
proc·ti'·tis
proc'·to·
proc'·to·cele
proc·toc'·ly·sis pl.
 ·ses
proc'·to·coc'·cy·pex'y
proc'·to·co·lec'·to·my
proc'·to·co·li'·tis
proc'·to·co'·lo·nos'·co·
 py

proc'·to·col'·po·plas'·
 ty
proc'·to·cys'·to·cele
proc'·to·cys'·to·plas'·ty
proc'·to·cys·tot'·o·my
proc'·to·de'·um Brit.
 ·dae'·um
proc'·to·dyn'·ia
proc'·to·log'·ic also
 ·i·cal
proc·tol'·o·gist
proc·tol'·o·gy
proc'·to·pa·ral'·y·sis
proc'·to·per'·i·ne'·o·
 plas'·ty
proc'·to·per'·i·ne·or'·
 rha·phy
proc'·to·pex'y
proc'·to·plas'·ty
proc'·to·ple'·gia
proc'·top·to'·sis
proc'·tor·rha'·gia
proc'·tor·rhe'a Brit.
 ·rhoe'a
proc'·to·scope
proc'·to·scop'·ic
proc·tos'·co·py
proc'·to·sig'·moid·ec'·
 to·my
proc'·to·sig'·moid·i'·tis
proc'·to·sig·moi'·do·
 pex'y
proc'·to·sig·moi'·do·
 scope
proc'·to·sig'·moid·os'·
 co·py
proc'·to·stat
proc'·to·ste·no'·sis
proc·tos'·to·my
proc·tot'·o·my
proc'·to·val·vot'·o·my
pro·cum'·bent
pro'·cur·si'·va
pro·cur'·sive
pro'·cur·va'·tion
pro·cy'·cli·dine
pro'·dro·ma pl. pro·
 dro'·ma·ta; var. of
 prodrome

pro·dro′·mal
pro′·drome
prod′·uct
pro·duc′·tion
pro·duc′·tive
pro′·elas′·tase
pro·e′mi·al
pro′·en·ceph′·a·ly
pro′·en·keph′·a·lin
pro·en′·zyme
pro′·eryth′·ro·blast
pro·es′·trus   *also*   ·trum
pro·fes′·sion·al
pro′·fi′·bri·no·ly′·sin
pro′·fil·ac′·tin
pro′·file
pro·fi′·lin
pro·fla′·vine   *also*   ·vin
pro′·flu·ens
pro·flu′·vi·um
pro·fun′·da   *fem. of*
   profundus; *pl. & gen.*
   sg. ·dae
pro·fun′·da·plas′·ty
pro·fun′·dum   *neut. of*
   profundus
pro·fun′·dus   *pl. &*
   gen. sg. ·di
pro·gas′·trin
pro·ge′·nia
pro·gen′·i·ta′·lis
pro·gen′·i·tor
prog′·e·ny
pro·ge′·ria [·ger′·ia]
pro′·ges·ta′·tion·al
pro·ges′·ter·one
pro·ges′·tin
pro·ges′·to·gen
pro·glot′·tid
pro·glot′·tis   *pl.*   ·ti·
   des; *var. of* proglottid
prog′·na·this′m
prog′·na·thous   *also*
   prog·nath′·ic
prog·nose′   ·nosed′,
   ·nos′·ing
prog·no′·sis   *pl.*   ·ses
prog·nos′·tic

prog·nos′·ti·cate   ·cat′·
   ed, ·cat′·ing
pro′·go·no′·ma
pro′·gram   *n. & v.*
   ·gramed *or* ·grammed,
   ·gram·ing *or* ·gram·ming
pro·gran′·u·lo·cyte
pro·gran′·u·lo·cyt′·ic
pro·grav′·id
prog′·ress   *n.*
pro·gress′   *v.*
pro·gres′·sion
pro′·gres·si′·va
pro·gres′·sive
pro·gua′·nil
pro·hor′·mone
pro·in′·su·lin
pro·jec′·tion
pro·kar′y·ote
pro·kar′y·ot′·ic
pro·la′·bi·um
pro·lac′·tin
pro′·lapse   *n.*
pro·lapse′   *n. & v.*
   ·lapsed, ·laps′·ing
pro·lap′·sus
pro·lep′·tic
pro·leu′·ko·cyte
pro·lif′·er·ans
pro·lif′·er·ate   ·at′·ed,
   ·at′·ing
pro·lif′·er·a′·tion
pro·lif′·er·a·tive
pro·lif′·er·ous
pro·lif′·ic
pro′·line
pro′·lin·e′·mia   *Brit.*
   ·ae′·mia
pro′·lo·ther′·a·py
pro′·lyl
pro·lym′·pho·cyte
pro′·lym′·pho·cyt′·ic
pro·mas′·ti·gote
pro′·ma·zine
pro′·meg′a·kar′y·o·cyte
pro·meg′·a·lo·blast
pro·met′a·phase
pro·meth′·a·zine

pro′·meth·es′·trol
   [·meth′·es·trol]
   Brit. ·oes′·trol
pro·me′·thi·um
prom′·i·nence
prom′·i·nens
prom′·i·nen′·tia   *pl. &*
   gen. sg. ·ti·ae
pro·mon′·o·cyte
prom′·on·to′·ri·um
   gen. ·rii
prom′·on·to′·ry
pro·mot′·er
pro·mox′·o·lane
pro·my′·e·lo·cyte
pro′·my′·e·lo·cyt′·ic
pro′·nase
pro′·nate   ·nat·ed, ·nat·
   ing
pro·na′·tion
pro·na′·to·flex′·or
pro′·na·tor   *gen.* pro′·
   na·to′·ris
prone
pro·neph′·ric
pro′·neph′·ro·gen′·ic
pro·neph′·ron
pro·neph′·ros   *pl.* ·roi
pro′·ne·phrot′·ic
pro′·no·grade
pro·nor′·mo·blast
pro·nu′·cle·us   *pl.* ·clei
pro·oes′·trus   *Brit.*
   spel. of proestrus
prop′·a·gate   ·gat′·ed,
   ·gat′·ing
prop′·a·ga′·tion
pro·pal′·i·nal
pro′·pane
pro′·pa·nol
pro·pan′·the·line
pro·par′·a·caine
pro′·par′a·thy′·roid
pro′·pene
prop′·er
pro·per′·din
pro·per′·i·to·ne′·al
pro′·phage

pro′·phase
pro′·phen·py·rid′·a·
  mine
pro′·phy·lac′·tic
pro′·phy·lax′·is
pro′·pi·cil′·lin
pro′·pio·lac′·tone
pro′·pi·o·nate
pro′·pi·on′i·bac′·ter
  [·o′ni·]
Pro′·pi·on′i·bac·te′·ri·
  um [·o′ni·]
  P. ac′·nes
pro′·pi·on′·ic
pro′·pi·o·nyl
pro·plas′·tid
pro′·pons
pro·por′·tion·ate
pro·pos′·i·ta fem. of
  propositus; pl. ·tae
pro·pos′·i·tus pl. ·ti
pro·pox′·y·caine
pro·pran′·o·lol
pro′·pria fem. of
  proprius; pl. & gen. sg.
  ·pri·ae
pro·pri′·etar′y
pro′·prii pl. & gen. sg.
  of proprius
pro′·pri·o·cep′·tion
pro′·pri·o·cep′·tive
pro′·pri·o·cep′·tor
pro′·prio·spi′·nal
pro′·pri·um neut. of
  proprius
pro′·pri·us pl. & gen.
  sg. ·prii
prop·tom′·e·ter
prop·to′·sis [pro·pto′·]
pro′·pyl
pro′·pyl·ene
pro′·pyl·hex′·e·drine
pro′·pyl·thi′o·u′ra·cil
pro re′ na′·ta
pro·ren′·nin
pro·ru′·bri·cyte
pro′·scil·lar′·i·din
pro′·se·cre′·tion

pro·sec′·tion
pro·sec′·tor
pros′·en′·ce·phal′·ic
pros′·en·ceph′·a·lon
pros′o·
pros′·o·branch
pros′·o·dem′·ic
pros′·op·ag·no′·sia
pros′·o·pal′·gia
pros′·o·pla′·sia
pros′·o·po·
pros′·o·po·di·ple′·gia
pros′·o·po·dys·mor′·
  phia
pros′·o·pop′·a·gus
pros′·o·pos′·chi·sis
pros′·o·po·tho′·ra·cop′·
  a·gus
pro·spec′·tive
pros′·ta·cy′·clin
pros′·ta·glan′·din
pros′·ta·no′·ic
pros′·ta·noid
pros′·ta·ta gen. ·ta·tae
pros′·ta·tal′·gia
pros′·tate
pros′·ta·tec′·to·my
pros·tat′·ic
pros·tat′·i·ca fem. of
  prostaticus
pros·tat′·i·co·ves′·i·cal
pros·tat′·i·cus pl. &
  gen. sg. ·ci
pros′·ta·tis′m
pros′·ta·ti′·tis
pros′·ta·to·
pros′·ta·to·cys·ti′·tis
pros′·ta·to·cys·tot′·o·
  my
pros′·ta·to·lith
pros′·ta·to·li·thot′·o·my
pros′·ta·to·meg′·a·ly
pros′·ta·to·my′·o·mec′·
  to·my
pros′·ta·tor·rhe′a
  Brit. ·rhoe′a
pros′·ta·tot′·o·my
  also prostat′·o·my

pros′·ta·to·ve·sic′·u·
  lec′·to·my
pros′·ta·to·ve·sic′·u·li′·
  tis
pros·the′·sis pl. ·ses
pros·thet′·ic
pros·thet′·ics
pros′·the·tist
pros′·thi·on
pros′·tho·don′·tia
pros′·tho·don′·tics
pros′·tho·don′·tist
pros′·tho·ker′·a·to·
  plas′·ty
pros·tra′·tion
pro′·tac·tin′·i·um
pro′·ta·mine
pro′·tan
pro·tan′·drous
prot′·anom′·a·lous
prot′·anom′·a·ly
pro′·tan·ope
pro′·tan·o′·pia also
  ·op′·sia
pro′·tan·o′·pic
pro′·te·an assuming
  different forms: Cf.
  protein
pro′·te·ase
pro·tec′·tin
pro·tec′·tion
pro·tec′·tive
pro·tec′·tor
pro′·tein substance
  composed of amino
  acids: Cf. protean
pro′·tein·a′·ceous
pro′·tein·ase
pro′·tein·o′·sis
pro′·tein·u′·ria
pro′·tein·u′·ric
pro′·te·o·gly′·can
pro′·te·ol′·y·sis
pro′·te·o·lyt′·ic
pro′·teo·me·tab′·o·
  lis′m
pro′·te·o·mor′·phic
pro′·te·o·pep′·sis

pro'·teo·pep'·tic
pro'·te·o·pex'·ic *also*
  ·pec'·tic
pro'·te·o·pex'y *also*
  pro'·te·o·pex'·is
pro'·te·o·se'·mia *Brit.*
  ·sae'·
pro'·ter·o·glyph'·ic
pro'·test
Pro'·te·us
proth'·e·sis *var. of*
  prosthesis
pro·thet'·ic *var. of*
  prosthetic
pro'·thi·pen'·dyl
pro·throm'·bin
pro·throm'·bin·ase
pro·throm'·bin·o·gen
pro·throm'·bin·o·pe'·nia
pro'·tide
pro'·tist
Pro·tis'·ta
pro'·ti·um
pro'·to·
pro'·to·ac·tin'·i·um
  var. of protactinium
pro'·to·blast
pro'·to·chlo'·ro·phyll
pro'·to·chon'·dri·um
pro'·to·chor'·dal
  [·chord'·al]
pro'·to·chor'·date
pro'·to·col
pro'·to·cone
pro'·to·co'·nid
pro'·to·cop'·ro·por·phyr'·ia
pro'·to·di·as'·to·le
pro'·to·di'·a·stol'·ic
pro'·to·du'·o·de'·num
pro'·to·elas'·tin
pro'·to·fi'·bril
pro'·to·fil'·a·ment
pro'·to·gon'·o·cyte
pro'·to·heme *Brit.*
  ·haem

pro'·to·he'·min *Brit.*
  ·hae'·min
pro'·to·ky'·lol
pro·tom'·e·ter
pro'·ton
pro'·to·nate [·ton·ate]
  ·nat'·ed, ·nat'·ing
pro'·to·on'·co·gene
pro'·to·path'·ic
pro'·to·pi'·a·no'·ma
  [·an·o'·ma]
pro'·to·pine
pro'·to·plas'm
pro'·to·plas'·mic *also*
  ·plas·mat'·ic
pro'·to·plas·mol'·y·sis
pro'·to·plast
pro'·to·por·phyr'·ia
pro'·to·por'·phy·rin
pro·top'·sis
pro'·to·spore
pro'·to·sul'·fate *Brit.*
  ·phate
pro'·to·syph'·i·lis
pro'·to·tax'·ic
pro'·to·the·co'·sis
pro'·to·troph
pro'·to·tro'·phic
  [·troph'·ic] *lacking a specific growth requirement: Cf.* prototropic
pro·tot'·ro·phy
pro'·to·tro'·pic [·trop'·ic] *acting upon proteins: Cf.* prototrophic
pro·tot'·ro·py
pro'·to·type
pro'·to·ver'·a·trine
pro'·to·ver'·ine
pro'·to·ver'·te·bra
Pro'·to·zo'a
pro'·to·zo'a *pl. of*
  protozoon
pro'·to·zo'·ag·glu'·ti·nin
pro'·to·zo'·al

pro'·to·zo'·an
pro'·to·zo·i'·a·sis *also*
  ·zo·o'·sis
pro'·to·zo'·icide *also*
  ·zo'·a·cide
pro'·to·zo·ol'·o·gy
pro'·to·zo'·on *pl.* ·zoa
pro'·to·zo'·o·phage
pro'·to·zo'o·ther'·a·py
pro·tract'
pro·trac'·tion
pro·trac'·tor
pro·trud'·ed
pro·tru'·sio
pro·tru'·sion
pro·tru'·sive
pro·tryp'·sin
pro·tu'·ber·ance
pro·tu'·ber·an'·tia
Prov'·i·den'·cia
pro·vid'·er
pro'·vi'·ral
pro'·vi'·rus
pro'·vi'·ta·min
prov'·o·ca'·tion
pro·voc'·a·tive
Pro'·wa·zek'·ia
prox·e'·mics
prox'·i·mad
prox'·i·mal
prox'·i·ma'·lis
prox'·i·mate
prox'·i·mo·
pro'·zon·al
pro'·zone
pru·rig'·i·no'·sa
pru·rig'·i·nous
pru·ri'·go
pru·rit'·ic
pru·ri'·tus
prus'·si·ate
prus'·sic
psal·te'·ri·um *gen.* ·rii
psam'·mo·
psam·mo'·ma *pl.* ·mas
  or ·ma·ta
psam·mom'·a·tous
  [·mo'·ma·]

psam'·mo·ther'·a·py
psau·os'·co·py
psel'·lism
pseud'·acou'·sis
pseud'·agraph'·ia *var.*
  of pseudoagraphia
pseud'·al·bu'·min·u'·ria
  [·mi·nu'·]
Pseud·al'·les·che'·ria
  P. boyd'·ii
pseud·al'·les·che·ri'·a·sis
pseud'·am·ne'·sia
pseud'·an·ky·lo'·sis
pseud'·arth·ro'·sis *pl.*
  ·ses
Pseu·de'·chis
pseud'·es·the'·sia
  Brit. ·aes·the'·
pseu'·di·no'·ma
pseu'·do·
pseu'·do·ac'·an·tho'·sis
pseu'·do·achon'·dro·plas'·tic
pseu'·do·ac'·ti·no·my·co'·sis
pseu'·do·ag·glu'·ti·na'·tion
pseu'·do·ag·gres'·sion
pseu'·do·agraph'·ia
pseu'·do·al·lele'
pseu'·do·al·le'·lic
pseu'·do·al·lel'·ism
pseu'·do·amen'·or·rhe'a *Brit.* ·rhoe'a
pseu'·do·an'a·phy·lax'·is
pseu'·do·an'·eu·rys'm
pseu'·do·an·gi'·na
  [·an'·gi·]
pseu'·do·an'·ky·lo'·sis
  var. of pseudankylosis
pseu'·do·an·tag'·o·nist
pseu'·do·ap·pen'·di·ci'·tis
pseu'·do·ar·thro'·sis
  var. of pseudarthrosis
pseu'·do·ath'·e·to'·sis

pseu'·do·at'·ro·pho·der'·ma
pseu'·do·bul'·bar
pseu'·do·car'·ti·lage
pseu'·do·car'·ti·lag'·i·nous
pseu'·do·cele *var. of*
  pseudocoele
pseu'·do·ceph'·a·lo·cele
pseu'·do·chan'·cre
pseu'·do·cho·les'·te·a·to'·ma
pseu'·do·cho'·lin·es'·ter·ase
pseu'·do·chrom'·es·the'·sia *Brit.* ·aes·the'·
pseu'·do·chy'·lous
pseu'·do·cir·rho'·sis
pseu'·do·clau'·di·ca'·tion
pseu'·do·co'·arc·ta'·tion
pseu'·do·coele *also*
  ·coel
pseu'·do·coe'·lo·mate
pseu'·do·cow'·pox
pseu'·do·cri'·sis
pseu'·do·croup
pseu'·do·crypt·or'·chi·dis'm *also* ·or'·chism
pseu'·do·cy·e'·sis
pseu'·do·cyst
pseu'·do·de·cid'·ua
pseu'·do·de·men'·tia
pseu'·do·dex'·tro·car'·dia
pseu'·do·di'·a·be'·tes
pseu'·do·dom'·i·nance
pseu'·do·ede'·ma
  Brit. ·do-oe·de'·
pseu'·do·elas'·tin
pseu'·do·ephed'·rine
pseu'·do·ep'·i·lep'·sy
pseu'·do·epiph'·y·sis

pseu'·do·ep'·i·the'·li·o'·ma·tous [·om'a·]
pseu'·do·ero'·sion
pseu'·do·es·the'·sia
  var. of pseudesthesia;
  Brit. ·aes·the'·
pseu'·do·ex·fo'·li·a·tive
pseu'·do·fol·lic'·u·lar
pseu'·do·fol·lic'·u·li'·tis
pseu'·do·gan'·gli·on
pseu'·do·gene
pseu'·do·geu'·sia
pseu'·do·gli·o'·ma *pl.*
  ·mas *or* ·ma·ta
pseu'·do·glob'·u·lin
pseu'·do·gout
pseu'·do·gy'·ne·co·mas'·tia *Brit.* ·gy'·nae·co·
pseu'·do·hal·lu'·ci·na'·tion
pseu'·do·hem'·ag·glu'·ti·na'·tion *Brit.* ·haem'·
pseu'·do·he'·ma·tu'·ria
  Brit. ·hae'·
pseu'·do·he·mop'·ty·sis
  Brit. ·hae·
pseu'·do·her·maph'·ro·dite
pseu'·do·her·maph'·ro·dit·is'm *also* ·ro·dis'm
pseu'·do·hy'·dro·ceph'·a·lus
pseu'·do·hy'·per·ka·le'·mia *Brit.* ·lae'·
pseu'·do·hy'·per·tro'·phic [·troph'·ic]
pseu'·do·hy·per'·tro·phy
pseu'·do·hy'·po·al·dos'·ter·on·is'm [·al'·do·ster'·on·]
pseu'·do·hy'·po·na·tre'·mia *Brit.* ·trae'·
pseu'·do·hy'·po·par'a·thy'·roid·is'm

pseu′·do·hy′·po·thy′·roid·is′m
pseu′·do·ic′·ter·us
pseu′·do·in′·flu·en′·za
pseu′·do·in′·ti·ma
pseu′·do·in′·tra·lig′·a·men′·tous
pseu′·do·i′so·chro·mat′·ic
pseu′·do·jaun′·dice
pseu′·do·ker′·a·tin
pseu′·do·le·prom′·a·tous [·pro′·ma·]
pseu′·do·li·po′·ma
pseu′·do·li·thi′·a·sis
pseu′·do·lym·pho′·ma *pl.* ·mas *or* ·ma·ta
pseu′·do·meg′a·co′·lon
pseu′·do·me′·lia
pseu′·do·mem′·brane
pseu′·do·mem′·bra·nous
pseu′·do·men′·in·gi′·tis
pseu′·do·men′·stru·a′·tion
pseu′·do·met′·a·tro′·pic [·trop′·ic]
pseu′·do·mi′·cro·ceph′·a·ly
pseu′·do·mil′·i·um
pseu′·do·mo′·nad
Pseu′·do·mo′·na·da′·ce·ae
Pseu′·do·mo′·nas [*Pseu·dom′·o·nas*]
P. ae·ru′·gi·no′·sa
P. fluo·res′·cens
P. mal′·lei
P. pseu′·do·mal′·lei
pseu′·do·mo′·ti·va′·tion
pseu′·do·mo′·tor
pseu′·do·mu′·ci·nous
pseu′·do·mus′·cu·lar
pseu′·do·my′·as·the′·nia
pseu′·do·my·ce′·li·um
pseu′·do·my·i′·a·sis
pseu′·do·my′·o·to′·nia

pseu′·do·my′·o·ton′·ic
pseu′·do·myx·o′·ma
pseu′·do·myx′o·vi′·rus
pseu′·do·ne′·o·plas′m
pseu′·do·neu·rot′·ic
pseu′·do·nu·cle′·o·lus
pseu′·do·nys·tag′·mus
pseu′·do-ob·struc′·tion
pseu′·do-o′chro·no′·sis
pseu′·do-o′vum
pseu′·do·pa·pil′·le·de′·ma *Brit.* ·pil′·loe·
pseu′·do·pa·ral′y·sis
pseu′·do·par′·a·lyt′·i·ca
pseu′·do·par′·a·site
pseu′·do·par′·kin·son·is′m
pseu′·do·pe·lade′
pseu′·do·pha′·kia
pseu′·do·phleg′·mon
pseu′·do·phyl′·lid *also* ·phyl·lid′·e·an
Pseu′·do·phyl·lid′·ea
pseu′·do·ple′·gia
pseu′·do·pock′·et
pseu′·do·pod
pseu′·do·po′·di·um *pl.* ·dia
pseu′·do·pol′y·me′·lia
pseu′·do·pol′·yp
pseu′·do·pol′·yp·o′·sis
pseu′·do·por′·en·ceph′·a·ly
pseu′·do·preg′·nan·cy
pseu′·do·pseu′·do·hy′·po·par′a·thy′·roid·is′m
pseu′·do·pto′·sis
pseu′·do·pty′·a·lis′m
pseu′·do·pu′·ber·ty
pseu′·do·py·lo′·ric
pseu′·do·ra′·bies
pseu′·do·re·ac′·tion
pseu′·do·ret′·i·ni′·tis
pseu′·do·rick′·ets
pseu′·do·ro·sette′
pseu′·do·sar·co′·ma

pseu′·do·sar·com′a·tous [·co′·ma·]
pseu′·do·scar′·la·ti′·na
pseu′·do·scler′·o·der′·ma
pseu′·do·scle·ro′·sis
pseu′·do·scro′·tum
pseu·dos′·to·ma [pseu′·do·sto′·ma]
pseu′·do·stra·bis′·mus
pseu′·do·strat′·i·fied
pseu′·do·struc′·ture
pseu′·do·ta′·bes
pseu′·do·ta·bet′·ic
pseu′·do·tet′·a·nus
pseu′·do·tra·cho′·ma
pseu′·do·tris′·mus
pseu′·do·tu′·ber·cle
pseu′·do·tu·ber′·cu·lo′·ma
pseu′·do·tu·ber′·cu·lo′·sis
pseu′·do·tu·ber′·cu·lous
pseu′·do·tu′·bule
pseu′·do·tu′·mor *Brit.* ·mour
pseu′·do·tym′·pa·ni′·tes
pseu′·do·u′·ri·dine
pseu′·do·urid′·y·late
pseu′·do·u′·ri·dyl′·ic
pseu′·do·vac′·u·ole
pseu′·do·ven′·tri·cle
pseu′·do·ver′·mi·cule
pseu′·do·ver·mic′·u·lus *pl.* ·li
pseu′·do·vil′·lus *pl.* ·li
pseu′·do·vi′·ri·on
pseu′·do·xan·tho′·ma *pl.* ·mas *or* ·ma·ta
psi′·lo·cin
psi′·lo·cy′·bin
psi·lo′·sis
psit′·ta·co′·sis
pso′·as *pl.* pso′·ai
psoph′·o·gen′·ic

pso′·ra·len
psor′·en′·ter·i′·tis
pso′·ri·as′·i·form
pso·ri′·a·sis
pso′·ri·at′·ic
pso′·ri·at′·i·cum
psor′·oph·thal′·mia
psy′·cha·go′·gy
psy·chal′·gia
psych′·an·op′·sia
psych′·as·the′·nia
psy′·che
psy′·che·del′·ic
psych·er′·go·graph
psy′·chi·at′·ric
psy·chi′·a·trist
psy·chi′·a·try
psy′·chic *also* ·chi·cal
psy′·cho·
psy′·cho·acous′·tics
psy′·cho·ac′·ti·va′·tor
psy′·cho·ac′·tive
psy′·cho·an′·a·lep′·tic
psy′·cho·anal′·y·sis
 pl. ·ses
psy′·cho·an′·a·lyst
psy′·cho·an′·a·lyt′·ic
 also ·i·cal
psy′·cho·bi′·o·log′·ic
 also ·i·cal
psy′·cho·bi·ol′·o·gy
psy′·cho·car′·di·ac
psy′·cho·ca·thar′·sis
 pl. ·ses
psy′·cho·chem′·is·try
psy′·cho·di′·ag·no′·sis
 pl. ·ses
psy′·cho·di′·ag·nos′·tics
psy′·cho·dra′·ma
psy′·cho·dy·nam′·ics
psy′·cho·gal·van′·ic
psy′·cho·gal′·va·nom′·e·ter
psy′·cho·gen′·der
psy′·cho·gen′·ic
psy′·cho·ger′·i·a·tri′·cian

psy′·cho·ger′·i·at′·rics
psy′·cho·gram
psy′·cho·graph
psy′·cho·his′·to·ry
psy′·cho·ki·ne′·sis
psy′·cho·lep′·sy
psy′·cho·lep′·tic
psy′·cho·lin·guis′·tics
psy′·cho·log′·i·cal
 also ·log′·ic
psy·chol′·o·gist
psy·chol′·o·gy
psy′·cho·met′·ric
psy′·cho·me·tri′·cian
psy′·cho·met′·rics
 also psy·chom′·e·try
psy′·cho·mo′·tor
psy′·cho·neu·ro′·sis
 pl. ·ses
psy′·cho·nom′·ics
psy′·cho·path
psy′·cho·path′·ia
psy′·cho·path′·ic
psy′·cho·pa·thol′·o·gy
psy·chop′·a·thy
psy′·cho·phar′·ma·col′·o·gy
psy′·cho·phys′·i·cal
psy′·cho·phys′·ics
psy′·cho·phys′·i·o·log′·ic *also* ·i·cal
psy′·cho·phys′·i·ol′·o·gy
psy′·cho·pro′·phy·lax′·is
psy′·cho·sex′·u·al
psy′·cho·sex′·u·al′·i·ty
psy′·cho·sine
psy·cho′·sis *pl.* ·ses;
 mental disorder: Cf.
 sycosis
psy′·cho·so′·cial
psy′·cho·so·mat′·ic
psy′·cho·sur′·gery
psy′·cho·syn′·drome
psy′·cho·syn′·the·sis
psy′·cho·tech′·nics

psy′·cho·ther′·a·peu′·tic
psy′·cho·ther′·a·pist
psy′·cho·ther′·a·py
psy·chot′·ic
psy·chot′·o·gen
psy·chot′·o·gen′·ic
psy·chot′o·mi·met′·ic
psy′·cho·tro′·pic
 [·trop′·ic]
psy′·chro·
psy′·chro·es·the′·sia
 Brit. ·aes·
psy·chrom′·e·ter
psy′·chro·phil′·ic
psyl′·li·um
ptar′·mic
pter′·i·dine
pter′·in
pter′·i·on
pter′o·
pte·ro′·ic
pter′·o·yl
pter′·o·yl·glu·tam′·ic
pte·ryg′·i·um *pl.* ·ia
pter′·y·go·
pter′·y·go·a′lar
pter′·y·goid
pter′·y·goi′·dea *fem.*
 of pterygoideus
pter′·y·goi′·de·us *pl.*
 & gen. sg. ·dei
pter′·y·go·man·dib′·u·la′·ris
pter′·y·go·man·dib′·u·lar
pter′·i·go·max′·il·la′·ris
pter′·y·go·max′·il·lar′y
pter′·y·go·pal′·a·ti′·na
 fem. of pterygopalatinus
pter′·y·go·pal′·a·tine
pter′·y·go·pal′·a·ti′·num *neut. of* ptery·gopalatinus
pter′·y·go·pal′·a·ti′·nus
 pl. & gen. sg. ·ni
pter′·y·go·pha·ryn′·gea

pter'·y·go·quad'·rate
pter'·y·go·spi·na'·lis
  neut. ·le
pter'·y·go·spi·no'·sus
pter'·y·go·spi'·nous
pthi·ri'·a·sis
Pthi'·rus[42] also Pthi'·ri·us
P. pu'·bis
pto'·maine
pto·mat'·ro·pine
pto·mat'·ro·pis'm
ptosed
pto'·sis
ptot'·ic
pty'·a·lec'·ta·sis
pty'·a·lis'm
pty'·a·lo·
pty'·a·log'·ra·phy
pty'·a·lo·li·thi'·a·sis
pty'·a·lo·li·thot'·o·my
pty'·a·lor·rhe'a Brit. ·rhoe'a
pty·oc'·ri·nous
pu'·bar·che [pu·bar'·che]
pu'·ber·pho'·nia
pu'·ber·tal also pu'·ber·al
pu'·ber·tas
pu'·ber·ty
pu'·ber·u'·lic
pu·ber'·u·lon'·ic
pu'·bes[43] gen. ·bis
pu·bes'·cence
pu·bes'·cent
pu'·bic
pu'·bi·cus fem. ·ca, neut. ·cum

pu'·bi·ot'·o·my
pu'·bis gen. of pubes
pu'·bo·ad·duc'·tor
pu'·bo·cap'·su·lar
pu'·bo·cav'·er·no'·sus
pu'·bo·coc·cyg'·e·al
pu'·bo·coc·cyg'·e·us
pu'·bo·fem'·o·ral
pu'·bo·fem'·o·ra'·le
pu'·bo·per'·i·to'·ne·a'·lis
pu'·bo·pros·tat'·ic
pu'·bo·pros·tat'·i·cus
  fem. ·ca, neut. ·cum
pu'·bo·rec'·tal
pu'·bo·rec·ta'·lis
pu'·bo·trans'·ver·sa'·lis
pu'·bo·tu'·ber·ous
pu'·bo·ure'·thral
pu'·bo·vag'·i·na'·lis
pu'·bo·ves'·i·cal
pu'·bo·ves'·i·ca'·lis
  neut. ·le
pu·den'·da pl. of pudendum & fem. sg. of pudendus; pl. & gen. sg. ·dae
pu'·den·dag'·ra
pu·den'·dal
pu'·den·da'·lis
pu·den'·dum pl. ·da, gen. sg. ·di
pu·den'·dus
pu'·dic
pu'·eri·cul'·ture [pu·er'i·]
pu·er'·per·al
pu'·er·pe'·ri·um
puff'·er

puits' de De·ver·gie'
Pu'·lex
  P. ir'·ri·tans
Pu·lic'·i·dae
pu'·li·cide also pu·lic'·i·cide
pu'·li·co'·sis
pul'·ley
pul'·lu·late ·lat'·ed, ·lat'·ing
pul'·lu·la'·tion
pul'·mo pl. pul·mo'·nes, gen. sg. pul·mo'·nis, gen. pl. pul·mo'·num
pul'·mo·
pul'·mo·aor'·tic
pul'·mo·lith
pul·mom'·e·ter
pul·mom'·e·try
pul'·mo·na'·le neut. of pulmonalis
pul'·mo·na'·lis pl. ·les, gen. pl. ·li·um
pul'·mo·nar'y
pul'·mo·nate
pul'·mo·nec'·to·my
pul·mon'·ic
pul·mo'·nis gen. of pulmo
pul'·mo·ni'·tis
pul'·mo·no·
pul'·mo·no·cor'·o·nar'y
pul'·mo·nol'·o·gist
pul'·mo·nol'·o·gy
pul'·mo·tor
pul'·pa gen. ·pae
pulp'·al
pulp·ec'·to·my [pul·pec'·]

---

[42] *Pthirus* is the official spelling for the genus of the pubic louse although *Phthirus* is linguistically more correct. In derived words, a fine but unreliable distinction is sometimes made, as for example between *pthiriasis* (infestation with *Pthirus pubis*) and *phthiriasis* (infestation with lice of any kind).

[43] This Latin singular noun means "the pubic region," and *pubis* is its genitive. In English, on the other hand, *pubis* usually means *os pubis*, "the bone of the pubic region," and functions as an ordinary noun with *pubes* as its plural. This use of *pubes* is not Latin, however. The Latin plural of *os pubis* is *ossa pubis*.

pulp′·i·form
pulp·i′·tis
pulp′·less
pulp·ot′·o·my
pul′·sate   ·sat·ed, ·sat·ing
pul′·sa·tile
pul·sat′·i·lis
pul·sa′·tion
pul′·sa·tor
pulse
pulse′·less
pul·sel′·lum   pl.   ·la
pul′·sion
pul′·sus   pl.   pulsus
pul′·ver·i·za′·tion
pul′·ver·ize   ·ized, ·iz′·ing
pul·ver′·u·lent
pul′·vi·nar
pul′·vis
pu′·na
punch′-drunk
punc·ta′·ta
punc′·tate
punc′·tu·ate
punc′·tum   pl.   ·ta
punc·tu′·ra
punc′·ture
pun′·gent
pu′·pa   pl.   ·pae
pu′·pal
pu′·pate   ·pat·ed, ·pat·ing
pu′·pil
pu·pil′·la   pl. & gen. sg.   ·lae
pu′·pil·la′·ris
pu′·pil·lar′·y
pu′·pil·la·to′·nia
pu′·pil·lo· [pu·pil′·lo·]
pu′·pil·lo·con·stric′·tion
pu·pil′·lo·graph
pu′·pil·log′·ra·phy
pu′·pil·lom′·e·ter
pu′·pil·lo·mo′·tor
pu′·pil·lo·ple′·gia

pu′·pil·lo·sta·tom′·e·ter
pu′·pil·lo·to′·nia
pu′·pil·lo·ton′·ic
Pu·pip′·a·ra
pu·pip′·a·rous
pu·piv′·o·rous
pur·ga′·tion
pur′·ga·tive
purge   purged, purg′·ing
pu′·ri·form
pu′·rine
pu′·ri·ne′·mia [·rin·e′·]   Brit.   ·nae′·
pu′·ri·ty
pu′·ro·my′·cin
pur′·ple
pur′·pu·ra
pur·pu′·rea·gly′·co·side
pur·pu′·ric
pur′·pu·rin
purse′·string
pu′·ru·lence
pu′·ru·lent
pu′·rum
pus
pus′·tu·lant
pus′·tu·lar
pus′·tu·late   ·lat′·ed, ·lat′·ing
pus′·tu·la′·tion
pus′·tule
pus′·tu·lo′·sa
pus′·tu·lo′·sis
pu·ta′·men
pu′·tre·fac′·tion
pu′·tre·fac′·tive
pu′·tre·fy   ·fied, ·fy′·ing
pu·tres′·cent
pu′·tre·scen′·tia
pu·tres′·cine
pu′·trid
py·ae′·mia   Brit. spel.   of pyemia
py·ae′·mi·cus
py′·ar·thro′·sis
pyc′·no·   var. of   pykno-

py′·e·lec′·ta·sis
py′·e·lit′·ic
py′·e·li′·tis
py′·e·lo·
py′·e·lo·cal′·i·ce′·al   [·ca′·li·]   also   ·cal′·y·
py′·e·lo·cal′·i·ec′·ta·sis   [·ca′·li·]   also   ·cal′·y·
py′·e·lo·cys·ti′·tis
py′·e·lo·cys′·to·sto·mo′·sis
py′·e·lo·gen′·ic
py′·e·lo·gram
py′·e·log′·ra·phy
py′·e·lo·il′·eo·cu·ta′·ne·ous
py′·e·lo·li·thot′·o·my
py′·e·lo·lym·phat′·ic
py′·e·lo·ne·phri′·tis
py′·e·lo·ne·phro′·sis
py′·e·lo·plas′·ty
py′·e·lo·re′·nal
py′·e·lo·si′·nus
py′·e·los′·to·my
py′·e·lot′·o·my
py′·e·lo·tu′·bu·lar
py′·e·lo·ure′·ter·al
py′·e·lo·ure′·ter·ec′·ta·sis
py′·e·lo·ure′·ter·og′·ra·phy
py′·e·lo·ure′·ter·ol′·y·sis
py′·e·lo·ure′·ter·o·plas′·ty
py′·e·lo·ve′·nous
py′·e·lo·ves′·i·cal
py·em′·e·sis
py·e′·mia   Brit.   ·ae′·mia
py·e′·mic   Brit.   ·ae′·mic
Py′·e·mo′·tes
py′·en·ceph′·a·lus
py′·gal
pyg′·my
py′·go·
py·gom′·e·lus

py·gop′·a·gus
pyk′·nic
pyk′·no·
pyk′·no·cyte
pyk′·no·cy·to′·sis
pyk′·no·dys′·os·to′·sis
pyk′·no·lep′·sy
pyk·nom′·e·ter
pyk·nom′·e·try
pyk′·no·mor′·phic
   also ·phous
pyk·no′·sis
pyk′·no·so·mat′·ic
pyk·not′·ic
py′·la
py′·lar
py′·le·
py′·le·phle·bit′·ic
py′·le·phle·bi′·tis
py′·lic
py′·lon
py′·lo·ral′·gia
py′·lo·rec′·to·my
py·lo′·ri *gen. of*
   pylorus
py·lo′·ric
py·lo′·ri·ca *fem. of*
   pyloricus; *pl.* ·cae
py·lo′·ri·cum *neut. of*
   pyloricus
py·lo′·ri·cus *pl.* ·ci
py′·lo·ri′·tis
py·lo′·ro·
py·lo′·ro·di′·la·tor
py·lo′·ro·di·o′·sis
py·lo′·ro·du′·o·de′·nal
py·lo′·ro·du′·o·de·ni′·tis
py·lo′·ro·gas·trec′·to·my
py·lo′·ro·my·ot′·o·my
py·lo′·ro·plas′·ty
py·lo′·ro·spas′m
py′·lo·ros′·to·my
py′·lo·rot′·o·my
py·lo′·rus *gen.* ·ri
py′·o·

py′·o·ar·thro′·sis *var.*
   of pyarthrosis
py′·o·ca′·lix
py′·o·cele
py′·o·ceph′·a·lus
py′·o·col′·po·cele
py′·o·col′·pos
py′·o·cy′·a·nin
py′·o·cy·a·no′·sis
py′·o·cys′·tis
py′·o·cyte
py′·o·der′·ma *also*
   ·der′·mia
py′·o·der′·ma·ti′·tis
   also ·der·mi′·tis
py′·o·der′·ma·to′·sis
py′·o·em′·e·sis *var. of*
   pyemesis
py′·o·gen′·e·sis
py′·o·gen′·ic
py·og′·e·nous
py′·o·he′·mo·tho′·rax
   Brit. ·hae′·mo·
py′·oid
py′·o·me′·tra
py′·o·me·tri′·tis
py′·o·my′·o·si′·tis
py′·o·ne·phri′·tis
py′·o·neph′·ro·li·thi′·a·sis
py′·o·ne·phro′·sis
py′·o·ne·phrot′·ic
py′·o·ovar′·i·um
py′·o·per′·i·car′·di·um
py′·oph·thal′·mia
py′·o·phy·lac′·tic
py′·o·phy′·so·me′·tra
py′·o·pneu′·mo·cyst
py′·o·pneu′·mo·per′·i·car′·di·um
py′·o·pneu′·mo·per′·i·to·ne′·um
py′·o·pneu′·mo·tho′·rax
py′·o·poi·e′·sis
py′·o·poi·et′·ic
py·op′·ty·sis
py′·or·rhe′a *Brit.*
   ·rhoe′a

py′·o·sal′·pin·gi′·tis
py′·o·sal·pin′·go-o′o·pho·ri′·tis
py′·o·sal′·pinx
py′·o·sep′·ti·ce′·mia
   Brit. ·cae′·
py·o′·sis
py′·o·sper′·mia
py′·o·stat′·ic
py′·o·tho′·rax
py′·o·um·bil′·i·cus
py′·o·u′ra·chus
py′·o·ure′·ter
py′·ra·hex′·yl
pyr′·a·mid
py·ram′·i·dal
py·ram′·i·da′·lis *neut.*
   ·le
py·ram′·i·do·an·te′·ri·or
py·ram′·i·do·lat′·er·al
py·ram′·i·dot′·o·my
pyr′·a·mis *pl.* py·ram′·i·des, *gen. sg.* py·ram′·i·dis, *gen. pl.* py·ram′·i·dum
py′·ran
py′·ra·nose [pyr′·a·]
py′·ra·no·side′ [py·ran′·o·]
py·ran′·tel
py′·ra·zin′·a·mide
   [pyr′·a·]
py′·ra·zine [pyr′·a·]
py·raz′·o·line
py·rec′·tic *var. of*
   pyretic
py′·rene
py′·re·nol′·y·sis
py′·re·ther′·a·py *var.*
   of pyretotherapy
py·re′·thrin
py·re′·thrum
py·ret′·ic
py′·re·to·
py′·re·to·gen′·ic
py′·re·tol′·y·sis
py′·re·to·ther′·a·py

py·rex′·ia
py·rex′·i·al
py·rex′·in
pyr′·i·dine
pyr′·i·do·stig′·mine
pyr′·i·dox′·al
pyr·i·dox′·a·mine
pyr′·i·dox′·ic
pyr′·i·dox′·ine
pyr′·i·dox′·ol
pyr′·i·form *var. of* piriform
py·ril′·a·mine
pyr′i·meth′·a·mine [py′ri·]
py·rim′·i·dine
pyr′·i·thi′·one
py′·ro·
py′·ro·cat′·e·chol
py′·ro·gal′·lol
py′·ro·gen
py′·ro·ge·net′·ic
py′·ro·gen′·ic *also* ·ge·net′·ic *or* py·rog′·e·nous
py′·ro·glob′·u·lin
py′·ro·glu·tam′·ic
py·rol′·y·sis
py′·ro·ma′·nia
py·rom′·e·ter
py′·rone
py′·ro·nine
py′·ro·ni′·no·phil′·ia
py′·ro·ni′·no·phil′·ic
py′·ro·pho′·bia
py′·ro·phos
py′·ro·phos′·pha·tase
py′·ro·phos′·phate
py′·ro·phos′·pho·me·val′·o·nate
py′·ro·phos·pho′·ric
py′·ro·phos′·pho·rol′·y·sis
py′·ro·phos·pho′·ry·lase
Py′·ro·plas′·ma
py·ro′·sis
Py′·ro·so′·ma

py′·ro·sul′·fite *Brit.* ·phite
py·rot′·ic
pyr′·ro·bu′·ta·mine
pyr′·ro·lase
pyr′·role
pyr·rol′·i·dine
pyr′·ro·lo·por·phyr′·ia
py′·ru·vate [py·ru′·vate]
py′·ru·ve′·mia *Brit.* ·vae′·
py·ru′·vic
pyr·vin′·i·um
py′·tho·gen′·ic
py·u′·ria

Q

quack
quack′·ery
qua·dran′·gu·lar
qua·dran′·gu·la′·ris
quad′·rant
quad′·rant·an·o′·pia *also* ·op′·sia
quad′·ran·tec′·to·my [·rant·ec′·]
qua·dran′·tic *also* ·tal
qua·dra′·ta *fem. of* quadratus
quad′·rate
qua·dra′·tum *neut. of* quadratus
qua·dra′·tus *pl. & gen. sg.* ·ti
quad′·ri·
quad′·ri·ceps
quad′·ri·cus′·pid
quad′·ri·gem′·i·na *neut. pl. & fem. sg. of* quadrigeminus; *gen. sg.* ·nae
quad′·ri·gem′·i·nal
quad′·ri·gem′·i·num *neut. of* quadrigeminus; *pl.* ·na

quad′·ri·gem′·i·nus *pl. & gen. sg.* ·ni
quad′·ri·lat′·er·al
quad′·ri·loc′·u·lar
qua·drip′·a·ra
quad′·ri·par′·i·ty
quad′·ri·ple′·gia
quad′·ri·ple′·gic
quad′·ri·po′·lar
quad′·ri·sect
quad′·ri·va′·lent
quad′·ru·ped
quad′·ru·ped′·al [qua·dru′·pe·dal]
qua·dru′·ple
qua·dru′·plet
qual′·i·ta′·tive
quan′·ta *pl. of* quantum
quan′·tal
quan′·ti·tate
quan′·ti·ta′·tive
quan′·ti·za′·tion
quan′·tized
quan′·tum *pl.* ·ta
quar′·an·tin′·a·ble
quar′·an·tine
quar′·tan
quar·ta′·na
quar′·tile
quar′·tus
quartz
qua′·si·
qua′·si·con·tin′·u·ous
qua′·si·dom′·i·nance
qua′·si·dom′·i·nant
quas′·sia
quat′·er in di′e
qua′·ter·nar′y [qua·ter′·na·ry]
que·bra′·cho
quel′·lung
quench′·ing
quer′·ce·tin
quick′·en
quick′·lime
quick′·sil′·ver
qui·es′·cent

quil·la′·ia *also* ·la·ja
quin′·a·crine
quin·al′·dic
quin·al′·dine [quin′·al·]
quin·hy′·drone
quin′·i·dine
qui′·nine [qui·nine′]
qui′·nin·is′m
qui′·nin·ize ·ized, ·iz′·ing
quin′·o·cide
quin′·o·line
quin′·o·lone
qui·none′ [quin′·one]
quin′·o·noid
quin′·que·cus′·pid
quin′·que·va′·lent
quin·qui′·na
quin′·sy
quin′·tan
quin·ta′·na
quin′·tile
quin·tip′·a·ra
quin·tup′·let
quin′·tus
quo·tid′·i·an
quo′·tient

R

rab′·bit·pox
rab′·e·lai′·sin
ra′·bic
ra′·bi·cid′·al [·ci′·dal]
rab′·id
ra′·bies
ra′·ce·mase [rac′·e·]
ra′·ce·mate [rac′·e·]
ra′·ce·me·thi′·o·nine
ra·ce′·mic
ra′·ce·mi·za′·tion [rac′·e·]
rac′·e·mose
ra′·chi· *also* ra′·chio·
ra′·chi·al
ra′·chi·cen·te′·sis
 also ra′·chio·
ra·chid′·i·an *also* ·al
ra·chil′·y·sis
ra′·chi·o·camp′·sis
ra′·chio·ky·pho′·sis
 also ·cy·pho′·sis
ra′·chi·op′·a·gus
ra′·chi·o·tome
ra′·chi·ot′·o·my
ra′·chi·re·sis′·tance
ra′·chis *pl.* ra′·chi·des
ra·chis′·chi·sis
ra·chit′·ic
ra·chi′·tis
rach′·i·tis′m
rach′·i·to·gen′·ic
ra′·chi·tome [rach′·i·]
  var. of rachiotome
ra·chit′·o·my *var. of* rachiotomy
ra′·cial
rad
ra′·dar·ky′·mo·gram
ra′·dar·ky·mog′·ra·phy
ra·dec′·to·my
ra′·di·a·bil′·i·ty
ra′·di·a·ble
ra′·di·ad
ra′·di·al
ra′·di·a′·le *neut. of* radialis
ra′·di·a′·lis *pl.* ·les,
  gen. pl. ·li·um
ra′·di·an
ra′·di·ant
ra′·di·a′·ta *pl. of* radiatum, *fem. of* radiatus; *pl. & gen. sg.* ·tae
ra′·di·ate ·at′·ed, ·at′·ing
ra′·di·a′·tio *pl.* ·a′·ti·o′·nes, *gen. sg.* ·o′·nis
ra′·di·a′·tion
ra′·di·a′·tum *neut. of* radiatus; *pl.* ·ta
ra′·di·a′·tus
rad′·i·cal *attacking the root cause; also,*

chemical group: Cf. radicle
ra′·di·ces [ra·di′·] *pl. of* radix
ra′·di·cis [ra·di′·]
  gen. of radix
rad′·i·cle *small rootlike anatomic structure: Cf.* radical
rad′·i·cot′·o·my
ra·dic′·u·la *pl.* ·lae
ra·dic′·u·lar
ra·dic′·u·la′·re *neut.*
  of radicularis; *pl.* ·ria
ra·dic′·u·la′·ris
ra·dic′·u·lec′·to·my
ra·dic′·u·li′·tis
ra·dic′·u·lo·
ra·dic′·u·lo·den′·tal
ra·dic′·u·lo·gan′·gli·on·i′·tis
ra·dic′·u·lo·med′·ul·lar′y
ra·dic′·u·lo·me·nin′·go·my′·e·li′·tis
ra·dic′·u·lo·my′·e·lop′·a·thy
ra·dic′·u·lo·neu·rit′·ic
ra·dic′·u·lo·neu·ri′·tis
ra·dic′·u·lo·neu·rop′·a·thy
ra·dic′·u·lop′·a·thy
ra′·dii *pl. & gen. sg. of* radius
ra′·dio·
ra′·dio·ab·la′·tion
ra′·dio·ac′·tive
ra′·dio·ac·tiv′·i·ty
ra′·dio·al′·ler·go·sor′·bent
ra′·dio·au′·to·gram
 also ·graph
ra′·dio·au·tog′·ra·phy
ra′·dio·bi·cip′·i·tal
ra′·dio·bi·ol′·o·gist
ra′·dio·bi·ol′·o·gy
ra′·dio·car′·bon

ra'·dio·car'·ci·no·gen'·e·sis
ra'·dio·car'·di·og'·ra·phy
ra'·dio·car'·pal
ra'·dio·car·pa'·lis *neut.* ·le
ra'·dio·ce·phal'·ic
ra'·dio·chem'·is·try
ra'·dio·co'·balt
ra'·dio·col'·loid
ra'·di·ode
ra'·dio·dense'
ra'·dio·den'·si·ty
ra'·dio·der'·ma·ti'·tis
ra'·dio·di'·ag·no'·sis *pl.* ·ses
ra'·dio·dig'·i·tal
ra'·dio·do·sim'·e·try
ra'·dio·ecol'·o·gy
ra'·dio·el'·e·ment
ra'·dio·ep'·i·the'·li·o'·ma
ra'·dio·fre'·quen·cy
ra'·dio·gal'·li·um
ra'·di·o·gen'·ic
ra'·dio·gold'
ra'·di·o·graph
ra'·di·o·graph'·ic
ra'·di·og'·ra·phy
ra'·dio·hu'·mer·al
ra'·dio·im'·mu·no·as·say' [·as'·say]
ra'·dio·im'·mu·no·dif·fu'·sion
ra'·dio·im'·mu·no·elec'·tro·pho·re'·sis
ra'·dio·im'·mu·no·pre·cip'·i·ta'·tion
ra'·dio·im'·mu·no·sor'·bent
ra'·dio·in'·di·ca'·tor
ra'·dio·i'o·di·nat'·ed
ra'·dio·i'o·dine
ra'·dio·i'ron
ra'·dio·i'so·tope
ra'·dio·lead'
ra'·dio·lig'·and [·li'·gand]
ra'·di·o·log'·ic *also* ·i·cal
ra'·di·ol'·o·gist
ra'·di·ol'·o·gy
ra'·dio·lu'·cent
ra·di'·o·lus *pl.* ·li
ra'·di·ol'·y·sis
ra'·di·om'·e·ter
ra'·dio·met'·ric
ra'·dio·mi·crom'·e·ter
ra'·dio·mi·met'·ic
ra'·dio·mu·ta'·tion
ra'·dio·ne·cro'·sis
ra'·dio·ne·phrog'·ra·phy
ra'·dio·neu·ri'·tis
ra'·dio·nu'·clide
ra'·dio·nu·clid'·ic
ra'·di·opac'·i·ty *also* ra'·dio·opac'·i·ty
ra'·dio·pal'·mar
ra'·di·opaque'
ra·di·o·par'·ent
ra'·dio·per'·i·os'·te·al
ra'·dio·phar'·ma·ceu'·ti·cal[44]
ra'·dio·phar'·ma·col'·o·gy
ra'·dio·po·ten'·ti·a'·tion
ra'·dio·pro'·na·tor
ra'·dio·re·cep'·tor
ra'·dio·re·nog'·ra·phy
ra'·dio·re·sis'·tant
ra'·dio·sen'·si·tive
ra'·dio·sen'·si·tiv'·i·ty
ra'·dio·so'·di·um
ra'·dio·spi·rom'·e·try
ra'·dio·ste'·reo·as'·say [·ster'·eo·, ·as·say']
ra'·dio·ste'·re·os'·co·py [·ster'·e·]
ra'·dio·stron'·ti·um
ra'·dio·sul'·fur
ra'·dio·sur'·gery
ra'·dio·te·lem'·e·try
ra'·dio·ther'·a·peu'·tic
ra'·dio·ther'·a·pist
ra'·dio·ther'·a·py
ra'·di·o·ther'·my
ra'·dio·thy'·roid·ec'·to·my
ra'·dio·tox·e'·mia *Brit.* ·ae'·mia
ra'·dio·trac'·er
ra'·dio·trans·par'·ent
ra'·dio·ul'·nar
ra'·dio·ul·na'·ris
ra'·dio·xe'·non [·xen'·on]
ra'·di·um
ra'·di·us *pl. & gen. sg.* ·dii
ra'·dix *pl.* ra'·di·ces, *gen. sg.* ra'·di·cis
ra'·don
raf'·fi·nose
rag'·o·cyte
rag'·weed
Rail'·li·e·ti'·na
rale *also* râle
ra'·mal
ra'·mex *pl.* ra'·mi·ces
ra'·mi *pl. & gen.sg. of* ramus
ram'·i·cot'·o·my
ram'·i·fi·ca'·tion
ram'·i·form
ram'·i·fy ·fied, ·fy'·ing
ram'·i·sec'·tion
ram'·i·sec'·to·my

---

[44] Radiopharmaceuticals with officially approved names are written with the full name of the radioactive compound followed by the symbol (element plus atomic weight) of the radionuclide it contains: ferrous citrate Fe 59.

ra″·mose
ram″·u·lus *pl.* ·li
ra″·mus *pl. & gen. sg.*
  ·mi, *ablative* ·mo, *gen.*
  pl. ra·mo″·rum
ran″·dom·i·za″·tion
ran″·dom·ize ·ized,
  ·iz′·ing
ra″·nine
ra·ni″·ti·dine
ran″·u·la
ran″·u·lar
ra″·phe *pl.* ·phae
rap·port′
rap″·tus *pl.* raptus
rar′·e·fac″·tion
ra·sce″·ta
rash
ras″·pa·to′·ry
ra″·tio
ra″·tion
ra″·tio·nal [·tion·al]
ra″·tio·nal·i·za″·tion
  [·tion·al·]
rat′·tle·snake
Rat′·tus
rau·wol″·fia
re′·ab·sorp″·tion *var.*
  of resorption
re′·ab·sorp″·tive
re·ac″·tance
re·ac″·tant
re·ac″·tion
re·ac″·ti·vate ·vat′·ed,
  ·vat′·ing
re·ac″·ti·va″·tion
re·ac″·tive
re′·ac″·tiv″·i·ty
re·ac″·tor
read′·i·ness
read′·ing
read′·out
read′·through
re·a′gent
re′·ag″·gre·ga″·tion
re·a′gin
ream′·er
re′·am″·pu·ta″·tion

re·an″·i·mate ·mat′·
  ed, ·mat″·ing
re″·as·so″·ci·a″·tion
re′·at·tach″·ment
Ré·au·mur′
re·base′ ·based′,
  ·bas″·ing
re″·bound
re·breath″·ing
re·cal″·ci·fi·ca″·tion
re″·call [re·call′]
re″·can″·a·li·za″·tion
re″·ca·pit′·u·la″·tion
re·cel″·lens
re″·cep·tac″·u·lum *pl.*
  ·la
re·cep″·tive
re·cep″·tor
re″·cess [re·cess″]
re·ces″·sive
re·ces″·sus *pl. & gen.*
  sg. recessus
re·cid″·i·va″·tion
re·cid″·i·vis″m
re·cid″·i·vist
re·cip″·i·ent
re·ĉip″·ro·cal
re·cip″·ro·cat″·ing
re·cip″·ro·ca″·tion
rec′·i·proc″·i·ty
re″·li·na″·tion
re″·og·ni″·tion
re″·coil
re·com″·bi·nant
re·com″·bi·na″·tion
re″·com·pres″·sion
re″·con·di″·tion
re·con″·sti·tu″·tion
re″·con·struc″·tion
re″·con·struc″·tive
re″·con·struc″·tor
re·con″·tour
rec″·ord *n.*
re·cord′ *v.*
re·cord″·er
re·cov″·ery
rec″·re·ment
re″·cru·des″·cence

re′·cru·des″·cent
re·cruit″·ment
rec″·ta *neut. pl. &*
  fem. sg. of rectus; *pl.*
  & gen. sg. ·tae
rec″·tal
rec·ta″·lis *pl.* ·les
rec·tec″·to·my
rec″·ti *pl. of* rectus,
  gen. sg. of rectus *&*
  rectum
rec″·ti·fi·ca″·tion
rec″·ti·fi′·er
rec″·ti·fy ·fied, ·fy′·ing
rec′·ti·lin″·e·ar
rec″·to·
rec′·to·ab·dom″·i·nal
rec′·to·a″nal
rec′·to·cele
rec′·to·coc·cyg″·e·us
rec′·to·coc″·cy·pex′y
rec′·to·cys·tot″·o·my
rec′·to·per″·i·ne·or′·
  rha·phy
rec′·to·pex′y
rec′·to·ro·man″·o·scope
rec′·to·ro′·ma·nos″·co·
  py
rec·tor″·rha·phy
rec″·to·scope
rec·tos″·co·py
rec′·to·sig″·moid
rec′·to·sig·moid·ec″·to·
  my
rec′·to·sig″·moid·i″·tis
rec′·to·sig″·moi·dos″·
  co·py [·moid·os″·]
rec′·to·ste·no″·sis
rec·tos″·to·my
rec·tot″·o·my
rec′·to·ure″·thral
rec′·to·u″·re·thra″·lis
rec′·to·u″·ter·ine
rec′·to·u″·ter·i″·nus
  fem. ·na
rec′·to·vag″·i·nal
rec′·to·vag″·i·na″·lis
  neut. ·le

rec′·to·ves′·i·cal
rec′·to·ves′·i·ca′·lis
   neut. ·le
rec′·tum *gen.* ·ti
rec′·tus *pl. & gen. sg.*
  ·ti
re·cum′·ben·cy
re·cum′·bent
re·cu′·per·ate ·at′·ed,
  ·at′·ing
re·cu′·per·a′·tion
re·cu′·per·a·tive
re·cur′·rence
re·cur′·rens *gen.* re′·
  cur·ren′·tis
re·cur′·rent
re′·cur·va′·tion
re′·cur·va′·tum
re·cur′·vus
re′·dia *pl.* ·di·ae
re′·dif′·fer·en′·ti·a′·tion
red·in′·te·gra′·tion
re·dis′·lo·ca′·tion
red′·out
re′·dox [red′·ox]
re·duce′ ·duced′,
  ·duc′·ing
re·du′·ci·ble
re·duc′·tant
re·duc′·tase
re·duc′·tion
re·dun′·dan·cy
re·dun′·dant
re·du′·pli·cate ·cat′·
  ed, ·cat′·ing
re·du′·pli·ca′·tion
re·du′·vi·id
Red′·u·vi′·idae
Re·du′·vi·us
  R. per′·so·na′·tus
reef′·ing
re·en′·trant
re·en′·try
re′·ep′i·the′·li·al·i·za′·
  tion
re′·ex′·ci·ta′·tion
re′·ex·pand′
re·fec′·tion

re·fer′ ·ferred′, ·fer′·
  ring
ref′·er·ence
re·fer′·ral
re·flect′
re·flec′·tion *Brit.*
  flex′·ion
re·flec′·tor
re′·flex
re·flex′·io
re·flex′·o·gen′·ic
re·flex′·o·graph
re′·flex·ol′·o·gy
re′·flex·om′·e·try
re·flex′·um
re′·flux
re·fract′
re·frac′·tile
re·frac′·tion
re·frac′·tive
re′·frac′·tiv′·i·ty
re′·frac′·tom′·e·ter
re′·frac′·tom′·e·try
re·frac′·tor
re·frac′·to·ry
re′·frac′·ture *n. & v.*
  ·tured, ·tur·ing
re·fran′·gi·bil′′·i·ty
re·fran′·gi·ble
re·frin′·gent
re·fu′·sion
re·gen′·er·ate ·at′·ed,
  ·at′·ing
re·gen′·er·a′·tion
re·gen′·er·a·tive
reg′·i·men
re′·gio *pl.* re′·gi·o′·
  nes, *gen. sg.* ·o′·nis
re′·gion
re′·gion·al
reg′·is·ter
reg′·is·tra′·tion
reg′·is·try
re·gress′
re·gres′·sion
re·gres′·sive
reg′·u·la′·tion
reg′·u·la′·tive

reg′·u·la′·tor
reg′·u·la·to′·ry
reg′·u·lon
re·gur′·gi·tant
re·gur′·gi·tate ·tat′·ed,
  ·tat′·ing
re·gur′·gi·ta′·tion
re′·ha·bil′·i·tate ·tat′·
  ed, ·tat′·ing
re′·ha·bil′·i·ta′·tion
re′·ha·bil′·i·tee′
re′·ha·la′·tion
re′·hy·dra′·tion
re′·im·plant′
re′·im′·plan·ta′·tion
re′·in·fec′·tion
re′·in·force′·ment
re′·in·forc′·er
re′·in·forc′·ing
re′·in·fu′·sion
re′·in′·ner·va′·tion
re′·in·oc′·u·la′·tion
re′·in′·te·gra′·tion
re′·in·ver′·sion
re·jec′·tion
re·lapse′ *v. & n.*
  ·lapsed′, ·laps′·ing
re′·lapse *n.*
re·lat′·ed
re·la′·tion
re·la′·tion·al
re·la′·tion·ship
rel′·a·tive
re·lax′
re·lax′·ant
re′·lax·a′·tion
re·lax′·in
re′·learn′·ing
re·lease′ ·leased′,
  ·leas′·ing
re·lief′
re·lieve′ ·lieved,
  ·liev′·ing
re·line′ ·lined′. ·lin′·
  ing
re·lu′·cence
re·me′·di·al
rem′·e·dy

re′·min′·er·al·i·za′·tion
re·mis′·sion
re·mit′ ·mit′·ted,
  ·mit′·ting
re·mit′·tence
re·mit′·tent
rem′·nant
re·mov′·al
re′·my′·e·lin·a′·tion
ren pl. re′·nes, gen.
  sg. re′·nis
re′·nal
re·na′·le neut. of
  renalis; pl. ·lia
re·na′·lis pl. ·les
re′·na′·tur·a′·tion
ren′·cu·lus pl. ·li; var.
  of reniculus
ren′·i· [re′·ni·] var. of
  reno-
re·nic′·u·lus pl. ·li
ren′·i·form [re′·ni·]
re′·nin [ren′·in]
re′·nin·o′·ma [ren′·in·]
re′·nis gen. of ren
ren′·net
ren′·nin[45]
ren·nin′·o·gen
re′·no·
re′·no·gen′·ic
re′·no·gram
re·nog′·ra·phy
re′·no·in·tes′·ti·nal
re′·no·pri′·val
re′·no·re′·nal
re′·no·tro′·phic
  [·troph′·ic]
re′·no·tro′·pic [·trop′·
  ic]
re′·no·ure′·ter·al
re′·no·vas′·cu·lar
Re′·o·vi′·ri·dae
re′·o·vi′·rus
re·pair′

re·par′·a·tive
re·peat′
re·pel′·lent also ·lant
re·pel′·ler
re′·pens
re′·per·cus′·sion
re′·per·cus′·sive
rep′·e·ta′·tur
re·place′·ment
re·plant′
re′·plan·ta′·tion
re·ple′·tion
rep′·li·case
rep′·li·cate
rep′·li·ca′·tion
rep′·li·ca′·tive
rep′·li·con
re·po′·lar·i·za′·tion
re·port′·a·ble
re′·po·si′·tion
re·pos′·i·tor
re·pos′·i·to′·ry
re·pres′·sion
re·pres′·sive
re·pres′·sor
re′·pro·duc′·tion
re′·pro·duc′·tive
rep′·ti·lase
re·pul′·sion
res·cin′·na·mine
re·sect′
re·sect′·a·ble
re·sec′·tion
re·sec′·to·scope
re·ser′·pine
res′·er·va′·tus
re·serve′
res′·er·voir
res′·i·den·cy
res′·i·dent
re·sid′·u·al
res′·i·due
re·sid′·u·um pl. ·sid′·
  ua

re·sil′·ien·cy also
  ·ience
re·sil′·ient
res′·in
res′·in·ous
res′ ip′·sa lo′·qui·tur
re·sis′·tance [·sist′·
  ance]
re·sis′·tant [·sist′·ant]
re·sis′·tive
re′·sis·tiv′·i·ty
re·sis′·tor
res′·o·lu′·tion
re·solve′ ·solved′,
  ·solv′·ing
re·sol′·vent
res′·o·nance
res′·o·nant
res′·o·na′·tor
re·sorb′
re·sor′·bent [·sorb′·ent]
res·or′·cin
res·or′·cin·ol
re·sorp′·tion
re·sorp′·tive
re·spi′·ra·ble [res′·pi·]
res′·pi·ra′·tion
res′·pi·ra′·tor
res′·pi·ra·to′·ria fem.
  of respiratorius
res′·pi·ra·to′·ri·um
  neut. of respiratorius
res′·pi·ra·to′·ri·us pl.
  ·rii
res′·pi·ra·to′·ry [re·
  spi′·]
re·spire′ ·spired′,
  ·spir′·ing
res′·pi·rom′·e·ter
res′·pi·rom′·e·try
re·spon′·de·at
re·spon′·dent [·spond′·
  ent]
re·spond′·er

---

[45] The name of this enzyme, produced in the stomachs of animals, has been replaced by *chymosin* to avoid confusion with *renin*, an enzyme produced in the kidney.

re·sponse′
re·spon′·sive
re′·ste·no′·sis
res′·ti·form
res′·ti·for′·me
res′·ti·tu′·tion
res′·to·ra′·tion
re·stor′·a·tive
re·stor′·er
re·straint′
re·sus′·ci·ta′·tion
re·sus′·ci·ta′·tor
re·tain′·er
re·tard′
re′·tar·da′·ta
re·tar′·date
re′·tar·da′·tion
retch
re′·te *pl.* re′·tia, *gen. sg.* re′·tis
re·ten′·tion
re′·ti·al
re·tic′·u·la *pl. of* reticulum
re·tic′·u·lar
re·tic′·u·la′·ris *neut.* ·re
re·tic′·u·late *also* ·lat′·ed
re·tic′·u·la′·tion
re·tic′·u·lin
re·tic′·u·li′·tis
re·tic′·u·lo·
re·tic′·u·lo·cyte
re·tic′·u·lo·cy′·to·pe′·nia
re·tic′·u·lo·cy·to′·sis
re·tic′·u·lo·en′·do·the′·li·al
re·tic′·u·lo·en′·do·the′·li·o′·sis
re·tic′·u·lo·en′·do·the′·li·um
re·tic′·u·lo·his′·ti·o·cyt′·ic
re·tic′·u·lo·his′·ti·o·cy·to′·ma

re·tic′·u·lo·his′·ti·o·cy·to′·sis
re·tic′·u·loid
re·tic′·u·lo-ol′·i·var′y
re·tic′·u·lo·pe′·nia
re·tic′·u·lo·plas′·mo·cy·to′·ma
re·tic′·u·lo·re·tic′·u·lar
re·tic′·u·lo′·sis
re·tic′·u·lo·spi′·nal
re·tic′·u·lo·spi·na′·lis
re·tic′·u·lo·teg·men′·tal
re·tic′·u·lo·the′·li·um
re·tic′·u·lot′·o·my
re·tic′·u·lum *pl.* ·la, *gen. sg.* ·li
re′·ti·form
ret′·i·na *L. pl. & gen. sg.* ·nae
ret′·i·nac′·u·lum *pl.* ·la
ret′·i·nal
ret′·in·al′·de·hyde
ret′·i·na·scope *var. of* retinoscope
ret′·i·nene
ret′·i·ni′·tis
ret′·i·no·
ret′·i·no·blas·to′·ma *pl.* ·mas *or* ·ma·ta
ret′·i·no·cho′·roid·i′·tis
ret′·i·no·cor′·ti·cal
ret′·i·no·di·al′·y·sis
ret′·i·no′·ic
ret′·i·noid
ret′·i·nol
ret′·i·no·pap′·il·li′·tis
ret′·i·nop′·a·thy
ret′·i·no·pex′y
ret′·i·no·pi·e′sis
ret′·i·nos′·chi·sis
ret′·i·no·scope
ret′·i·nos′·co·py
ret′·i·no·top′·ic
re′·to·per′·i·the′·li·um
re·tort′
Re′·tor·tam′·o·nas
re·tract′

re·trac′·tile
re·trac′·tion
re·trac′·tor
re′·trad [ret′·rad]
ret′·ra·hens
ret′·ro·
ret′·ro·ac′·tive
ret′·ro·aor′·tic
ret′·ro·au·ric′·u·lar
ret′·ro·bul′·bar
ret′·ro·cae·ca′·lis *pl.* ·les
ret′·ro·cal·ca′·ne·al
ret′·ro·cal·ca′·neo·bur·si′·tis
ret′·ro·cath′·e·ter·is′m
ret′·ro·ca′·val
ret′·ro·ce′·cal *Brit.* ·cae·
ret′·ro·ce′·dent
ret′·ro·cen′·tral
ret′·ro·ces′·sion
ret′·ro·cli·na′·tion
ret′·ro·coch′·le·ar
ret′·ro·co′·lic
  occurring behind the colon: Cf. retrocollic
ret′·ro·col′·lic *relating to retrocollis: Cf.* retrocolic
ret′·ro·col′·lis
ret′·ro·con·duc′·tion
ret′·ro·cos′·tal
ret′·ro·cur′·sive
ret′·ro·de′·vi·a′·tion
ret′·ro·dis′·cal
ret′·ro·dis·place′·ment
ret′·ro·du′·o·de′·nal
ret′·ro·du′·o·de·na′·lis *pl.* ·les
ret′·ro·du′·ral
ret′·ro·fill′·ing
ret′·ro·flex′·ion
ret′·ro·flex′·us
ret′·ro·gas·se′·ri·an
ret′·ro·gnath′·ism *also* ·gnath′·ia
ret′·ro·grade

re·trog′·ra·phy
ret′·ro·gres′·sion
ret′·ro·gres′·sive
ret′·ro·hy·oi′·dea
ret′·ro·il′i·ac
ret′·ro·il·lu′·mi·na′·tion
ret′·ro·in·fec′·tion
ret′·ro·jec′·tion
ret′·ro·len′·tal
ret′·ro·len·tic′·u·lar
ret′·ro·len′·ti·for′·mis
ret′·ro·lin′·gual
ret′·ro·mal′·le·ar
ret′·ro·mam′·ma·ry
ret′·ro·man·dib′·u·lar
ret′·ro·man·dib′·u·la′·ris
ret′·ro·mas′·toid
ret′·ro·max′·il·lar′y
ret′·ro·mo′·lar
ret′·ro·my′·lo·hy′·oid
ret′·ro-oc′·u·lar
ret′·ro-or′·bi·tal
ret′·ro·pa·rot′·id
ret′·ro·pa·tel′·lar
ret′·ro·per·fu′·sion
ret′·ro·per′·i·to·ne′·al
ret′·ro·per′·i·to·ne·a′·le
ret′·ro·per′·i·to·ne′·um
ret′·ro·per′·i·to·ni′·tis
ret′·ro·pha·ryn′·ge·al
ret′·ro·pha·ryn′·ge·a′·lis pl. ·les
ret′·ro·pha·ryn′·ge·um
ret′·ro·phar′·ynx
ret′·ro·po·si′·tion
ret′·ro·pu′·bic
ret′·ro·pu′·bi·cum
ret′·ro·pul′·sion
ret′·ro·pul′·sive
re·tror′·sine
ret′·ro·si′·nus
ret′·ro·spec′·tive
ret′·ro·sple′·ni·al
ret′·ro·spon′·dy·lo·lis·the′·sis
ret′·ro·stal′·sis
ret′·ro·ster′·nal

ret′·ro·sub′·tha·lam′·ic
ret′·ro·tar′·sal
ret′·ro·ton′·sil·lar
ret′·ro·ure′·thral
ret′·ro·u″ter·ine
ret′·ro·ver′·sio·flex′·ion
ret′·ro·ver′·sion
Ret′·ro·vi′·ri·dae
ret′·ro·vi′·rus
re·trude′ ·trud′·ed, ·trud′·ing
re·tru′·sion
re·tru′·sive
re·u′ni·ens
re′·vac′·ci·na′·tion
re′·vas′·cu·lar·i·za′·tion
rev′·e·hent [re·ve′·]
rev′·e·hens pl. rev′·e·hen″·tes
re·ver′·sal
re·verse′ adj. & v. ·versed′, ·vers″·ing
re·vers′·i·ble
re·ver′·sion
re·ver′·tant
re·view′
re·viv′·al
re·viv′·i·fi·ca′·tion
rev′·o·lute
re·vul′·sant
re·vul′·sion
re·ward′
re·warm′·ing
rhab·dit′·ic
rhab·dit′·i·form
Rhab·di′·tis
rhab′·di·toid
rhab′·do·
rhab′·do·cyte
rhab′·do·my′·o·blast
rhab′·do·my′·o·chon·dro′·ma pl. ·mas or ·ma·ta
rhab′·do·my·ol′·y·sis
rhab′·do·my·o′·ma pl. ·mas or ·ma·ta
rhab′·do·my′·o·sar·co′·ma pl. ·mas or ·ma·ta

Rhab′·do·ne′·ma
rhab′·do·sphinc′·ter
Rhab′·do·vi′·ri·dae
rhab′·do·vi′·rus
rha′·chi· var. of rachi-
rha′·cous
rha·gad′·i·form
rhag′·i·o·crine
rham′·nose
rha′·phe var. of raphe
rhe′·bo·cra′·nia Brit. rhae′·
rheg′·ma·tog′·e·nous
rhe′·ni·um
rhe′o·
rhe″o·base
rhe′o·ba′·sic
rhe′o·en·ceph′·a·log′·ra·phy
rhe·ol′·o·gy
rhe·om′·e·ter
rhe·om′·e·try
rhe′·o·nome
rhe′·o·stat
rhe·os·to′·sis
rhe′o·tax′·is
rhe′·ot′·ro·pis′m
rhe′·sus
rheum
rheu·mat′·ic
rheu·mat′·i·cus fem. ·ca, neut. ·cum
rheu′·ma·tis′m
rheu′·ma·tis′·mal
rheu′·ma·to·gen′·ic
rheu′·ma·toid
rheu′·ma·to·log′·ic
rheu′·ma·tol′·o·gist
rheu′·ma·tol′·o·gy
rhex′·is
rhi′·nal
rhi·na′·lis
rhi·nec′·to·my
rhin′·en·ce·phal′·ic
rhin′·en·ceph′·a·lon
rhin′·es·the′·sia Brit. ·aes·
rhi′·nism

rhi·ni′·tis
rhi′·no·
rhi′·no·can·thec′·to·my
rhi′·no·ceph′·a·ly
rhi′·no·chei′·lo·plas′·ty
rhi′·no·coele *also*
 ·cele
rhi′·no·dym′·ia
rhi′·no·en′·to·moph′·
 tho·ro·my·co′·sis
Rhi′·noes′·trus
rhi·nog′·e·nous *also*
 rhi′·no·gen′·ic
rhi′·no·la′·lia
rhi′·no·lar′·yn·gol′·o·gy
rhi′·no·lith
rhi′·no·li·thi′·a·sis
rhi·nol′·o·gist
rhi·nol′·o·gy
rhi′·no·ma·nom′·e·ter
rhi′·no·ma·nom′·e·try
rhi′·nom·mec′·to·my
rhi·nop′·a·thy *also*
 rhi′·no·path′·ia
rhi′·no·pha·ryn′·ge·al
rhi′·no·phar′·yn·gi′·tis
rhi′·no·phar′·ynx
rhi′·no·pho′·nia
rhi′·no·phy′·co·my·co′·
 sis
rhi′·no·phy′·ma
rhi′·no·plas′·tic
rhi′·no·plas′·ty
rhi′·nor·rhe′a *Brit.*
 ·rhoe′a
rhi′·no·scle·ro′·ma
 pl. ·mas *or* ·ma·ta
rhi′·no·scope
rhi′·no·scop′·ic
rhi·nos′·co·py
rhi′·no·spo·rid′·i·o′·sis
Rhi′·no·spo·rid′·i·um
rhi′·no·ste·no′·sis
rhi·not′·o·my
rhi′·no·tra′·che·i′tis
rhi′·no·vi′·rus
Rhi′·pi·ceph′·a·lus
 R. san·guin′·e·us

rhit′·i·do′·sis *var. of*
 rhytidosis
rhiz′·an·es·the′·sia
 Brit. ·aes·
rhi′·zo·
Rhi·zog′·ly·phus
rhi′·zoid
rhi·zoi′·dal
rhi′·zo·me′·lia
rhi′·zo·mel′·ic [·me′·
 lic]
rhi′·zo·me·nin′·go·my′·
 e·li′·tis
rhi′·zo·pod
Rhi·zop′·o·da
rhi′·zo·po′·di·um *pl.*
 ·dia
Rhi′·zo·pus
rhi·zot′·o·my
rho′·da·mine
rho′·da·nese
rho′·di·um
Rhod′·ni·us
rho′·do·
rho′·do·gen′·e·sis
rho′·do·my′·cin
rho′·do·phy·lac′·tic
rho′·do·phy·lax′·is
rho·dop′·sin
Rho′·do·tor′·u·la
 R. ru′·bra
rho′·do·tor′·u·lo′·sis
rho′·do·tox′·in
rhomb′·en′·ce·phal′·ic
rhomb′·en·ceph′·a·lon
rhom′·bic
rhom′·boid
rhom·boi′·dea *fem. of*
 rhomboideus; *gen.* ·de·
 ae
rhom·boi′·de·us
rhon′·chal *also* ·chi·al
rhon′·chus *pl.* ·chi
rhop′·try
rho′·ta·cis′m
Rhus
rhyth′m
rhyth′·mic

rhyth·mic′·i·ty
rhyt′·i·dec′·to·my
rhyt′·i·do·plas′·ty
rhyt′·i·do′·sis
ri′·ba·vi′·rin
rib′·bon
ri′·bi·tol
ri′·bo·
ri′·bo·fla′·vin [ri′·bo·
 fla′·vin]
ri′·bo·fu′·ra·nose
ri′·bo·fu·ran′·o·syl·ad′·
 e·nine
ri′·bo·fu·ran′·o·syl·cy′·
 to·sine
ri′·bo·fu·ran′·o·syl·
 gua′·nine
ri′·bo·nu′·cle·ase
ri′·bo·nu·cle′·ic
ri′·bo·nu′·cleo·pro′·tein
ri′·bo·nu′·cle·o·side
ri′·bo·nu′·cle·o·tide
ri′·bose
ri′·bose·phos′·phate
ri′·bo·side
ri′·bo·som′·al [·so′·
 mal]
ri′·bo·some
ri′·bos·u′·ria [·bo·su′·]
ri′·bo·syl
ri′·bo·syl·thy′·mine
ri′·bo·thy′·mi·dine
ri′·bo·vi′·rus
ri′·bo·zyme
ri′·bu·lose [rib′·u·]
ri′·bu·lose·phos′·phate
ri′·cin [ric′·in]
ri′·cin·is′m [ric′·in·]
ri′·cin·ole′·ic
rick′·ets
rick′·ett·se′·mia *Brit.*
 ·sae′·
Rick·ett′·sia
 R. ak′·a·ri
 R. aus·tra′·lis
 R. bur·net′·ii
 R. pro′·wa·zek′·ii
 R. rick·ett′·sii

R. tsu′·tsu·ga′·mu·
    shi
R. ty′·phi
rick·ett′·sia pl. ·si·ae
rick·ett′·si·al
rick·ett′·si·al·pox′
rick·ett′·si·cid′·al [·ci′·
    dal]
rick·ett′·si·ol′·o·gy
rick·ett′·si·o′·sis also
    ·si′·a·sis
rick·ett′·si·o·stat′·ic
rick′·ety
ric′·tal
ric′·tus
ridge
ridg′·ing
rid′·it
rif′·a·mide
rif·am′·pin also rif·
    am′·pi·cin
rif′·a·my′·cin
right′-hand′·ed
rig′·id
ri·gid′·i·ty
rig′·i·dus
rig′·or
ri′·ma pl. & gen. sg.
    ·mae
ri′·mal
ri·man′·ta·dine
rim′·i·ter′·ol
ri′·mose also ·mous
rim′·u·la pl. ·lae
ring′·bin′·den
ring′·worm
ri′·o·mit′·sin
ri′·pa
ri·par′·i·an
ris′·to·ce′·tin
ri′·sus
rit′·o·drine
rit′·u·al
ri′·val·ry
ri·vin′·i·an
ri′·vus pl. ·vi
roach
rob′·o·rant

ro·bust′ [ro′·bust]
Ro′·cha·li·mae′a
R. quin·ta′·na
ro′·dent
Ro·den′·tia
ro·den′·ti·cide
roent′·gen
roent′·gen·ky′·mo·
    graph
roent′·gen·ky·mog′·ra·
    phy
roent′·geno·
roent′·geno·car′·di·o·
    gram
roent′·gen·o·gram
roent′·gen·o·graph
roent′·gen·o·graph′·ic
roent′·gen·og′·ra·phy
roent′·gen·o·log′·ic
roent′·gen·ol′·o·gist
roent′·gen·ol′·o·gy
roent′·gen·om′·e·ter
roent′·gen·om′·e·try
roent′·geno·ther′·a·py
    also ·gen·ther′·a·py
roe′·teln var. of rö′·
    teln
ro·flu′·rane
ro·lan′·dic
ro·lan′·di·cus fem. ·ca
rolf′·ing
ro′·li·tet′·ra·cy′·cline
roll′·er
ro·man′·o·pex′y
ro·man′·o·scope
ron·geur′
rönt′·gen var. of
    roentgen
rönt′·gen·og′·ra·phy
    var. of roentgenography
room′·ing-in′
root′·let
rop′y   rop′·i·er, rop′·i·
    est
ro·sa′·cea
ros·an′·i·line
ro′·sa·ry
rose′ ben·gal′

ro′·sea
ro′·se·o′·la [ro·se′·o·la]
ro′·se·o′·lar [ro·se′·o·
    lar]
ro·sette′
ros′·in
ro·sol′·ic
ros·tel′·lum pl. ·la
ros′·trad
ros′·tral
ros·tra′·lis
ros′·trate
ros′·trum pl. ·tra
ro·tam′·e·ter [ro′·ta·
    me′·ter]
ro′·ta·ry
ro′·tate ·tat·ed, ·tat·ing
ro·ta′·tion
ro·ta′·tion·al
ro′·ta·tor L. pl. ro′·ta·
    to′·res
ro′·ta·to′·ry
ro′·ta·vi′·rus
rö′·teln
ro′·te·none
ro·tex′·ion
ro′·to·sco′·li·o′·sis
ro·tox′·a·mine
rot′·u·la pl. ·lae
rot′·u·lad
ro·tun′·da
rouge
rough
rough′·age
rou·leau′ pl. ·leaux′
round′·worm
rub′·ber
ru′·be·fa′·cient
ru′·be·fac′·tion
ru·bel′·la
ru·bel′·li·form
ru′·be·o′·la
ru′·be·o′·sis
ru′·ber fem. ·bra, neut.
    ·brum
ru·bes′·cent
ru·bid′·i·um
ru′·bin

ru′·bi·vi′·rus
ru″·bor
ru″·bra *fem. of* ruber
ru·bres′·er·ine
ru″·bri·blast
ru″·bri·cyte
ru″·bro·
ru″·bro·bul′·bar
ru″·bro·cer′·e·bel′·lar
ru″·bro·gli·o·cla″·din
ru″·bro·ol′·i·var′y
ru″·bro·re·tic″·u·lar
ru″·bro·re·tic″·u·lo·spi′·nal
ru″·bro·spi′·nal
ru″·bro·spi·na′·lis
ru″·bro·tha·lam′·ic
ru″·brum *neut. of* ruber
ruc″·tus
ru″·di·ment
ru″·di·men″·ta·ry
ru″·di·men″·tum
rue
ru″·fo·chro′·mo·my′·cin
ru″·fous
ru″·ga *pl.* ·gae, *gen. pl.*
 ru·ga″·rum
ru″·gi·tus
ru″·gose *also* ·gous
ru·gos″·i·ty
rum′·ble
ru″·men
ru″·mi·nant
ru″·mi·na″·tion
run″·around *also* run″·round
run″·off
ru″·pia
ru″·pi·al
ru″·pi·oid
rup″·ture *n. & v.*
 ·tured, ·tur·ing
ru·the′·ni·um
ruth′·er·ford
ru″·ti·do′·sis *var. of*
 rhytidosis
ru″·tin
ru″·to·side

S

Sa·be′·thes
sab′·u·lous
sab′·u·lum
sa·bur″·ra
sa·bur″·ral
sac
sac·cade′
sac·cad′·ic
sac″·cha·rate
sac″·cha·ri *var. of*
 saccharo-
sac″·cha·ride
sac·char′·i·fi·ca″·tion
sac″·cha·rim″·e·ter
 also ·rom″·e·ter
sac″·cha·rin *food sweetener: Cf.* saccharine
sac″·cha·rine *relating to sugar: Cf.* saccharin
sac″·cha·ro·
sac″·cha·ro·lyt″·ic
Sac″·cha·ro·my″·ces
sac″·cha·rum
sac″·ci *pl. & gen. sg. of* saccus
sac″·ci·form
sac′·ci·for′·mis
sac′·cu·lar
sac′·cu·la′·ris
sacc″·u·lat′·ed
sacc″·u·la″·tion
sac″·cule
sac″·cu·li·form
sac″·cu·lo·coch″·le·ar
sac″·cu·lo·utric″·u·lar
sac″·cu·lus *pl. & gen. sg.* ·li
sac″·cus *pl. & gen. sg.* ·ci
sa″·crad
sa″·cral
sa·cra′·le *neut. of*
 sacralis; *pl.* ·lia
sa·cral″·gia
sa·cra″·lis *pl.* ·les, *gen. pl.* ·li·um

sa′·cral·i·za″·tion
sa·crec′·to·my
sa″·cri *gen. of* sacrum
sa′·cro· [sac′·ro·]
sa″·cro·coc·cyg″·e·al
sa″·cro·coc·cyg″·e·us
 fem. ·cyg″·ea, *neut.*
 ·cyg″·e·um
sa″·cro·coc″·cyx
sa″·cro·cox·al″·gia
sa″·cro·cox·i′·tis
sa″·cro·il″·i·ac
sa″·cro·ili″·a·ca
sa″·cro·il′i·i′tis
sa″·cro·lis·the″·sis
sa″·cro·pel″·vic
sa″·cro·pel″·vi·ca
sa″·cro·sci·at″·ic
sa″·cro·spi″·nal
sa″·cro·spi·na″·lis
 neut. ·le
sa·crot″·o·my
sa″·cro·tu″·ber·a″·lis
 neut. ·le
sa″·cro·tu″·ber·ous
 also ·ber·al
sa″·cro·u″ter·ine
sa″·crum *gen.* sa″·cri
sac″·to·sal″·pinx
sad′·dle
sad′·dle·nose
sa″·dism [sad′·ism]
sa″·dist [sad′·ist]
sa·dis″·tic
sa″·do·mas″·och·is′m
sa″·do·mas″·och·is″·tic
saf′·ra·nine
saf″·ra·no·phil″·ic
saf″·role
sag′·it·tal
sag″·it·ta″·lis
sal
sal′·abra″·sion
sal″·acet″·a·mide [sal·ac′·et·am′·ide]
sal″·azo·sul″·fa·pyr″·i·dine *Brit.* ·sul′·pha·
sal′·i·cyl·al′·de·hyde
sal′·i·cyl″·a·mide

sa·lic′·y·late
sal′·i·cyl·a′zo·sul′·fa·
 pyr′·i·dine *Brit.*
 ·sul′·pha·
sal′·i·cyl′·ic
sal′·i·cyl·is′m
sal′·i·cyl·sul·fon′·ic
 Brit. ·phon′·ic
sal′·i·cyl·u′ric
sa′·lient
sa·lim′·e·ter
sa′·line
sa·lin′·i·ty
sal′·i·nom′·e·ter [sa′·
 li·] *var. of* salimeter
sa·li′·va
sal′·i·va′·ria *pl.* ·ri·ae
sal′·i·var′y
sal′·i·vate ·vat′·ed,
 ·vat′·ing
sal′·i·va′·tion
sal′·i·va·to′·ry
Sal′·mo·nel′·la
 S. en′·ter·it′·i·dis
 S. ty′·phi
 S. ty′·phi·mu′·ri·um
sal′·mo·nel′·la *pl.* ·lae
sal′·mo·nel·lo′·sis
sal′·ol
sal·pin′·ge·al *also* sal·
 pin′·gi·an
sal′·pin·gec′·to·my
sal·pin′·ges *pl. of*
 salpinx
sal·pin′·gi·on
sal′·pin·gi′·tis
sal·pin′·go·
sal·pin′·go·cele
sal·pin′·go·gram
sal′·pin·gog′·ra·phy
sal′·pin·go·li·thi′·a·sis
sal′·pin·gol′·y·sis
sal·pin′·go-o′o·pho·
 rec′·to·my
sal·pin′·go-o′o·pho·ri′·
 tis
sal·pin′·go-ooph′·o·ro·
 cele

sal·pin′·go-o′o·the·
 cec′·to·my
sal·pin′·go-o′o·the·ci′·
 tis
sal·pin′·go-o′o·the′·co·
 cele
sal·pin′·go-ovar′·i·ec′·
 to·my
sal·pin′·go-ovar′·i·ot′·
 o·my
sal·pin′·go·pal′·a·ti′·na
sal·pin′·go·pal′·a·tine
 also ·tal
sal·pin′·go·pex′y
sal·pin′·go·pha·ryn′·ge·
 al
sal·pin′·go·pha·ryn′·ge·
 us *fem.* ·gea
sal·pin′·go·plas′·ty
sal′·pin·gor′·rha·phy
sal·pin′·go·sal′·pin·
 gos′·to·my
sal′·pin·gos′·to·my
sal·pin′·go·the′·cal
sal′·pin·got′·o·my
sal′·pinx *pl.* sal·pin′·
 ges, *gen. sg.* sal·pin′·
 gis
sal′·sa·late
sal·ta′·tion
sal′·ta·to′·ry
salt′·ing-in′
salt′·ing-out′
salt·pe′·ter *Brit.* ·tre
sa·lu′·bri·ous
sal′·ure′·sis
sal′·uret′·ic
sal′·u·tar′y
sal′·vage ·vaged, ·vag·
 ing
sal′·var·san′
salve
sal′·y·sal
sa·mar′·i·um
sam′·ple
sam′·pler
sam′·pling
san′·a·to′·ri·um *pl.*
 ·ria *or* ·ri·ums

san′·a·to′·ry
san·cy′·cline
san′·da·rac
sand′·fly *also* sand fly
sand′·worm
san′·gui·
san·guic′·o·lous
san·guif′·er·ous
san′·gui·mo′·tor *also*
 ·to·ry
San′·gui·nar′·ia
san′·gui·na′·ri·us
san′·guine
san·guin′·e·ous *also*
 san′·gui·nous
san·guin′·e·us *fem.*
 ·guin′·ea
san′·gui·no· *var. of*
 sangui-
san·guin′·o·lent
san′·gui·no·poi·et′·ic
san′·gui·no·pu′·ru·lent
san′·guis *gen.* san′·
 gui·nis
San′·gui·su′·ga
san′·gui·su′·ga
sa′·ni·es *pl.* sanies
sa′·nio·pu′·ru·lent
sa′·nio·se′·rous
sa′·ni·ous
san′·i·tar′·i·an
san′·i·tar′·i·um *pl.* ·ia
 or ·i·ums
san′·i·tar′y
san′·i·ta′·tion
san′·i·ti·za′·tion
san′·i·tize ·tized, ·tiz′·
 ing
san′·i·ty
san·ton′·i·ca
sa·phe′·na *fem. of*
 saphenus; *pl. & gen.
 sg.* ·nae
saph′·e·nec′·to·my
sa·phe′·no·fem′·o·ral
sa·phe′·nous
sa·phe′·nus *pl. & gen.
 sg.* ·ni
sap′·id

sa'·pi·en'·tia [sap'·i·]
   gen. ·ti·ae
sa'·po gen. sa·po'·nis
sap'·o·gen'·in
sap'·o·na'·ceous
sap'·o·nat'·ed
sa·pon'·i·fi'·a·ble
sa·pon'·i·fi·ca'·tion
sa·pon'·i·fy ·fied, ·fy'·ing
sap'·o·nin
sap'·o·ros'·i·ty
sap'·phism
Sap·pin'·ia di·ploi'·dea
sa·pre'·mia *Brit.*
  ·prae'·
sap'·ro·
sap'·robe
sap'·ro·gen'·ic *also*
  sa·prog'·e·nous
sa·proph'·a·gous
sap'·ro·phyte
sap'·ro·phyt'·ic
sap'·ro·troph
sap'·ro·zo'·ic
sap'·ro·zo'·ite
sap'·ro·zo'·o·no'·sis
sar·al'·a·sin
Sar'·ci·na
sar'·co·
sar'·co·blast
sar'·co·cele
sar'·co·cyst
Sar'·co·cys'·ti·dae
Sar'·co·cys'·tis
  S. hom'·i·nis
  S. lin'·de·man'·ni
  S. su'i·hom'·i·nis
sar'·co·cys·to'·sis
Sar'·co·di'·na
sar'·co·gen'·ic
sar'·coid
sar'·coi·do'·sis
sar'·co·lac'·tic
sar'·co·lem'·ma
sar'·co·lem'·mic *also*
  ·mal
sar·col'·y·sis

sar'·co·lyte
sar'·co·lyt'·ic
sar·co'·ma *pl.* ·mas *or*
  ·ma·ta
sar·co'·ma·toid
sar'·co·ma·to'·sis
sar·com'a·tous
  [·co'ma·]
sar'·co·mere
Sar·coph'·a·ga
Sar'·co·phag'·i·dae
sar'·co·plas'm
sar'·co·plas'·mic
sar'·co·plast
Sar·cop'·tes
  S. sca'·bi·e'i
sar·cop'·tic
Sar·cop'·ti·dae
sar'·cop·ti·do'·sis
sar'·co·sine
sar'·co·sin·e'·mia
  Brit. ·ae'·mia
sar'·co·some
sar'·co·spo·rid'·i·an
sar'·co·spo·rid'·i·o'·sis
  also ·spo'·ri·di'·a·sis
sar'·cos·to'·sis
sar'·co·tu'·bu·lar
sar'·co·tu'·bule
sar'·cous
sar·don'·i·cus
sa'·rin [sa·rin']
sar·men'·to·gen'·in
sar·to'·ri·us *pl. &*
  gen. sg. ·rii
sas'·sa·fras
sat'·el·lite
sat'·el·li·to'·sis
sa'·ti·a'·tion
sa·ti'·ety
sat'·u·rate ·rat'·ed,
  ·rat'·ing
sat'·u·ra'·tion
sat'·ur·nine
sat'·ur·ni'·nus
sat'·ur·nis'm [·urn·is'm]
sat'·y·ri'·a·sis

sat'·yr·is'm
sau·cer·i·za'·tion
sau'·cer·ize ·ized, ·iz'·ing
sax·if'·ra·gant
sax'i·tox'·in
scab
sca'·bi·cide
sca'·bies
sca'·bi·et'·ic *also* sca·bet'·ic
sca'·bi·ous
sca'·la *pl. & gen. sg.*
  ·lae
scald
scale *n. & v.* scaled,
  scal'·ing
sca'·lene
sca'·le·nec'·to·my
sca'·le·not'·o·my
sca·le'·nus *pl. & gen.*
  sg. ·ni
scal'·er
scall
scal'·lop·ing
scalp
scal'·pel
scalp'·ing
scal'·prum
scal'y scal'·i·er, scal'·i·est
scan *n. & v.* scanned,
  scan'·ning
scan'·di·um
scan'·ner
scan·og'·ra·phy
scan·so'·ri·us
scaph'a [sca'·pha] *pl.*
  & gen. sg. scaph'·ae
scaph'o·
scaph'o·ce·phal'·ic
scaph'o·ceph'·a·ly
scaph'o·hy'·dro·ceph'·a·ly
scaph'·oid
sca·phoi'·dea *fem. of*
  scaphoideus

sca·phoi′·de·um *neut.*
of scaphoideus; *gen.*
·dei
sca·phoi′·de·us
scaph′·oid·i′·tis
Scap′·to·co′·sa rap·to′·ria
scap′·u·la *pl. & gen. sg.* ·lae
scap′·u·lar
scap′·u·la′·ris
scap′·u·lar′y
scap′·u·lec′·to·my
scap′·u·lo·an·te′·ri·or
scap′·u·lo·cla·vic′·u·lar
scap′·u·lo·cos′·tal
scap′·u·lo·hu′·mer·al
scap′·u·lo·per′·o·ne′·al
scap′·u·lo·pex′y
scap′·u·lo·pos·te′·ri·or
sca′·pus *pl.* ·pi
scar *n. & v.* scarred, scar′·ring
scar′·a·bi′·a·sis
scar′·i·fi·ca′·tion
scar′·i·fi′·er
scar′·i·fy ·fied, ·fy′·ing
scar′·la·ti′·na
scar′·la·ti′·nal
scar′·la·tin′′·i·form [·ti′·ni·]
scar′·let
sca·te′·mia *Brit.* ·tae′·
scat′o·
scat′·o·log′·ic *also* ·i·cal
sca·tol′·o·gy
sca·to′·ma *pl.* ·mas *or* ·ma·ta
sca·toph′·a·gy
scat′·ter
scat′·u·la
scav′·en·ger
schar′·lach
sched′·ule
sche′·ma *pl.* ·ma·ta
sche·mat′·ic
sche·mat′·o·gram

sche·mat′·o·graph
scheme
schin′·dy·le′·sis
schis′·ta·sis
schis′·ten·ceph′·a·ly
  var. of schizencephaly
schis′·to·
schis′·to·ce′·lia *also*
  ·coe′·
schis′·to·ceph′·a·lus
schis′·to·cor′·mia
schis′·to·cys′·tis
schis′·to·cyte *var. of* schizocyte
schis′·to·cy·to′·sis
  var. of schizocytosis
schis′·to·glos′·sia
schis′·to·me′·lia
schis′·to·pro·so′·pia
schis·tor′·rha·chis
  also schis′·to·ra′·chis
Schis′·to·so′·ma
S. *hae′·ma·to′·bi·um*
S. *ja·pon′·i·cum*
S. *man·so′·ni*
schis′·to·so′·ma·cid′·al
  [·ci′·dal] *var. of* schistosomicidal
schis′·to·so′·ma·cide
  var. of schistosomicide
schis′·to·so′·mal
Schis′·to·so·ma′·ti·um
S. *dou′·thit·ti*
Schis′·to·so′·ma·toi′·dea
schis′·to·some
schis′·to·so′·mia
schis′·to·so·mi′·a·sis
schis′·to·so′·mi·cid′·al
  [·ci′·dal]
schis′·to·so′·mi·cide
schis′·to·ster′·nia
schis′·to·tho′·rax
schis′·to·tra·che′·lus
  [·trach′·e·lus]
schiz·am′·ni·on
schiz′·en·ceph′·a·ly
schiz′o·

schiz′o·af·fec′·tive
schiz′o·ce·phal′·ic
schiz′·o·coel′·ic
schiz′o·cor′·tex
schiz′·o·cyte
schiz′·o·cy·to′·sis
schiz′o·gen′·e·sis
schi·zog′·e·nous
schi·zog′·o·ny
schiz′·o·gy′·ria
schiz′·oid
schiz′o·ki·ne′·sis
schiz′o·my′·cete [·my·cete′′]
Sciz′o·my·ce′·tes
schiz′o·my·co′·sis
schiz′·ont
schi·zont′·ti·cide
schiz′·o·pha′·sia
schiz′·o·phre′·nia
schiz′·o·phren′·ic
schiz′·o·phren′·i·form
schiz′o·pro·so′·pia
  var. of schistoprosopia
schiz′o·tho′·rax *var. of* schistothorax
schiz′o·thy′·mic
schiz′·o·to′·nia
schiz′·o·tro′·pic
  [·trop′·ic]
schiz′·o·try′·pa·no′·sis
schiz′o·try·pan′·o·so·mi′′·a·sis
Schiz′·o·try′·pa·num cru′·zi
schiz′·o·zo′·ite
schlaf′·krank′·heit
schlaf′·sucht
schlep′·per
schnei·der′·i·an
Schoen·gas′·tia
schwan′·no·gli·o′·ma
  pl. ·mas *or* ·ma·ta
schwan·no′·ma *pl.*
  ·mas *or* ·ma·ta
schwel′·le
sci′a· *var. of* skia·
sci·al′′·y·scope

sciatic / scrotoplasty

sci·at′·ic
sci·at′·i·ca
sci′·ence
sci′·en·tif′·ic
sci′·en·tist
scil′·la
scin′·ti·
scin′·ti·an′·gi·og′·ra·phy
scin′·ti·gram
scin·tig′·ra·phy
scin′·til·lant
scin′·til·lat′·ing
scin′·til·la′·tion
scin′·til·la′·tor
scin′·ti·pho·tog′·ra·phy
scin′·ti·scan
scin′·ti·scan′·ner
sci′·on
scir′·rhoid
scir·rho′·ma   *pl.* ·mas *or* ·ma·ta
scir′·rhous
scir′·rhus
scis′·sile
scis′·sion
scis′·sors
scis·su′·ra
scis′·su·ral
scle′·ra   *pl. & gen. sg.* ·rae
scler′·ad·e·ni′·tis
scle′·ral
scle·rec′·to·ir′i·do·di·al′·y·sis
scle·rec′·tome
scle·rec′·to·my
scler′·ede′·ma   *Brit.* ·oe·de′·
scle·re′·ma
scler′·irit′·o·my
scle·rit′·ic
scle·ri′·tis
scle′·ro· [scler′·o·]
scle′·ro·blas·te′·ma
scle′·ro·cho′·roid·i′·tis
scle′·ro·con′·junc·ti′·val

scle′·ro·con·junc′·ti·vi′·tis
scle′·ro·cor′·nea
scle′·ro·cor′·ne·al
scle′·ro·cys′·tic
scle′·ro·dac′·ty·ly   also ·dac·tyl′·ia
scle′·ro·der′·ma
scle′·ro·der′·ma·ti′·tis
scle′·ro·der′·ma·to·my′·o·si′·tis
scle′·ro·der′·ma·tous
scle′·ro·gum′·ma·tous
scle′·roid
scle′·ro·iri′·tis
scle′·ro·ker′·a·ti′·tis
scle′·ro·ker′·a·to·iri′·tis
scle·ro′·ma
scle′·ro·ma·la′·cia
scle′·ro·mere
scle·rom′·e·ter
scle′·ro·o′o·pho·ri′·tis
scler′·oph·thal′·mia
scle′·ro·pro′·tein
scle·ro′·sal
scle·rose′   ·rosed′, ·ros′·ing
scle·ro′·sis
scle′·ro·skel′·e·ton
scle′·ro·ste·no′·sis
scler·os′·te·o′·sis
scle·ros′·to·my
scle′·ro·ther′·a·py
scle·rot′·ic
scle·rot′·i·ca
scle·rot′·i·cec′·to·my
scle·rot′·i·cot′·o·my
scle′·ro·ti′·tis
scle·ro′·ti·um   *pl.* ·tia
scle′·ro·tized
scle′·ro·tome
scle′·ro·tom′·ic [·to′·mic]
scle·rot′·o·my
scle′·rous
sco′·le·coid
sco′·lex   *pl.* sco′·le·ces *or* sco′·li·ces

sco′·lio·
sco′·lio·ky·pho′·sis
sco′·lio·lor·do′·sis
sco′·li·o′·sis
sco′·li·ot′·ic
Sco′·lo·pen′·dra
sco′·po·la   also sco·po′·lia
sco′·po·lag′·nia
sco·pol′·a·mine
sco·pom′·e·ter
sco′·po·phil′·ia
scor·bu′·tic
scor·bu′·ti·ca
scor·bu′·ti·gen′·ic
scor·bu′·tus
Scor′·pio
scor′·pi·on
sco′·to·
sco′·to·chro′·mo·gen
sco·to′·ma   *pl.* ·mas *or* ·ma·ta
sco·to′·ma·graph
sco·to′·ma·tous   [·tom′a·]
sco·tom′·e·ter
sco·tom′·e·try
sco′·to·mi·za′·tion
sco·to′·pia
sco·to′·pic [·top′·ic]
sco·top′·sin
sco·tos′·co·py
scrap′·er
scra′·pie
scrap′·ing
scratch
screen′·ing
screw′·worm
scro·bic′·u·late
scro·bic′·u·lus   *pl.* ·li
scrof′·u·la
scrof′·u·lo·der′·ma
scrof′·u·lous
scro′·tal
scro·ta′·lis   *pl.* ·les
scro·tec′·to·my
scro′·to·cele
scro′·to·plas′·ty

scro'·tum L. pl. ·ta,
  gen. sg. ·ti
scrub scrubbed,
  scrub'·bing
scru'·ple
scul·te'·tus
scurf
scurf'y
scur'·vy
scu'·tate
scute
scu'·ti·form
Scu·tig'·era
scu'·tu·lum pl. ·la
scu'·tum pl. ·ta
scyb'·a·lous
scyb'·a·lum pl. ·la
scy'·phi·form
scy'·phoid
Scy'·ta·lid'·i·um hy'·a·li'·num
seal'·ant
seal'·er
seal'·ing
sea'·sick·ness also
  sea sickness
seat'·worm
se·ba'·cea pl. ·ce·ae
se·ba'·ceous
se'·bi·a·gog'·ic [seb'i·]
se'·bo· [seb'o·] also
  se'·bi·
se'·bo·poi·e'·sis
seb'·or·rhe'a Brit.
  ·rhoe'a
seb'·or·rhe'·ic also
  ·rhe'·al; Brit. ·rhoe'·
seb'·or·rhe'·ica Brit.
  ·rhoe'·
seb'·or·rhe'·id Brit.
  ·rhoe'·
se'·bo·tro'·phic
  [·troph'·ic]
se'·bum
Se'·cer·nen'·tea
se·clu'·sio
se'·co·bar'·bi·tal
se'·co·dont

sec'·ond
sec'·ond·ar'·ies
sec'·ond·ar'y
se'·co·ste'·roid
se·cre'·ta
se·cre'·ta·gogue
se·crete' ·cret'·ed,
  ·cret'·ing
se·cre'·tin
se·cre'·tion
secretogogue
  misspelling of secretagogue
se·cre'·to·in·hib'·i·to'·ry
se·cre'·to·mo'·tor
  also ·to·ry or ·mo·to'·ric
se·cre'·tor
se·cre'·to·ry
sec'·tile
sec'·tio pl. sec'·ti·o'·nes
sec'·tion
sec'·tion·al
sec'·tor
sec·to'·ri·al
se·cun'da fem. of
  secundus
sec'·un·da'·ri·us pl.
  & gen. sg. ·rii
se·cun'·di·grav'·i·da
sec'·un·dines
sec'·un·dip'·a·ra
se·cun'·dus fem. ·da,
  neut. ·dum
se·date' ·dat'·ed,
  ·dat'·ing
se·da'·tion
sed'·a·tive
sed'·en·tar'y
se'·des gen. ·dis
se·dig'·i·tate
sed'·i·ment
sed'·i·men'·ta·ry
sed'·i·men·ta'·tion
sed'·i·men·tom'·e·ter
se'·dis gen. of sedes

se'·do·hep'·tu·lose
seg'·ment
seg·men'·tal also
  seg'·men·tar'y
seg'·men·ta'·lis pl.
  ·les
seg'·men·ta'·tion
seg'·ment·ed
seg'·ment·er
seg·men'·tum pl. ·ta,
  gen. sg. ·ti
seg'·re·ga'·tion
seg'·re·ga'·tor
seg'·re·some
seis'·es·the'·sia Brit.
  ·aes·
seis'·mes·the'·sia
  Brit. ·maes·
seis'·mo·gen'·ic
sei'·zure
se·junc'·tion
se·lec'·tion
se·lec'·tive
se·le'·ne pl. ·nai or
  ·nae
se·le'·nic
sel'·e·nite
se·le'·ni·um
sel'·e·no·cys'·te·ine
sel'·e·no·me·thi'·o·nine
sel'·e·no'·sis
self'-ab·sorp'·tion
self'-con'·scious·ness
self'-dif'·fer·en'·ti·a'·tion
self'-di·ges'·tion
self'-ex·tinc'·tion
self'-fer'·til·i·za'·tion
self'-hyp·no'·sis
self'-im'·age
self'-in·duc'·tance
self'·ing
self'-lim'·it·ing also
  -lim'·it·ed
self'·ness
self'-rec'·og·ni'·tion
self'-tol'·er·ance
self'·wise

sel′·la *pl. & gen. sg.*
·lae
sel′·lar
sel·la′·ris
se·man′·tic
se′·mei·og′·ra·phy
se′·mei·ol′·o·gy
se′·mei·ot′·ic
sem′·el·in′·ci·dent
se′·men *gen.* se′·mi·nis
se′·men·u′·ri·a *var. of* seminuria
sem′i·
sem′i·al′·de·hyde
sem′i·ap′o·chro′·mat
sem′i·ap′o·chro·mat′·ic
sem′i·ca·nal′
sem′i·ca·na′·lis *pl.*
·les
sem′i·car′·ba·zide
sem′i·car′·ba·zone
sem′i·car′·ti·lag′·i·nous
sem′i·cir′·cu·lar
sem′i·cir′·cu·la′·ris *pl.* ·res
sem′i·co′·ma
sem′i·co′·ma·tose
sem′i·con·duc′·tor
sem′i·con′·scious
sem′i·cris′·ta
sem′i·de′·cus·sa′·tion
sem′i·dom′·i·nance
sem′i·dom′·i·nant
sem′i·flex′·ion
sem′i·lu′·nar
sem′i·lu·na′·re *neut. of* semilunaris
sem′i·lu·na′·ris *pl.*
·res, *gen. pl.* ·ri·um
sem′i·lux·a′·tion
sem′i·mem′·bra·no′·sus *pl. & gen. sg.* ·si
sem′i·mem′·bra·nous
sem′·i·nal
sem′·i·na′·lis
sem′·i·na′·tion
sem′·i·nif′·er·ous

sem′·i·nif′·er·us *pl.*
·eri
sem′·i·no′·ma *pl.*
·mas *or* ·ma·ta
sem′·i·nu′·ria
se′·mi·og′·ra·phy *var. of* semeiography
se′·mi·ol′·o·gy *var. of* semeiology
sem′i·o′pen
se′·mi·ot′·ic *var. of* semeiotic
sem′i·o′val
sem′i·ova′·lis *neut.*
·le
sem′i·par′·a·site
sem′i·pen′·ni·form
sem′i·per′·me·able
sem′i·pri′·vate
sem′i·pro·na′·tion
sem′i·prone′
sem′i·qui·none′ [·quin′·one]
sem′i·re·cum′·bent
se′·mis
sem′i·spi′·nal
sem′i·spi·na′·lis
sem′i·su′·pi·na′·tion
sem′i·su′·pine
sem′i·syn′·thet′·ic
sem′i·sys′·tem·at′·ic
sem′i·ten′·di·no′·sus
sem′i·ten′·di·nous
sem′i·ter′·tian
sem′i·triv′·i·al
Se·ne′·cio
se·ne′·ci·o′·sis
sen′·e·ga
sen′·e·gen′·in
se·nes′·cence
se·nes′·cent
se′·nile
se·ni′·lis
se·nil′·i·ty
se′·ni·um
sen′·na
se·nog′·ra·phy
se·no′·pia

sen·sa′·tion
sense
sen′·si·bil′·i·ty
sen′·si·bil·i·za′·tion
sen′·si·ble
sen′·si·tive
sen′·si·tiv′·i·ty
sen′·si·ti·za′·tion
sen′·si·tize ·tized,
·tiz′·ing
sen′·si·tiz′·er
sen′·so·mo′·tor *var. of* sensorimotor
sen′·so·pa·ral′·y·sis
sen′·sor
sen·so′·ria *fem. of* sensorius, *pl. of* sensorium
sen·so′·ri·al
sen′·so·ri·glan′·du·lar
sen′·so·rim′·e·try
sen′·so·ri·mo′·tor
sen′·so·ri·mus′·cu·lar
sen′·so·ri·neu′·ral
sen·so′·ri·um *pl.* ·ria
sen·so′·ri·us *pl.* ·rii
sen′·so·ry
sen′·su·al
sen′·su·al·is′m
sen′·tient
sen′·ti·nel
sep′·a·rans
sep′·a·ra′·tion
sep′·a·ra′·tor
sep′·sis
sep′·ta *pl. of* septum
sep′·tal
sep·ta′·lis *pl.* ·les
sep′·tan
sep′·tate
sep·ta′·tion
sep·tec′·to·my
sep·te′·mia *var. of* septicemia; *Brit.* ·tae′·
sep′·ti *gen. of* septum
sep′·ti·
sep′·tic

sep'·ti·ce'·mia *Brit.*
  ·cae'·
sep'·ti·ce'·mic *Brit.*
  ·cae'·
sep'·ti·co·
sep'·ti·co·py·e'·mia
  Brit. ·ae'·mia
sep'·ti·co·py·e'·mic
  Brit. ·ae'·mic
sep'·ti·form
sep'·tile
sep'·ti·me·tri'·tis
sep'·to·
sep'·to·ha·ben'·u·lar
sep'·to·mar'·gi·nal
sep'·to·mar'·gi·na'·lis
sep'·to·plas'·ty
sep'·to·rhi'·no·plas'·ty
sep·tos'·to·my
sep'·tu·lum *pl.* ·la
sep'·tum *pl.* ·ta, *gen.*
  sg. ·ti
sep·tup'·let
sep'·tus
se'·quel
se·quel'a *pl.* se·quel'·
  ae
se'·quence *n. & v.*
  ·quenced, ·quenc·ing
se·quen'·tial
se·ques'·ter
se·ques'·tral
se'·ques·tra'·tion
se'·ques·trec'·to·my
se·ques'·trum *pl.* ·tra
se'·quoi·o'·sis
se'·ra *pl. of* serum
se'·ran·gi'·tis
ser'·apher·e'·sis
  [·apher'·e·]
se·rem'·pi·on
se·re'·na
se'·ri·al
se'·ri·al'·o·graph
Ser'·i·co·pel'·ma
  S. com·mu'·nis
se'·ries *pl.* series
ser'·ine [se'·rine]

ser'i·scis'·sion
se'·ro·
se'·ro·al·bu'·mi·nous
se'·ro·co·li'·tis
se'·ro·con·ver'·sion
se'·ro·cys'·tic
se'·ro·di'·ag·no'·sis
  pl. ·ses
se'·ro·en'·ter·i'·tis
se'·ro·ep'·i·de'·mi·o·
  log'·ic
se'·ro·ep'·i·de'·mi·ol'·
  o·gy
se'·ro·fi'·bri·nous
se'·ro·floc'·cu·la'·tion
se'·ro·flu'·id
se'·ro·hem'·or·rhag'·ic
  Brit. ·haem'·
se'·ro·li'·pase
se'·ro·log'·ic *also*
  ·i·cal
se·rol'·o·gist
se·rol'·o·gy
se'·rol'·y·sin
se'·ro·mem'·bra·nous
se'·ro·mu'·coid
se'·ro·mu·co'·sa
se'·ro·mu'·cous
se'·ro·mus'·cu·lar
se'·ro·neg'·a·tive
se'·ro·neg'·a·tiv'·i·ty
se'·ro·per'·i·to·ne'·um
se'·ro·pher·e'·sis *var.*
  of serapheresis
se'·ro·pneu'·mo·tho'·
  rax
se'·ro·pos'·i·tive
se'·ro·pos'·i·tiv'·i·ty
se'·ro·prog·no'·sis
se'·ro·pu'·ru·lent
se'·ro·pus'
se'·ro·re·ac'·tion
se'·ro·re·sis'·tance
se'·ro·re·sis'·tant
se'·ro·re·ver'·sal
se·ro'·sa *pl. & gen.*
  sg. ·sae
se'·ro·san·guin'·e·ous

se'·ro·se'·rous
'se'·ro·si'·tis
se'·ro·syn'·o·vi'·tis
se'·ro·ther'·a·py
se'·ro·tho'·rax
se·ro'·ti·nus [se'·ro·ti'·
  nus] *pl.* ·ni
se'·ro·to·ner'·gic
se'·ro·to'·nin
se'·ro·type
se'·rous
se'·ro·vac'·ci·na'·tion
se'·ro·var
se'·ro·zyme
ser'·pen·tar'·ia
ser'·pen·tine
ser·pig'·i·no'·sa
ser·pig'·i·nous
ser·ra'·ta *fem. of*
  serratus
ser'·rate *also* ·rat·ed
Ser·ra'·tia mar·ces'·
  cens
ser·ra'·tion
ser·ra'·tus *pl. & gen.*
  sg. ·ti
serre·fine'
ser'·ru·late
se'·rum *pl.* ·ra *or*
  ·rums
se'·rum·al
ser'·vice
ser'·vo·mech'·a·nis'm
ses'·a·moid
ses'·a·moi'·dea
ses'·qui·
ses'·qui·ho'·ra
ses'·qui·ter'·pene
ses'·sile
set *n. & v.* set, set'·
  ting
se'·ta *pl.* ·tae
se·ta'·ceous
set'·back
se·tif'·er·ous
se'·ton
set'·up
se'·vo·flu'·rane

se′·vum
sex·dig′·i·tate
sex·duc′·tion
sex′-link′·age
sex′-linked
sex′·tan
sex′·ti·grav′·i·da
sex·tip′·a·ra
sex·tup′·let
sex′·u·al
sex′·u·al′·i·ty
sex′·u·al·i·za′·tion
shad′·ow-cast′·ing
shank
shap′·ing
shears
sheath
sheathed
shell′·shocked
shi·a′·tsu
shield
Shi·gel′·la
  S. boyd′·ii
  S. dys′·en·ter′·i·ae
  S. flex′·neri
  S. son′·nei
shi·gel′·la *pl.* ·lae
shig′·el·lo′·sis
shi·kim′·ic
shi′·ma·mu′·shi
shin′·bone
shin′·gles
shin′·splints *also* shin splints
shock
short′·sight′·ed
short′·sight′·ed·ness
short′-wind′·ed
short′-wind′·ed·ness
shot′·ty
shoul′·der
shunt
si′·al·ad′·e·nec′·to·my
  var. of sialoadenectomy
si′·al·ad·e·ni′·tis
si′·al·ad′·e·nog′·ra·phy
si′·al·ad′·e·not′·o·my
  var. of sialoadenotomy

si′·a·la·gog′·ic
si·al′·a·gogue
si′·a·lec′·ta·sis *also*
  ·lec·ta′·sia
si·al′·ic
si·al′·i·dase
si′·a·lis′m
si′·a·lo·
si′·a·lo·ad′·e·nec′·to·my
si′·a·lo·ad′·e·ni′·tis
  var. of sialadenitis
si′·a·lo·ad′·e·nog′·ra·phy *var. of* sialadenography
si′·a·lo·ad′·e·not′·o·my
si′·a·lo·aer′·o·pha′·gia
si′·a·lo·an′·gi·ec′·ta·sis
si′·a·lo·an′·gi·i′tis
si′·a·lo·an′·gi·og′·ra·phy
si′·a·lo·do·chi′·tis
si′·a·lo·do′·cho·li·thi′·a·sis
si′·a·lo·do′·cho·plas′·ty
sialogogic *misspelling of* sialagogic
sialogogue *misspelling of* sialagogue
si·al′·o·gram
si′·a·log′·ra·phy
si·al′·o·lith
si′·a·lo·li·thi′·a·sis
si′·a·lo·li·thot′·o·my
si′·a·lom′·e·ter
si′·a·lom′·e·try
si′·a·lo·pha′·gia
si′·a·lor·rhe′a Brit. ·rhoe′a
si′·a·lo′·sis
si′·a·lo·ste·no′·sis
sib′·i·lant
sib′·ling
sib′·ship
sic′·cant
sic′·co·la′·bile
sic′·co·sta′·bile
sic′·cus *fem.* ·ca

sick′·le *n. & v.* ·led, ·ling
sick·le′·mia *Brit.* ·lae′·
sick·le′·mic *Brit.* ·lae′·
sick′·ler
sick′·ness
side′-ef·fect′ *also* side effect
sid′·er·a·mine
si′·der·ans
sid′·ero·
sid′·er·o·blast
sid′·er·o·blas′·tic
sid′·er·o·chrome
sid′·er·o·cyte
sid′·er·o·cy·to′·sis
sid′·er·o·der′·ma
sid′·ero·fi·bro′·sis
sid′·er·og′·e·nous
sid′·er·o·my′·cin
sid′·er·o·pe′·nia
sid′·er·o·pe′·nic
sid′·er·o·phil *also* ·phile
sid′·er·oph′·i·lous
sid′·er·o·phore
sid′·er·o·scope
sid′·ero·sil′·i·co′·sis
sid′·er·o′·sis
sid′·er·ot′·ic
side′-shift
side′·wind′·er
sie′·mens
sieve
sie′·vert
sigh′·ing
sight′·ed
sig′·ma
sig′·moid
sig·moi′·dea *fem. of* sigmoideus; *pl. & gen. sg.* ·de·ae
sig′·moid·ec′·to·my
sig·moi′·de·um *neut. of* sigmoideus; *gen.* ·dei

sig·moi'·de·us *pl. &*
   gen. sg. ·dei
sig'·moid·i'·tis
sig·moi'·do·pex'y
sig·moi'·do·proc·tos'·
   to·my
sig·moi'·do·rec·tos'·to·
   my
sig·moi'·do·scope
sig'·moid·os'·co·py
sig·moi'·do·sig'·moid·
   os'·to·my
sig'·moid·os'·to·my
sig'·moid·ot'·o·my
sign
sig'·na
sig'·nal
sig'·na·ture
sig·nif'·i·cance
si'·gua·ter'a *var. of*
   ciguatera
si'·lent
si'·lex
sil'·i·ca
sil'·i·cate
sil'·i·ca·to'·sis *var. of*
   silicosis
si·li'·ceous *also* ·cious
sil'·i·co·flu'o·ride
sil'·i·con
sil'·i·cone
sil'·i·co·no'·ma
sil'·i·co·sid'·er·o'·sis
sil'·i·co'·sis
sil'·i·cot'·ic
sil'·i·co·tu·ber'·cu·lo'·
   sis
sil'·i·qua
sil'·ver
Sil'·vi·us
si·meth'·i·cone
sim'·i·an
*Si·mo'·nea fol·lic'·u·
   lo'·rum*

sim'·ple
sim'·plex
sim'·ul
sim'·u·la'·tion
sim'·u·la'·tor
Sim'·u·li'·idae
Si·mu'·li·um
   S. dam·no'·sum
   S. nea'·vei
   S. ochra'·ce·um
si'·mul·tan'·ag·no'·sia
si'·mul·ta'·ne·ous
*Sin·an'·thro·pus pe'·ki·
   nen'·sis*
sin'·a·pis'm
sin'·ca·lide
sin·cip'·i·tal
sin'·ci·put
sin'e
sin'·ew
sin'·gle-blind'
sin'·gu·la'·re
sin'·gul·ta'·tion
sin·gul'·tus *pl.*
   singultus
si·nis'·ter[46] [sin'·is·]
   gen. ·tri
si·nis'·tra *fem. of*
   sinister; *gen.* ·trae
sin'·is·trad
sin'·is·tral
sin'·is·tral'·i·ty
sin'·is·tra'·tion
si·nis'·tri *gen. of*
   sinister & sinistrum
sin'·is·tro· [si·nis'·tro·]
sin'·is·tro·car'·dia
sin'·is·tro·cer'·e·bral
sin'·is·troc'·u·lar
sin'·is·tro·tor'·sion
sin'·is·trous
si·nis'·trum *neut. of*
   sinister; *gen.* ·tri
si'·no·a'tri·al *var. of*
   sinuatrial

si'·no·au·ric'·u·lar
si'·no·ca·rot'·id
si'·no·du'·ral
si'·no·gram
si·nog'·ra·phy
si'·no·spi'·ral
si'·no·vag'·i·nal
si'·no·ven·tric'·u·lar
sin'·ter
si'·nu·a'tri·al
si'·nu·a'tri·a'·lis
si'·nu·au·ric'·u·lar
   var. of sinoauricular
sin'·u·os'·i·ty
sin'·u·ous
si'·nus *L. pl. & gen.
   sg.* sinus, *gen. pl.* si'·
   nu·um
si'·nus·al
si'·nus·i'·tis
si'·nu·soid
si'·nu·soi'·dal
si·nu·soi'·dal·i·za'·tion
si'·nus·ot'·o·my
si'·nu·um *gen. pl. of*
   sinus
si'·nu·ven·tric'·u·lar
   var. of sinoventricular
si'·nu·ver'·te·bral
si'·phon
si'·phon·age
*Si·phun'·cu·li'·na
   S. fu·nic'·o·la*
si·ren'·i·form *also* ·o·
   form
si'·ren·o·me'·lia
si're·nom'·e·lus
sir'·up *var. of* syrup
sis'·o·my'·cin
Sis·tru'·rus
site
si'·to·
si·tos'·ter·ol
si'·to·ther'·a·py

---

[46] As a Latin word for "left," *sinister* is best accented on the middle syllable and divided accordingly.

si·tot'·ro·pis'm
sit'·u·a'·tion
sit'·u·a'·tion·al
si'·tus *pl. & gen. sg.*
  situs, *ablative* si'·tu
skat'o· *var. of* scato-
skat'·ole
skat'·o·log'·ic *var. of*
  scatologic
ska·tol'·o·gy *var. of*
  scatology
skein
skel'·e·tal
skel'·e·ti *gen. of*
  skeleton
skel'·e·to·den'·tal
skel'·e·to·fu'·si·mo'·tor
skel'·e·tog'·e·nous
skel'·e·tog'·e·ny
skel'·e·to·mo'·tor
skel'·e·ton *gen.* ·e·ti
skene·i'tis *also* ske·
  ni'·tis
skene'·oscope *also*
  ske'·no·scope
skew'·foot
skew'·ness
ski'a·
ski·ag'·ra·phy
ski·am'·e·try
ski'·a·po·res'·co·py
ski'·a·scope
ski·as'·co·py
ski'a·sco·tom'·e·try
skin'·fold
skle'·ro· [skler'o·]
  var. of sclero-
skull
skull'·cap
sleep *n. & v.* slept,
  sleep'·ing
sleep'·walk·ing
slid'·ing
slough
sludge sludged, sludg'·
  ing
slur'·ry
small'·pox

smear
smeg'·ma
smeg·mat'·ic
smeg'·mo·lith
smell'-brain
smok'·er
smok'·ing
snake'·bite
snake'·root
snare
sneeze sneezed,
  sneez'·ing
snore snored, snor'·ing
snow'·blind'·ness
  also snow blindness
snuff'·box
snuff'·les
soap'·stone
sob'·bing
so'·cia
so'·cial
so'·cio·
so'·cio·acu'·sis *also*
  so'·ci·
so'·cio·bi·ol'·o·gy
so'·cio·dra'·ma
so'·cio·med'·i·cal
so'·ci·o·path
so'·ci·op'·a·thy
so'·cio·ther'·a·py
sock'·et
so'·da
so'·dio·
so'·di·um
so'·do·ko'·sis
so'·do·ku
sod'·om·ite *also* ·ist
sod'·omy
soft'·en·ing
so·ko'·sho
sol
so·lan'·i·dine
so'·la·nine
so'·la·nis'm
so'·la·noid *resembling*
  raw potato: Cf.
  solenoid
So·la'·num

so·lap'·sone
so'·lar
so·la'·ris
so·lar'·i·um
so'·la·so'·dine
so'·la·sul'·fone
sol'·der
sole
so'·le·al
so'·lei *gen. of* soleus
so'le·no·
So'·le·nog'·ly·pha
so'·le·no·glyph'·ic
so'·le·noid *helical*
  electric wire: Cf.
  solanoid
so'·le·no·nych'·ia
so'·le·nop'·sin
So'·le·nop'·sis
so'·le·us *gen.* ·lei
sol'·id
sol'·ip·sis'm
sol'·ip·sis'·tic
sol'·i·ta'·ri·us
sol'·i·tar'y
sol'·u·bil'·i·ty
sol'·u·ble
so'·lum
sol'·ute
so·lu'·tion
sol'·vate
sol·va'·tion
sol'·ven·cy
sol'·vent
sol·vol'·y·sis
so'·ma
so'·mal
so'·ma·plas'm *var. of*
  somatoplasm
so'·mat·ag·no'·sia
so'·mat·es·the'·sia
  Brit. ·aes·the'·
so'·mat·es·thet'·ic
  Brit. ·aes·thet'·
so·mat'·ic
so·mat'·i·co· *var. of*
  somato-
so'·ma·ti·za'·tion

so′·ma·to [so·mat′o·]
so·mat′·o·blast
so·mat′·o·chrome
so′·ma·to·dym′·ia
so·mat′·o·form
so′·ma·to·gen′·e·sis
so′·ma·to·gen′·ic [so·mat′·o·]
so′·ma·to·in·tes′·ti·nal
so′·ma·tol′·o·gy
so′·ma·to·mam′·mo·tro′·pin
so′·ma·to·me′·din
so′·ma·to·meg′·a·ly
so′·ma·tom′·e·try
so′·ma·to·mo′·tor
so′·ma·top′·a·gus
so′·ma·to·path′·ic
so·mat′·o·plas′m [so′·ma·to·]
so·mat′·o·pleure [so′·ma·to·]
so′·ma·to·psy′·chic
so′·ma·tos′·chi·sis
so′·ma·to·sen′·so·ry [so·mat′o·]
so′·ma·to·stat′·in
so′·ma·to·stat′·in·o′·ma
so′·ma·to·ther′·a·py
so′·ma·to·top′·ag·no′·sia
so′·ma·to·top′·ic
so·mat′·o·troph
so′·ma·to·tro′·pic [·trop′·ic] *also* ·tro′·phic
so′·ma·to·tro′·pin *also* ·tro′·phin
so·mat′·o·type [so′·ma·to·]
som′·es·the′·sia *Brit.* ·aes·
som′·es·thet′·ic *Brit.* ·aes·

so′·mite
so·mit′·ic
som·nam′·bu·lis′m
som·nam′·bu·lis′·tic
som′·ni·
som′·ni·fa′·cient
som·nif′·er·ous
som·nif′·ic
som′·no·lence
som′·no·len′·tia
so′·nar
sone
son′·ic
son′·i·cate ·cat′·ed, ·cat′·ing
son′·i·ca′·tion
son′·o·gram
so·nog′·ra·pher
so·nog′·ra·phy
so′·no·in·ver′·sion
so·nol′·o·gy
so·phis′·ti·cate ·cat′·ed, ·cat′·ing
so·phis′·ti·ca′·tion
so′·por
sop⌐·o·rif′·er·ous [so′·po·]
sop′·o·rif′·ic [so′·po·]
sor′·bate
sor′·be·fa′·cient
sor′·bic
sor′·bi·tol
sor′·bose
sor′·des
sore
so·ro′·che
sorp′·tion
souf′·fle
sound
spac′·er
spal·la′·tion
spar′·er
spar′·ga·no′·sis
spar′·ga·num *pl.* ·na

spar′·ing
spar′·so·my′·cin
spar′·te·ine
spar′·tism
spas′m
spas′·mo·
spas·mod′·ic
spas·mod′·i·cus *fem.* ·ca
spas′·mo·gen
spas′·mo·gen′·ic
spas′·mo·lyg′·mus
spas·mol′·y·sis
spas′·mo·lyt′·ic
spas′·mus
spas′·tic
spas′·ti·ca
spas·tic′·i·ty
spa′·tial
spa′·ti·um *pl.* ·tia, *gen. sg.* ·tii
spat′·u·la
spat′·u·late
spat′·u·la′·tion
spay
spe′·cial·ist
spe′·cial·i·za′·tion
spe′·cial·ize ·ized, ·iz′·ing
spe′·cial·ty
spe′·ci·a′·tion
spe′·cies[47] *pl.* species
spe·cif′·ic
spec′·i·fic′·i·ty
spe·cil′·lum
spec′·i·men
speck′·le
spec′·ta·cles
spec′·ti·no·my′·cin
spec′·tra *pl. of* spectrum
spec′·tral
spec′·trin
spec′·tro·

---

[47] The singular of *species* is abbreviated: sp. The plural is abbreviated: spp. Species names are italicized.

spec′·tro·col′·or·im′·e·
ter
spec′·tro·fluo·rom′·e·
ter
spec′·tro·gram
spec′·tro·graph
spec·trog′·ra·phy
spec·trom′·e·ter
spec·trom′·e·try
spec′·tro·pho′·to·fluo·
rom′·e·ter
spec′·tro·pho·tom′·e·
ter
spec′·tro·pho·tom′·e·
try
spec′·tro·po′·lar·im′·e·
ter
spec′·tro·scope
spec′·tro·scop′·ic
spec·tros′·co·py
spec′·trum pl. ·tra
spec′·u·lar
spec′·u·lum pl. ·la or
·lums
spel′·en·ce·pha′·lia
sperm
sper′·ma
sper′·ma·ce′·ti
sper′·ma·cra′·sia also
sper′·ma·ta·
sperm′·ag·glu′·ti·na′·
tion
sper′·ma·tel′·e·o′·sis
sper′·ma·tem·phrax′·is
sper·mat′·ic
sper·mat′·i·ca fem. of
spermaticus
sper·mat′·i·cid′·al [·ci′·
dal]
sper·mat′·i·cide
sper·mat′·i·cus pl. &
gen. sg. ·ci
sper′·ma·tid
sper′·ma·tis′m
sper′·ma·ti′·tis
sper′·ma·to· [sper·
mat′o·]

sper′·ma·to·cele′ [sper·
mat′·o·cele]
sper′·ma·to·ce·lec′·to·
my
sper·mat′·o·cid′·al
[·ci′·dal] var. of
spermaticidal
sper·mat′·o·cide var.
of spermaticide
sper′·ma·to·cyst′ [sper·
mat′o·]
sper′·ma·to·cys·tec′·to·
my
sper′·ma·to·cys·ti′·tis
sper′·ma·to·cys·tot′·o·
my
sper·mat′·o·cyte [sper′·
ma·to·]
sper′·ma·to·cyt′·ic
sper′·ma·to·cy′·to·gen′·
e·sis
sper′·ma·to·gen′·e·sis
sper′·ma·to·gen′·ic
sper′·ma·tog′·e·nous
sper′·ma·to·go′·ni·al
sper′·ma·to·go′·ni·um
pl. ·nia
sper′·ma·tol′·y·sin
sper′·ma·tol′·y·sis
sper′·ma·to·lyt′·ic
sper′·ma·tor·rhe′a
Brit. ·rhoe′a
sper′·ma·to·tox′·in
also sper′·ma·tox′·in
sper′·mat·o′·vum
sper′·ma·to·zo′·on
pl. ·zo′a
sper′·ma·tu′·ria
sper·mec′·to·my
sper′·mi·a′·tion
sper′·mi·cid′·al [·ci′·
dal]
sper′·mi·cide
sper′·mi·dine
sper′·mi·duct
sper′·mine
sper′·mio·gen′·e·sis
sper′·mio·tel′·e·o′·sis

sper′·mo·
sper′·mo·cy·to′·ma
sper′·mo·lith
sper′·mo·lo′·ro·pex′y
also ·lo′·ro·pex′·is
sper·mol′·y·sin var.
of spermatolysin
sper·mol′·y·sis var. of
spermatolysis
sper′·mo·lyt′·ic var.
of spermatolytic
sper′·mo·phleb′·ec·ta′·
sia
sper′·mo·plas′m
sper′·mor·rhe′a var.
of spermatorrhea; Brit.
·rhoe′a
sper′·mo·sphere
sper′·mo·tox′·in var.
of spermatotoxin
spes
sphac′·e·late ·lat′·ed,
·lat′·ing
sphac′·e·la′·tion
sphac′·e·lin′·ic
sphac′·e·lis′m
sphac′·e·loid
sphac′·e·lous
sphac′·e·lus pl. ·li
spha′·gi·as′·mus
sphen·eth′·moid var.
of sphenoethmoid
sphe′·nic
sphe′·no·
sphe′·no·bas′·i·lar
sphen′·oc·cip′·i·tal
var. of spheno-occipital
sphe′·no·ceph′·a·ly
sphe′·no·eth′·moid
also ·eth·moi′·dal
sphe′·no·eth′·moi·da′·
lis
sphe′·no·fron′·tal
sphe′·no·fron·ta′·lis
sphe′·noid
sphe·noi′·dal
sphe′·noi·da′·le neut.
of sphenoidalis

sphe′·noi·da′·lis *pl.*
 ·les, *gen. pl.* ·li·um
sphe′·noid·i′·tis
sphe′·noid·os′·to·my
sphe′·noid·ot′·o·my
sphe′·no·man·dib′·u·
 la′·ris *neut.* ·re
sphe′·no·man·dib′·u·lar
sphe′·no·max′·il·la′·ris
sphe′·no·max′·il·lar′y
sphe′·no-oc·cip′·i·tal
sphe′·no-oc·cip′·i·ta′·
 lis
sphe′·no·pal′·a·tine
sphe′·no·pal′·a·ti′·nus
 fem. ·na, *neut.* ·num
sphe′·no·pa·ri′·etal
sphe′·no·pa·ri′·eta′·lis
sphe′·no·pe·tro′·sa
sphe′·no·pe·tro′·sal
sphe′·no·pha·ryn′·ge·al
sphe·no′·sis
sphe′·no·squa·mo′·sa
sphe′·no·squa·mo′·sal
sphe·no′·tic
sphe′·no·tribe
sphe′·no·trip′·sy
sphe′·no·tur′·bi·nal
sphe′·no·vo·mer′·i·a′·
 na
sphe′·no·vo′·mer·ine
 also ·vo·mer′·i·an
sphe′·no·zy′·go·mat′·ic
sphe′·no·zy′·go·mat′·i·
 ca
spher′·i·cus [sphe′·ri·]
sphe′·ro· [spher′o·]
sphe′·ro·cyl′·in·der
sphe′·ro·cyte
sphe′·ro·cyt′·ic
sphe′·ro·cy·to′·sis
sphe′·roid [spher′·oid]
sphe·roi′·dal
sphe·roi′·dea
sphe·rom′·e·ter
sphe′·ro·pha′·kia
sphe′·ro·plast
spher′·ule

sphinc′·ter *gen.*
 sphinc·ter′·is
sphinc′·ter·al *also*
 sphinc·ter′·ic
sphinc′·ter·al′·gia
sphinc′·ter·ec′·to·my
sphinc′·ter·is′·mus
sphinc′·ter·i′·tis
sphinc′·ter·o·plas′·ty
sphinc′·ter·o·scope
sphinc′·ter·o·tome
sphinc′·ter·ot′·o·my
sphin′·ga·nine
sphin′·go·
sphin′·go·lip′·id
sphin′·go·lip′·i·do′·sis
 pl. ·ses
sphin′·go·my′·e·lin
sphin′·go·my′·e·lin·ase
sphin′·go·sine
sphyg′·mic
sphyg′·mo·
sphyg′·mo·chron′·o·
 graph
sphyg′·mo·chro·nog′·
 ra·phy
sphyg′·mo·dy′·na·
 mom′·e·ter
sphyg′·mo·gram
sphyg′·mo·graph
sphyg′·mo·graph′·ic
sphyg·mog′·ra·phy
sphyg′·mo·ma·nom′·e·
 ter
sphyg′·mo·ma·nom′·e·
 try
sphyg·mom′·e·ter
sphyg′·mo·scope
sphyg′·mus
spi′·ca
spic′·ule
spic′·u·lum *pl.* ·la
spi′·der
spi·ge′·li·an
spike
spill′·way
spi′·lus

spi′·na *pl. & gen. sg.*
 ·nae
spi′·nal
spi·na′·le *neut. of*
 spinalis; *pl.* ·lia
spi·nal′·gia
spi·na′·lis *pl.* ·les,
 gen. pl. ·li·um
spin′·dle
spine
spi′·ni·form
spi·nif′·u·gal
spi·nip′·e·tal
spinn′·bar·keit′
spi′·no·
spi′·no-ad·duc′·tor
spi′·no·bul′·bar
spi′·no·cer′·e·bel′·lar
spi′·no·cer′·e·bel·la′·ris
spi′·no·cer′·vi·co·tha·
 lam′·ic
spi′·no·cos·ta′·lis
spi′·no·gen′·i·tal
spi′·no·gle′·noid
spi′·no-ol′·i·var′y
spi′·no·pon′·tine
spi·no′·sal
spi′·nose
spi·no′·sus *fem.* ·sa,
 neut. ·sum
spi′·no·tec′·tal
spi′·no·tec·ta′·lis
spi′·no·tha·lam′·ic
spi′·no·tha·lam′·i·cus
spi′·no·trans′·ver·sa′·
 ri·us
spi′·nous
spin·thar′·i·con
spin′·ther·is′m
spi′·nu·lo′·sa
spi′·ra·cle
spir·ad′·e·no′·ma
spi′·ral
spi·ra′·lis *neut.* ·le
spi′·ra·my′·cin
spi′·reme
spi·ril′·lar *also* spi′·ril·
 lar′y

spi'·ril·lo'·sis
Spi·ril'·lum
spi·ril'·lum   pl.   ·la
spir'·it
spir'·i·tus
spi'·ro·
Spi'·ro·chae'·ta
Spi'·ro·chae·ta'·ce·ae
spi'·ro·che'·tal [·chet'·
  al]   also   ·chae'·tal
spi'·ro·chete   also
  ·chaete
spi'·ro·che·to'·sis
  [·chet·o'·]   also
  ·chae·
spi'·ro·gram
spi'·ro·graph
spi·rog'·ra·phy
spi·rom'·e·ter
Spi'·ro·me'·tra
  S. man·so'·ni
  S. man'·so·noi'·des
spi'·ro·met'·ric
spi·rom'·e·try
spi'·ro·no·lac'·tone
spi'·ro·scope
spi'·ru·roid
spit   n. & v.   spit or
  spat, spit'·ting
spit'·tle
splanch'·na·po·phys'·i·
  al
splanch'·na·poph'·y·sis
splanch'·nec·to'·pia
splanch'·nes·the'·sia
  Brit. ·naes·the'·
splanch'·nic
splanch'·ni·cec'·to·my
splanch'·ni·cot'·o·my
splanch'·ni·cum   neut.
  of splanchnicus
splanch'·ni·cus   pl.   ·ci
splanch'·no·   also
  splanch'·ni·
splanch'·no·cele
  visceral herniation: Cf.
  splanchnocoele
splanch'·no·coele
  embryonic cavity: Cf.
  splanchnocele

splanch'·no·cra'·ni·um
splanch·nog'·ra·phy
splanch'·no·lith
splanch'·no·lo'·gia
splanch·nol'·o·gy
splanch'·no·meg'·a·ly
  also ·me·ga'·lia
splanch'·no·mi'·cria
splanch·nop'·a·thy
splanch'·no·pleure
splanch'·nop·to'·sis
splanch'·no·skel'·e·ton
splanch'·no·so·mat'·ic
splanch·not'·o·my
S'-plas·ty
splay
splay'·foot   also splay
  foot
spleen
splen   gen.   sple'·nis
sple·nal'·gia
sple·naux'e
splen'·cu·lus
sple·nec'·to·mize
  mized, ·miz'·ing
sple·nec'·to·my
sple·ne'·o·lus
sple·net'·ic
sple'·ni·al
splen'·ic
splen'·i·ca   fem.   of
  splenicus; pl. & gen.
  sg. ·cae
sple·nic'·u·lus
splen'·i·cum   neut.   of
  splenicus
splen'·i·cus   pl. & gen.
  sg. ·ci
splen'·i·form
sple'·nin
sple'·nis   gen.   of splen
sple'·ni·ser'·rate
  [splen'i·]
sple·ni'·tis
sple'·ni·um
sple'·ni·us
sple'·ni·za'·tion
  [splen'·i·]
sple'·no··[splen'o·]

sple'·no·blast
sple'·no·cele
sple'·no·clei'·sis
sple'·no·co'·lic
sple'·no·cyte
splen'·o·dyn'·ia
sple·nog'·e·nous
sple'·no·gran'·u·lo'·ma·
  to'·sis
sple·nog'·ra·phy
sple'·no·hep'·a·to·
  meg'·a·ly
sple'·noid
sple'·no·lap'·a·rot'·o·
  my
sple·nol'·o·gy
sple'·no·lymph
sple'·no·lym·phat'·ic
sple·nol'·y·sin
sple·nol'·y·sis
sple·no'·ma   pl.   ·mas
  or ·ma·ta
sple'·no·ma·la'·cia
sple'·no·med'·ul·lar'y
sple'·no·me·gal'·ic
sple'·no·meg'·a·ly
sple'·no·my'·e·log'·e·
  nous
sple'·no·my'·e·lo·ma·
  la'·cia
sple'·no·pan'·cre·at'·ic
sple·nop'·a·thy
sple'·no·pex'y [splen'·
  o·]
sple'·no·por'·to·gram
sple'·no·por·tog'·ra·
  phy
sple'·nop·to'·sis
  [splen'·op·]
splen'o·re'·nal [sple'·
  no·]
splen'o·re·na'·le
splen'o·re'·no·pex'y
  [sple'·no·]
splen'·or·rha'·gia
  [sple'·nor·]
sple·nor'·rha·phy
sple·not'·o·my
sple'·no·tox'·in

splen'·ule
splen'·u·lus
splice n. & v. spliced,
   splic'·ing
splint'·age
splin'·ter
splint'·ing
split adj. & v. split,
   split'·ting
split'·ter
spo'·dio·my'·e·li'·tis
spo·dog'·e·nous
spod'·o·gram [spo'·do·]
spo·dog'·ra·phy
spoke'·shave
spon'·dyl·ar·thri'·tis
spon'·dyl·ar·thro'·sis
spon'·dy·lit'·ic
spon'·dy·li'·tis
spon'·dy·lo·
spon'·dy·lod'·e·sis [·lo·
   de'·sis]
spon'·dy·lo·di·dym'·ia
spon'·dy·lo·ep'·i·phys'·
   e·al [·epiph'·y·se'·al]
spon'·dy·lo·lis·the'·sis
spon'·dy·lo·lis·thet'·ic
spon'·dy·lol'·y·sis
spon'·dy·lo·ma·la'·cia
spon'·dy·lo·met'a·ep'·i·
   phys'·e·al [·epiph'·y·
   se'·al]
spon'·dy·lop'·a·thy
spon'·dy·lop·to'·sis
   [·lo·pto'·sis]
spon'·dy·los'·chi·sis
spon'·dy·lo'·sis
spon'·dy·lo·syn'·de·sis
   [·syn·de'·sis]
spon'·dy·lot'·o·my
spon'·dy·lus pl. &
   gen. sg. ·li
sponge
spon'·ge·i'tis var. of
   spongiositis
spon'·gia
spon'·gi·form
spon'·gi·i'tis var. of
   spongiositis

spon'·gio·
spon'·gi·o·blast
spon'·gi·o·blas·to'·ma
spon'·gi·o·cyte
spon'·gi·o·cy·to'·ma
spon'·gi·oid
spon'·gi·o'·sa fem. of
   spongiosus
spon'·gi·ose
spon'·gi·o'·sis
spon'·gi·o·si'·tis
spon'·gi·o'·sum neut.
   of spongiosus; gen. ·si
spon'·gi·o'·sus pl. &
   gen. sg. ·si
spong'y spong'·i·er,
   spong'·i·est
spo·rad'·ic
spo·ran'·gi·al
spo·ran'·gi·um pl. ·gia
spore
spo'·ri·cid'·al [·ci'·dal]
spo'·ri·cide
spo'·ro·
spo'·ro·ag·glu'·ti·na'·
   tion
spo'·ro·blast
spo'·ro·cyst
spo'·ro·gen'·e·sis
spo'·ro·gen'·ic
spo·rog'·e·nous
spo·rog'·e·ny
spo'·ro·gon'·ic
spo·rog'·o·ny
spo'·ront
spo'·ro·phyte
spo'·ro·plas'm
spo'·ro·the'·ca pl.
   ·cae
Spo'·ro·thrix
spo'·ro·tri·cho'·sis
spo'·ro·tri·chot'·ic
Spo·rot'·ri·chum
Spo'·ro·zo'a
spo'·ro·zo'a pl. of
   sporozoon
spo'·ro·zo'·an
Spo'·ro·zo'·ea
spo'·ro·zo'·ite

spo'·ro·zo'·oid
spo'·ro·zo'·on pl.
   ·zo'a
spor'·u·lar
spor'·u·la'·tion
spor'·ule
spot'·ted
sprain
sprue
Spu'·ma·vi'·ri·nae
spu'·ma·vi'·rus
spur
spu'·ria fem. of
   spurius; pl. ·ri·ae
spu'·ri·ous
spu'·ri·us fem. ·ria,
   neut. ·ri·um
spu'·tum pl. ·ta
squa'·lene
squa'·ma pl. ·mae
squa'·mate
squa'·ma·ti·za'·tion
squame
squa'·mo·
squa'·mo·co·lum'·nar
squa'·mo·fron'·tal
squa'·mo·man·dib'·u·
   lar
squa'·mo·mas'·toid
squa'·mo-oc·cip'·i·tal
squa'·mo·pa·ri'·etal
squa'·mo'·sa fem. of
   squamosus; gen. ·sae
squa·mo'·sal
squa·mo'·so·mas·toi'·
   dea
squa·mo'·sus fem.
   ·sa, neut. ·sum
squa'·mo·tem'·po·ral
squa'·mo·tym·pan'·ic
squa'·mous
squa'·mo·zy'·go·mat'·
   ic
squash'-bite
squill
squint
stab stabbed, stab'·
   bing

sta′·bile
sta′·bi·lim′·e·ter
sta·bil′·i·ty
sta′·bi·li·za′·tion
sta′·bi·liz′·er
sta′·ble
stach′·y·drine
stach′·y·ose
stac·tom′·e·ter
sta′·di·um *pl.* ·dia,
    gen. sg. ·dii
stag′·ing
stain′·a·ble
stain′·a·bil′·i·ty
stair′·case
stal′·ag·mom′·e·ter
stam′·i·na
stam′·mer
stanch
stan′·dard
stan·dard·i·za′·tion
stan′·dard·ize
stand′·still
stan′·nic
stan·no′·sis
stan′·nous
stan′·o·lone
stan·o′·zo·lol
sta′·pe·dec′·to·my
sta·pe′·di·al
sta·pe′·di·a′·lis
sta·pe′·di·ol′·y·sis
sta·pe′·dio·te·not′·o·my
sta·pe′·dio·ves·tib′·u·
    lar
sta·pe′·di·us
sta′·pes *pl.* sta·pe′·
    des, *gen. sg.* sta·pe′·dis
staph′·y·lec′·to·my
staph′·y·line
staph′·y·li′·nus
staph′·y·lo·
staph′·y·lo·co·ag′·u·
    lase
staph′·y·lo·coc′·cal
staph′·y·lo·coc·ce′·mia
    Brit. ·cae′·

staph′·y·lo·coc·col′·y·
    sin
staph′·y·lo·coc·co′·sis
Staph′·y·lo·coc′·cus
    S. au′·re·us
    S. ep′·i·der′·mi·dis
    S. sap′·ro·phyt′·i·cus
staph′·y·lo·coc′·cus
    pl. ·ci
staph′·y·lo·der′·ma
staph′·y·lo·he′·mia
    Brit. ·hae′·
staph′·y·lo·he·mol′·y·
    sin *Brit.* ·hae·
staph′·y·lo·leu′·ko·ci′·
    din
staph′·y·lol′·y·sin
staph′·y·lo′·ma *pl.*
    ·mas *or* ·ma·ta
staph′·y·lo′·ma·tous
    [·lom′a·]
staph′·y·lo·plas′·ty
staph′·y·lor′·rha·phy
staph′·y·los′·chi·sis
staph′·y·lot′·o·my
starch
start′·er
star·va′·tion
starve starved, starv′·
    ing
stas′·i·mor′·phy *also*
    stas′·i·mor′·phia
sta′·sis *pl.* sta′·ses
state′·ment
stat′·es·the′·sia *Brit.*
    ·aes·the′·
stat′·ic
stat′·im
sta′·tion
sta·tis′·tic
sta·tis′·ti·cal
sta·tis′·tics
stat′o·
stat′·o·co′·nia *sg.*
    ·co′·ni·um, *gen. pl.*
    ·co′·ni·o′·rum
stat′·o·co′·nic
stat′o·cyst

stat′o·ki·net′·ic
stat′·o·lith
stat′·o·lon
sta·tom′·e·ter
stat′o·re·cep′·tor
stat′·o·ton′·ic
stat′·ur·al
stat′·ure
sta′·tus *L. pl. & gen.*
    sg. status
staunch *var. of* stanch
stau′·ri·on
stau′·ro·co·nid′·i·um
    pl. ·nid′·ia
stau′·ro·ple′·gia
stau′·ro·spore
steal
ste′a·rate
ste·ar′·ic [ste′a·ric]
ste′a·ro·
ste′·at·ad′·e·no′·ma
    pl. ·mas *or* ·ma·ta
ste′·ati′·tis
ste′·ato·
ste′·ato·cele [ste·at′o·]
ste′·ato·cys·to′·ma
    pl. ·mas *or* ·ma·ta
ste′·atoid
ste′·atol′·y·sis
ste′·ato·lyt′·ic
ste′·ato′·ma *pl.* ·mas
    or ·ma·ta
ste′·ato′·ma·to′·sis
ste′·ato′·ma·tous
ste′·ato·pyg′·ia [·py′·
    gia]
ste′·ato·pyg′·ic *also*
    ·py′·gous
ste′·ator·rhe′a *Brit.*
    ·rhoe′a
ste′·ato′·sis
Steg′·o·my′·ia
stel′·la *pl.* ·lae
stel′·lar
stel·la′·ta *fem. of*
    stellatus; *pl.* ·tae
stel′·late

stel·la′·tus *fem.* ·ta,
  neut. ·tum
stel·lec′·to·my
stel′·lu·la *pl.* ·lae
sten′o·
sten′o·breg·mat′·ic
sten′·o·car′·dia
sten′o·ceph′·a·ly
sten′o·com·pres′·sor
sten′·o·co·ri′·a·sis
sten′·o·crot′·a·phy
ste·nog′·a·mous
sten′·o·pe′·ic *Brit.*
  ·pae′·ic; *also* ·pa′·ic
ste·no′·sal
ste·nose′ ·nosed′,
  ·nos′·ing
ste·no′·sis *pl.* ·ses
sten′o·tho′·rax
ste·not′·ic
sten′·o·tro′·phic
  [·troph′·ic]
ste·nox′·e·nous
stent
ste·pha′·ni·al
ste·pha′·ni·on
step′·page
ste·ra′·di·an
ster′·co·
ster′·co·bi′·lin
ster′·co·bi·lin′·o·gen
ster′·co·lith
ster′·co·ra′·ceous
ster′·co·ral *also* ·rous
ster′·co·ro′·ma
ster·cu′·lia
ste′·reo· [ster′·eo·]
ste′·reo·ag·no′·sis
ste′·reo·an′·es·the′·sia
  Brit. ·aes·
ste′·reo·cam·pim′·e·ter
ste′·reo·chem′·i·cal
ste′·reo·chem′·is·try
ste′·reo·cil′·i·um *pl.*
  ·cil′·ia
ste′·reo·col′·po·gram
ste′·reo·col′·po·scope

ste′·reo·en·ceph′·a·lo·
  tome
ste′·reo·en·ceph′·a·lot′·
  o·my
ste′·re·og·no′·sis
ste′·re·og·nos′·tic
ste′·re·o·gram
ste′·re·o·graph
ste′·reo·i′so·mer
ste′·reo·isom′·er·is′m
ste′·re·ol′·o·gy
ste′·re·om′·e·try
ste′·reo·mon′·o·scope
ste′·reo·phan′·to·scope
ste′·reo·pho·rom′·e·ter
ste′·re·op′·sis
ste′·reo·ra′·di·og′·ra·
  phy
ste′·reo·roent′·gen·og′·
  ra·phy
ste′·re·o·scope
ste′·re·o·scop′·ic
ste′·re·os′·co·py
ste′·reo·spe·cif′·ic
ste′·reo·spec′·i·fic′·i·ty
ste′·re·o·tac′·tic *also*
  ·tax′·ic
ste′·reo·tax′·is
ste′·re·o·tax′y
ste′·re·o·tro′·pic
  [·trop′·ic]
ste′·reo·tro′·pism
ste′·re·o·ty′·py
ste′·ric
ste·rig′·ma *pl.* ·ma·ta
ster′·il·ant [·i·lant]
ster′·ile
ste·ril′·i·ty
ster′·il·i·za′·tion
ster′·il·ize   ·ized, ·iz′·
  ing
ster′·il·iz′·er
ster′·nad
ster′·nal
ster·na′·lis *pl.* ·les
ster′·ne·bra *pl.* ·brae
ster′·ne·bral

ster′·ni *gen. of*
  sternum
ster′·no·
ster′·no·bra′·chi·al
ster′·no·chon′·dral
ster′·no·cla·vic′·u·lar
ster′·no·cla·vic′·u·la′·
  ris *neut.* ·re
ster′·no·clei′·dal
ster′·no·clei′·do·mas′·
  toid
ster′·no·clei′·do·mas·
  toi′·dea *fem. of*
  sternocleidomastoideus
ster′·no·clei′·do·mas·
  toi′·de·us *pl.* &
  gen. sg. ·dei
ster′·no·cos′·tal
ster′·no·cos·ta′·le
  neut. of sternocostalis;
  pl. ·lia
ster′·no·cos·ta′·lis *pl.*
  ·les
ster·nod′·y·mus
ster′·no·hy′·oid
ster′·no·hy·oi′·de·us
ster′·no·mas′·toid
ster·nop′·a·gus
ster′·no·per′i·car·di′·a·
  ca
ster′·no·per′i·car′·di·al
  also ·di·ac
ster′·no·thy′·roid
ster′·no·thy·roi′·de·us
ster·not′·o·my
ster′·no·tra′·che·al
ster′·no·xi·phop′·a·gus
ster′·num *pl.* ·ni
ster′·nu·ta′·tor
ster·nu′·ta·to′·ry
ste′·roid
ste·roi′·dal
ste·roi′·do·gen′·e·sis
ste·roi′·do·gen′·ic
ste′·rol
ster′·tor
ster′·to·rous
steth·al′·gia

steth'o·
steth'o·cyr'·to·graph
　also ·kyr'·to·
steth'o·go'·ni·om'·e·ter
steth'·o·graph
steth'·o·phone
steth'·o·scope
steth'·o·scop'·ic
ste·thos'·co·py
sthen'·ic
sthen'o·
sthe·nom'·e·ter
sthe·nom'·e·try
stib'·a·mine
stib'·e·nyl
stib'·i·al·is'm
stib'·i·at'·ed
stib'·ine
sti·bin'·ic
stib'·o·cap'·tate
stib'·o·phen
stiff'·ness
sti'·fle
stig'·ma pl. stig·ma'·ta
stig·mas'·ter·ol
stig·ma'·ta [stig'·ma·ta]
　pl. of stigma
stig·mat'·ic
stig'·ma·tis'm
stig'·ma·ti·za'·tion
stil·al'·gin
stil·baz'·i·um
stil'·bene
stil·bes'·trol Brit.
　·boes'·
sti'·let [sti·let'] var.
　of stylet; also ·lette'
still'·birth
still'·born
stil'·li·cid'·i·um
stil·lin'·gia
sti'·lus pl. ·li; var. of
　stylus
stim'·u·lant
stim'·u·late ·lat'·ed,
　·lat'·ing
stim'·u·la'·tion
stim'·u·la'·tor

stim'·u·lus pl. ·li
sting
sting'·ray
stip'·ple ·pled, ·pling
stir'·rup
stitch
Sti·va'·li·us
sto·chas'·tic
stock'·i·net' also
　·nette'
stoi'·chi·o·met'·ric
　also stoi'·chei·
stoi'·chi·om'·e·try
　also stoi'·chei·
sto'·ma pl. ·mas or
　·ma·ta
stom'·ach
stom'·ach·ache'
stom'·ach·al
sto·mach'·ic
sto'·mal also sto'·ma·
　tal
sto'·ma·ta pl. of stoma
sto'·ma·tal'·gia
sto·mat'·ic
sto'·ma·ti'·tis
sto'·ma·to·
sto'·ma·to·cyte
sto'·ma·to·cy·to'·sis
sto'·ma·to·de'·um
　var. of stomodeum;
　Brit. ·dae'·um
sto'·ma·to·gas'·tric
sto'·ma·to·glos·si'·tis
sto'·ma·to·gnath'·ic
sto'·ma·to·log'·ic also
　·i·cal
sto'·ma·tol'·o·gist
sto'·ma·tol'·o·gy
sto'·ma·to·me'·nia
sto'·ma·to·my·co'·sis
sto'·ma·to·ne·cro'·sis
sto'·ma·top'·a·thy
sto'·ma·to·plas'·tic
sto'·ma·to·plas'·ty
sto'·ma·tor·rha'·gia
sto'·ma·to'·sis
sto'·ma·to·ty'·phus

sto'·mo·ceph'·a·lus
sto'·mo·de'·um Brit.
　·dae'·um
sto·mos'·chi·sis
Sto·mox'·ys
　S. cal'·ci·trans
stool
stop'·ping
stor'·age
sto'·rax
sto'·re·sin
sto·res'·in·ol
sto'·ri·form
stra·bis'·mic also ·mal
strab'·is·mom'·e·ter
　also stra·bom'·e·ter
stra·bis'·mus
stra·bot'·o·my
strain
strain'·er
strait
strait'·jack'·et also
　straight'·
stra·mo'·ni·um
stran'·gle ·gled, ·gling
stran'·gu·lat'·ed
stran'·gu·la'·tion
stran'·gu·ry
stra'·ta pl. of stratum
strat'·i·fi·ca'·tion
strat'·i·fied
strat'·i·form
stra·tig'·ra·phy
stra'·tum pl. ·ta
stream
streph'·en'·o·po'·dia
streph'·ex'·o·po'·dia
streph'·o·po'·dia
streph'o·sym·bo'·lia
strep'·i·tus
strep'·ti·ce'·mia Brit.
　·cae'·
strep'·ti·dine
strep'·to·
strep'·to·bac'·il·lar'y
　[·ba·cil'·la·ry]
Strep'·to·ba·cil'·lus
　mo·nil'·i·for'·mis

strep'·to·cer·ci'·a·sis
strep'·to·coc'·cal
strep'·to·coc·ce'·mia
  Brit. ·cae'·
strep'·to·coc·co'·sis
Strep'·to·coc'·cus
  S. fae·ca'·lis
  S. mi'·tis
  S. mu'·tans
  S. pneu·mo'·ni·ae
  S. py·og'·e·nes
strep'·to·coc'·cus *pl.*
  ·ci
strep'·to·dor'·nase
strep'·to·gen'·in
strep'·to·ki'·nase
strep'·to·ly'·di·gin
strep'·to·ly'·sin [strep·
  tol'·y·sin]
Strep'·to·my'·ces
strep'·to·my'·cete
strep'·to·my'·cin
strep'·to·my·co'·sis
strep'·to·ni'·grin
strep'·tose
strep'·to·thri'·cin
strep'·to·tri·cho'·sis
stress
stres'·sor
stretch'·er
stri'a *pl.* stri'·ae
stri·a'·ta *fem. of*
  striatus, *pl. of* striatum
stri·a'·tal
stri'·ate
stri'·at·ed
stri·a'·tion
stri·a'·to·ni'·gral
stri·a'·to·pal'·li·dal
stri·a'·to·tha·lam'·ic
stri·a'·tum *neut. of*
  striatus; *pl.* ·ta, *gen.*
  sg. ·ti
stri·a'·tus *pl. & gen.*
  sg. ·ti
stric'·ture
stric'·tur·ot'·o·my
stri'·dor

strid'·u·lous
stri'o·cer'·e·bel'·lar
stri'o·cor'·ti·cal
stri'o·mo'·tor
stri'o·ni'·gral
stri'o·pal'·li·dal
stri'o·ru'·bral
strip *n. & v.* stripped,
  strip'·ping
strip'·per
stro·bi'·la *pl.* ·lae
stro'·bi·la'·tion
stro'·bi·lo·cer'·cus
  pl. ·ci
stro'·bi·loid
stro'·bo·scope
stro'·bo·scop'·ic
stroke
stro'·ma *pl.* ·ma·ta
stro'·mal
stro·mat'·ic
stro'·ma·tog'·e·nous
stro'·muhr [strom'·uhr]
stron'·gyle
Stron·gyl'·i·da
stron·gyl'·i·form
stron'·gy·lo·
Stron'·gy·loi'·dea
Stron'·gy·loi'·des
stron'·gy·loi·di'·a·sis
  also ·loi·do'·sis
Stron'·gy·lus
stron'·ti·um
stro·phan'·thi·din
stro·phan'·thin
stroph'o·ceph'·a·ly
stroph'·u·lus
struc'·tur·al
struc'·ture
stru'·ma *pl.* ·mae *or*
  ·mas
stru·mec'·to·my
stru'·mi·form
stru·mi'·tis
stru'·mous
stru'·vite
strych'·nine

strych'·nin·is'm *also*
  strych'·nism
strych·nin·i·za'·tion
stupe
stu'·pe·fa'·cient
stu'·pe·fac'·tive
stu'·por
stu'·por·ous *also* ·ose
stut'·ter
stut'·ter·ing
stye *also* sty
sty'·let
sty'·li·form
sty'·lo·
sty'·lo·glos'·sal
sty'·lo·glos'·sus
sty'·lo·hy'·al
sty'·lo·hy'·oid
sty'·lo·hy·oi'·de·us
  neut. ·de·um
sty'·loid
sty·loi'·dea *fem. of*
  styloideus
sty·loi'·de·us *pl. &*
  gen. sg. ·dei
sty'·loid·i'·tis
sty'·lo·man·dib'·u·lar
sty'·lo·man·dib'·u·la'·
  re
sty'·lo·mas'·toid
sty'·lo·mas·toi'·de·us
  fem. ·dea, *neut.* ·de·um
sty'·lo·max'·il·lar'y
sty'·lo·pha·ryn'·ge·al
sty'·lo·pha·ryn'·ge·us
  pl. & gen. sg. ·gei
sty'·lo·po'·di·um
sty'·lo·ra'·di·al
styl·os'·te·o·phyte
sty'·lo·stix'·is
sty'·lus *pl.* ·li
sty'·ma·to'·sis
styp'·age [sty·page']
stype
styp'·sis
styp'·tic
sty'·ra·mate
sty'·rene *also* ·rol

sty′·ryl
sub′·ab·dom′·i·nal
sub′·ab·dom′·i·no·per′·
  i·to·ne′·al
sub′·ac′·e·tab′·u·lar
sub′·acro′·mi·al
sub′·acro′·mi·a′·lis
sub′·acro′·mio·del′·toid
sub′·acute′
sub·ad′·ven·ti′·tial
sub′·al′·i·men·ta′·tion
sub·am′·bi·ent
sub′·an·co′·ne·us
sub·ap′i·cal [·a′pi·]
sub′·ap′·o·neu·rot′·ic
sub′·arach′·noid *also*
  arach·noi′·dal
sub′·arach·noi′·dea
sub′·arach·noi′·de·a′·le
  neut. of subarach-
  noidealis
sub′·arach·noi′·de·a′·lis
  pl. ·les
sub′·arach′·noid·i′·tis
sub·ar′·cu·a′·ta
sub·ar′·cu·ate
sub′·are′·o·lar
sub′·atom′·ic
sub′·au·ra′·le
sub′·au·ric′·u·lar
sub·ba′·sal
sub·bra′·chi·al
sub·cal′·ca·rine
sub′·cal·lo′·sal
sub′·cal·lo′·sus *fem.*
  ·sa, *neut.* ·sum
sub·cap′·i·tal
sub·cap′·su·lar
sub·car′·di·nal
sub·car′·ti·lag′·i·nous
sub·ce′·cal *Brit.* ·cae′·
sub′·cer′·e·bel′·lar
sub·cer′·e·bral
sub·cer′·vi·cal
sub·chlo′·ride
sub·chon′·dral
sub·cho′·ri·al
sub·cho′·ri·a′·lis

sub·chron′·ic
sub′·class
sub·cla′·via *fem. of*
  subclavius; *pl. & gen.*
  sg. ·vi·ae
sub·cla′·vi·an
sub′·cla·vic′·u·lar
sub·cla′·vi·us *pl. &*
  gen. sg. ·vii
sub·clin′·i·cal
sub·cli′·noid
sub′·col·lat′·er·al
sub·co′·ma
sub′·com·mis′·su·ral
  [·com′·mis·su′·ral]
sub′·con′·junc·ti′·val
sub·con′·scious
sub·cor′·a·coid
sub·cor′·a·coi′·dea
sub·cor′·ne·al
sub·cor′·tex
sub·cor′·ti·cal
sub·cos′·tal
sub′·cos·ta′·lis *pl.* ·les
sub·cra′·ni·al
sub·crep′·i·tant
sub·cres′·tal
sub′·cul′·ture
sub·cu′·ra·tive
sub′·cu·ta′·nea *pl.*
  ·ne·ae
sub′·cu·ta′·ne·ous
sub′·cu·tic′·u·lar
sub·cu′·tis
sub·del′·toid
sub′·del·toi′·dea
sub·der′·mal
sub′·di′·a·phrag·mat′·ic
sub′·duct′
sub·duc′·tion
sub·du′·ral
sub′·du·ra′·lis *neut.*
  ·le
sub·du′·ro·per′·i·to·ne′·
  al
sub·du′·ro·pleu′·ral
sub′·en′·do·car′·di·al
  also ·di·ac

sub′·en′·do·the′·li·al
sub′·en′·do·the′·li·a′·lis
  neut. ·le
sub′·ep·en′·dy·mal
sub′·ep·en′·dy·mo′·ma
sub·ep′·i·car′·di·al
sub·ep′i·cra′·ni·al
sub′·ep′·i·der′·mal
sub′·ep′·i·the′·li·al
su′·ber·o′·sis
sub·fal′·ci·al
sub′·fam′·i·ly
sub·fas′·cial
sub·fas′·ci·a′·lis
sub′·fe·cun′·di·ty
sub′·fer·til′·i·ty
sub′·fis′·sure
sub·fo′·li·ar
sub·fo′·li·um *pl.* ·lia
sub·for′·ni·cal
sub·fron′·tal
sub′·fron·ta′·lis
sub·ga′·le·al
sub·gal′·late
sub′·ge′·nus *pl.* ·gen′·
  era
sub·ger′·mi·nal
sub·gin′·gi·val
sub·gle′·noid
sub·glot′·tic
sub·glot′·tis
sub′·gy′·rus [sub′·gy′·
  rus] *pl.* ·ri
sub′·he·pat′·ic
sub′·he·pat′·i·cus *pl.*
  ·ci
sub·hy′·a·loid
sub·hy′·oid *also* ·hy·
  oi′·de·an
sub′·ic·ter′·ic
su·bic′·u·lar
su·bic′·u·lum *pl.* ·la
sub·il′·i·ac
sub·in′·gui·nal
sub·in′·tern
sub·in′·ti·mal
sub′·in·vo·lu′·tion
su′·bi·tum

sub·ja′·cent
sub′·ject
sub·jec′·tive
sub′·jec·tiv′·i·ty
sub·la′·tio
sub·la′·tion
sub·len′·ti·for′·mis
sub·le′·thal
sub′·leu·ke′·mic Brit.
·kae′·
sub′·li·mate n. & v.
·mat′·ed, ·mat′·ing
sub′·li·ma′·tion
sub·lime′ ·limed′,
·lim′·ing
sub·lim′·i·nal
sub·li′·mis
sub·lin′·gual
sub′·lin·gua′·le neut.
of sublingualis
sub′·lin·gua′·lis pl.
·les
sub·lob′·u·lar
sub·lux′·at·ed
sub′·lux·a′·tion
sub′·mal·le′·o·lar
sub·mam′·ma·ry
sub′·man·dib′·u·lar
sub′·man·dib′·u·la′·re
neut. of submandibu-
laris
sub′·man·dib′·u·la′·ris
pl. ·res
sub·mar′·gi·nal
sub·max′·il·la′·ris
sub·max′·il·lar′y
sub·me′·di·al
sub′·me·nin′·ge·al
sub·men′·tal
sub′·men·ta′·le neut.
of submentalis
sub′·men·ta′·lis pl.
·les
sub′·met′a·cen′·tric
sub′·mi·cro·scop′·ic
sub′·mi·to·chon′·dri·al
sub′·mu·co′·sa
sub′·mu·co′·sal

sub′·mu·co′·sus fem.
·sa, neut. ·sum
sub·mu′·cous
sub·na′·sal
sub·na′·tant
sub·neu′·ral
sub·nor′·mal
sub′·nor·mal′·i·ty
sub·nu′·cle·us
sub′·oc·cip′·i·tal
sub′·oc·cip′·i·ta′·lis
sub′·oc·cip′·i·to·breg·
mat′·ic
sub′·oc·cip′·i·to·fron′·
tal
sub′·odon′·to·blas′·tic
sub′·oper′·cu·lum
sub·op′·tic
sub·op′·ti·mal
sub·or′·bi·tal
sub′·or·der
sub′·pap′·il·la′·ris
neut. ·re
sub·pap′·il·lar′y
sub·pa·ri′·etal
sub′·pa·ri′·eta′·lis
sub′·pa·tel′·lar
sub′·pe·dun′·cu·lar
sub′·per′·i·car′·di·al
sub·pe′·ri·od′·ic
sub′·per′i·os′·te·al
sub′·per′·i·to·ne′·al
sub′·pe·tro′·sal
sub·phren′·ic
sub·phren′·i·cus pl.
·ci
sub′·phy·lum pl. ·la
sub·pi′·al
sub′·pla·cen′·tal
sub·pleu′·ral
sub·pon′·tine also
·tile
sub′·pop·lit′·e·al
[·pop′·li·te′·al]
sub′·pop′·li·te′·us
sub′·pop′·u·la′·tion
sub·pu′·bic
sub·pu′·bi·cus

sub·pul′·mo·nar′y
sub′·py·ram′·i·dal
sub·ret′·i·nal
sub·ros′·tral
sub′·sa·lic′·y·late
sub′·sar·to′·ri·al
sub′·sar·to′·ri·a′·lis
sub·scap′·u·lar
sub·scap′·u·la′·ris pl.
·res
sub′·scle·rot′·ic
sub·scrip′·tion
sub·sep′·tus
sub′·se·ro′·sus fem.
·sa, neut. ·sum
sub·se′·rous
sub·sig′·moid
sub·son′·ic
sub·spe′·cial·ty
sub′·spe′·cies pl.
subspecies
sub·spi′·nous
sub·sple′·ni·al
sub′·stance
sub·stan′·tia pl. &
gen. sg. ·ti·ae
sub′·stan·tive [sub·
stan′·tive]
sub·ster′·nal
sub·stit′·u·ent
sub′·sti·tute
sub′·sti·tu′·tion
sub′·strate
sub′·stra·tum pl. ·ta
sub′·struc·ture
sub·sul′·cus
sub·syl′·vi·an
sub′·syn·ap′·tic
sub′·sy·no′·vi·al [·syn·
o′·]
sub·ta′·lar
sub′·ta·la′·ris
sub·tem′·po·ral
sub′·ten·din′·ea pl.
·e·ae
sub·ten′·di·nous
sub·ter′·tian
sub′·te·tan′·ic

sub′·tha·lam′·ic
sub′·tha·lam′·i·cus
   fem. ·ca, *neut.* ·cum
sub·thal′·a·mus   *pl.*
   ·mi
sub·thresh′·old
sub′·ti·lin
sub·til′·i·sin
sub·to′·tal
sub′·tra·pe′·zi·al
sub′·tra·pe′·zi·us
sub·tri′·go·nal [·trig′·o·]
sub′·tro′·chan·ter′·ic
sub′·um·bil′·i·cal
sub·un′·gual
sub′·un·gua′·lis
sub′·u′nit
sub·vag′·i·nal
sub·val′·vu·lar
sub·ver′·te·bral
sub·vi′·ral
sub′·vi′·ta·min·o′·sis
   pl. ·ses
sub′·vo·lu′·tion
sub·zo′·nal [·zon′·al]
suc′·ca·gogue
suc′·ce·da′·ne·ous
suc′·ce·da′·ne·us
   fem. ·nea, *neut.* ·ne·um
suc′·cen·tu′·ri·ate
suc·ces′·sion
suc′·ci·nate
suc·cin′·ic
suc·cin′·i·mide
suc′·ci·nyl
suc′·ci·nyl·cho′·line
suc′·ci·nyl·sul′·fa·thi′·a·zole   *Brit.* ·sul′·pha·
suc′·cor·rhe′a   *Brit.* ·rhoe′a
suc′·cu·lence
suc′·cu·lent
suc′·cus
suc·cus′·sion
suck′·er
suck′·le   ·led, ·ling

su′·crase
su′·crose
su′·cros·e′·mia [·cro·se′·]   *Brit.* ·ae′·mia
su′·cros·u′·ria [·cro·su′·]
suc′·tion
suc·to′·ri·al
su·da′·men   *pl.* su·dam′·i·na
Su·dan′
su·dan′·o·phil
su·dan′·o·phil′·ia
su·dan′·o·phil′·ic
su·da′·tion
su′·da·to′·ry
su′·do·gram
su′·do·mo′·tor
su′·dor
su′·do·ral
su′·do·rif′·era   *fem. of* sudoriferus; *pl.* ·er·ae
su′·do·rif′·er·ous
su′·do·rif′·er·us
su′·do·rif′·ic
su′·do·rip′·a·rous
su′·do·rom′·e·ter
su′·et
suf′·fo·cant
suf′·fo·cate   ·cat′·ed, ·cat′·ing
suf′·fo·ca′·tion
suf′·fo·ca′·tive
suf·fo′·di·ens
suf·fuse′   ·fused′, ·fus′·ing
suf·fu′·sion
sug′·ar
sug·ges′·ti·bil′·i·ty
sug·ges′·tion
sug′·gil·la′·tion
su′·i·cid′·al [·ci′·dal]
su′·i·cide
su′·i·cid·ol′·o·gy [·ci·dol′·]
su′i·gen′·der·is′m
suit
sul′·cal

sul′·cate
sul·ca′·tion
sul′·ci·form
sul′·co·mar′·gi·nal
sul′·co·mar′·gi·na′·lis
sul′·cu·lus   *pl.* ·li
sul′·cus   *pl. & gen. sg.* ·ci
sulf- *Words beginning thus have the British spelling* sulph-
sul′·fa   *Brit.* ·pha
sul′·fa·cet′·a·mide
sul′·fa·cy′·tine
sul′·fa·di′·a·zine
sul′·fa·di′·me·thox′·ine
sul′·fa·di′·mi·dine
sul′·fa·eth′·i·dole
sul′·fa·mer′·a·zine
sul′·fa·meth′·a·zine
sul′·fa·meth·ox′·a·zole
sul′·fa·me·thox′y·py·rid′·a·zine
sul′·fan
sul′·fa·nil′·a·mide
sul′·fa·nil′·ic
sul·fan′·i·lyl·sul′·fa·nil′·a·mide
sulf′·an·u′·ria
sul′·fa·pyr′·a·zine
sul′·fa·pyr′·i·dine
sul′·fa·py·rim′·i·dine
sul′·fa·sal′·a·zine
sul′·fa·tase
sul′·fate
sul′·fa·thi′·a·zole
sul′·fa·tide
sul′·fa·ti·do′·sis
sul·fa′·tion
sulf·he′·mo·glo′·bin   *Brit.* sul·phae′·mo·glo′·bin
sulf·he′·mo·glo′·bin·e′·mia [·bi·ne′·]   *Brit.* sul·phae·, ·ae′·mia
sulf·hy′·dryl
sul′·fide
sul·fin′·ic

sul′·fin·pyr′·a·zone
sul′·fi·nyl
sul′·fi·som′·i·dine
sul′·fi·sox′·a·zole
sul′·fite
sulf′·met·he′·mo·glo′·
 bin *Brit.* sulph′·met·
 hae′·mo·glo′·bin
sul′·fo· *Brit.* ·pho·
sul′·fo·ami′·no
sul′·fo·bro′·mo·phtha′·
 lein [·phthal′·ein]
sul′·fo·mu′·cin
sul·fon′·a·mide
sul′·fo·nate
sul′·fone
sul·fon′·ic
sul·fo′·ni·um
sul′·fon·meth′·ane
sul′·fo·nyl·
sul′·fo·nyl·ure′a
sul′·fo·sal′·i·cyl′·ic
sul′·fo·trans′·fer·ase
sulf·ox′·ide
sulf·ox′·ism
sul′·fur
sul′·fu·rate ·rat′·ed,
 ·rat′·ing
sul′·fu·ret′·ted
sul·fu′·ric
sul·fu′·rous *denoting
 sulfur in its lower
 valence*
sul′·fur·ous
 *containing or resem-
 bling sulfur*
sul′·pho· *Brit. spel. of
 sulfo-*
sul′·phur *Brit. spel. of
 sulfur*
su′·mac *also* ·mach
sum·ma′·tion
sun′·burn
sun′·screen
sun′·stroke
su′·per·
su′·per·ac′·id
su′·per·acute′

su′·per·al′·i·men·ta′·
 tion
su′·per·an′·ti·gen
su′·per·cal·lo′·sal
 var. of supracallosal
su′·per·cil′·ia
su′·per·cil′·i·a′·ris
su′·per·cil′·i·ar′y
su′·per·cil′·i·um *pl.*
 ·cil′·ia, *gen. sg.* ·cil′·ii
su′·per·coil
sup′·er·duc′·tion *var.
 of* supraduction
sup′·er·e′go
su′·per·fam′·i·ly
su′·per·fe′·cun·da′·tion
su′·per·fe·ta′·tion
su′·per·fi′·cial
su′·per·fi′·ci·a′·le
 neut. of superficialis;
 pl. ·lia
su′·per·fi′·ci·a′·lis *pl.*
 ·les
su′·per·fi′·ci·es
su′·per·gene
su′·per·he′·lix
su′·per·in·duce′
 ·duced′, ·duc′·ing
su′·per·in·duc′·tion
su′·per·in·fec′·tion
su′·per·in′·vo·lu′·tion
su·pe′·ri·or *pl.* su·pe′·
 ri·o′·res, *gen. sg.* su·
 pe′·ri·o′·ris, *gen. pl.*
 su·pe′·ri·o′·rum
su·pe′·ri·us *neut. of*
 superior
su′·per·ja′·cent
su′·per·lac·ta′·tion
su′·per·le′·thal
su′·per·li·ga′·men
su′·per·me′·di·al *var.
 of* superomedial
su′·per·na′·tant
su′·per·nu′·mer·ar′y
su′·per·nu·tri′·tion
su′·per·oc·cip′·i·tal
 var. of supraoccipital

su′·pero·in·fe′·ri·or
su′·pero·lat′·er·al
su′·pero·lat′·er·a′·lis
su′·pero·me′·di·al
su′·per·ov′u·la′·tion
 [·o′vu·]
su′·per·ox′·ide
su′·per·par′·a·site
su′·per·par′·a·sit·is′m
su′·per·phos′·phate
su′·per·sat′·u·rate
 ·rat′·ed, ·rat′·ing
su′·per·scrip′·tion
su′·per·se·cre′·tion
su′·per·sen′·si·tive
su′·per·son′·ic
su′·per·spe′·cies *pl.*
 superspecies
su′·per·sphe′·noid
su′·per·struc′·ture
su′·per·sul′·cus
su′·per·tem′·po·ral
su′·per·ven′·tion
su′·per·vi′·ta·min·o′·sis
 pl. ·ses
su′·pi·nate ·nat′·ed,
 ·nat′·ing
su′·pi·na′·tion
su′·pi·na′·tor
su·pine′
sup′·ple·men′·tal
sup′·ple·men′·ta·ry
sup′·ple·men·ta′·tion
sup·port′·er
sup·port′·ing
sup·por′·tive
sup·pos′·i·to′·ry
sup·pres′·sant
sup·pressed′
sup·pres′·sion
sup·pres′·sor
sup′·pu·rant
sup′·pu·rate ·rat′·ed,
 ·rat′·ing
sup′·pu·ra′·tion
sup′·pu·ra·ti′′·va
sup′·pu·ra′·tive
su′·pra·

su'·pra-aor'·tic
su'·pra-ar'·y·te'·noid
su'·pra·bon'y
su'·pra·cal·lo'·sal
su'·pra·cal·lo'·sus
su'·pra·cer'·e·bel'·lar
su'·pra·cer'·vi·cal
su'·pra·cho'·roid *also*
 ·cho·roi'·dal
su'·pra·cho·roi'·dea
su'·pra·cil'·i·ar'y *var.
 of* superciliary
su'·pra·cla·vic'·u·lar
su'·pra·cla·vic'·u·la'·ris
 pl. ·res
su'·pra·cli'·noid
su'·pra·clu'·sion
su'·pra·con'·dy·lar
 also ·loid
su'·pra·cres'·tal
su'·pra·di'·a·phrag·
 mat'·ic
su'·pra·duc'·tion
su'·pra·du'·o·de'·nal
su'·pra·du·o'·de·na'·lis
su'·pra·ep'i·con'·dy·la'·
 ris
su'·pra·ep'i·troch'·le·ar
su'·pra·ge·nic'·u·late
su'·pra·gin'·gi·val [·gin·
 gi'·]
su'·pra·gle'·noid
su'·pra·gle'·noi·da'·le
su'·pra·glot'·tic
su'·pra·gran'·u·lar
su'·pra·hy'·oid
su'·pra·hy·oi'·dea
 fem. of suprahyoideus;
 pl. ·de·ae
su'·pra·hy·oi'·de·us
 pl. ·dei
su'·pra·le'·thal
su'·pra·le·va'·tor
su'·pra·lim'·i·nal
su'·pra·mal'·le·o·la'·ris
su'·pra·mam'·il·lar'y
su'·pra·mar'·gi·nal
su'·pra·mar'·gi·na'·lis

su'·pra·mas'·toid
su'·pra·max'·il·lar'y
su'·pra·max'·i·mal
su'·pra·me·a'tal
su'·pra·me·at'i·ca
su'·pra·nod'·al
su'·pra·nu'·cle·ar
su'·pra·oc·cip'·i·tal
su'·pra·oc·clu'·sion
 var. of supraclusion
su'·pra·omen'·tal
su'·pra·op'·tic
su'·pra·op'·ti·ca *fem.
 of* supraopticus; *pl.*
 ·cae
su'·pra·op'·ti·co·hy'·
 po·phys'·i·al
su'·pra·op'·ti·cus
su'·pra·op'·ti·mum
su'·pra·or'·bit·al
su'·pra·or'·bi·ta'·lis
 neut. ·le
su'·pra·pa·tel'·lar
su'·pra·pat'·el·la'·ris
su'·pra·pin'·e·al [·pi'·
 ne·]
su'·pra·pin'·e·a'·lis
 [·pi'·ne·]
su'·pra·pleu'·ral
su'·pra·pleu·ra'·lis
su'·pra·pon'·tine
su'·pra·prom'·on·to'·ri·
 al
su'·pra·pu'·bic
su'·pra·ra'·di·al
su'·pra·re'·nal
su'·pra·re·na'·lis *pl.*
 ·les
su'·pra·re'·no·tro'·pic
 [·trop'·ic]
su'·pra·scap'·u·la
su'·pra·scap'·u·lar
su'·pra·scap'·u·la'·ris
su'·pra·scle'·ral
su'·pra·seg·men'·tal
su'·pra·sel'·lar
su'·pra·spi'·nal *also*
 ·nous

su'·pra·spi·na'·le *pl.*
 ·lia
su'·pra·spi·na'·tus
 fem. ·ta, *neut.* ·tum
su'·pra·sple'·ni·al
su'·pra·ster'·nal
su'·pra·ster·na'·le *pl.*
 ·lia
su'·pra·syl'·vi·an
su'·pra·tem'·po·ral
su'·pra·ten·to'·ri·al
su'·pra·ton'·sil·lar
su'·pra·ton'·sil·la'·ris
su'·pra·tra'·gic
su'·pra·trag'·i·cum
su'·pra·troch'·le·ar
su'·pra·troch'·le·a'·ris
 pl. ·res
su'·pra·tur'·bi·nal
su'·pra·um·bil'·i·cal
su'·pra·vag'·i·nal
su'·pra·val'·vu·lar
su'·pra·vas'·cu·lo'·sum
su'·pra·ven·tric'·u·lar
su'·pra·ver'·gence
su'·pra·ver'·sion
su'·pra·ves'·i·ca'·lis
su'·pra·vi'·tal
su·pre'·ma *pl.* ·mae
su·preme'
su'·ra *pl. & gen. sg.*
 ·rae
su'·ral
sur'·al'·i·men·ta'·tion
su·ra'·lis *pl.* ·les
su'·ra·min
sur'·di·mut'·ism
sur'·di·ty
sur'·do·car'·di·ac
sur'·face
sur'·face-ac'·tive
sur·fac'·tant
sur'·geon
sur'·gery
sur'·gi·cal
sur'·ro·gate
sur'·sum·duc'·tion
sur'·sum·ver'·gence

sur'·sum·ver'·sion
sur·veil'·lance
sur·vey'·or
sur·viv'·al
sur·vi'·vor·ship
sus·cep'·ti·bil'·i·ty
sus·cep'·ti·ble
sus·pen'·si·om'·e·ter
sus·pen'·sion
sus'·pen·so'·ri·um
   neut. of suspensorius;
   pl. ·ria
sus'·pen·so'·ri·us   pl.
   & gen. sg. ·rii
sus·pen'·so·ry
sus·pi'·ri·ous
sus'·ten·tac'·u·lar
sus'·ten·tac'·u·lum
su'·sur·ra'·tion
su·sur'·rus
su'·ti·ka
su·tu'·ra
su'·tur·al
su'·tu·ra'·le   pl. ·lia
su'·ture
sux'a·me·tho'·ni·um
sved'·berg
swab n. & v.
   swabbed, swab'·bing
swad'·dler
swage   swaged, swag'·ing
swal'·low
swarm'·ing
sway'·back   also sway back
sweat n. & v.   sweat or sweat'·ed, sweat'·ing
sweat'y
sweet'·en·er
sweet'·gum
swell'·ing
swing'-bed
switch
sy·ceph'·a·lus   var. of syncephalus
sych·nu'·ria

sy·co'·si·form
sy·co'·sis   infection of hair follicles: Cf. psychosis
syl'·van
syl·vat'·ic
syl'·vi·an
sym·bal'·lo·phone
sym'·bi·o·gen'·ic
sym·bi·ol'·o·gy
sym'·bi·ont   also ·ote
sym'·bi·o'·sis
sym'·bi·ot'·ic   also ·on'·ic
sym·bleph'·a·ron
sym·bleph'·a·ro·pte·ryg'·i·um
sym'·bol
sym'·bol·is'm
sym'·bol·i·za'·tion
sym·brach'y·dac'·ty·ly   also ·dac·tyl'·ia or ·dac'·tyl·is'm
sym·me'·lia
sym'·me·lus
sym·met'·ri·cal   also ·met'·ric
sym'·me·try
sym'·pa·thec'·to·my   also ·the·tec'·
sym'·pa·thet'·ic
sym'·pa·thet'·i·co·   var. of sympatho-
sym·pa·thet'·i·co·mi·met'·ic
sym'·pa·thet'·i·co·par'·a·lyt'·ic
sym'·pa·thet'·i·co·to'·nia
sym'·pa·thet'·i·co·ton'·ic
sym'·pa·thet'·i·cus   fem. ·ca, neut. ·cum
sym·pa·thet'·o·blast   var. of sympathoblast
sym·path'·ic   var. of sympathetic

sym·path'·i·ca   fem. of sympathicus; pl. & gen. sg. ·cae
sym·path'·i·cec'·to·my   var. of sympathectomy
sym·path'·i·ci   pl. & gen. sg. of sympathicus
sym·path'·i·co·   var. of sympatho-
sym·path'·i·co·blast   var. of sympathoblast
sym·path'·i·co·blas·to'·ma   var. of sympathoblastoma
sym·path'·i·co·gen'·ic
sym·path'·i·co·lyt'·ic
sym·path'·i·co·mi·met'·ic
sym·path'·i·co·neu·ri'·tis
sym·path'·i·co'·rum   gen. pl. of sympathicus
sym·path'·i·co·ther'·a·py
sym·path'·i·co·to'·nia
sym·path'·i·co·ton'·ic
sym·path'·i·co·trip'·sy
sym·path'·i·co·tro'·pic [·trop'·ic]
sym·path'·i·cus   pl. & gen. sg. ·ci, gen. pl. sym·path'·i·co'·rum
sym'·pa·thin
sym'·pa·thiz'·er
sym'·pa·tho·
sym'·pa·tho·adre'·nal
sym'·pa·tho·blast'
sym'·pa·tho·blas'·tic
sym'·pa·tho·blas·to'·ma   pl. ·mas or ·ma·ta
sym'·pa·tho·go'·nia   sg. ·ni·um
sym'·pa·tho·go'·ni·o'·ma
sym'·pa·tho·lyt'·ic
sym'·pa·tho·mi·met'·ic

sym'·pa·tho·par'·a·lyt'·ic
sym'·pa·tho·tro'·pic [·trop'·ic]
sym'·pa·thy
sym·per'·i·to·ne'·al
sym·phal'·an·gy *also* ·gis'm
sym·phys'·e·al [sym'·phy·se'·al] *var. of* symphysial
sym·phys'·i·al
sym·phys'·i·a'·lis
sym·phys'i·ec'·to·my
sym·phys'·i·on
sym·phys'·i·ot'·o·my
sym'·phy·sis *pl.* ·ses
sym'·phy·so·dac'·ty·ly
sym'·phy·tum
sym'·plasm *also* ·plast
sym·plas'·tic
sym·po'·dia
sym'·port
symp'·tom
symp'·to·mat'·ic
symp'·to·ma·tol'·o·gy
symp'·to·mat'·o·lyt'·ic *also* symp'·to·mo·lyt'·ic
sym·pto'·sis
symp'·to·ther'·mal
sym'·pus
syn'·adel'·phus
syn·al'·gia
syn·al'·gic
syn'·anas'·to·mo'·sis
syn'·an·throp'·ic
syn'·apse
syn·ap'·sis *pl.* ·ses
syn·ap'·tene
syn·ap'·tic
syn·ap'·tol'·o·gy
syn·ap'·to·ne'·mal *also* ·ap'·ti·
syn·ap'·to·some
syn'·ar·thro'·di·al
syn'·ar·throph'·y·sis
syn'·ar·thro'·sis *pl.* ·ses

syn'·caine
syn·can'·thus
syn·ceph'·a·lus
syn·chei'·lia
syn'·che·sis *var. of* synchysis
syn·chi'·ria
syn'·chon·drec'·to·my
syn'·chon·dro'·se·ot'·o·my
syn'·chon·dro'·sis *pl.* ·ses
syn'·chon·drot'·o·my
syn·cho'·ri·al
syn'·chro·nis'm
syn'·chro·ni·za'·tion
syn'·chro·nous
syn'·chro·ny
syn'·chy·sis
synciput *misspelling of* sinciput
syn·cli'·nal
syn'·cli·tis'm
syn'·co·pal *also* syn·cop'·ic
syn'·co·pe
syn·cy'·tial
syn·cy'·ti·o'·ma
syn·cy'·tio·tox'·in
syn·cy'·tio·tro'·pho·blast
syn·cy'·ti·um *pl.* ·tia
syn·dac'·tyl *also* ·ty·lous
syn·dac'·ty·ly *also* ·lis'm
syn'·de·sine
syn'·de·sis [syn·de'·sis]
syn'·des·mec'·to·my
syn'·des·mi'·tis
syn·des'·mo·
syn·des'·mo·cho'·ri·al
syn·des'·mo·di·as'·ta·sis
syn'·des·mol'·o·gy
syn·des'·mo·phyte
syn'·des·mo'·sis *pl.* ·ses

syn'·des·mot'·o·my
syn'·drome
syn·drom'·ic
syn'·dro·mol'·o·gist
syn'·dro·mol'·o·gy
syn·ech'·ia *pl.* ·i·ae
syn'·e·chot'·o·my
syn'·en·ceph'·a·lo·cele
syn'·en·ceph'·a·ly
syn·er'·e·sis
syn·er'·get'·ic
syn·er'·gic
syn·er'·gis'm
syn·er'·gist
syn·er'·gis'·tic
syn·er'·gy
syn'·es·the'·sia Brit. ·aes·
syn'·es·thet'·ic Brit. ·aes·
syn·gam'·ic
syn'·ga·mous
syn'·ga·my
syn'·ge·ne'·ic *also* syn·gen'·ic
syn'·ge·ne'·sio·graft
syn'·ge·ne'·si·o·plas'·tic
syn·gen'·e·sis
syn'·ge·net'·ic
syn·gnath'·ia
syn'·graft
syn·hex'·yl
syn'·hi·dro'·sis *also* syn'·i·
syn'·i·ze'·sis
syn·kar'y·on
syn'·ki·ne'·sis *also* ·sia
syn'·ki·net'·ic
syn·ne'·ma·tin
syn'·o·nych'·ia
syn'·o·nym
syn·on'·y·mize ·mized, ·miz'·ing
syn·oph'·rys *also* syn'·o·phrid'·ia

syn′·oph·thal′·mia
    also ·mus
syn·op′·to·phore
syn·or′·chi·dis′m   also
    ·or′·chism
syn·os′·che·os
syn·os′·te·ol′·o·gy
syn′·os·to′·sis   also
    ·os′·te·o′·sis
syn′·os·tot′·ic   also
    ·os′·te·ot′·ic
syn·o′·tia
syn′·o·vec′·to·my
sy·no′·via [syn·o′·]
sy·no′·vi·al [syn·o′·]
sy·no′·vi·a′·le   neut.
    of synovialis
sy·no′·vi·a′·lis   pl.   ·les
sy·no′·vi·o′·ma   also
    ·vi·al·o′·ma; pl. ·mas or
    ·ma·ta
sy·no′·vi·or·tho′·sis
syn′·o·vip′·a·rous
syn′·o·vi′·tis [sy′·no·]
sy·no′·vi·um [syn·o′·]
syn′·pneu·mon′·ic
syn·tac′·ti·cal
syn′·ta·sis
syn·tax′·is
syn·te′·nic
syn·te·ny
syn·tex′·is
syn′·thase
syn·ther′·mal
syn′·the·sis   pl.   ·ses
syn′·the·size   ·sized,
    ·siz′·ing
syn′·the·siz′·er
syn′·the·tase
syn·thet′·ic
syn′·the·tis′m
syn·ton′·ic
syn·top′·ic
syn′·to·py   also   ·pie
syn′·tro·phis′m
syn·tro′·pho·blast
syn·tro′·pic [·trop′·ic]
syn′·tro·py

Sy·nu′·ra
Sy·pha′·cia
syph′·i·le′·mia   Brit.
    ·lae′·
syph′·i·lid   also   ·lide
syph′·i·lid·oph·thal′·
    mia
syph′·i·lis
syph′·i·lit′·ic
syph′·i·lit′·i·cus   fem.
    ·ca, neut. ·cum
syph′·i·lo·
syph′·i·lol′·o·gist
syph′·i·lo′·ma   pl.
    ·mas or ·ma·ta
syph′·i·lo′ma·tous
    [·lom′a·]
syph′·i·lo·nych′·ia
syr′·ing·ad′·e·no′·ma
    pl. ·mas or ·ma·ta
syr′·ing·ad′·e·no′·sus
syr′·ing·ad′·e·nous
sy·ringe′
syr′·in·gec′·to·my
sy·rin′·go·
sy·rin′·go·bul′·bia
sy·rin′·go·car′·ci·no′·
    ma   pl. ·mas or ·ma·
    ta
sy·rin′·go·cele
sy·rin′·go·cyst′·ad′·e·
    no′·ma   pl. ·mas or
    ·ma·ta
sy·rin′·go·cyst·ad′·e·
    no′·sus
sy·rin′·go·cys·to′·ma
    pl. ·mas or ·ma·ta
sy·rin′·goid
syr′·in·go′·ma   pl.
    ·mas or ·ma·ta
sy·rin′·go·me·nin′·go·
    cele
sy·rin′·go·my·e′·lia
sy·rin′·go·my·e′·lic
sy·rin′·go·my′·e·lo·
    bul′·bia
sy·rin′·go·my′·e·lo·cele
sy·rin′·go·my′·e·lus

syr′·in·got′·o·my
syr′·inx   pl.   sy·rin′·ges
syr′·o·sin′·go·pine
syr′·up
syr′·u·pus
sys·tal′·tic
sys′·tem
sys·te′·ma   gen.   ·ma·
    tis
sys′·tem·at′·ic
sys·tem′·ic
sys′·to·le
sys·tol′·ic
sys·trem′·ma
sy·zyg′·i·al
sy·zyg′·i·ol′·o·gy
syz′·y·gy   also   sy·zyg′·
    i·um

T

tab′·a·cis′m   also
    ·gis′m
tab′·a·co′·sis
tab′·a·nid
Ta·ban′·i·dae
Ta·ba′·nus
ta·ba·tière′ ana·to·
    mique′
ta·bel′·la   pl.   ·lae
ta′·bes
ta·bes′·cent
ta·bet′·ic
ta·bet′·i·form
tab′·la·ture
ta′·ble
tab′·let
ta′·bo·pa·ral′·y·sis
ta′·bo·pa·re′·sis
tab′·u·la   pl.   ·lae
tab′·u·lar
ta′·bun
tache
ta·chis′·to·scope
tach′·is·tos′·co·py
ta·chom′·e·ter
tach′y·

tach′y·ar·rhyth′·mia
tach′y·aux·e′·sis
tach′y·car′·dia
tach′y·car′·di·ac
ta·chym′·e·ter
tach′y·phe′·mia
tach′y·phy·lac′·tic
tach′y·phy·lax′·is
tach′y·pne′a   *Brit.*
 ·pnoe′a
tach′y·rhyth′·mia
ta·chys′·ter·ol
tach′y·zo′·ite
tac′·tile
tac′·ti·lis   *pl.* ·les
tac′·tor
tac′·tu·al
tac′·tus   *gen.* tactus
Tae′·nia
  T. sag′·i·na′·ta
  T. so′·li·um
tae′·nia   *pl.* ·ni·ae; *also*
  te′·
tae′·nia·cide
tae′·nia·fu′·gal
tae′·nia·fuge
tae′·ni·al   *also* te′·
Tae′·nia·rhyn′·chus
  genus of tapeworms:
  Cf. Taeniorhynchus
tae·ni′·a·sis
tae′·ni·form
tae′·ni·id
Tae·ni′·idae
tae′·ni·oid
tae·ni′·o·la
Tae′·nio·rhyn′·chus
  genus of mosquitoes:
  Cf. Taeniarhynchus
tag   *n. & v.* tagged,
  tag′·ging
ta′·glia·co′·tian
tag′·ma   *pl.* ·ma·ta
tail′·gut
tai′·pan
ta′·lar
ta·la′·ris

tal′·bot
tal′·bu·tal
talc
tal·co′·sis
tal′·cum
ta·lec′·to·my
ta′·li   *pl. & gen. sg. of*
  talus
tal′·i·ped
tal′·i·pes
tal′·i·po·man′·us
ta′·lo·cal·ca′·ne·al
ta′·lo·cal·ca′·ne·a′·ris
  neut. ·re
ta′·lo·cal·ca′·neo·na·
  vic′·u·lar
ta′·lo·cal·ca′·neo·na·
  vic′·u·la′·ris
ta′·lo·cal·ca′·ne·us
  neut. ·ne·um
ta′·lo·cru′·ral
ta′·lo·cru·ra′·lis
ta′·lo·fib′·u·la′·ris
  neut. ·re
tal′·on
ta′·lo·na·vic′·u·lar
ta′·lo·na·vic′·u·la′·ris
  neut. ·re
tal′·o·nid
ta′·lo·tib′·i·al
ta′·lo·tib′·io·fib′·u·lar
ta′·lus   *pl. & gen. sg.*
  ·li
tam′·bour
ta·mox′·i·fen
tam′·pan
tam′·pon
tam′·pon·ade′
tam·pon′·ment
tan   *n. & v.* tanned,
  tan′·ning
ta′·na·pox
tan·gen′·tial
tan·gen′·ti·al′·i·ty
tan′·go·re·cep′·tor
tan′·nic
tan′·nin

tan′·no·phil
tan′·ta·lum
tan′·trum
ta·pe′·tal
ta·pe′·to·cho·roi′·dal
ta·pe′·to·ret′·i·nal
ta·pe′·tum   *pl.* ·ta
tape′·worm
ta·pote′·ment
tar′·an·tis′m   *also* tar′·
  en·
ta·ran′·tu·la
tar′·dive
tar′·dus   *fem.* ·da
tare
tar′·get
tar′·get·ing
tar′·i·cha·tox′·in
Ta·ri′·ni   *gen. of*
  Tarinus
tars′·ad′·e·ni′·tis
tar′·sal
tar·sa′·le   *neut. of*
  tarsalis; *pl.* ·lia
tar·sal′·gia
tar·sa′·lis   *pl.* ·les
tar·sec′·to·my
tar′·si   *gen. of* tarsus
tar·si′·tis
tar′·so·
tar′·so·chei′·lo·plas′·ty
tar·soc′·la·sis
tar′·so·meg′·a·ly
tar′·so·met′a·tar′·sal
tar′·so·met′a·tar·sa′·le
  neut. of tarsometatar-
  salis; *pl.* ·lia
tar′·so·met′a·tar·sa′·lis
  pl. ·les
tar′·so·pla′·sia
tar′·so·plas′·ty
tar′·sop·to′·sis
tar·sor′·rha·phy
tar·sot′·o·my
tar′·sus   *pl. & gen. sg.*
  ·si
tar′·tar

tar·tar′·ic
tar′·trate
tast′·er
tat·too′
tau′·rine
tau′·ro·cho′·late
tau′·ro·cho·le′·mia
　Brit. ·lae′·
tau′·ro·cho′·lic
tau′·ro·cy′·a·mine
tau′·ro·don′·tism
tau′·to·
tau′·to·mer
tau′·tom′·er·al
tau·tom′·er·ase
tau′·to·mer′·ic
tau·tom′·er·is′m
tax′·is　pl. ·es
tax′·on　pl. tax′a
tax′·o·nom′·ic
tax·on′·o·mist
tax·on′·o·my
tear　n. & v.　tore,
　torn, tear′·ing
teart
tease　teased, teas′·ing
teat
teb′·u·tate
tech·ne′·tium
tech′·ni·cal
tech·ni′·cian
tech·nique′　also tech′·
　nic
tech′·no·log′·ic　also
　·i·cal
tech·nol′·o·gist
tech·nol′·o·gy
tec′·ta　pl. of tectum
tec′·tal
tec′·to·
tec′·to·bul′·bar
tec′·to·ceph′·a·ly
tec′·to·cer′·e·bel′·lar
tec·tol′·o·gy
tec·ton′·ic
tec·to′·ria
tec·to′·ri·al

tec·to′·ri·um　pl. ·ria
tec′·to·ru′·bral
tec′·to·sep′·tal
tec′·to·spi′·nal
tec′·to·teg·men′·tal
tec′·to·tha·lam′·ic
tec′·tum　pl. ·ta, gen.
　sg. ·ti
teeth　pl. of tooth
teeth′·ing
tef′·lu·rane
teg′·men　pl. teg′·mi·na
teg·men′·tal
teg′·men·ta′·lis
teg·men′·to-ol′·i·var′y
teg·men′·to·spi′·nal
teg·men′·tum　pl. ·ta,
　gen. sg. ·ti, gen. pl.
　teg′·men·to′·rum
teg′·u·ment
teg′·u·men′·tal
teg′·u·men′·ta·ry
tei·cho′·ic
tei·chop′·sia
tei′·co·plan′·in
tei′·no·dyn′·ia
te′·la　pl. & gen. sg.
　·lae
tel·al′·gia
tel·an′·gi·ec·ta′·sia
　also ·ec′·ta·sis
tel·an′·gi·ec·tat′·ic
tel·an′·gi·ec·tat′·i·cum
tel·an′·gi·ec·to′·des
tel·an′·gi·on
te′·lar
tel′·e·
tel′·e·bin·oc′·u·lar
tel′·e·can′·thus
tel′·e·car′·di·o·gram
tel′·e·car′·di·og′·ra·phy
tel′·e·car′·di·o·phone
tel′·e·cep′·tor
tel′·e·co′·balt
tel′·e·den′·drite
tel′·e·den′·dron　var. of
　telodendron

tel′·e·di′·ag·no′·sis
tel′·e·fluo·ros′·co·py
tel′·e·gram′·ma·tis′m
tel′·e·ir·ra′·di·a′·tion
tel′·e·ki·ne′·sis　psychic
　control of objects at a
　distance: Cf. telokinesis
te·lem′·e·ter [tel′·e·me′·
　ter]
te·lem′·e·try
tel′·en′·ce·phal′·ic
tel′·en·ceph′·a·li·za′·
　tion
tel′·en·ceph′·a·lon
tel′·e·neu′·rite
tel′·e·neu′·ron
tel′·e·ra′·di·og′·ra·phy
tel′·e·ra′·dio·ther′·a·py
tel′·e·roent′·gen·og′·ra·
　phy
tel′·e·roent′·gen·ther′·a·
　py
tel′·e·steth′·o·scope
tel′·es·the′·sia　Brit.
　·aes·
tel′·e·ther′·a·py
tel′·lu·ris′m
tcl′·lu·rite
tel·lu′·ri·um
tel′·o·
tel′·o·cen′·tric
tel′·o·ci·ne′·sis　var. of
　telokinesis
tel′·o·den′·dron　also
　·den′·dri·on
tel′·o·gen
te·log′·lia
tel′·o·ki·ne′·sis　end
　phase of cell division:
　Cf. telekinesis
tel′·o·lec′·i·thal
tel′·o·mere
tel′·o·pep′·tide
tel′·o·phase
tem′·per·a·ment

tem′·per·a·ture[48]
tem′·plate
tem′·ple
tem′·po·la′·bile
tem′·po·ra   *pl. of*
  tempus
tem′·po·ral
tem′·po·ra′·le   *neut. of*
  temporalis
tem′·po·ra′·lis   *pl.* ·les
tem′·po·ris   *gen. of*
  tempus
tem′·po·ro·
tem′·po·ro·man·dib′·u·
  lar
tem′·po·ro·man·dib′·u·
  la′·ris   *pl.* ·res
tem′·po·ro·max′·il·lar′·y
tem′·po·ro-oc·cip′·i·tal
tem′·po·ro·pa·ri′·etal
tem′·po·ro·pa·ri′·eta′·
  lis
tem′·po·ro·pon′·tine
  also ·tile
tem′·po·ro·zy·go·mat′·
  ic
tem′·po·ro·zy·go·mat′·
  i·ca
tem′·po·sta′·bile
tem′·pus   *pl.* ·po·ra,
  gen. sg. ·po·ris
te·nac′·i·ty
te·nac′·u·lum   *pl.* ·la
ten′·den·cy
ten′·der·ness
ten·din′·ea   *fem. of*
  tendineus; *pl.* ·e·ae
ten′·di·nes   *pl. of*
  tendo
ten·din′·e·um   *neut. of*
  tendineus
ten·din′·e·us
ten′·di·ni′·tis
ten′·di·no·plas′·ty
  var. of tenoplasty

ten′·di·no·su′·ture
ten′·di·nous
ten′·do   *pl.* ·di·nes,
  gen. sg. ·di·nis, *gen. pl.*
  ·di·num
ten′·do·   *var. of* teno-
ten·dol′·y·sis   *var. of*
  tenolysis
ten′·don
ten′·don·i′·tis   *var. of*
  tendinitis
ten′·do·plas′·ty   *var.*
  of tenoplasty
ten′·do·syn′·o·vi′·tis
  [·sy′·no·]   *var. of*
  tenosynovitis
ten′·do·vag′·i·nal
ten′·do·vag′·i·ni′·tis
te·nec′·to·my
te·nes′·mus
te′·nia   *var. of* taenia
te′·nia·cide   *var. of*
  taeniacide
te′·nia·fu′·gal   *var. of*
  taeniafugal
te′·nia·fuge   *also* te′·
  ni·fuge; *var. of* tae-
  niafuge
te·ni′·a·sis   *var. of*
  taeniasis
te′·ni·form   *var. of*
  taeniform
te·nif′·u·gal   *var. of*
  taeniafugal
te′·ni·oid   *var. of*
  taenioid
te·ni′·o·la   *var. of*
  taeniola
ten′·o·
te·nod′·e·sis [ten′·o·
  de′·sis]
ten′·o·dyn′·ia
te·nol′·y·sis
ten′·o·my′·o·plas′·ty

ten′·o·my·ot′·o·my
ten′·o·nec′·to·my
ten′·on·os·to′·sis   *var.*
  of tenostosis
te·non′·to·   *var. of*
  teno-
te·non′·to·dyn′·ia
  var. of tenodynia
ten′·on·tol′·o·gy
te·nop′·a·thy
ten′·o·phyte
ten′·o·plas′·tic
ten′·o·plas′·ty   *also* te·
  non′·to·
ten′·o·re·cep′·tor
te·nor′·rha·phy
ten′·os·to′·sis
ten′·o·sus·pen′·sion
ten′·o·su′·ture   *var. of*
  tendinosuture
ten′·o·syn′·o·vec′·to·my
ten′·o·syn′·o·vi′·tis
  [·sy′·no·]
ten′·o·tome
te·not′·o·my
ten′·o·vag′·i·ni′·tis
  var. of tendovaginitis
ten′·si·om′·e·ter
ten′·sion
ten′·sor   *L. pl.* ten·so′·
  res, *gen. sg.* ten·so′·ris
ten·to′·ri·al
ten·to′·ri·um   *pl.* ·ria,
  gen. sg. ·rii
ten′·u·is   *neut.* ten′·ue
tep′·id
ter′a·
ter′·as   *pl.* ter′·a·ta
te·rat′·ic
ter′·a·tis′m
ter′·a·to·
ter′·a·to·blas·to′·ma
  pl. ·mas *or* ·ma·ta
ter′·a·to·car′·ci·no′·ma
  pl. ·mas *or* ·ma·ta

---

[48] When indicating degrees of a temperature scale, there is no space between the degree sign and the scale symbol: 90°C, 36°F.

ter′·a·to·gen
ter′·a·to·gen′·e·sis
ter′·a·to·gen′·ic also
  ·ge·net′·ic or ·tog′·e·
  nous
ter′·a·to·ge·nic′·i·ty
ter′·a·tog′·e·ny
ter′·a·toid
ter′·a·to·log′·ic also
  ·i·cal
ter′·a·tol′·o·gist
ter′·a·tol′·o·gy
ter′·a·to′·ma pl. ·mas
  or ·ma·ta
ter′·a·to′·ma·tous
  [·tom′a·]
ter′·a·to′·sis
ter′·a·to·sper′·mia
ter′·bi·um
ter′e
ter′·e·binth
ter′·e·bin′·thi·nis′m
  [·thin·is′m]
ter′·e·brant
ter′·e·bra′·tion
ter′·es masc. & fem.
  pl. ter′·e·tes, neut. pl.
  te·re′·tia, gen. sg. ter′·
  e·tis
ter′·ete
ter′·gal
ter′·mi·nad
ter′·mi·nai·son′
ter′·mi·nal
ter′·mi·na′·le neut. of
  terminalis; pl. ·lia
ter′·mi·na′·lis pl. ·les
ter′·mi·nal·i·za′·tion
ter′·mi·na′·tio pl.
  ·na′·ti·o′·nes
ter′·mi·na′·tion
ter′·mi·na′·tor
ter′·mi·no·ter′·mi·nal
ter′·mi·nus pl. & gen.
  sg. ·ni
ter′·na·ry
Ter′·ni·dens
ter′·pene

ter′·pen·is′m
ter′·pin
ter·pin′·e·ol
ter′·ra
ter·res′·tri·al
ter·res′·tric
ter′·ror
ter′·tian
ter′·ti·ar′y [·tia·ry]
ter·tip′·a·ra
ter′·ti·us gen. ·tii
tes′·la
tes′·sel·lat′·ed
tes′·ta pl. ·tae
tes·ta′·ceous
tes·tal′·gia
test′·cross
tes·tec′·to·my
tes′·ter
tes′·tes pl. of testis
tes′·ti·cle
tes·tic′·u·lar
tes·tic′·u·la′·ris
tes·tic′·u·lus pl. ·li
test′·ing
tes′·tis pl. ·tes, gen.
  sg. testis
tes·ti′·tis
tes′·toid
tes′·to·lac′·tone
tes·top′·a·thy
tes·tos′·ter·one
tet′·a·nal
te·ta′·nia
te·tan′·ic
te·tan′·i·form
tet′·a·ni·za′·tion
tet′·a·nize ·nized,
  ·niz′·ing
tet′·a·no·
tet′·a·node
tet′·a·noid
tet′·a·nol′·y·sin
tet′·a·no·spas′·min
tet′·a·nus gen. ·ni
tet′·a·ny
te·tar′·ta·nope

te·tar′·ta·no′·pia also
  ·nop′·sia
te·tar′·ta·no′·pic
te·tar′·to·cone also
  tet′·ar·cone
te·tar′·to·co′·nid
tet′·ra·
tet′·ra-ame′·lia
tet′·ra·blas′·tic
tet′·ra·bra′·chi·us
tet′·ra·bro′·mo·phe′·nol
tet′·rac
tet′·ra·caine
tet′·ra·chi′·rus
tet′·ra·chlor·eth′·ane
tet′·ra·chlor·eth′·yl·ene
  also ·chlo′·ro·eth′·
tet′·ra·chlo′·ride
tet′·ra·chrome
tet′·ra·chro′·mic
tet′·ra·cy′·cline
tet′·rad
tet′·ra·dac′·ty·ly
tet′·ra·eth′·yl
tet′·ra·eth′·yl·am·mo′·
  ni·um
tet′·ra·eth′·yl·mon′o·
  thi′·o·no·py′·ro·
  phos′·phate
tet′·ra·eth′·yl·thi′·u·
  ram
tet′·ra·gly′·cine
tet′·ra·go′·num
tet′·ra·go′·nus
tet′·ra·he′·dron
tet′·ra·hy′·dro·can·
  nab′·i·nol
tet′·ra·hy′·dro·fo′·late
tet′·ra·hy′·dro·fo′·lic
tet′·ra·hy′·droz′·o·line
Tet′·ra·hy′·me·na
  T. pyr′·i·for′·mis
te·tral′·o·gy
te·tram′·e·lus
tet′·ra·mer
tet′·ra·mer′·ic
tet′·ra·meth′·yl·am·
  mo′·ni·um

tet'·ra·meth'·yl·ene·di'·a·mine
tet'·ra·meth'·yl·rho'·da·mine
Te·tram'·i·tus
tet'·ran·op'·sia
Te·tran'·y·chus
tet'·ra·o'·don
tet'·ra·o'·don·tox'·in
  var. of tetrodotoxin
tet'·ra·o'·don·tox'·ism
  var. of tetrodontoxism
tet'·ra·pa·re'·sis
tet'·ra·pep'·tide
tet'·ra·pho'·co·me'·lia
tet'·ra·ple'·gia
tet'·ra·ploid
tet'·ra·ploi'·dy
tet'·ra·pod
tet'·ra·so'·mic
tet'·ra·so'·my
tet·ras'·ter [tet'·ras·]
tet'·ra·sti·chi'·a·sis
tet'·ra·va'·lent
tet'·ra·zo'·li·um
tet'·ro·do·tox'·in
tet'·ro·do·tox'·ism
tet'·rose
tet·rox'·ide
tet'·ter
tex'·ti·form
tex'·tus pl. & gen. sg.
  textus
thal'·a·mec'·to·my
thal'·a·mi pl. & gen.
  sg. of thalamus
tha·lam'·ic
tha·lam'·i·cus
thal'·a·mo·
thal'·a·mo·cor'·ti·cal
thal'·a·mo·cru'·ral
thal'·a·mo·ge·nic'·u·late
thal'·a·mo·hy'·po·tha·lam'·ic
thal'·a·mo·len·tic'·u·lar
thal'·a·mo·mam'·il·lar'y

thal'·a·mo·oc·cip'·i·tal
thal'·a·mo·ol'·i·var'y
thal'·a·mo·pa·ri'·etal
thal'·a·mo·pe·dun'·cu·lar
thal'·a·mo·per'·fo·rate
thal'·a·mo·stri'·ate
thal'·a·mo·teg·men'·tal
thal'·a·mo·tem'·po·ral
thal'·a·mot'·o·my
thal'·a·mus pl. & gen. sg. ·mi
thal'·as·sa·ne'·mia
  Brit. ·nae·; var. of thalassemia
thal'·as·se'·mia Brit. ·sae'·
tha·lid'·o·mide
thal'·li·um
thal'·lus pl. ·li
than'·a·to·
than'·a·to·gno·mon'·ic
than'·a·tol'·o·gy
than'·a·to·pho'·bia
than'·a·to·pho'·ric
than'·a·tos also
  Thanatos
the'·a
the'·a·is'm
the·ba'·ine
the·be'·si·an
the'·ca pl. & gen. sg. ·cae
the'·cal
the·ci'·tis
the·co'·ma pl. ·mas or ·ma·ta
the'·co·ma·to'·sis
the'·co·steg·no'·sis
Thei·le'·ria
thei'·le·ri'·a·sis
the'·lar·che
The·la'·zia
the'·le·plas'·ty
thel·er'·e·this'm
the·li'·tis
the'·lo·
the'·lor·rha'·gia

the'·ly·blast
the·lyt'·o·ky
the·mat'·ic
the'·nad
the'·nar
The'·o·bal'·dia
the'·o·bro'·mine
the·oph'·yl·line
the'·o·rem
the'·o·ry
thèque
ther'·a·peu'·sis
ther'·a·peu'·tic
ther'·a·peu'·tics
Ther'·a·pho'·si·dae
ther'·a·pi'a
ther'·a·pist
ther'·a·py
ther'·i·ac
Ther'·i·di'·idae
ther'·ma·co·gen'·e·sis
ther'·mal
therm'·al·ge'·sia var. of thermoalgesia
ther·mal'·gia
therm'·an·al·ge'·sia
therm'·an·es·the'·sia
  var. of thermoanesthesia; Brit. ·aes·the'·
therm'·es·the'·sia
  Brit. ·aes·the'·
therm'·es·the'·si·om'·e·ter Brit. ·aes·the'·
therm'·hy'·per·es·the'·sia Brit. ·aes·the'·
therm'·hyp'·es·the'·sia Brit. ·aes·the'·
ther'·mic
ther'·mi·on
ther'·mi·on'·ic
therm·is'·tor
ther'·mo·
ther'·mo·al·ge'·sia
ther'·mo·an'·al·ge'·sia
ther'·mo·an'·es·the'·sia
  Brit. ·aes·the'·
ther'·mo·asym'·me·try

ther'·mo·cau'·ter·ec'·
 to·my
ther'·mo·cau'·tery
ther'·mo·chem'·i·cal
ther'·mo·chro'·ic
ther'·mo·chro'·ism
ther'·mo·co·ag'·u·la'·
 tion
ther'·mo·cou'·ple
ther'·mo·di·lu'·tion
ther'·mo·du'·ric
ther'·mo·dy·nam'·ic
ther'·mo·dy·nam'·ics
ther'·mo·elec'·tric
ther'·mo·elec'·tric'·i·ty
ther'·mo·es·the'·sia
 var. of thermesthesia;
 Brit. ·aes·the'·
ther'·mo·es·the'·si·om'·
 e·ter var. of therm-
 esthesiometer; Brit.
 ·aes·the'·
ther'·mo·gen'·e·sis
ther'·mo·gen'·ic also
 ·ge·net'·ic
ther'·mo·gram
ther'·mo·graph
ther'·mo·graph'·ic
ther·mog'·ra·phy
ther'·mo·hy'·per·al·ge'·
 sia
ther'·mo·hy'·per·es·
 the'·sia var. of
 thermhyperesthesia;
 Brit. ·aes·the'·
ther'·mo·hyp'·es·the'·
 sia var. of thermhyp-
 esthesia; also ·hy'·po·;
 Brit. ·aes·the'·
ther'·mo·in'·te·gra'·tor
ther'·mo·junc'·tion
ther'·mo·la'·bile
ther·mol'·o·gy
ther'·mo·lu'·mi·nes'·
 cence
ther'·mo·lu'·mi·nes'·
 cent
ther·mol'·y·sin

ther·mol'·y·sis
ther'·mo·lyt'·ic
ther'·mo·mas·sage'
ther'·mom'·e·ter
ther'·mom'·e·try
ther'·mo·pen'·e·tra'·
 tion
ther'·mo·phile
ther'·mo·phore
ther'·mo·pile
ther'·mo·plac'·en·tog'·
 ra·phy
ther'·mo·ple'·gia
ther'·mo·pol'·y·pne'a
 Brit. ·pnoe'a
ther'·mo·ra'·dio·ther'·
 a·py
ther'·mo·re·cep'·tor
ther'·mo·reg'·u·la'·tor
ther'·mo·reg'·u·la·to'·
 ry
ther'·mo·scope
ther'·mo·stat
ther'·mo·stro'·muhr
 [·strom'·uhr]
ther'·mo·sys'·tal·tis'm
ther'·mo·tac'·tic also
 ·tax'·ic
ther'·mo·tax'·is
ther'·mo·ther'·a·py
ther·mot'·ics
ther'·mo·tox'·in
ther'·mo·tro'·pic
 [·trop'·ic]
ther·mot'·ro·pis'm
the'·ro·morph
the·sau'·ris·mo'·sis
 also the'·sau·ro'·sis
the'·ta
thev'·e·tin
thi'·a·ben'·da·zole
thi'·a·cet'·a·zone
thi'·am·bu'·to·sine
thi'·a·mine also ·min
thi'·a·mi·nase
thi·am'·y·lal
Thi·a'·ra
thi'·a·zide

thi'·a·zine
thi'·a·zole
thi'·a·zo'·li·um
thick'·ness
thi·e'·na·my'·cin
thigh
thig'·mes·the'·sia
 Brit. ·maes·
thig'·mo·
thig'·mo·tac'·tic
thig'·mo·tax'·is
thig'·mo·tro'·pic
 [·trop'·ic]
thig·mot'·ro·pis'm
thi·hex'·i·nol
thim'·ble
thi·mer'·o·sal
thi'o·
thi'o·ac'·id also thio
 acid
thi'o·ar'·se·nite
thi'o·bar'·bi·tu'·ric
thi'·o·chrome
thi·oc'·tic
thi'o·cy·a·nate
thi'o·es'·ter
thi'o·e'ther
thi'o·glu'·cose
thi'o·gly'·co·late also
 ·col·late
thi'o·gly·col'·ic also
 ·col'·lic
thi'o·gua'·nine
thi'o·ki'·nase
thi'·ol
thi'·o·late
thi'o·mer'·sa·late
thi'·o·ne'·ine
thi·on'·ic
thi'·o·nine
thi'·o·pan'·ic
thi'o·pen'·tal
thi'o·pen'·tone
thi'o·pro'·pa·zate
thi'·o·re·dox'·in
thi'·o·rid'·a·zine
thi'o·sem'i·car'·ba·
 zone

thi'o·strep'·ton
thi'o·sul'·fate
thi'o·u'ra·cil
thi'o·ure′a
thi'o·xan'·thene
thix'·o·tro'·pic [·trop'·ic]
thix·ot'·ro·py *also* ·pis'm
thon·zyl'·a·mine
tho'·ra·ca'·lis
tho'·ra·cec'·to·my
tho'·ra·cen·te'·sis
tho·rac'·ic
tho·rac'·i·ca *fem. of* thoracicus; *pl. & gen. sg.* ·i·cae
tho·rac'·i·co· *var. of* thoraco-
tho·rac'·i·co·lum'·bar *var. of* thoracolumbar
tho·rac'·i·cus *pl. & gen. sg.* ·i·ci; *gen. pl.* tho·rac'·i·co'·rum
tho'·ra·cis [tho·ra'·cis] *gen. of* thorax
tho'·ra·co·
tho'·ra·co·ab·dom'·i·nal *also* tho·rac'·i·co·
tho'·ra·co·acro'·mi·al *also* tho·rac'·i·co·
tho'·ra·co·acro'·mi·a'·lis
tho'·ra·co·ce·los'·chi·sis *also* ·coe·los'·
tho'·ra·co·cen·te'·sis *var. of* thoracentesis
tho'·ra·co·dor'·sal
tho'·ra·co·dor·sa'·lis
tho'·ra·co·dyn'·ia
tho'·ra·co·ep'i·gas'·tric
tho'·ra·co·ep'i·gas'·tri·ca *pl.* ·cae
tho'·ra·co·gas·trop'·a·gus
tho'·ra·co·lap'·a·rot'·o·my

tho'·ra·co·lum·ba'·lis
tho'·ra·co·lum'·bar
tho'·ra·col'·y·sis
tho'·ra·com'·e·lus
tho'·ra·co·my'·o·dyn'·ia
tho'·ra·cop'·a·gus
tho'·ra·co·plas'·ty
tho'·ra·cos'·chi·sis
tho·ra'·co·scope [·rac'o·]
tho'·ra·cos'·co·py
tho'·ra·cos'·to·my
tho'·ra·cot'·o·my
tho'·rax *pl.* ·rax·es *or* ·ra·ces, *gen. sg.* ·ra·cis
tho'·ri·um
tho'·ron
thread'·worm
thre'·o·nine
thre'·ose
thresh'·old
thrill
thrix
throat
throe
throm'·bas·the'·nia
throm·bec'·to·my
throm'·bi *pl. of* thrombus
throm'·bin
throm'·bo·
throm'·bo·an'·gi·i'tis
throm'·bo·ar'·ter·i'·tis
throm·boc'·la·sis
throm'·bo·clas'·tic
throm'·bo·cyt'·apher·e'·sis [·apher'·e·]
throm'·bo·cyte
throm'·bo·cy·the'·mia *Brit.* ·thae'·
throm'·bo·cy'·to·crit
throm'·bo·cy·tol'·y·sis
throm'·bo·cy'·to·path'·ic
throm'·bo·cy·top'·a·thy
throm'·bo·cy'·to·pe'·nia

throm'·bo·cy'·to·pe'·nic
throm'·bo·cy'·to·poi·e'·sis
throm'·bo·cy'·to·poi·et'·ic
throm'·bo·cy·to'·sis
throm'·bo·elas'·to·graph
throm'·bo·em'·bo·lec'·to·my
throm'·bo·em'·bo·lis'm
throm'·bo·end·ar'·ter·ec'·to·my
throm'·bo·gen'·e·sis
throm'·bo·gen'·ic
throm'·boid
throm'·bo·ki'·nase
throm'·bo·ki·ne'·sis
throm·bol'·y·sis
throm'·bo·lyt'·ic
throm'·bo·path'·ic
throm'·bo·pe'·nia
throm'·bo·pe'·nic
throm'·bo·phil'·ia
throm'·bo·phle·bit'·ic
throm'·bo·phle·bi'·tis
throm'·bo·plas'·tic
throm'·bo·plas'·tin
throm'·bo·poi·e'·sis
throm'·bo·poi·et'·ic
throm'·bose ·bosed, ·bos·ing
throm·bo'·sis *pl.* ·ses
throm'·bo·sthe'·nin
throm'·bo·test'
throm·bot'·ic
throm·box'·ane
throm'·bus *pl.* ·bi
throw'·back
thrush
thu'·jone
thu'·li·um
thumb
thumb'-suck'·ing
thy'·la·ken'·trin
thy·mec'·to·my
thy'·mi *gen. of* thymus

thy'·mic
thy'·mi·ca *fem. of*
    thymicus; *pl.* ·cae
thy'·mi·cus *pl.* ·ci
thy'·mi·co·lym·phat'·ic
thy'·mi·dine
thy'·mi·dyl'·ate
thy'·mi·dyl'·ic
thy'·min *hormone: Cf.*
    thymine
thy'·mine *DNA base:*
    Cf. thymin
thy·mi'·tis
thy'·mo·
thy'·mo·cyte
thy'·mol
thy'·mol·ize
thy'·mol·phtha''·lein
thy'·mol·sul'·fon·
    phtha''·lein
thy·mol'·y·sis
thy'·mo·lyt'·ic
thy·mo'·ma *pl.* ·mas
    or ·ma·ta
thy'·mo·pha·ryn'·ge·al
thy'·mo·poi''·e·tin
thy'·mo·pri''·vous
    also ·priv'·ic
thy'·mo·sin
thy'·mus *gen.* ·mi
thy'·mus·ec''·to·my
    var. of thymectomy
thy'·ro· *also* thy'·reo·
thy'·ro·ac''·tive
thy'·ro·ar''·y·te''·noid
thy'·ro·ar''·y·te·noi''·de·
    us
thy'·ro·cal''·ci·to''·nin
thy'·ro·car''·di·ac
thy'·ro·car·di''·tis
thy'·ro·cer''·vi·cal
thy'·ro·cer''·vi·ca''·lis
thy'·ro·chon·drot''·o·
    my
thy'·ro·cri·cot''·o·my
thy'·ro·ep'i·glot''·tic
thy'·ro·ep'i·glot''·ti·cus
    neut. ·cum

thy'·ro·fis''·sure
thy'·ro·gen''·ic
thy·rog''·e·nous
thy'·ro·glob''·u·lin
thy'·ro·glos''·sal
thy'·ro·hy''·al
thy'·ro·hy''·oid
thy'·ro·hy·oi''·de·us
    fem. ·dea, *neut.* ·de·um
thy'·roid
thy·roi''·dea *fem. of*
    thyroideus; *pl. & gen.*
    sg. ·de·ae
thy'·roid·ec''·to·my
thy·roi''·de·um *neut.*
    of thyroideus
thy·roi''·de·us *pl.* ·dei
thy'·roid·is'm
thy'·roid·i''·tis
thy·roi'·do·ther''·a·py
thy'·roid·ot''·o·my
thy'·ro·la·ryn''·ge·al
thy'·ro·lin''·gual
thy'·ro·lyt''·ic
thy'·ro·meg''·a·ly
thy'·ro·nine
thy'·ro·par'a·thy''·roid·
    ec''·to·my
thy'·ro·pe''·nia
thy'·ro·pha·ryn''·gea
thy'·ro·pha·ryn''·ge·al
thy'·ro·pri''·val *also*
    ·priv'·ic
thy'·ro·priv''·ia
thy'·rop·to''·sis
thy'·ro·ther''·a·py
thy'·ro·tome
thy·rot''·o·my
thy'·ro·tox''·ic
thy'·ro·tox'·i·co''·sis
thy'·ro·trope
thy'·ro·troph
thy'·ro·tro''·phic
    [·troph''·ic] *var. of*
    thyrotropic
thy'·ro·tro''·pic [·trop''·
    ic]

thy'·ro·tro''·pin *also*
    ·phin
thy·rox''·ine *also* ·in
tib'·ia *L. pl. & gen.*
    sg. ·i·ae
tib'·i·ad
tib'·i·al
tib'·i·a''·le *neut. of*
    tibialis
tib'·i·a''·lis *pl.* ·les
tib'·io·ad·duc''·tor
tib'·io·cal·ca''·nea
tib'·io·fem''·o·ral
tib'·io·fib''·u·lar
tib'·io·fib''·u·la''·ris
    neut. ·re
tib'·io·na·vic''·u·lar
tib'·io·na·vic''·u·la''·ris
tib'·io·ta·la''·ris
tic *muscle twitch: Cf.*
    tick
ti'·car·cil''·lin
tick *parasite: Cf.* tic
tick'·le *n. & v.* ·led,
    ·ling
ti·clo''·pi·dine
tic'·po·lon''·ga
tid'·al
tig'·lic
ti'·groid
ti·grol''·y·sis
til·tom''·e·ter
tim'·bre
tinc·ta·ble
tinc·to''·ri·al
tinc·tu''·ra
tinc'·tu·ra''·tion
tinc'·ture
tin'·ea
tin'·gi·ble
ti·nid''·a·zole
tin·ni''·tus
ti·sane'
tis''·sue
tis''·su·lar
ti·ta''·ni·um
ti'·ter *also* ·tre
ti'·trant

ti′·trat·a·ble
ti′·trate ·trat·ed, ·trat·ing
ti·tra′·tion
ti′·tri·met′·ric
ti·trim′·e·try
tit′·u·bat′·ing
tit′·u·ba′·tion
Tit′·y·us
to·bac′·co
to·bac′·co·is′m
to′·bra·my′·cin
to′·co·
to′·co·dy′·na·mom′·e·ter
to·cog′·ra·phy
to′·col
to·col′·o·gy
to·col′·y·sis
to′·co·lyt′·ic
to·com′·e·ter
to·coph′·er·ol
to·coph′·er·ol·qui·none′
toe′·nail
To′·ga·vi′·ri·dae
to′·ga·vi′·rus
toi′·let
to′·ko·   var. of toco-
to′·ko·dy′·na·mom′·e·ter   var. of tocodynamometer
to·laz′·a·mide
to·laz′·o·line
tol·bu′·ta·mide
tol′·er·ance
tol′·er·ant
tol′·er·o·gen
tol′·er·o·gen′·ic
to′·li·dine
tol′·me·tin
tol·naf′·tate
tol′·u·ene
tol·u′·ic
tol·u′·i·dine
tom′·a·tine
to′·mo·
to′·mo·gram
to′·mo·graph
to′·mo·graph′·ic
to·mog′·ra·phy
to′·mo·lev′·el
tongue
tongue′-tie′
ton′·ic
to·nic′·i·ty
ton′·i·co·clon′·ic
ton′·o·clon′·ic
ton′·o·fi′·bril
ton′·o·fil′·a·ment
to′·no·gram
to·nog′·ra·phy
to·nom′·e·ter
to·nom′·e·try
to′·no·scope
ton′·sil
ton·sil′·la *pl.* ·lae
ton′·sil·lar
ton′·sil·la′·ris *pl.* ·res
ton′·sil·lec′·to·my
ton′·sil·lit′·ic
ton′·sil·li′·tis
ton′·sil·lo·ad′·e·noid·ec′·to·my
ton·sil′·lo·lith *also*
ton′·sil·lith
ton′·sil·lo·phar′·yn·gi′·tis
ton·sil′·lo·tome
ton′·sil·lot′·o·my
to′·nus
tooth *pl.* teeth
tooth′·ache
tooth′·brush′·ing
toothed
tooth′·pick
top′·ag·no′·sia *also* ·sis
to·pal′·gia
to·pec′·to·my
top′·es·the′·sia *Brit.* ·aes·the′·
to·pha′·ceous
to′·phic
to′·phus *pl.* ·phi
top′·i·cal
top′·o· [to′·po·]
top′·o·al′·gia [to′·po·]
top′·o·an′·es·the′·sia *Brit.* ·aes·the′·
top′·o·es·the′·sia [to′·po·] *Brit.* ·aes·the′·
top′·o·graph′·ic *also* ·i·cal
to·pog′·ra·phy
top′·o·isom′·er·ase [to′·po·]
top′·o·log′·i·cal
to·pol′·o·gy
top′·o·nym
to·pon′·y·my
top′·o·phy·lax′·is [to′·po·]
top′·o·therm′·es·the′·si·om′·e·ter *Brit.* ·aes·the′·
tor′·cu·lar
to′·ri *pl. of* torus
to′·ric
to′·rose *also* ·rous
tor′·pent
tor′·pid
tor·pid′·i·ty
tor′·pi·tude
tor′·por
torque
torr
tor′·re·fac′·tion
tor′·re·fy ·fied, ·fy′·ing
tor·sade′ de pointes′
tor′·si·oc·clu′·sion *also* tor′·so·clu′· *or* tor′·so-oc·
tor′·sion
tor′·sion·al
tor′·sion·om′·e·ter
tor′·si·ver′·sion
tor′·so *pl.* ·sos *or* ·si
tor′·tus *pl.* tor′·ti
tor′·ti·col′·lis
tor′·ti·pel′·vis
tor′·tua
tor′·tu·ous

tor′·u·la
tor′·u·lar
tor′·u·loid
Tor′·u·lop′·sis
 T. gla·bra′·ta
tor′·u·lop·so′·sis
tor′·u·lo′·sis
tor′·u·lus pl. ·li
to′·rus
to·ta′·lis
to·tip′·o·ten·cy [to′·ti·po′·] also ·tence
to′·tip′·o·tent also
to′·ti·po·ten′·tial
to′·ti·po·ten′·ti·al′·i·ty
touch
tour′·ni·quet
tox′·al·bu′·min
tox′·ane′·mia Brit. ·anae′·
tox′·a·phene
Tox·as′·ca·ris
 T. le′·o·ni′·na
tox·e′·mia Brit. ·ae′·mia
tox·e′·mic Brit. ·ae′·mic
tox·en′·zyme
tox′i·
tox′·ic
tox′·i·cant
tox′·i·ce′·mia var. of toxemia; Brit. ·cae′·
tox′·i·cide
tox·ic′·i·ty
tox′·i·co·
tox′·i·co·den′·drol
tox′·i·co·der′·ma·ti′·tis
tox′·i·co·gen′·ic
tox′·i·coid
tox′·i·co·ki·net′·ics
tox′·i·co·log′·ic also ·i·cal
tox′·i·col′·o·gist
tox′·i·col′·o·gy
tox′·i·co·ma′·nia
tox′·i·co·path′·ic
tox′·i·cop′·a·thy

tox′·i·co′·sis
tox′·i·cum
tox·if′·er·ine
tox·if′·er·ous
tox′·i·gen′·ic also tox·ig′·e·nous
tox′·i·ge·nic′·i·ty
tox′·ig·nom′·ic [·no′·mic]
tox·im′·e·try
tox′·in
tox′·in·e′·mia Brit. ·ae′·mia
tox′·in·o·gen′·ic var. of toxigenic
tox′·in·o·ge·nic′·i·ty var. of toxigenicity
tox′·i·no′·sis
tox′·i·path′·ic var. of toxicopathic
tox·ip′·a·thy var. of toxicopathy
tox·is′·ter·ol
tox′o·
Tox′·o·car′a
tox′·o·ca·ri′·a·sis
tox′·o·gen
tox′·oid
tox′o·lec′·i·thin also ·thid
tox′·o·neme
tox′·o·no′·sis
tox′·o·phore
Tox′·o·plas′·ma
Tox′·o·plas·mat′·i·dae
tox′·o·plas′·mic also ·plas·mat′·ic
tox′·o·plas′·min
tox′·o·plas·mo′·sis
tra·bec′·u·la pl. ·lae
tra·bec′·u·lar also ·late or ·lat′·ed
tra·bec′·u·la′·ris neut. ·re
tra·bec′·u·la′·tion
tra·bec′·u·lec′·to·my
trabs pl. tra′·bes
trac′·er

tra′·chea gen. ·che·ae
tra′·che·al
tra′·che·a′·le neut. of trachealis; pl. ·lia
tra′·che·a′·lis pl. ·les
tra′·che·i′tis
trach′·e·lag′·ra
trach′·e·lec′·to·my
trach′·e·lis′·mus
trach′·e·li′·tis
trach′·e·lo·
trach′·e·lo·cele
trach′·e·lo·cys·ti′·tis
trach′·e·lo·dyn′·ia
trach′·e·lo·mas′·toid
trach′·e·lo·pex′y
trach′·e·lo·plas′·ty
trach′·e·lor′·rha·phy
trach′·e·los′·chi·sis
trach′·e·lo·syr′·in·gor′·rha·phy
trach′·e·lot′·o·my
tra′·cheo·
tra′·cheo·bron′·chi·al
tra′·cheo·bron′·chi·a′·lis pl. ·les
tra′·cheo·bron·chi′·tis
tra′·cheo·bron′·cho·meg′·a·ly
tra′·cheo·bron·chos′·co·py
tra′·che·o·cele
tra′·cheo·esoph′·a·ge′·al Brit. ·cheo·oe·soph′·
tra′·che·og′·ra·phy
tra′·cheo·lar′·yn·got′·o·my
tra′·cheo·ma·la′·cia
tra′·che·op′·a·thy also ·o·path′·ia
tra′·cheo·pha·ryn′·ge·al
tra′·che·o·plas′·ty
tra′·che·or′·rha·phy
tra′·che·os′·chi·sis
tra′·che·o·scope
tra′·che·os′·co·py
tra′·cheo·ste·no′·sis

tra′·che·o·stome *also*
  tra′·che·os′·to·ma
  tra′·che·os′·to·my
  tra′·che·ot′·o·my
tra·cho′·ma
tra·cho′·ma·tous
trac′·ing
tract
trac′·tion
trac·tol′·o·gy
trac′·tor
trac·tot′·o·my
trac′·tus *pl. & gen.
  sg.* tractus
trag′·a·canth
tra′·gal
trag′·i·cus
tra·goph′·o·ny
tra′·gus *pl. & gen. sg.*
  ·gi
train′·a·ble
trait
trance
tran′·ex·am′·ic
tran′·quil·iz′·er *also*
  ·quil·liz′·
trans′·ab·dom′·i·nal
trans′·acet′·y·lase
trans·ac′·yl·ase
trans·al′·do·lase
trans·am′·i·da′·tion
trans·am′·i·di·nase
trans·am′·i·nase
trans·am′·i·na′·tion
trans·an′·i·ma′·tion
trans·an′·tral
trans′·aor′·tic
trans·a′tri·al
trans·ax′·o·nal
trans·ca′·lent
trans′·car·bam′·o·yl·
  ase
trans·cav′·i·tar′·y
trans·cel′·lu·lar
trans·cer′·vi·cal
trans′·co·bal′·a·min
trans′·co·lon′·ic
trans·con′·dy·lar

trans·cor′·ti·cal
trans·cor′·tin
trans·cra′·ni·al
tran·scrip′·tase
tran·scrip′·tion
trans′·cu·ta′·ne·ous
trans·duc′·er
trans·duc′·tant
trans·duc′·tion
trans·du′·o·de′·nal
tran·sect′
tran·sec′·tion
trans′·ep′·i·der′·mal
trans′·ep′·i·the′·li·al
tran·sep′·tal *var. of*
  transseptal
trans′·esoph′·a·ge′·al
  Brit. ·oe·soph′·
trans·eth·moi′·dal
trans·fau·na′·tion
trans·fec′·tion
trans′·fer *n.*
trans·fer′ *v.* ·ferred′,
  ·fer′·ring
trans′·fer·ase
trans·fer′·ence
trans·fer′·rin
trans·fix′·ion
trans′·for·ma′·tion
trans·form′·er
trans′·for·mim′·i·nase
trans·fuse′   fused′,
  ·fus′·ing
trans·fu′·sion
trans·fu′·sion·al
trans·gen′·ic
trans′·he′·mo·phil′·in
  Brit. ·hae′·mo·
trans′·hi·a′·tal
trans·hy′·dro·gen·ase′
trans·hy′·oid
tran′·sient
tran·sil′·i·ent
trans′·il·lu′·mi·na′·tion
tran·sis′·tor
tran·si′·tion
tran·si′·tion·al
tran′·si·to′·ry

tran′·si·to·zo′·o·no′·sis
trans·ke′·to·lase
trans·la′·tion
trans·lin′·gual
trans·lo′·case
trans′·lo·ca′·tion
trans·lu′·cent
trans·lum′·bar
trans·lu′·mi·nal
trans′·me·a′tal
trans·mem′·brane
trans′·mes′·en·ter′·ic
trans·meth′·yl·ase
trans·meth′·yl·a′·tion
trans′·mi·gra′·tion
trans·mis′·si·bil′·i·ty
trans·mis′·si·ble
trans·mis′·sion
trans·mit′·tance
trans·mit′·ter
trans·mu′·ral
trans′·mu·ta′·tion
trans·or′·bit·al
trans′·ovar′·i·al *also*
  ·an
trans·par′·en·cy
trans·par′·ent
trans′·pep′·ti·da′·tion
trans′·per′·i·to·ne′·al
trans′·pha·lan′·ge·al
trans′·phos′·pho·ryl·a′·
  tion
tran′·spi·ra′·tion
tran·spire′   ·spired′,
  ·spir′·ing
trans′·pla·cen′·tal
trans′·plant *n.*
trans·plant′ *v.*
trans′·plan·ta′·tion
trans·pleu′·ral
trans′·port
trans·pos′·a·ble
trans·po′·sase
trans·pose′   ·posed′,
  ·pos′·ing
trans′·po·si′·tion
trans·po′·son
trans′·py·lo′·ric

trans·sa′·cral
trans·sec′·tion *var. of*
  transection
trans·sep′·tal
trans·sex′·u·al
trans·sex′·u·al·is′m
trans′·sphe·noi′·dal
trans·sta′·di·al *also*
  tran·sta′·
trans′·syn·ap′·tic
trans·tem′·po·ral
trans′·ten·to′·ri·al
trans′·tho·rac′·ic
trans′·thy·ret′·in
trans·tra′·che·al
trans′·tro′·chan·ter′·ic
trans·tru′·sion
trans′·tu·ber′·cu·lar
trans′·tym·pan′·ic
tran′·su·date
tran′·su·da′·tion
trans′·uran′·ic *also*
  ·ura′·ni·an
trans′·ure′·tero·ure′·ter·al
trans′·ure′·tero·ure′·ter·os′·to·my
trans′·ure′·thral
trans·vag′·i·nal
trans′·va·ter′·i·an
trans·vec′·tor
trans·ve′·nous
trans′·ven·tric′·u·lar
trans·ver′·sa *fem. of*
  transversus; *pl.* ·sae
trans′·ver·sa′·lis *pl.*
  ·les
trans·verse′ [trans′·verse]
trans′·ver·sec′·to·my
trans·ver′·sion
trans·ver′·so·pla′·nus
trans·ver′·so·spi·na′·lis *pl.* ·les
trans·ver′·sum *neut.*
  of transversus
trans·ver′·sus *pl. &*
  gen. sg. ·si

trans·ves′·i·cal
trans·ves′·tism *also*
  ·ti·tism
trans·ves′·tite
tran′·yl·cy′·pro·mine
  [·cyp′·ro·]
tra·pe′·zi·um *neut. of*
  trapezius; *pl.* ·zia, *gen.*
  sg. ·zii
tra·pe′·zi·us *pl. &*
  gen. sg. ·zii
trap′·e·zoid
trap′·e·zoi′·de·um
trau′·ma *pl.* ·mas *or*
  ·ma·ta
trau·mat′·ic
trau′·ma·tis′m
trau′·ma·tize ·tized,
  ·tiz′·ing
trau′·ma·to·
trau′·ma·to·gen′·ic
trau′·ma·tol′·o·gist
trau′·ma·tol′·o·gy
trea′·cle
treat′·ment
Tre·cho′·na
tre·ha′·lose [tre′·ha·]
tre′·ma *pl.* ·ma·ta
Trem′·a·to′·da
trem′·a·tode
trem′·a·to·di′·a·sis
trem′·a·toid
tre′·mens [trem′·ens]
trem′·e·tol *also* trem′·a·tole *or* trem′·e·tone
trem′·o·gram *also*
  trem′·or·
trem′·o·graph *also*
  trem′·or·
trem′o·la′·bile
tre·mom′·e·ter
trem′·or
trem′·or·ine
trem′o·sta′·ble
trem′·u·lous
tre·pan′ *n. & v.*
  ·panned′, ·pan′·ning
trep′·a·na′·tion

treph′·i·na′·tion
tre·phine′ *n. & v.*
  ·phined′, ·phin′·ing
treph′·o·cyte *var. of*
  trophocyte
trep′·i·dant
trep′·i·da′·tio
trep′·i·da′·tion
Trep′·o·ne′·ma
  T. ca·ra′·te·um
  T. pal′·li·dum
  T. per·ten′·ue
trep′·o·ne′·mal
trep′·o·ne′·ma·to′·sis
trep′·o·neme
trep′·o·ne·mi′·a·sis
trep′·o·ne′·mi·ci′·dal
  [·cid′·al]
tres′·to·lone
tret′·i·noin [tret′·i·no′in]
tri′·ac
tri·acan′·thine
tri·ac′·e·tate
tri′·ace′·tin
tri·ace′·tyl·o′le·an′·do·my′·cin
tri′·ad
tri′·ad·i′·tis
tri·age′
tri′·al
tri′·a·lis′m
tri′·a·lis′·tic
tri′·am·cin′·o·lone
tri·am′·ter·ene
tri′·an·gle
tri·an′·gu·la′·ris *neut.*
  ·re
Tri·at′·o·ma
  T. san′·gui·su′·ga
Tri′·a·tom′·i·nae
tri·a′tri·al
tri·ba′·sic
tri·bas′·i·lar
tri·bas′·i·la′·re
tri·bol′·o·gy
tri·bra′·chi·al
tri·bra′·chi·us

tri′·bro′·mo·eth′·a·nol
 also tri′·brom·eth′·a·nol
tri′·bro′·mo·eth′·yl
tri′·car′·box·yl′·ic
tri′·ceps gen. tri·cip′·i·tis
tri·chi′·a·sis
trich′·i·lem′·mal
trich′·i·lem·mo′·ma
 var. of tricholemmoma
tri·chi′·na pl. ·nae
Trich′·i·nel′·la
 T. spi·ra′·lis
trich′·i·nel·li′·a·sis
Trich′·i·nel·loi′·dea
trich′·i·nel·lo′·sis
trich′·i·ni′·a·sis
trich′·i·ni·za′·tion
trich′·i·no·scope [tri·chi′·no·]
trich′·i·nosed
trich′·i·no′·sis
trich′·i·not′·ic
trich′·i·nous
tri·chlo′·ride
tri′·chlor′·me·thi′·a·zide
tri′·chlo′·ro·ace′·tic
tri′·chlo′·ro·eth′·yl·ene
tri′·chlo′·ro·meth′·ane
tri′·chlo′·ro·meth′·yl·chlo′·ro·for′·mate
tri′·chlo′·ro·phe′·nol
tri′·chlo′·ro·phen·ox′y·ace′·tic
tri′·chlo′·ro·tri′·vi′·nyl·ar′·sine
trich′o·
trich′o·be′·zoar
Trich′o·bil·har′·zia
trich′o·ceph′·a·li′·a·sis
Trich′o·ceph′·a·lus
tri·choc′·la·sis also trich′·o·cla′·sia
trich′o·cyst
Trich′·o·der′·ma
trich′o·ep′·i·the′·li·o′·ma pl. ·mas or ·ma·ta

trich′o·es·the′·sia
 var. of trichesthesia;
 Brit. ·aes·
trich′o·fol·lic′·u·lo′·ma
trich′o·hy′·a·lin
trich′·oid
trich′o·lem·mo′·ma
 pl. ·mas or ·ma·ta
tri·chol′·o·gy
trich′o·ma·la′·cia
tri′·chome [trich′·ome]
trich′o·meg′·a·ly
trich′·o·mo′·na·cid′·al [·ci′·dal]
trich′·o·mo′·na·cide
trich′·o·mo′·nad
Trich′·o·mo·nad′·i·da
trich′·o·mo′·nal
Trich′·o·mo′·nas
 T. ten′·ax
 T. vag′·i·na′·lis
trich′·o·mo·ni′·a·sis
 also ·mo·no′·sis
trich′o·my·co′·sis
trich′·o·no·car′·di·o′·sis
tri·chop′·a·thy
trich′·o·phyt′·ic
trich′·o·phy′·tid also ·tide
trich′·o·phy′·tin
trich′·o·phy′·to·be′·zoar
Tri·choph′·y·ton [Trich′·o·phy′·ton]
 T. ec′·to·thrix
 T. en′·do·thrix
 T. men·tag′·ro·phy′·tes
 T. ru′·brum
 T. ton′·su·rans
trich′·o·phy·to′·sis
Tri·chop′·tera
trich′o·pti·lo′·sis
trich′o·rhi′·no·pha·lan′·ge·al
trich′·or·rhex′·is
tri·chos′·chi·sis

trich′o·sid′·er·in
tri·cho′·sis
Trich′·o·spo′·ron
trich′·o·spo·ro′·sis
tri·chos′·ta·sis
trich′o·stron′·gyle
Trich′o·stron·gyl′·i·dae
trich′o·stron′·gy·lo′·sis
Trich′o·stron′·gy·lus
trich′o·thi′o·dys′·tro·phy
trich′o·til′·lo·ma′·nia
tri·chot′·o·my
tri·chro′·ic
tri·chro′·ism
tri·chro′·mat
tri′·chro·mat′·ic
tri·chro′·ma·tis′m
tri′·chro′·ma·top′·sia
tri′·chrome
tri·chro′·mic var. of trichromatic
trich′·ter·brust′
trich′·u·ri′·a·sis
Trich·u′·ris
 T. trich′·i·u′·ra
Trich′·u·roi′·dea
tri·cip′·i·tal
tri·cip′·i·tis gen. of triceps
tri′·clo′·bi·so′·ni·um
tri·clo′·san
tri·cor′·nute
tri·cre′·sol
tri·cres′·yl
tri·crot′·ic
tri′·cro·tis′m
tri·cus′·pid also ·pi·dal or ·pi·date
tri·cy′·cla·mol
tri·cy′·clic
tri·dac′·ty·lous
tri′·dent
tri·der′·mic also ·mal
tri·dig′·i·tate
tri′·di′·hex′·eth′·yl
trid′·y·mus
tri·es′·ter

tri′·eth′·a·nol′·a·mine
tri·eth′·yl·ene·mel′·a·mine
tri·eth′·yl·ene·phos·phor′·a·mide
tri·eth′·yl·ene·thi′o·phos·phor′·a·mide
tri·fa′·cial
tri′·fid
tri′·flu·o·per′·a·zine
tri′·flu·per′·i·dol
tri′·flu·pro′·ma·zine
tri·flu′·ri·dine
tri·fo′·cal
tri·fur′·cate [tri′·fur·]
tri′·fur·ca′·tion
tri·gas′·tric
tri·gas′·tri·cus
tri·gem′·i·na *fem. of* trigeminus
tri·gem′·i·nal
tri·gem′·i·no·cer′·vi·cal
tri·gem′·i·na′·lis *neut.* ·le
tri·gem′·i·no·fa′·cial
tri·gem′·i·no·tha·lam′·ic
tri·gem′·i·nus *pl. & gen. sg.* ·ni
tri·gem′·i·ny
tri·glyc′·er·ide
tri′·gly·col′·la·mate
tri·go′·na *pl. of* trigonum
tri′·go·nal [trig′·o·]
tri′·gone
tri′·go·nec′·to·my
trig′·o·nel′·line
tri′·go·nid [tri·gon′·id]
tri′·go·ni′·tis [trig′·o·]
tri′·go·no·ce·phal′·ic [trig′·o·]
tri′·go·no·ceph′·a·ly [trig′·o·]
tri·go′·num *pl.* ·na, *gen. sg.* ·ni
tri·hex′·o·side
tri′·hex′y·phen′·i·dyl
tri·hy′·brid
tri′·hy·drox′y·es′·trin
tri′·i′o·do·meth′·ane
tri′·i′o·do·thy′·ro·nine
tri′·labe
tri·lam′·i·nar
tri·lat′·er·al
tri·lo′·bate
tri′·lobed
tri·loc′·u·lar
tril′·o·gy
tri′·mal·le′·o·lar
Tri·mas′·ti·ga·moe′·ba
tri·mas′·ti·gote
tri·mep′·ra·zine
tri′·mer
Trim′·er·e·su′·rus
tri·mer′·ic
tri·mes′·ter
tri′·meth′·a·di′·one
tri·meth′·a·phan
tri·meth′o·ben′·za·mide
tri·meth′·o·prim
tri·meth′·yl·ac′·e·tate
tri·meth′·yl·ene
tri′·me·trex′·ate
tri·mip′·ra·mine
tri·mor′·phism
Tri·mor′·pho·don
tri·mor′·phous *also* ·phic
tri·ni′·trin
tri′·ni′·tro·glyc′·er·in *also* ·er·ol
tri·ni′·trol
tri′·ni′·tro·tol′·u·ene
tri·no′·mi·al
tri·nu′·cle·ate
tri·nu′·cle·o·tide
tri′o·ceph′·a·lus
tri′·ode
tri′·oph·thal′·mos
tri·or′·chid
tri′·ose
tri·o′·tus
tri·ox′·sa·len
tri·pal′·mi·tin
trip′·a·ra
tri·par′·tite
tri′·pel·en′·na·mine
tri′·pha·lan′·gia *also* ·gism
tri·phar′·ma·con *also* ·cum
tri·pha′·sic
tri′·phen′·yl·chlor·eth′·yl·ene
tri′·phen′·yl·eth′·yl·ene
tri·phos′·pha·tase
tri·phos′·phate
tri′·phos′·pho·pyr′·i·dine
tri′·phos·pho′·ric
tri′·phyl·lom′·a·tous
tri·ple′·gia
trip′·let
trip′·lex [trip′·plex]
trip′·lo·blas′·tic
trip′·loid
trip′·loi·dy
trip·lo′·pia
tri′·pod
tri·po′·dia
tri·pro′·li·dine
trip′·sis
tri′·pus
tri·que′·tral
tri·que′·trous
tri·que′·trum
tri·ra′·di·ate
tri·ra′·di·us
tri·sac′·cha·ride
tri·sil′·i·cate
tris′·mic
tris′·moid
tris′·mus
tri′·so·my
tri·splanch′·nic
tri·stich′·ia
tri·sul′·cate
trit′·anom′·a·ly
tri′·tan·ope
tri′·tan·o′·pia *also* ·op′·sia
tri′·tan·o′·pic
tri′·ti·at′·ed

tri·ti′·ce·al
tri·tic′·e·us *fem.* ·ea,
  neut. ·e·um
trit′·i·um
tri′·to·cone
tri′·to·co′·nid
tri·tu·ber′·cu·lar
trit′·u·ra·ble
trit′·u·rate   ·rat′·ed,
  ·rat′·ing
trit′·u·ra′·tion
trit′·u·ra′·tor
tri·va′·lent
triv′·i·al
tri·zon′·al [·zo′·nal]
tro′·car
tro·chan′·ter
tro′·chan·ter′·ic
tro′·chan·ter′·i·ca
tro·chan′·ter·i′·tis
tro·chan′·ter·plas′·ty
tro′·che
tro′·chis·ca′·tion
tro·chis′·cus *pl.* ·ci
troch′·lea *pl. & gen.*
  sg. ·le·ae
troch′·le·ar
troch′·le·ar′·i·form
troch′·le·a′·ris *pl.*
  ·les, *gen. pl.* ·ri·um
tro′·cho·car′·dia
  [troch′·o·]
tro′·cho·ceph′·a·ly
  [troch′o·]
tro′·choid
tro·choi′·dea
tro′·land
tro′·le·an′·do·my′·cin
trol·ni′·trate
Trom·bic′·u·la

T. al′·fred·du·ge′·si
T. au′·tum·na′·lis
trom·bic′·u·li′·a·sis
  also ·lo′·sis
trom·bic′·u·lid
Trom′·bi·cu′·li·dae
Trom′·bi·di′·idae
Trom·bid′·i·um
trom′·o·pho′·nia
tro·pae′·o·lin *also*
  ·pe′·o·
tro′·pe·ine
tro·pe′·in·is′m
troph·ec′·to·derm
troph′·ede′·ma *Brit.*
  ·oe·de′·
tro′·phic[49] [troph′·ic]
tro′·pho· [troph′·o·]
tro′·pho·blast
tro′·pho·blas′·tic
tro′·pho·blas·to′·ma
  pl. ·mas *or* ·ma·ta
tro′·pho·cyte
tro′·pho·derm
troph′·oe·de′·ma *Brit.*
  spel. of trophedema
tro′·pho·neu·ro′·sis
tro′·pho·neu·rot′·ic
tro′·pho·nu′·cle·us
tro′·pho·plast
tro′·pho·spon′·gi·um
  pl. ·gia
tro′·pho·tax′·is
tro′·pho·tro′·pic
  [·trop′·ic]
tro·phot′·ro·pis′m [tro′·
  pho·tro′·pism]
tro′·pho·zo′·ite
tro′·pia
tro′·pic[50]

trop′·i·ca
trop′·i·cal
tro·pic′·a·mide
tro′·pine
tro′·pism
tro′·po·col′·la·gen
tro′·po·elas′·tin
tro·pom′·e·ter
tro′·po·my′·o·sin
tro′·po·nin
trough
trox′·i·done
trun′·cal
trun′·cate   ·cat′·ed,
  ·cat′·ing
trun′·cus *pl. & gen.*
  sg. ·ci
trunk
tru′·sion
truss
tryp′·an
try′·pa·nid
try·pan′·o·cid′·al [·ci′·
  dal]
try·pan′·o·cide *also*
  ·i·cide
try·pan′·o·lyt′·ic
Try·pan′·o·so′·ma
  T. bru′·cei
  T. cru′·zi
  T. gam′·bi·en′·se
  T. ran′·geli
  T. rho·de′·si·en′·se
try·pan′·o·so′·mal
try·pan′·o·so′·ma·tid
*Try·pan′·o·so·mat′·i·
  dae*
try·pan′·o·some
try·pan′·o·so·mi′·a·sis
try·pan′·o·so′·mic

---

49 See note at *tropic*.
50 The alphabetic sequences *tropic* and *trophic* also occur as word-endings which should be carefully distinguished from one another. The ending *-tropic* has to do with orientation or attraction, while *-trophic* concerns nutrition, growth, or source of energy. Compare *phototropic* (moving in response to light) with *phototrophic* (deriving energy from light). However, in many terms the two forms tend to be confused; for example, *lymphotrophic* is often used in the sense of *lymphotropic* (attracted to lymphocytes).

try·pan′·o·so′·mi·cid′·al [·ci′·dal]
try·pan′·o·so′·mi·cide
try·pan′·o·so′·mid
tryp·ars′·a·mide
try′·po·chete
try′·po·mas′·ti·gote
try′·po·nar′·syl
try′·po·tan
tryp′·sin
tryp′·sin·ize ·ized, ·iz′·ing
tryp·sin′·o·gen
tryp′·ta·mine
tryp′·tic
tryp′·tone
tryp′·to·phan also ·phane
tryp′·to·pha·nase′
tryp′·t.)·phan·u′·ria [·pha·nu′·]
tryp′·to·phyl
tset′·se
tsu′·tsu·ga′·mu·shi [·ga·mu′·]
tu′·ami′·no·hep′·tane [·am′i·no·]
tu′·ba pl. & gen. sg. ·bae, accusative ·bam
tub′·al [tu′·bal]
tu·ba′·ria fem. of tubarius; pl. ·ri·ae
tu·ba′·ri·us
tub′·ba also ·boe
tube
tu·bec′·to·my
tu′·ber pl. ·bera, gen. sg. ·ber·is
tu′·ber·a′·lis
tu′·ber·cle
tu·ber′·cu·la pl. of tuberculum
tu·ber′·cu·lar
tu·ber′·cu·late also ·lat′·ed
tu·ber′·cu·la′·tion
tu·ber′·cu·li gen. of tuberculum

tu·ber′·cu·lid also ·lide
tu·ber′·cu·lin
tu·ber′·cu·lin·i·za′·tion also ·lin·a′·tion
tu·ber′·cu·li′·num
tu·ber′·cu·li·za′·tion
tu·ber′·cu·lo·
tu·ber′·cu·lo·cele
tu·ber′·cu·lo·cid′·al [·ci′·dal]
tu·ber′·cu·lo·cide
tu·ber′·cu·lo·derm also tu·ber′·cu·lo·der′·ma
tu·ber′·cu·loid
tu·ber′·cu·loi′·din
tu·ber′·cu·lo′·ma pl. ·mas or ·ma·ta
tu·ber′·cu·lo·pro′·tein
tu·ber′·cu·lo′·sa
tu·ber′·cu·lose
tu·ber′·cu·lo·sil′·i·co′·sis
tu·ber′·cu·lo′·sis
tu·ber′·cu·lo·stat′·ic
tu·ber′·cu·lot′·ic
tu·ber′·cu·lo·tox′·in
tu·ber′·cu·lous
tu·ber′·cu·lum pl. ·la, gen. sg. ·li
tu′·ber·is gen. of tuber
tu′·bero·hy′·po·phys′·i·al
tu′·bero·in′·fun·dib′·u·lar
tu′·ber·o′·si·tas pl. ·o′·si·ta′·tes, gen. sg. ·o′·si·ta′·tis
tu′·ber·os′·i·ty
tu′·ber·o′·sus fem. ·sa, neut. ·sum
tu′·ber·ous also ·ose
tu′·bo·
tu′·bo·ab·dom′·i·nal
tu′·bo·cu·ra′·rine
tu′·bo·gas·tros′·to·my
tu′·bo-ovar′·i·an
tu′·bo-ovar′·i·ec′·to·my

tu′·bo-ovar′·i·ot′·o·my
tu′·bo-o′va·ri′·tis
tu′·bo·pha·ryn′·ge·al
tu′·bo·plas′·ty
tu′·bo·tym·pan′·ic also ·tym′·pa·nal
tu′·bo·tym·pan′·i·cus
tu′·bo·u′ter·ine
tu′·bu·lar
tu′·bule
tu′·bu·li pl. of tubulus
tu′·bu·lin
tu′·bu·li·za′·tion
tu′·bu·lo·ac′·i·nar also ·nous
tu′·bu·lo·cyst
tu′·bu·lo·in′·ter·sti′·tial
tu′·bu·lor·rhex′·is
tu′·bu·lous
tu′·bu·lo·vil′·lous
tu′·bu·lus pl. & gen. sg. ·li
tu′·bus pl. & gen. sg. ·bi
tuck′·ing
tuft′·ing
tug′·ging
tu′·la·re′·mia Brit. ·rae′·
tu′·la·re′·mic Brit. ·rae′·mic
tu′·la·rine
tulle′ gras′
tu′·me·fa′·cient
tu′·me·fac′·tion
tu′·me·fy ·fied, ·fy′·ing
tu·mes′·cence
tu·mes′·cent
tu′·mid
tu′·mor Brit. ·mour
tu′·mor·al
tu′·mor·i·cid′·al [·ci′·dal]
tu′·mori·gen′·e·sis
tu′·mor·i·gen′·ic
tu′·mor·let
tu′·mor·ous

tu′·mour Brit. spel. of tumor
Tun′·ga
  T. pen′·e·trans
tun·gi′·a·sis
tung′·sten
tu′·nic
tu′·ni·ca pl. & gen. sg. ·cae
tun′·nel
tur′·bid
tur′·bi·dim′·e·ter
tur′·bi·di·met′·ric
tur′·bi·dim′·e·try
tur·bid′·i·ty
tur′·bi·nate also ·nat′·ed or ·nal
tur′·bi·nec′·to·my
tur′·bi·no·tome
tur′·bi·not′·o·my
tur′·ci·ca gen. ·ci·cae
tur·ges′·cence
tur·ges′·cent
tur′·gid
tur′·gid·i·za′·tion
tur′·gor
tu·ris′·ta
tur′·mer·ic
tus′·sal
tus·sic′·u·lar
tus′·sis
tus′·sive
tu·ta′·men pl. tu·tam′·i·na
tweez′·ers
twin n. & v. twinned, twin′·ning
twitch
ty·lec′·to·my
ty·lo′·sis
ty·lot′·ic
tym′·pa·nal
tym′·pa·nec′·to·my
tym′·pa·ni gen. of tympanum
tym·pan′·ic
tym·pan′·i·ca fem. of tympanicus; pl. & gen. sg. ·cae

tym′·pa·nic′·i·ty
tym·pan′·i·cum neut. of tympanicus
tym·pan′·i·cus pl. & gen. sg. ·ci, ablative ·co
tym′·pa·ni′·tes
tym′·pa·nit′·ic
tym′·pa·no·
tym′·pa·no·gram
tym′·pa·no·hy′·al
tym′·pa·no·lab′·y·rin′·tho·pex′y
tym′·pa·no·mal′·le·al
tym′·pa·no·mas′·toid
tym′·pa·no·mas·toi′·dea
tym′·pa·no·mas′·toid·i′·tis
tym′·pa·nom′·e·try
tym′·pa·no·plas′·ty
tym′·pa·no·scle·ro′·sis
tym′·pa·no·squa·mo′·sa
tym′·pa·no·squa′·mous also ·squa·mo′·sal
tym′·pa·no·sta·pe′·dia
tym′·pa·no·sta·pe′·di·al
tym′·pa·nos′·to·my
tym′·pa·no·sym′·pa·thec′·to·my
tym′·pa·not′·o·my
tym′·pa·nous
tym′·pa·num pl. ·na, gen. sg. ·ni
tym′·pa·ny
type
ty·phe′·mia Brit. ·phae′·
typh·lec′·ta·sis
typh·lec′·to·my
typh·li′·tis
typh′·lo·
typh′·lo·ap·pen′·di·ci′·tis
typh′·lo·dic′·li·di′·tis
typh·lol′·o·gy
typh′·lo·pex′y also typh′·lo·pex′·ia

typh·los′·to·my
typh′·lo·ure′·ter·os′·to·my
ty′·pho·
ty′·phoid
ty·phoi′·dal
ty′·pho·ma·lar′·i·al
ty′·pho·ma′·nia
ty′·pho·par′a·ty′·phoid
ty′·pho·pneu·mo′·nia
ty′·phous
ty′·phus
typ′·i·cal
typ′·ing
ty′·po·dont
ty·pol′·o·gy
ty′·po·scope
ty′·pus
ty′·ra·mine
ty′·ro·
ty′·ro·ci′·dine
ty·rog′·e·nous
Ty·rog′·ly·phus [Ty′·ro·glyph′·us]
ty′·ro·pa·no′·ate
Ty·roph′·a·gus
ty′·ro·sin·ase [ty·ro′·si·nase]
ty′·ro·sine
ty′·ro·sin·e′·mia [·si·ne′·] Brit. ·ae′·mia
ty′·ro·si·no′·sis
ty′·ro·sin·u′·ria [·si·nu′·]
ty′·ro·sy·lu′·ria
ty′·ro·thri′·cin
ty′·ro·tox′·i·con
ty′·ro·tox′·i·co′·sis
ty′·ro·tox′·ism
ty′·son·i′·tis
tzet′·ze var. of tsetse

U

u′·ar·thri′·tis
u′·bi·chro′·ma·nol
u′·bi·chro′·me·nol

ubiq′·ui·nol
ubiq′·ui·none [u′bi·qui·none′]
ubiq′·ui·tin
u′la
ul′·cer
ul′·cera *pl. of* ulcus
ul′·cer·ate ·at′·ed, ·at′·ing
ul′·cer·a′·tion
ul′·cer·a·tive
ul′·ce·re *ablative of* ulcus
ul′·cer·o·gen′·ic *also* ·og′·e·nous
ul′·cero·glan′·du·lar
ul′·cero·mem′·bra·nous
ul′·cer·o′·sa
ul′·cer·ous
ul′·cus *pl.* ul′·cera
u′le·gy′·ria
ul′·er·y·the′·ma
ulex′·ine
uli′·tis
ul′·na *pl. & gen. sg.* ·nae
ul′·nad
ul′·nar
ul·na′·re *neut. of* ulnaris
ul·na′·ris *pl.* ·res, *ablative sg.* ·ri
ul′·no·car′·pal
ul′·no·car·pa′·le
u′lo·
u′lo·der′·ma·ti′·tis
u′lor·rha′·gia
u′lose
ulo′·sis
ul′·ti·mo·bran′·chi·al
ul′·tra·
ul′·tra·cen′·tri·fu·ga′·tion
ul′·tra·cen′·tri·fuge
ul·tra′·di·an
ul′·tra·fil′·ter
ul′·tra·fil′·trate
ul′·tra·fil·tra′·tion

ul′·tra·li·ga′·tion
ul′·tra·mi′·cro·pi·pet′
ul′·tra·mi′·cro·scope
ul′·tra·mi′·cro·scop′·ic
ul′·tra·mi·cros′·co·py
ul′·tra·mi′·cro·tome
ul′·tra·paque′
ul′·tra·phag′·o·cy·to′·sis
ul′·tra·pro′·phy·lax′·is
ul′·tra·son′·ic
ul′·tra·son′·ics
ul′·tra·son′·o·gram
ul′·tra·son′·o·graph
ul′·tra·son′·o·graph′·ic
ul′·tra·so·nog′·ra·phy
ul′·tra·son′·o·scope
ul′·tra·sound
ul′·tra·struc′·ture
ul′·tra·ter′·mi·nal
ul′·tra·thin′
ul′·tra·vi′·o·let
ul′·tra·vi′·rus
ul′·tra·vis′·i·ble
um′·bau·zo′·nen
um·bel′·la·tine
um′·bel·lif′·er·one
um′·ber
um′·bi·lec′·to·my
um·bil′·i·cal
um·bil′·i·ca′·lis *neut.* ·le
um·bil′·i·cate *also* ·cat′·ed
um·bil′·i·ca′·tion
um·bil′·i·co·il′i·ac
um·bil′·i·co·mam′·mil·lar′y
um·bil′·i·co·ves′·i·cal
um·bil′·i·cus *pl. & gen. sg.* ·ci
um′·bo *pl.* ·bos *or* um·bo′·nes
um′·bo·nate
um′·bra
un′·cal
un′·ci·form
Un′·ci·nar′·ia

un′·ci·nar′·i·al
un′·ci·na·ri′·a·sis
un′·ci·nate *also* ·nal
un′·ci·na′·tus
un·com′·pen·sat′·ed
un′·con·di′·tioned
un·con′·scious
un·con′·scious·ness
un′·co-os′·si·fied
un·cot′·o·my
un·cou′·pling
un′·co·ver′·te·bral
un·crossed′
unc′·tion
unc′·tu·ous
unc′·ture
un′·cus *pl.* ·ci
un·dec′·y·len′·ate [un·dec′·y·le·nate]
un·dec′·y·len′·ic
un′·der·achiev′·er
un′·der·cut′
un′·der·horn′
un′·der·ly′·ing
un′·der·nu·tri′·tion
un′·der·stain′
un′·der·toe′
un′·der·weight′
un′·des·cend′·ed
un′·di′·ag·nosed
un′·dif′fer·en′·ti·at′·ed
un′·dine
un′·di·nism
un·do′·ing
un′·du·lant
un′·du·late *adj. & v.* ·lat′·ed, ·lat′·ing
un′·du·la′·tion
un′·du·la·to′·ry
un′·en·cap′·su·lat′·ed
un·fer′·til·ized
un′·gual
un′·guent
un·guen′·tum
un·guic′·u·lus
un′·gui·nal
un′·guis *pl.* ·gues, *gen. pl.* ·gui·um

u'ni·
u'ni·ar·tic'·u·lar
u'ni·ax'·i·al
u'ni·cam'·er·al
u'ni·cel'·lu·lar
u'ni·ceps
u'ni·col'·lis
u'ni·cor'·nis
u'ni·cus'·pid
u'ni·di·rec'·tion·al
u'ni·flag'·el·late
u'ni·fo'·cal
u'ni·gem'·i·nal
u'ni·ger'·mi·nal
u'ni·grav'·i·da
u'ni·lam'·i·nar
u'ni·lat'·er·al
u'ni·lat'·er·a'·lis
u'ni·lo'·bar
u'ni·loc'·u·lar
un'·in·duc'·i·ble
u'ni·neme
u'ni·nu'·cle·ar *also*
·cle·ate
u'ni·oc'·u·lar
u'nion
un·i'on·ized *not*
ionized: Cf. u'nion·ized
(*organized in a union*)
u'ni·ov'u·lar [·o'vu·]
unip'·a·ra
unip'·a·rous
u'ni·pen'·nate
u'ni·pen·na'·tus
u'ni·po'·lar
u'ni·po'·ten·cy
unip'·o·tent
u'ni·po·ten'·tial
u'ni·sex'·u·al
un'·i·tar'·i·an
u'ni·tar'y
uni'·us
u'ni·va'·lent
u'ni·ver'·sal
u'ni·ver·sa'·lis
u'ni·vi·tel'·line
un·med'·ul·lat'·ed
un·my'·e·lin·at'·ed

un'·of·fi'·cial
un·or'·ga·nized
un'·phys'·i·o·log'·ic
also ·i·cal
un·primed'
un'·re·al'·i·ty
un'·re·sect'·a·ble
un'·re·solved'
un·sat'·u·rat'·ed
un·sta'·ble
un·stri'·at·ed
up'·gaze
up'·stream
up'·take
u'ra·chal
u'ra·cho·ves'·i·cal
u'ra·chus
u'ra·cil
urae'·mia *Brit. spel. of*
uremia
u'ra·nis'·co·
u'ra·nis'·co·plas'·ty
u'ra·nis·cor'·rha·phy
u'ra·nis'm
ura'·ni·um
u'ra·no·
u'ra·no·plas'·tic
u'ra·no·plas'·ty
u'ra·nor'·rha·phy
u'ra·nos'·chi·sis
u'ra·no·staph'·y·lo·
plas'·ty
u'ra·no·staph'·y·los'·
chi·sis
u'ran·os'·te·o·plas'·ty
u'ra·nyl
ur'·ar·thri'·tis
u'rate
u'ra·te'·mia *Brit.*
·tae'·
urat'·ic
u'ra·to'·sis
u'ra·tu'·ria
ur'-de·fense'
ure'a
Ure'·a·plas'·ma
u're·ase
urec'·chy·sis

u're·ide
ure'·mia *Brit.* urae'·
ure'·mic *Brit.* urae'·
ure'·mi·gen'·ic *Brit.*
urae'·
u'reo·
u're·ol'·y·sis
u're·o·lyt'·ic
u're·o·tel'·ic
ure'·ter *gen.* ·ter·is
ure'·ter·al
ure'·ter·al'·gia
ure'·ter·ec'·ta·sis
ure'·ter·ec'·to·my
u're·ter'·ic
u're·ter'·i·cus *pl.* ·ci
ure'·ter·is [u're·ter'·is]
gen. of ureter
ure'·ter·i'·tis
ure'·tero·
ure'·ter·o·cele
ure'·ter·o·ce·lec'·to·my
ure'·tero·co'·lic
ure'·tero·co·los'·to·my
ure'·tero·cu·ta'·ne·os'·
to·my
ure'·tero·cyst'·anas'·to·
mo'·sis
ure'·tero·cys'·tic
ure'·tero·cys'·to·ne·
os'·to·my
ure'·tero·cys·tos'·to·
my
ure'·tero·en'·ter·os'·to·
my
ure'·ter·og'·ra·phy
ure'·tero·hem'i·ne·
phrec'·to·my
ure'·tero·il'·e·al
ure'·tero·il'·eo·cu·ta'·
ne·ous
ure'·tero·il'·e·os'·to·my
ure'·ter·o·lith
ure'·tero·li·thot'·o·my
ure'·ter·ol'·y·sis
ure'·tero·me'·atot'·o·
my

ure′·tero·ne′o·cys·tos′·to·my
ure′·tero·ne′o·py′·e·los′·to·my
ure′·tero·ne·phrec′·to·my
ure′·ter·op′·a·thy
ure′·tero·pel′·vic
ure′·tero·pel′·vio·ne·os′·to·my
ure′·tero·pel′·vi·o·plas′·ty
ure′·ter·o·plas′·ty
ure′·tero·proc·tos′·to·my
ure′·tero·py′·e·li′·tis
ure′·tero·py′·e·log′·ra·phy
ure′·tero·py′·e·lo·ne·os′·to·my
ure′·tero·py′·e·lo·plas′·ty
ure′·tero·py′·e·los′·to·my
ure′·tero·rec·tos′·to·my
ure′·ter·or·rha′·gia
ure′·ter·or′·rha·phy
ure′·ter·os′·co·py
ure′·tero·sig′·moid·os′·to·my
ure′·tero·ste·no′·sis
ure′·ter·os′·to·ma
ure′·ter·os′·to·my
ure′·tero·the′·cal
ure′·ter·ot′·o·my
ure′·tero·tri′·go·nal
ure′·tero·tri′·go·no·en′·ter·os′·to·my
ure′·tero·tri′·go·no·sig′·moid·os′·to·my
ure′·tero·tub′·al [tu′·bal]
ure′·tero·ure′·ter·al
ure′·tero·ure′·ter·os′·to·my
ure′·tero·ves′·i·cal
ure′·tero·ves′·i·co·plas′·ty
ure′·tero·ves′·i·cos′·to·my
u′re·thane *also* ·than
ure′·thra *gen.* ·thrae
ure′·thral
u′re·thral′·gia
u′re·thra′·lis *pl.* ·les
ure′·thra·scope *var. of* urethroscope
ure′·thra·tre′·sia
u′re·threc′·to·my
ure′·threm·phrax′·is
u′re·thri′·tis
ure′·thro·
ure′·thro·cele
ure′·thro·cys·ti′·tis
ure′·thro·cys′·to·cele
ure′·thro·cys·tog′·ra·phy
ure′·thro·cys·tom′·e·try
ure′·thro·cys′·to·pex′y
ure′·thro·dyn′·ia
ure′·thro·gram
u′re·throg′·ra·phy
u′re·throm′·e·ter
u′re·throm′·e·try
ure′·thro·pex′y
ure′·thro·plas′·ty
ure′·thror·rha′·gia
u′re·thror′·rha·phy
ure′·thror·rhe′a *Brit.* ·rhoe′a
ure′·thro·scope
u′re·thros′·co·py
ure′·thro·scro′·tal
ure′·thro·spas′m
ure′·thro·ste·no′·sis
u′re·thros′·to·my
ure′·thro·tome
u′re·throt′·o·my
ure′·thro·tri′·go·ni′·tis [·trig′·o·]
ure′·thro·vag′·i·nal
ur′·gen·cy
ur′·hi·dro′·sis
u′ric
u′ric·ac′·id·e′·mia *Brit.* ·ae′·mia
u′ri·case
u′ri·ce′·mia *Brit.* ·cae′·
ur′i·ce′·mic *Brit.* ·cae′·
u′ri·co·
u′ri·co·poi·e′·sis
u′ri·co·su′·ria
u′ri·co·su′·ric
u′ri·co·tel′·ic
u′ri·dine
ur′·i·dro′·sis *var. of* urhidrodis
u′ri·dyl′·ic
u′ri·dyl′·yl·trans′·fer·ase
u′ri·nal
u′ri·nal′·y·sis
u′ri·na′·ria *pl.* ·ri·ae
u′ri·nar′y
u′ri·nate ·nat′·ed, ·nat′·ing
u′ri·na′·tion
u′rine
u′rin·i·dro′·sis *var. of* urhidrosis
u′ri·nif′·er·ous
u′ri·no·
u′ri·no·gen′·i·tal *var. of* urogenital
u′ri·nog′·e·nous
u′ri·no′·ma *pl.* ·mas *or* ·ma·ta
u′ri·nom′·e·ter
u′ri·nom′·e·try
u′ri·nose
u′ri·nous
u′ro·
u′ro·bi′·lin
u′ro·bi·lin′·o·gen
u′ro·bi·lin′·o·gen·u′·ria
u′ro·ca·nate
u′ro·can′·ic
u′ro·cele
u′ro·che′·zia
u′ro·chrome
u′ro·clep′·sia

u′ro·cop′·ro·por·phyr′·ia
u′ro·cys·ti′·tis
u′ro·de′·um
u′ro·di·al′·y·sis
u′ro·dy·nam′·ics
u′ro·dyn′·ia
u′ro·dys·func′·tion
u′ro·flow′·me·ter
u′ro·gas′·trone
u′ro·gen′·i·tal
u′ro·gen′·i·ta′·lis neut. ·le
urog′·e·nous
u′ro·gram
urog′·ra·phy
u′ro·gra·vim′·e·ter
u′ro·ki′·nase
u′ro·lag′·nia
u′ro·lith
u′ro·li·thi′·a·sis
u′ro·lith′·ic
u′ro·li·thot′·o·my
u′ro·log′·ic also ·i·cal
urol′·o·gist
urol′·o·gy
u′ro·lyt′·ic
urom′·e·ter
uron′·cus
uron′·ic
urop′·a·thy
u′ro·phan′·ic
u′ro·phil′·ia
u′ro·pod
u′ro·poi·e′sis
u′ro·poi·et′·ic
u′ro·por′·phy·rin
u′ro·por′·phy·rin′·o·gen
u′ro·psam′·mus
u′ro·pter′·in
u′ro·rec′·tal
uros′·che·o·cele
u′ro·the′·li·um
u′ro·tox·ic′·i·ty
u′ro·tox′·in
ur′o·ure′·ter
ur′·ti·cant

ur′·ti·car′·ia
ur′·ti·car′·i·al
ur′·ti·car′·i·o·gen′·ic
uru′·shi·ol
us′·nic
us′·ti·lag′·i·nis′m
Us′·ti·la′·go
us′·tion
us′·tu·la′·tion
u′ta
u′teri pl. & gen. sg. of uterus
u′ter·i′·na fem. of uterinus; pl. & gen. sg. ·nae
u′ter·ine
u′ter·i′·num neut. of uterinus
u′ter·i′·nus
u′tero ablative of uterus
u′tero·
u′tero·fix·a′·tion
u′tero·ges·ta′·tion
u′ter·og′·ra·phy
u′ter·o·lith
u′ter·om′·e·ter
u′tero-ovar′·i·an
u′tero·pel′·vic
u′ter·o·pex′y
u′tero·pla·cen′·tal
u′ter·o·plas′·ty
u′tero·sa′·cral
u′tero·sal′·pin·gog′·ra·phy
u′ter·o·scope
u′tero·ther·mom′·e·try
u′ter·ot′·o·my
u′tero·ton′·ic
u′ter·o·tro′·pic [·trop′·ic]
u′tero·tub′·al [·tu′·bal]
u′tero·tu·bog′·ra·phy
u′tero·vag′·i·nal
u′tero·vag′·i·na′·lis
u′tero·ves′·i·cal
u′ter·us pl. & gen. sg. u′teri, ablative u′tero

u′tri·cle
utric′·u·lar
utric′·u·la′·ris
utric′·u·li pl. & gen. sg. of utriculus
utric′·u·li′·tis
utric′·u·lo·am·pul′·lar
utric′·u·lo·am′·pul·la′·ris
utric′·u·lo·sac′·cu·lar
utric′·u·lo·sac′·cu·la′·ris
utric′·u·lus pl. & gen. sg. ·li
u′va ur′si
u′vea pl. & gen. sg. u′ve·ae
u′ve·al
u′ve·it′·ic
u′ve·i′tis
u′veo·lab′·y·rin·thi′·tis
u′veo·me·nin′·go·en·ceph′·a·li′·tis
u′veo·neu′·rax·i′·tis
u′veo·pa·rot′·id
u′veo·par′·o·ti′·tis
u′vio·fast′
u′vi·ol
u′vi·om′·e·ter
u′vio·re·sis′·tant [·sist′·ant]
u′vio·sen′·si·tive
u′vu·la gen. ·lae
u′vu·lar
u′·vu·la′·ris
u′vu·lec′·to·my
u′vu·lo·
u′vu·lo·nod′·u·lar
u′vu·lo·pal′·a·to·pha·ryn′·go·plas′·ty
u′vu·lot′·o·my

V

vac·ci′·na var. of vaccinia
vac′·ci·na·ble

vac′·ci·nal
vac′·ci·nate ·nat′·ed,
·nat′·ing
vac′·ci·na′·tion
vac′·ci·na′·tor
vac·cine′ [vac′·cine]
vac·cin′·ia
vac·cin′·i·al
vac′·ci·nid
vac·cin′·i·form
vac·cin′·i·o′·la
vac′·ci·noid
vac′·ci·no·ther′·a·py
vac·ci′·num
vac′·u·o′·lar
vac′·u·o·late adj. & v.
·lat′·ed, ·lat′·ing
vac′·u·o·la′·tion also
·li·za′·tion
vac′·u·ole
vac′·u·um
va′·dum
va′·gal
va·ga′·lis
va·gec′·to·my
va′·gi pl. & gen. sg. of
vagus
va·gi′·na L. pl. & gen.
sg. ·nae, accusative
·nam
vag′·i·nal [va·gi′·nal]
vag′·i·na·lec′·to·my
[·nal·ec′·]
vag′·i·na′·lis pl. ·les
vag′·i·na·li′·tis
vag′·i·na·pex′y [va·gi′·na·] var. of
vaginopexy
vag′·i·nate
vag′·i·nec′·to·my
vag′·i·nis′·mus
vag′·i·ni′·tis
vag′·i·no·
vag′·i·no·cele

vag′·i·no·dyn′·ia
vag′·i·no·fix·a′·tion
vag′·i·nog′·ra·phy
vag′·i·no·la′·bi·al
vag′·i·nom′·e·ter
vag′·i·nop′·a·thy
vag′·i·no·per′·i·ne·or′·rha·phy
vag′·i·no·per′·i·to·ne′·al
vag′·i·no·pex′y
vag′·i·no·plas′·ty
vag′·i·no·scope
vag′·i·nos′·co·py
vag′·i·not′·o·my
Va·gin′·u·lus ple·be′·ius
va′·go·
va′·go·ac′·ces·so′·ri·us
va′·go·ac·ces′·so·ry
va′·go·de·pres′·sor
va′·go·glos′·so·pha·ryn′·ge·al
va·gol′·y·sis
va′·go·lyt′·ic
va′·go·mi·met′·ic
va′·go·sym′·pa·thet′·ic
va·got′·o·my
va′·go·to′·nia also va·got′·o·ny
va′·go·ton′·ic
va′·go·to′·nin
va′·go·tro′·pic [·trop′·ic]
va·got′·ro·pis′m
va′·go·va′·gal
va′·grant
va′·gus pl. & gen. sg. ·gi
va′·lence[51] also va′·len·cy
val′·er·ate
va·le′·ri·an
va·le′·ric [va·ler′·ic]

val·eth′·a·mate
val′·e·tu′·di·nar′·i·an
val′·e·tu′·di·nar′·i·an·is′m
val′·gus fem. ·ga,
neut. ·gum
val′·i·da′·tion
va·lid′·i·ty
val′·ine
val′·i·ne′·mia [·in·e′·]
Brit. ·nae′·
val′·i·no·my′·cin
val′·late
val·lec′·u·la pl. ·lae
val·lec′·u·lar
val′·lum
val·pro′·ate
val′·ue
val′·va pl. & gen. sg.
·vae
val′·val also ·var
valve
val·vec′·to·my
val′·vo·plas′·ty
val′·vo·tome
val·vot′·o·my
val′·vu·la pl. & gen.
sg. ·lae, gen. pl. val′·vu·la′·rum
val′·vu·lar
val′·vu·late
val′·vule
val′·vu·lec′·to·my
var. of valvectomy
val′·vu·li′·tis
val′·vu·lo·plas′·ty
var. of valvoplasty
val′vu·lo·tome
val′·vu·lot′·o·my var.
of valvotomy
van′·a·date
va·nad′·ic [va·na′·dic]
va·na′·di·um
va·na′·di·um·is′m

---

[51] To indicate valence in chemical terms, use Roman numerals in parentheses. This follows without a space the name or symbol of an element: Cu(II), iron(III) oxide.

van′·co·my′·cin
va·nil′·la
va·nil′·lic
va·nil′·lin
va·nil′·lism [van′·il·is′m]
va·nil′·lyl·man·del′·ic
va′·po·cau′·ter·i·za′·tion
va′·po-cool′·ant
va′·por *Brit.* ·pour
va′·por·i·za′·tion
va′·por·ize ·ized, ·iz′·ing
va′·por·iz′·er
va′·po·ther′·a·py
va′·ra *fem. of* varus
var′·i·a·bil′·i·ty
var′·i·a·ble
var′·i·ance
var′·i·ant
var′·i·ate
var′·i·a′·tion
var′·i·cat′·ed
var′·i·ca′·tion
var′·i·ce′·al
var′·i·cec′·to·my
var′·i·cel′·la
var′·i·cel·la′·tion *also* ·li·za′·tion
var′·i·cel′·li·form
var′·i·cel·lo′·sus
var′·i·ces *pl. of* varix
var′·i·co·
var′·i·co·cele
var′·i·co·ce·lec′·to·my
var′·i·cog′·ra·phy
var′·i·co·phle·bi′·tis
var′·i·cose
var′·i·co′·sis
var′·i·cos′·i·ty
var′·i·cot′·o·my
va·ric′·u·la *pl.* ·lae
var′·i·e·ga′·ta
var′·i·egate
va·ri′·e·ty
va·ri′·o·la
va·ri′·o·lar

var′·i·o·la′·tion *also* ·li·za′·tion
var′·i·o′·li·form
var′·i·o′·li·for′·mis
var′·i·o·loid
var′·i·o·lo′·sa
va·ri′·o·lous
var′·ix *pl.* var′·i·ces
va·ro′·li·an
Va·ro′·lii *gen. of* Varolius
va′·rus *fem.* ·ra, *neut.* ·rum
vas *pl.* va′·sa, *gen. pl.* va·so′·rum
va′·sal
vas′·cu·lar
vas′·cu·la′·ris
vas′·cu·lar′·i·ty
vas′·cu·lar·i·za′·tion
vas′·cu·lar·ize ·ized, ·iz′·ing
vas′·cu·la·ture
vas′·cu·li′·tis
vas′·cu·lo·
vas′·cu·lo·car′·di·ac
vas′·cu·lo·gen′·e·sis
vas′·cu·lo′·sus *fem.* ·sa, *neut.* ·sum
vas′·cu·lo·sym′·pa·thet′·ic
vas′·cu·lo·tox′·ic
va·sec′·to·mize [vas·ec′·] ·mized, ·miz′·ing
va·sec′·to·my [vas·ec′·]
va′·si·form
va·si′·tis
va′·so [vas′o·]
va′·so·ac′·tive
va′·so·con·stric′·tion
va′·so·con·stric′·tive
va′·so·con·stric′·tor
va′·so·co·ro′·na
va′·so·de·pres′·sion
va′·so·de·pres′·sor

va′·so·dil′·a·ta′·tion *also* ·di·la′·tion
va′·so·di′·la·tor
va′·so·di′·la·to′·ry
va′·so·ep′·i·did′·y·mos′·to·my
va′·so·for′·ma·tive
va·sog′·ra·phy
va′·so·in·hib′·i·tor
va′·so·in·hib′·i·to′·ry
va′·so·la′·bile
va′·so·li·ga′·tion
va′·so·mo′·tion
va′·so·mo′·tor
va′·so·neu·rop′·a·thy
va′·so·neu·ro′·sis
va′·so-or′·chi·dos′·to·my
va′·so·pa·ral′·y·sis
va′·so·pres′·sin
va′·so·pres′·sor
va′·so·re′·flex
va′·so·re′·lax·a′·tion
va′·so·re·sec′·tion
va·sor′·rha·phy
va·so′·rum *gen. pl. of* vas
va′·so·sec′·tion
va′·so·spas′m
va′·so·spas′·mo·lyt′·ic
va′·so·spas′·tic
va′·so·stim′·u·lant
va·sos′·to·my
va·sot′·o·my
va′·so·to′·nia
va′·so·ton′·ic
va′·so·tribe
va′·so·tro′·pic [·trop′·ic]
va′·so·va′·gal
va′·so·va·sot′·o·my
va′·so·ve·sic′·u·lec′·to·my
va′·so·ve·sic′·u·li′·tis
vas′·tus *pl. & gen. sg.* ·ti
vault
vec′·tion

vec′·tor
vec′·tor·car′·di·o·gram
vec′·tor·car′·di·o·graph
vec′·tor·car′·di·og′·ra·phy
vec·to′·ri·al
veg′·an
veg′·e·tal
veg′·e·tans
veg′·e·tar′·i·an
veg′·e·tar′·i·an·is′m
veg′·e·ta′·tion
veg′·e·ta′·tive
ve′·hi·cle
veil
Veil′·lo·nel′·la
vein
ve′·la *pl. of* velum
ve·la′·men *pl.* ve·lam′·i·na
ve′·la·men′·tous
ve′·la·men′·tum *pl.* ·ta
ve′·lar
ve′·li *gen. of* velum
vel′·lus
vel′·o·cim′·e·try
ve·loc′·i·ty
ve′·lo·pal′·a·tine
ve′·lo·pha·ryn′·ge·al
ve′·lo·plas′·ty
ve′·lo·syn′·the·sis
ve·lour′
ve′·lum *pl.* ·la, *gen. sg.* ·li
ve′·na *pl. & gen. sg.* ·nae, *gen. pl.* ·na′·rum
ve′·na·ca·vog′·ra·phy
ve·na′·tion
ve′ne· [ven′e·]
ve′·nec·ta′·sia
ve·nec′·to·my
ve·neer′
ven′·e·na′·tion
ven′·ene
ven′·e·nif′·er·ous
ven′·e·nous *also* ·nose

ve′ne·punc′·ture [ven′e·] *var. of* venipuncture
ve·ne′·re·al
ve·ne′·re·ol′·o·gist
ve·ne′·re·ol′·o·gy
ven′·ery
ve′ne·sec′·tion [ven′e·]
ve′ne·su′·ture [ven′e·]
ve′ni· [ven′i·]
ve′ni·punc′·ture [ven′i·]
ve′ni·sec′·tion [ven′i·] *var. of* venesection
ve′ni·su′·ture [ven′i·] *var. of* venesuture
ve′·no·
ve′·no·a′·tri·al
ve·noc′·ly·sis
ve′·no·fi·bro′·sis
ve′·no·gram
ve·nog′·ra·phy
ven′·om
ven′·om·i·za′·tion
ve′·no·mo′·tor
ven′·om·ous
ve′·no-oc·clu′·sive
ve′·no·per′·i·to·ne·os′·to·my
ve′·no·pres′·sor
ve′·no·res′·pi·ra·to′·ry
ve·no′·sa *fem. of* venosus; *pl.* ·sae
ve′·no·scle·ro′·sis
ve′·nose
ve′·no·si′·nal
ve·nos′·i·ty
ve′·no·sta′·sis [ve·nos′·ta·sis]
ve·no′·sum *neut. of* venosus; *gen.* ·si
ve·no′·sus *pl. & gen. sg.* ·si
ve·not′·o·my
ve′·nous
ve′·no·ve·nos′·to·my
ven′·ter

ven′·ti·late ·lat′·ed, ·lat′·ing
ven′·ti·la′·tion
ven′·ti·la′·tor
ven′·til·a·to′·ry
ven′·ti·lom′·e·try
ven·to′·sa
vent′·plant
ven′·trad
ven′·tral
ven·tra′·le *neut. of* ventralis
ven·tra′·lis *pl.* ·les
ven′·tral·ward
ven′·tri· *var. of* ventro-
ven′·tri·cle
ven′·tri·cor′·nu
ven·tric′·u·lar
ven·tric′·u·lar·i·za′·tion
ven·tric′·u·la′·ris
ven·tric′·u·li *pl. & gen. sg. of* ventriculus
ven·tric′·u·li′·tis
ven·tric′·u·lo·
ven·tric′·u·lo·ar·te′·ri·al
ven·tric′·u·lo·a′·tri·al
ven·tric′·u·lo·a′·tri·os′·to·my
ven·tric′·u·lo·cis·ter′·nal
ven·tric′·u·lo·cis′·ter·nos′·to·my
ven·tric′·u·lo·gram
ven·tric′·u·log′·ra·phy
ven·tric′·u·lo·jug′·u·lar
ven·tric′·u·lom′·e·try
ven·tric′·u·lo·myot′·o·my
ven·tric′·u·lo·nec′·tor
ven·tric′·u·lo·per′·i·to·ne′·al
ven·tric′·u·lo·pha′·sic
ven·tric′·u·lo·plas′·ty
ven·tric′·u·lo·pleu′·ral
ven·tric′·u·lo·punc′·ture

ven·tric′·u·lo·ra′·di·al
ven·tric′·u·lo·scope
ven·tric′·u·los′·co·py
ven·tric′·u·los′·to·my
ven·tric′·u·lo·sub′·arach′·noid
ven·tric′·u·lot′·o·my
ven·tric′·u·lo·ve·nos′·to·my
ven·tric′·u·lo·ve′·nous
ven·tric′·u·lus *pl. & gen. sg.* ·li
ven′·tri·cum′·bent
ven′·tri·duc′·tion
ven′·tri·lat′·er·al *var. of* ventrolateral
ven′·tro-
ven′·tro·cys·tor′·rha·phy
ven′·tro·fix·a′·tion
ven′·tro·hys′·ter·o·pex′y
ven′·tro·lat′·er·al
ven′·tro·me′·di·al
ven′·tro·me′·di·an
ven′·tro·pto′·sis [·trop·to′·]
ven′·tro·sus·pen′·sion
ven·trot′·o·my
ven′·u·la [ve′·nu·] *pl.* ·lae
ven′·u·lar
ven′·ule [ve′·nule]
ven′·u·lous
ve′·ra *fem. of* verus; *pl. & gen. sg.* ·rae
ve·rap′·a·mil
ver′·a·trine
ve·ra′·trum
ver·big′·er·a′·tion
ver′·do·per·ox′·i·dase
verge
ver′·gence *also* ·gen·cy

ver′·mal *var. of* vermian
ver′·me·toid
ver′·mi·
ver′·mi·an
ver′·mi·cid′·al [·ci′·dal]
ver′·mi·cide
ver·mic′·u·lar
ver·mic′·u·late
ver′·mi·cule
ver·mic′·u·lous *also* ·lose
ver·mic′·u·lus *pl.* ·li
ver′·mi·form
ver′·mi·for′·mis
ver·mif′·u·gal
ver′·mi·fuge
ver·mil′·ion
ver·mil′·ion·ec′·to·my
ver′·min *pl.* vermin
ver′·mi·na′·tion
ver′·min·o′·sis
ver′·min·ous
ver′·mis
ver′·mix
ver·mog′·ra·phy
ver′·nal
ver′·ni·er
ver′·nix
ver·ru′·ca *pl.* ·cae
ver·ru′·ci·form
ver·ru′·ci·for′·mis
ver′·ru·coid
ver′·ru·cose
ver′·ru·co′·sis
ver′·ru·cos′·i·ty
ver′·ru·co′·sus *fem.* ·sa
ver·ru′·cous
ver·ru′·ga
ver′·si·col′·or
ver′·sion
ver′·sive

ver′·te·bra[52] *pl. & gen. sg.* ·brae, *gen. pl.* ver′·te·bra′·rum
ver′·te·bral
ver′·te·bra′·le *neut. of* vertebralis
ver′·te·bra′·lis *pl.* ·les
ver′·te·brar·te′·ri·al
ver′·te·brar·te′·ri·a′·lis *neut.* ·le
ver′·te·bra′·rum *gen. pl. of* vertebra
Ver′·te·bra′·ta
ver′·te·brate
ver′·te·brec′·to·my
ver′·te·bro·
ver′·te·bro·ar·te′·ri·al *var. of* vertebrarterial
ver′·te·bro·bas′·i·lar
ver′·te·bro·chon′·dral
ver′·te·bro·cos′·tal
ver′·te·bro·pel′·vic
ver′·te·bro·per′·i·car′·di·al
ver′·te·bro·sa′·cral
ver′·te·bro·ster′·nal
ver′·tex *pl.* ·ti·ces, *gen. sg.* ·ti·cis
ver′·ti·cal
ver′·ti·ca′·lis
ver′·ti·cil·la′·ta
ver′·ti·co·men′·tal
ver·tig′·i·nous
ver′·ti·go
ver′·u·mon′·ta·ni′·tis
ver′·u·mon·ta′·num
ve′·rus *fem.* ·ra, *neut.* ·rum
ve·sa′·li·an
ve·si′·ca *pl. & gen. sg.* ·cae
ves′·i·cal *of the urinary bladder: Cf.* vesicle

---

52 Vertebrae are designated C I–X (cervical), T I–X (thoracic), L I–XII (lumbar), and S I–X (sacral). Nomina Anatomica uses Roman numerals, but Arabic numbers are becoming increasingly common in texts.

ves′·i·ca′·lis *pl.* ·les
ves′·i·cant
ves′·i·cate
ves′·i·ca′·tion
ves′·i·ca·to′·ry
ves′·i·cle *sac or follicle: Cf.* vesical
ves′·i·co·
ves′·i·co·ab·dom′·i·nal
ves′·i·co·cer′·vi·cal
ves′·i·coc′·ly·sis
ves′·i·co·co·lon′·ic
ves′·i·co·fix·a′·tion
ves′·i·co·in·tes′·ti·nal
ves′·i·co·per′·i·ne′·al
ves′·i·co·pros·tat′·ic
ves′·i·co·rec′·tal
ves′·i·co·re′·nal
ves′·i·co·sig′·moid
ves′·i·co·sig′·moid·os′·to·my
ves′·i·cos′·to·my
ves′·i·cot′·o·my
ves′·i·co·um·bil′·i·cal
ves′·i·co·ure′·ter·al
ves′·i·co·ure′·thral
ves′·i·co·u′ter·ine
ves′·i·co·u′ter·i′·nus *fem.* ·na, *neut.* ·num
ves′·i·co·vag′·i·nal
ve·sic′·u·la *pl.* ·lae
ve·sic′·u·lar
ve·sic′·u·late *also* ·lat′·ed
ve·sic′·u·la′·tion
ve·sic′·u·lec′·to·my
ve·sic′·u·li′·tis
ve·sic′·u·lo·
ve·sic′·u·lo·bron′·chi·al
ve·sic′·u·lo·bul′·lous
ve·sic′·u·lo·cav′·ern·ous
ve·sic′·u·log′·ra·phy
ve·sic′·u·lo·pros′·ta·ti′·tis
ve·sic′·u·lo·pus′·tu·lar
ve·sic′·u·lo′·sa *pl.* ·sae

ve·sic′·u·lot′·o·my
ves′·sel
ves·tib′·u·la *pl. of* vestibulum
ves·tib′·u·lar
ves·tib′·u·la′·re *neut. of* vestibularis
ves·tib′·u·la′·ris *pl.* ·res
ves′·ti·bule
ves·tib′·u·lec′·to·my
ves·tib′·u·li *gen. of* ·lum
ves·tib′·u·lo·cer′·e·bel′·lar
ves·tib′·u·lo·cer′·e·bel′·lum
ves·tib′·u·lo·coch′·le·ar
ves·tib′·u·lo·coch′·le·a′·ris *neut.* ·re
ves·tib′·u·lo·e′qui·lib′·ra·to′·ry
ves·tib′·u·lo·oc′·u·lar
ves·tib′·u·lo·spi′·nal
ves·tib′·u·lot′·o·my
ves·tib′·u·lo·ure′·thral
ves·tib′·u·lo·vag′·i·nal
ves·tib′·u·lum *pl.* ·la, *gen. sg.* ·li
ves′·tige
ves·tig′·i·al
ves·tig′·i·um *pl.* ·ia
vet′·er·i·nar′·i·an
vet′·er·i·nar′y
vet′·u·la *gen. pl.* vet′·u·la′·rum
vi′a *pl. & gen. sg.* vi′·ae, *accusative pl.* vi′·as
vi′·a·bil′·i·ty
vi′·a·ble
vi′·al
vi′·be·sate
vi′·bex *pl.* vi′·bi·ces *or* vi·bi′·ces
vi′·brat·ing
vi·bra′·tion
vi′·bra·tor
vi′·bra·to′·ry

Vib′·rio
V. chol′·er·ae
V. par′a·hae·mo·lyt′·i·cus
vib′·rio *pl.* vib′·ri·os *or* vib′·ri·o′·nes
vib′·ri·o·cid′·al [·ci′·dal]
vib′·ri·ol′·y·sis
vib′·ri·on′·ic
vi·bris′·sae *sg.* ·sa
vi′·bro·mas·sage′
vi·car′·i·ous
vic′·i·nal
vid·ar′·a·bine
vid′·i·an
vig′·il
vig′·il·am′·bu·lis′m
vig′·or
vil′·li *pl. of* villus
vil′·li·form
vil′·lo·nod′·u·lar
vil·lo′·sa *fem. of* villosus; *pl.* ·sae
vil′·lose
vil′·lo·si′·tis
vil·los′·i·ty
vil·lo′·sus *fem.* ·sa, *neut.* ·sum
vil′·lous
vil′·lus *pl.* ·li
vil′·lus·ec′·to·my
vin·bar′·bi·tal
vin·blas′·tine
vin′·ca·leu′·ko·blas′·tine
vin·cris′·tine
vin′·cu·lum *pl.* ·la
vin′·e·gar
vi′·nyl
vi′·o·cid
vi′·o·la′·ceous
vi′·o·la′·tion
vi′·o·les′·cent
vi′·o·let
vi′·o·my′·cin
vi·os′·ter·ol
vi′·per

vi'·per·id
Vi·per'·i·dae
vi'·per·ine
vi·pryn'·i·um
vi'·ral
vir·chow'·i·an
vi·re'·mia Brit. ·rae'·
vir'·gin
vir'·gin·al
vir·gin'·i·ty
vi'·ri·cid'·al [·ci'·dal]
  var. of virucidal
vi'·ri·cide
vir'·i·din
vir'·ile
vi·ril'·ia
vir'·il·is'm
vi·ril'·i·ty
vir'·il·i·za'·tion
vir'·il·ize ·ized, ·iz'·ing
vi'·ri·on [vir'·i·on]
vi'·ro·cyte
vi'·ro·gene
vi'·roid
vi·rol'·o·gist
vi·rol'·o·gy
vi'·ro·pex'·is
vi'·rose also ·rous
vi'·ro·stat'·ic var. of virustatic
vir'·tu·al
vi'·ru·cid'·al [·ci'·dal]
vi'·ru·cide
vir'·u·lence
vir'·u·lent
vi·ru'·ria
vi'·rus
vi'·ru·stat'·ic
vis'·cera pl. of viscus
vis'·cer·ad
vis'·cer·al
vis'·cer·a'·le neut. of visceralis
vis'·cer·al'·gia
vis'·cer·a'·lis pl. ·les
vis'·ceri·mo'·tor var. of visceromotor

vis'·cero·
vis'·cero·car'·di·ac
vis'·cero·cra'·ni·um
vis'·cer·o·gen'·ic
vis'·cero·in·hib'·i·to'·ry
vis'·cero·meg'·a·ly
vis'·cero·mo'·tor
vis'·cer·op·to'·sis
vis'·cero·sen'·so·ry
vis'·cero·skel'·e·ton
vis'·cero·so·mat'·ic
vis'·cer·o·tome
vis'·cer·ot'·o·my
vis'·cer·o·tro'·phic [·troph'·ic]
vis'·cer·o·tro'·pic [·trop'·ic]
vis'·cid
vis·cid'·i·ty
vis'·co·elas'·tic'·i·ty
vis'·co·sim'·e·ter also vis·com'·e·ter
vis'·co·sim'·e·try also vis·com'·e·try
vis·cos'·i·ty
vis'·cous
vis'·cus pl. vis'·cera
vi'·sion
vis'·it
vis'·u·al
vis'·u·al·i·za'·tion
vis'·uo·cor'·ti·cal
vis'·uo·psy'·chic
vis'·uo·sen'·so·ry
vis'·uo·spa'·tial
vi'·sus gen. visus
vis'·u·scope
vi'·ta gen. ·tae
vi'·ta·glass
vi'·tal
vi·tal'·i·ty
vi'·tal·ize ·ized, iz'·ing
vi'·ta·mer
vi'·ta·min Brit. vit'·a·mine
vit'·el·lar'·i·um pl. ·lar'·ia
vi·tel'·li·form

vi·tel'·lin
vi·tel'·line
vit'·el·li'·nus fem. ·na
vi·tel'·lo·gen'·e·sis
vi·tel'·lo·gen'·ic
vi·tel'·lo·in·tes'·ti·nal
vi·tel'·lo·mes'·en·ter'·ic
vi·tel'·lus
vi'·ti·a'·tion
vit'·i·lig'·i·nes
vit'·i·lig'·i·nous
vit'·i·li'·go
vit'·i·li'·goid
vi'·ti·um pl. ·tia
vi'·to·dy·nam'·ics
vit·rec'·to·my
vit'·reo·ret'·i·nal
vit'·re·ous
vit'·re·us fem. ·rea, neut. ·re·um
vi·tri'·na
vit'·ri·ol
vi·var'·i·um pl. ·ia or ·ums
vi'·vax
viv'i·
vi'·vi·par'·i·ty [viv'i·]
vi·vip'·a·rous
viv'i·sect'
viv'i·sec'·tion
vo'·cal
vo·ca'·lis neut. ·le
vo'·cal·i·za'·tion
voice
void
vo'·la
vo'·lar
vo·la'·ris
vol'·a·tile
vol'·a·til·ize ·ized, ·iz'·ing
vol·e'·mic [vo·le'·]
  Brit. ae'·mic
vo·li'·tion
vo·li'·tion·al
vol'·ley
vol·sel'·la
volt'·age

vol·ta′·ic
volt·am′·me·ter
volt′·me·ter
vol′·ume
vol′·u·met′·ric
vol′·u·mom′·e·ter
   also ·me·nom′·e·ter
vol′·un·tar′y
vol′·un·to·mo′·to·ry
vo′·lute
vol′·u·tin [vo·lu′·tin]
vol′·vu·late ·lat′·ed,
  ·lat′·ing
vol′·vu·lo′·sis
vol′·vu·lus *pl.* ·li
vo′·mer *gen.* ·mer·is
vo′·mer·ine *also* vo·
  mer′·i·an
vo′·mero·na′·sal
vo′·mero·na·sa′·lis
  neut. ·le
vo′·mero·vag′·i·nal
vo′·mero·vag′·i·na′·lis
vom′·it
vo·mi′·tion
vom′·i·tive
vom′·i·to′·ry
vom′·i·tus
vor′·tex *pl.* ·ti·ces
vor′·ti·co′·sa *pl.* ·sae
vor′·ti·cose
vous·sure′
vox *gen.* vo′·cis
voy·eur′
voy′·eur·is′m
voy′·eur·is′·tic
vul·ga′·ris
vul′·ner·a·bil′·i·ty
vul′·ner·a·ble
vul′·ner·ar′y
vul·sel′·la *also* ·lum
vul′·va *gen.* ·vae
vul′·var *also* ·val
vul·vec′·to·my
vul·vi′·tis
vul′·vo·
vul·vop′·a·thy

vul′·vo·vag′·i·nal
vul′·vo·vag′·i·ni′·tis

W

wad′·ding
wa′·fer
waist
waist′·line
wake′·ful·ness
wal·le′·ri·an
wall′·eye
wan′·der·ing
wan′·der·lust
war′·fa·rin
warm′-blood′·ed
wart
wart′y wart′·i·er,
  wart′·i·est
wash′·ing
wash′·out
was′·ser·hel′·le
Was′·ser·mann-fast′
wast′·age
waste *n. & v.* wast′·
  ed, wast′·ing
wa′·ter
wa′·ter-bite
wa′·ter-borne
wa′·ter-brash
wa′·ter·shed
wa′·tery
*Wat·so′·ni·us wat′·so·
  ni*
watt
watt′·age
watt′·me′·ter
wave′·form
wave′·length
wave′·me′·ter
wave′·shape
wav′y wav′·i·er, wav′·
  i·est
wax′·ing
wax′y wax′·i·er, wax′·
  i·est
weal *var. of* wheal

wean
wean′·ling
wear
wea′·sand
webbed
web′·bing
we′·ber
web′-fin′·gered
web′·foot
wedge *n. & v.*
  wedged, wedg′·ing
weep wept, weep′·ing
weight
weis′·mann·is′m
well′·ness
wet′-nurse
wet′·ta·ble
wet′·ting
wheal
wheel′·chair
wheeze *n. & v.*
  wheezed, wheez′·ing
whey
whip′·lash
whip′·worm
whirl′·bone
whis′·per
whis′·tle *n. & v.* ·tled,
  ·tling
white′·head
white′·leg
white′·pox
whit′·low
whoop′·ing
whorl
wild′-type
wind′·lass
win′·dow
wind′·pipe
witch′·ha′·zel
with·draw′·al
wit′·zel·sucht
Wohl·fahr′·tia
wolff′·i·an
wolfs′·bane
womb
work′-up *also* work′
  up

worm
wor'·mi·an
worm'·wood
wound
wov'·en
W'-plas'·ty
wreath
wrin'·kle
wrist
wrist'·drop
wry'·neck
Wu'·cher·er'·ia
  W. ban·crof'·ti
wu'·cher·er·i'·a·sis
Wye'·o·my'·ia

X

xan'·thate
xan'·the·las'·ma
xan'·the·las'·ma·to'·sis
xan·the'·mia Brit.
 ·thae'·
xan'·thene
xan'·thine
xan'·thin·ox'·i·dase
 also xanthine oxidase
xan'·thin·u'·ria [·thi·nu'·]
xan'·thin·u'·ric [·thi·nu'·]
xan'·thism
xan'·tho·
xan'·tho·chro'·mia
xan'·tho·chro'·mic
 also ·chro·mat'·ic
xan'·tho·cyte
xan'·tho·fi·bro'·ma
 pl. ·mas or ·ma·ta
xan'·tho·gran'·u·lo'·ma
 pl. ·mas or ·ma·ta
xan'·tho·gran'·u·lo'·ma·tous [·lom'a·]
xan·tho'·ma pl. ·mas or ·ma·ta
xan·tho'·ma·to'·sis
xan·tho'ma·tous [·thom'a·]

xan'·thone
xan'·tho·phane
xan'·tho·phyll
xan·thop'·sia also ·tho'·pia
xan·thop'·sin
xan·thop'·ter·in
xan'·thor·rhe'a Brit. ·rhoe'a
xan'·tho·ru'·bin var. of xantorubin
xan'·tho·sar·co'·ma
xan'·tho·sine
xan·tho'·sis
xan'·tho·tox'·in
xan'·thous
xan'·thu·ren'·ic
xan·thu'·ria var. of xanthinuria
xan'·to·ru'·bin
xen'o·
xen'o·bi·ot'·ic
xen'o·di'·ag·no'·sis
xen'·o·ge·ne'·ic also ·gen'·ic
xen'o·gen'·e·sis
xe·nog'·e·nous
xen'o·graft
xe·nol'·o·gy
xe'·non [xen'·on]
xen'o·par'·a·site
xen'·o·plas'·ty
Xen'·o·psyl'·la
Xen'·o·pus
xen'o·rex'·ia
xen'o·tope
xen'·o·tro'·pic [·trop'·ic]
xe'·ro·
xe'·ro·chei'·lia
xe'·ro·der'·ma also ·der'·mia
xe'·ro·der·mat'·ic
xe·rog'·ra·phy
xe·ro'·ma
xe'·ro·me'·nia
xe'·ro·pha'·gia also xe·roph'·a·gy

xer'·oph·thal'·mia
xe'·ro·ra'·di·og'·ra·phy
xe·ro'·sis
xe'·ro·sto'·mia
xe·rot'·ic
xe·rot'·i·ca
xe'·ro·to'·cia
xiph'i·cos'·tal also xiph'o·
xiph'i·ster'·nal
xiph'i·ster'·num
xiph'o· also xiph'i·
xiph'o·did'·y·mus also xi·phod'·y·mus
xiph'·o·dyn'·ia
xiph'·oid [xi'·phoid]
xiph'·oid·al'·gia
xi·phoi'·de·us
xiph'·oid·i'·tis
xi·phop'·a·got'·o·my
xi·phop'·a·gus
X'-linked
x'-ra'·di·a'·tion
x ray n. also X ray
x-ray adj. & v. also X-ray
xy'·lan
xy'·lene
xy'·li·dine
xy'·li·tol
xy'·lo·
xy'·lo·ke'·tose
xy'·lo·me·taz'·o·line
xy'·lose
xy'·los·u'·ria [·lo·su'·ria]
xy'·lu·lose
xy'·lu·los·u'·ria
xy'·ro·spas'm
xys'·ma
xys'·ter

Y

yab'a·pox
ya·jé' also ya·gé'
yaw

yaws
yeast
yel′·low
yer′·ba
Yer·sin′·ia
yer·sin′·i·o′·sis
Y′-linked
yo′·chu·bio′
yo′·gurt
yo·him′·bine
yoke
yolk
Y′-plas′·ty
yt·ter′·bi·um
yt′·tri·um

Z

Ze′a mays′
ze′·a·tin
ze′·a·xan′·thin
ze′·in
zeis′·i·an
ze′·ism
zen′·ker·ize ·ized,
  ·iz′·ing
ze′·o·lite
zeug′·ma·tog′·ra·phy
zi·do′·vu·dine
zinc
zinc′·a·lis′m
zinc·un′·de·cate
zir·co′·ni·um
zo′·ac·an·tho′·sis
zo′·ite
zo′·na   pl. & gen. sg.
  ·nae
zo′·nal [zon′·al]
zo·na′·lis   neut. ·le
zon′·a·ry [zo′·na·]
zo′·nate [zon′·ate]
zon′·es·the′·sia   Brit.
  ·aes·
zo·nif′·u·gal
zo·nip′·e·tal
zo′·nu·la   pl. & gen.
  sg. ·lae

zo′·nu·lar [zon′·u·]
zo′·nu·la′·re   neut. of
  zonularis
zo′·nu·la′·ris   pl. ·res
zo′·nule
zo′·nu·li′·tis
zo′·nu·lot′·o·my
zo′·nu·ly′·sis   also
  ·lol′·y·sis
zo′o·
zo′o·an′·thro·po·no′·sis
zo′o·bi·ol′·o·gy
zo′·o·der′·mic
zo′o·dy·nam′·ics
zo′o·eras′·tia   also
  ·er′·as·ty
zo·og′·e·nous   also
  zo′·o·gen′·ic
zo′o·ge·og′·ra·phy
zo′·o·gle′a   Brit.
  ·gloe′a
zo′o·graft
zo′·o·log′·i·cal   also
  ·log′·ic
zo·ol′·o·gy
Zo′o·mas′·ti·go·pho′·
  rea
zo′·o·no′·sis   pl. ·no′·
  ses
zo′·o·not′·ic
zo′o·par′·a·site
zo′o·par′·a·sit′·ic
zo·oph′·a·gous
zo′·o·phile
zo′·o·phil′·ia
zo′·o·phil′·ic
zo′·o·sper′·mia
zo′o·spore
zo′o·tox′·in
zo′·o·tro′·phic [·troph′·
  ic]
zos′·ter
zos·ter′·i·form
zos′·ter·oid
Z′-plas′·ty
zuck′·er·guss
zwit′·ter·i′on
zy′·gal

zyg′·ap′·o·phys′·e·al
  [·apoph′·y·se′·al]
  var. of zygapophysial
zyg′·ap′·o·phys′·i·al
zyg′·ap·o·phys′·i·a′·lis
  pl. ·les
zyg′·apoph′·y·sis   pl.
  ·ses
zyg′·i·on   pl. ·gia
zy′·go·
zy·go′·ma   pl. ·mas or
  ·ma·ta
zy′·go·mat′·ic
zy′·go·mat′·i·ca   neut.
  pl. & fem. sg. of
  zygomaticus
zy′·go·mat′·i·ci   pl. of
  zygomaticus, gen. sg.
  of zygomaticus &
  zygomaticum
zy′·go·mat′·i·co
  ablative of zygomaticus
zy′·go·mat′·i·co·
zy′·go·mat′·i·co·au·
  ric′·u·lar
zy′·go·mat′·i·co·fa′·cial
zy′·go·mat′·i·co·fa′·ci·
  a′·lis   neut. ·le
zy′·go·mat′·i·co·fron′·
  tal
zy′·go·mat′·i·co·max′·
  il·la′·ris
zy′·go·mat′·i·co·max′·
  il·lar′y
zy′·go·mat′·i·co-or′·bit·
  al
zy′·go·mat′·i·co-or′·bi·
  ta′·lis   neut. ·le
zy′·go·mat′·i·co·sphe′·
  noid
zy′·go·mat′·i·co·tem′·
  po·ral
zy′·go·mat′·i·co·tem′·
  po·ra′·lis   neut. ·le
zy′·go·mat′·i·cum
  neut. of zygomaticus;
  pl. ·ca, gen. sg. ·ci

zy'·go·mat'·i·cus   *pl.*
   & gen. sg. ·ci
zy'·go·my·ce'·tous
zy'·go·my·co'·sis
zy'·go·ne'·ma
zy'·go·po'·di·um   *pl.*
   ·dia
zy·gos'·i·ty
zy'·go·spore
zy'·go·style
zy'·gote
zy'·go·tene
zy·got'·ic
zy'·mase
zy'·mo·
zy'·mo·gen
zy'·mo·gen'·e·sis
zy·mog'·e·nous   *also*
   zy'·mo·gen'·ic
zy'·mo·gram
zy'·mo·hy·drol'·y·sis
zy·mol'·y·sis
zy·mo'·sis
zy·mos'·ter·ol
zy·mot'·ic

MEDICAL EPONYMS

Surnames and their Pronunciations

An eponymous term is one containing the name of a person (for example, *Addison's disease*) or derived from a name (*parkinsonism, mendelian*). The person whose name is so used is called the *eponym*. A group of eponymous terms may represent several people with the same surname. If these surnames are all spelled and pronounced the same way, we do not distinguish them here.

Where two or more names may be confused because of slight spelling differences (e.g., *Clark* and *Clarke* or *Hofmann* and *Hoffmann*), or because although spelled alike the names are pronounced differently, terms they are associated with are given. Terms on the same line and separated by commas are associated with a single individual; terms on different lines are associated with different individuals:

Gart·ner   gärt′-nər
   cyst, duct
Gärt·ner   gert′-nər
   bacillus
   phenomenon

This means there are three different eponyms: one who lent his name to the terms *Gartner cyst* and *Gartner's duct*, one whose name is in the term *Gärtner's bacillus*, and another whose name is in the term *Gärtner's phenomenon*.

In contexts where words like *sign* or *syndrome* are insufficient clues for differentiating individuals, further information is given in the form of associated eponyms, or, if that is not possible, non-eponymous synonyms or explanatory material in parentheses:

Weil   vīl
   stain
   W.-Felix test
   disease (icteric
     leptospirosis)
   basal layer
Weill   vey
   sign (for pneumonia)
   W.-Reys-Adie syndrome

Some double or multi-part names in this list are surnames only, e.g., *Gilles de la Tourette*, but others represent a first or middle name plus surname as *Wier Mitchell* (middle and last name) or *Pierre Robin* (first and last name). Where only a surname is involved, all the syllables of the pronunciation are linked by hyphens, whereas a space rather than a hyphen appears between the syllables of first or middle names and surnames:

    Gilles de la Tou·rette   zhēl′-də-la-too-ret′
    Weir Mitch·ell   wēr′ mich′-əl

The pronunciations transcribed on this list approximate the original sounds of foreign names, but in many cases, the original pronunciation is followed by an anglicized version:

    Mar·fan   mar-fäN′; *angl.* mär′-fan

One person's name may have more than one correct spelling. Alternatives, such as *Müller* or *Mueller*, *Roth* or *Rot*, are provided when we have found them in the literature, but the reader may occasionally come across variants that do not appear in our list. One common type of variation occurs with the German umlauted vowels:

    ä / ae   Gräfe *or* Graefe
    ö / oe   Döhle *or* Doehle
    ü / ue   Hürtle *or* Huertle

Russian names are often transliterated into the Roman alphabet in different ways. One common variation is between *v*, *w*, and *ff*; for example, *Ivanov*, *Iwanow*, or *Iwanoff*. In English texts, the preferred modern spelling is usually with *v*, but for many medical eponyms earlier forms (often 19th-century German adaptations) remain firmly established. Other variations in the spelling of Russian names include *sh* and *sch*, *kh* and *ch*, *zh* and *j*, *ch* and *tsch*, and *-skii* and *-sky*:

    Bekhterev *or* Bechterew
    Darkshevich *or* Darkschewitsch
    Kozhevnikov *or* Kojewnikoff
    Kandinskii *or* Kandinsky

The forms on the left above are considered more modern or more accurate, or better adapted for use in English. However, in some cases (e.g., Darkschewitsch, Kandinsky) the forms on the right still predominate.

PRONUNCIATION KEY

VOWELS:

Symbol	Examples	Comparisons
a	*English* p**a**t, c**a**rrot; *French* p**a**tte, h**a**s**a**rd	The French *a* is somewhat farther back than the corresponding English sound, between the *a* of *gather* and the *a* of *father*.
ä	*English* f**a**ther, p**a**rt; *German* V**a**ter, M**a**nn; *Italian* p**a**dre, p**a**rte	The *a* sound of German, Italian, and various other languages is generally not as far back as the English *a* in *father*, but is farther back than the French *a* (see above).
ā	*English* f**a**ce, s**ay**; *French* **é**t**é**; *German* s**e**hen; *Italian* v**e**ro	The English *ā* sound ends with a *y*-like glide, while the corresponding sound in most other languages (usually spelled *e*) does not.
e	*English* b**e**t, s**ai**d, b**ea**r; *French* p**è**re, ch**ai**se, for**ê**t, servi**e**tte; *German* b**e**sser, b**ä**r; *Italian* m**e**zzo, mi**e**le	
ē	*English* f**ee**t, r**e**gion, mach**i**ne; *French* v**i**te; *German* w**ie**viel ; *Italian* z**i**t**i**	
ey	*French* v**ei**lle; *Dutch* d**ij**k; *Afrikaans* aparth**ei**d	A sound between *ā* as in *say* and *ī* as in *sigh*.
i	*English* b**i**t, w**i**lling, m**i**rror; *German* b**i**tte, W**i**rt	
ī	*English* s**i**te, m**y**, s**igh**, h**ei**ght; *German* Z**ei**t, M**ai**	

Continued

PRONUNCIATION KEY

VOWELS:

Symbol	Examples	Comparisons
o	British English p*o*t, b*o*ther; French ch*o*c, p*o*rte; German K*o*pf, S*o*nne; Italian n*o*tte, p*o*rta	These short *o* sounds vary considerably from one language to another, and are generally absent from American English, where the *ä* sound is used instead.
ô	English s*aw*, t*a*ll, f*o*rm; French f*o*rt; Italian r*o*sa	
ō	English n*o*se, b*oa*t, l*ow*; French c*ô*te, b*eau*; German R*o*se, S*oh*n; Italian s*o*le	The English *ō* sound ends with a *w*-like glide, while the corresponding sound in most other languages does not.
œ	French p*eu*, b*œu*f, c*œu*r; German sch*ö*n, K*ö*pfe, G*oe*the	These sounds, which do not occur in English, are like *ā* or *e* pronounced with rounded lips.
oi	English v*oi*ce, b*oy*; German L*eu*te, Fr*äu*lein; Italian p*oi*	
oo	English m*oo*n, r*u*le, m*o*ve; French b*ou*che; German g*u*t; Italian c*u*ra, virt*ù*	
ou	English h*ou*se, cr*ow*d, b*ou*t; German H*au*sfrau; Italian c*au*sa	
ow	Dutch geb*ouw*	A sound between *ō* as in *boat* and *ou* as in *bout*.
u	English c*u*p, m*o*ther, en*ou*gh, h*u*rry	
ᴜ	English b*oo*k, f*u*ll; German M*u*tter, K*u*rt	
Y	French l*u*ne, s*û*r, br*u*sque; German k*ü*hl, Schl*ü*ssel	These sounds, which do not occur in English, are like *ē* or *i* pronounced with rounded lips.

Continued

PRONUNCIATION KEY

VOWELS:

Symbol	Examples	Comparisons
ə	English about, sofa, second, sufficient; German Ende, gegen, Bezirk; French retenir, quatre-vingts	In English, German, etc. this "neutral" vowel sound occurs only in unstressed syllables. In French it tends to appear or disappear depending on the context of the word.
		The combination -ər as in *bitter* has various pronunciations. In most American English, it is just a syllabic *r*, but in most British English it is like ə without the *r*. In German it is a muffled *ä*-like sound.

CONSONANTS:

Symbol	Examples	Comparisons
ch	English child, lunch; German deutsch; Italian pace, ciao; Spanish muchacho	
g	English go, give	Not as in *gist* (= *j*). See also *ng*.
kh	German Bach, kochen; Spanish jota, mujer, ángel	This sound does not occur in ordinary English, though it may be heard in Scottish *loch*, *Sassenach*. It is similar to *h* but is produced with friction in the back of the mouth.
N	French bon /bôN/, vin /veN/, sans /säN/; Portuguese mãe /mīN/, mão /mouN/	This N is not a separate sound, but indicates nasalization of the preceding vowel or diphthong.
ng	English singer, hangar, sank	Compare *finger, anger*, which have an *ng* sound followed by a *g* sound.

Continued

PRONUNCIATION KEY

CONSONANTS:

Symbol	Examples	Comparisons
s	English sit, this	Not as in *his* (= z).
sh	English shop, machine, initial; French chercher; German Schule; Italian scendi; Portuguese baixa	
SH	German Licht, Mädchen	This sound does not occur in English. It is similar to *kh* but is produced farther forward in the mouth.
th	English think, path; Castilian Spanish cinco, paz	
TH	English this, father; Spanish nido, padre	
y	English yet, canyon	Not used here for a vowel sound (as in *dye*, *city*)
y	French signe /sēn^y/; Italian ogni /ōn$^{y\prime}$-ē/; Hungarian nagy /nod^y/; Russian Olga /ol$^{y\prime}$-gə/, Vladimir /vlä-d^{y}ē′-mir/	A small raised *y* is used in some cases instead of the regular *y* to emphasize the fact that it does not form an additional syllable, and/or to show a palatal (*y*-like) quality in the preceding consonant.
zh	English azure, vision; French jour, page, gigot	

All other letters used in the pronunciations—b, d, f, h, j, k, l, m, n, p, r, t, v, w, and z—represent their normal English sounds or similar sounds in other languages.

Doubled consonants When a consonant is shown doubled in the pronunciation, it is meant to be held longer than a single one: Italian *gnocchi* /nyok′-kē/, Spanish *rico* /rrē′-kō/.

MEDICAL EPONYMS

Ab·be	äb′-ə	Apert	a-per′
A.-Zeiss counting chamber		Ap·gar	ap′-gär
		Aran	a-räN′
Ab·be	ab′-ē	Aran·ti·us	ə-ran′-chē-əs
flap, operation		Ar·gyll Rob·ert·son	är′-gīl rob′-ərt-sən
Ab·bott	ab′-ət		
Abri·ko·sov	ä-brē-kô′-səf	Arlt	ärlt
Achard	a-shar′	Ar·man·ni	är-män′-nē
Ad·ams	ad′-əmz	Arndt	ärnt
Ad·dis	ad′-is	Ar·neth	är′-net
Ad·di·son	ad′-i-sən	Ar·nold	är′-nolt
Adie	ā′-dē	Ar·thus	ar-tys′
Ad·ler	ä′-dlər; *angl.* ad′-lər	Asch·heim	äsh′-hīm
Ahu·ma·da	ä′-oo-mä′-THä	Asch·off	äsh′-of
Ala·joua·nine	a-la-zhwa-nēn′	Au·er·bach	ou′-ər-bäkh
Al·ba·rrán	äl′-bä-rrän′	Aus·tin Flint	ôs′-tin flint′
Al·bers-Schön·berg	äl′-bərs-shœn′-berk	Avel·lis	ä-vel′-is
		Avo·ga·dro	ä′-vō-gä′-dro
Al·bert	äl′-bert	Ax·en·feld	äk′-sən-felt
Al·bright	ôl′-brīt	Ayer·za	ä-yer′-sä
Aes·cu·la·pi·us	es′-kyoo-lā′-pē-əs	Bab·cock	bab′-kok
Al·cock	ôl′-kok *or* al′-kok	Ba·bès	
Al·der	äl′-dər	or Ba·beş	French ba-bes′; Romanian bä′-besh
Al·drich	ôl′-drich		
Alez·zan·dri·ni	äl′-e-sän-drē′-nē	Ba·bin·ski	ba-bin′-skē; French ba-beN-skē′
Ali·bert	a-lē-ber′		
Al·len	al′-ən	Bail·lar·ger	bī-yar-zhā′
Al·lis	al′-is	Bain·bridge	bān′-brij
Al·mei·da	äl-mā′-də	Ba·ker	bā′-kər
Al·pers	al′-pərz	Ba·lint	
Al·port	ôl′-pôrt	or Bá·lint	bä′-lint
Alz·hei·mer	älts′-hī-mər; *angl.* alz′-	Baló	bol′-ō
An·der·sen disease	an′-dər-sən	Ban·croft	ban(g)′-kroft
		Ban·ti	bän′-tē
An·der·son test amputation	an′-dər-sən	Bá·rány	bä′-räny; *angl.* bä′-rä-nē
		Barr	bär
Anich·kov	ä-nēch′-kəf	Bar·ré	ba-rā′
An·ton	än′-tōn	Bar·rett	bar′-ət

Bar·sony	bär′-sō-nē; *Hungarian* -shōnʸ	Bi·chat	bē-sha′
		Biedl	bē′-dəl
Bar·tho·lin	bär′-tō-lin	Biel·schow·sky	bil-shof′-skē
Bar·ton bodies	bär′-ton	Big·e·low	big′-ə-lō
		Bi·gna·mi	bē-nyä′-mē
Bar·ton forceps, fracture	bär′-tən	Bil·harz	bil′-härts
		Bill·roth	bil′-rōt
Bart·ter	bär′-tər	Bi·net	bē-ne′
Ba·se·dow	bä′-zə-dō	Bing	bing
Bas·sen	bas′-ən	Bin·swang·er	bin′-sväng-ər
Bas·si·ni	bäs-sē′-nē	Biot	byō
Bat·ten	bat′-ən	Bi·tot	bē-tō′
Bau·hin	bō-eN′	Biz·zo·ze·ro	bid-dzod′-dze-ro
Baum·gar·ten	boum′-gär-tən	Bjer·rum	byer′-rʊm
Beck	bek	Björn·stad	byœrn′-städ
Beck·er	bek′-ər	Black·fan	blak′-fan
Beck·with	bek′-with	Blake·more	blāk′-môr
Beh·çet	beh-chet′	Bla·lock	blā′-lok
Behr	bār	Blaud	blō
Bé·késy	bā′-kāsh	Bles·sig	bles′-ik
Bekh·te·rev or Bech·te·rew	bekh′-tʸə-rʸəf	Bloch	blokh
		Blount	blount *or* blunt
Bell	bel	Bo·a·ri	bō-ä′-rē
Bel·li·ni	bel-lē′-nē	Boch·da·lek	bokh′-dä-lek
Bence Jones	bens′-jōnz′	Bo·dan·sky	bō-dan′-skē
Ben·e·dict Atwater-B. calorimeter method	ben′-ə-dikt	Boeck	bœk; *angl.* bek
		Boer·haa·ve	boor′-hä-və
		Bo·go·mo·lets	bə-gä-mô′-lʸəts
		Bohr	bōr
Be·ne·dikt syndrome	bā′-ne-dikt	Bonne·vie	bon-vē′
		Bor·det	bor-de′
Ben·nett	ben′-ət	Bor·rel	bo-rel′
Ber·ger rhythm	ber′-gər	Bött·cher	bœt′-sʜər
		Bou·chard	boo-shar′
Ber·ger disease amputation	ber-zhā′	Bouil·laud	boo-yō′
		Bouin	bweN
		Bour·ne·ville	boor-nə-vēl′
Ber·lin	ber-lēn′	Bou·ve·ret	boo-vre′
Ber·nard	ber-nar′	Bo·wen	bō′-ən
Bern·hardt	bern′-härt	Bow·man	bō′-mən
Bern·heim	ber-nem′	Boyle	boil
Ber·tin	ber-teN′	Boze·man	bōz′-mən
Ber·to·lot·ti	ber′-to-lot′-tē	Brad·ford	brad′-fərd
Bes·nier	bā-nyā′	Brain	brān
Betz	bets	Brau·ne	brou′-nə
Be·zold	bā′-tsolt	Brax·ton Hicks	braks′-tən hiks′
Bian·chi	byäng′-kē	Bren·ne·mann	bren′-ə-mən
Bi·ber	bē′-bər	Bren·ner	bren′-ər

Word Guide 317

Breu·er	broi'-ər	Bu·row	boo'-rō
Bright	brīt	Busch·ke	bush'-kə
Brill	bril	Bus·se	bus'-ə
Bri·quet	brē-ke'	By·wa·terz	bĭ'-wô-tərz
Bris·saud	brē-sō'	Cab·ot	kab'-ət
Broad·bent	brôd'-bent	Cac·chio·ne	käk-kyō'-ne
Bro·ca	bro-ka'	Caf·fey	kaf'-ē
Brock	brok	Cairns	kernz
operation, syndrome		Ca·jal	kä-khäl'
		Cald·well	kôld'-wel
Brock·en·brough	brok'-ən-brō	Ca·lle·ja	kä-l^yä'-khä or kä-yä'-hä
Brocq	brok		
sycosis, pseudopelade		Cal·mette	kal-met'
		Ca·lot	ka-lō'
Brö·del	brœ'dəl	Cal·vé	kal-vä'
Bro·die	brō'-dē	Cam·per	käm'-pər
Brod·mann	brōt'-män; angl. brod'-mən	Ca·mu·ra·ti	kä'-moo-rä'-tē
		Can·a·da	kan'-ə-də
Brøn·sted	brœn'-steтн	Can·a·van	kan'-ə-vən
Brown	broun	Can·non	kan'-ən
Brown-Sé·quard	bron'-sā-kwar' or broon'-	Cap·gras	kab-grä'
		Cap·lan	kap'-lən
Bru·dzin·ski	broo-jin'-skē; angl. -dzin'-	Ca·ro·li	ka-ro-lē'
		Car·rel	ka-rel'
Brug	brukh	Ca·rrión	kä-rryon'; angl. kar'-ē-ōn'
Brunn	brun		
Brun·ner	brun'-ər	Car·va·llo	kär-vä'-l^yo
Bruns	broons	Ca·sal	kä-säl'
Brush·field	brush'-fēld	Ca·so·ni	kä-sō'-nē
Bru·ton	broo'-tən	Cas·ser	kas'-ər
Buch·ner	bukh'-nər	or Cas·se·rio	käs-se'-rē-o
tuberculin, extract		Cas·tel·la·ni	käs'-tel-lä'-nē
		Caze·nave	kaz-nav'
Büch·ner	bysн'-nər	Ces·tan	ses-tän'
funnel		Cha·gas	shä'-gəs
Bucky	buk'-ē	Cham·ber·land	chäm'-bər-lənd
Bu·cy	byoo'-sē	Chan·dler	chand'-lər
Budd	bud	Char·cot	shar-kō'
Buer·ger	byoor'-gər	Charles	chärlz
Büng·ner	byng'-nər	Char·lin	chär-lēn'
Bun·nell	bun'-əl	Chas·sai·gnac	sha-se-nyak'
Bun·sen	bun'-zən; angl. bun'-sən	Chauf·fard	shō-far'
		Ché·diak	shä-dyak'
Bur·dach	bur'-dakh	Che·nais	shə-ne'
Bür·ger	byr'-gər	Cheyne	chān or chā'-nē
Bur·kitt	bur'-kit	Chi·a·ri	kē-ä'-rē
Bur·nett	bur-net'	Cho·part	sho-par'
Burns	burnz	Christ	krist

Medical Eponyms

Chris·tian	kris(h)'-chən	Creutz·feldt	kroits'-felt
Churg	churg	Crig·ler	krig'-lər
Chvos·tek	khvos'-tek	Crohn	krōn
Ci·tel·li	chē-tel'-lē	Cronk·hite	krongk'-(h)īt
Ci·vi·ni·ni	chē-vē-nē'-nē	Crou·zon	kroo-zôN'
Cla·do	klä'-THō; *French* kla-dō'	Cru·veil·hier	krY-ve-yā'
		Cruz	kroos
Clark	klärk	Cu·rie	kY-rē'; *angl.* kyUr'-ē
sign		Cur·ling	kur'-ling
rule		Cush·ing	kUsh'-ing
method		Cu·vier	kY-vyā'
chamber		Cy·on	tsi-ôn'
electode		Czer·ny	cher'-nē
Clarke	klärk	Daae	dô'-ə
C.-Hadfield syndrome		Da·Cos·ta	də-kos'-tə
nucleus, column		Da·ma·shek	da-mäsh'-ek
		Dan·dy	dan'-dē
Clau·dius	klou'-dyUs	Dan·los	däN-los'
Clé·ram·bault	klä-räN-bō'	Da·nysz	dä'-nish
Clo·quet	klo-ke'	Da·rier	da-ryā'
Clut·ton	klut'-ən	Dark·sche·witsch or ·she·vich	därk-shä'-vich
Coats	kōts		
Cock·ayne	kok-ān'	Dau·ben·ton	dō-bänN-tôN'
Cof·fey	kof'-ē	De·bré	də-brā'
Co·gan	kō'-gən	Dei·ters	dī'-tərs
Cohn·heim	kōn'-hīm	Dé·je·rine	dāzh-(ə)-rēn'
Col·les	kol'-əs	de Lange	də-läng'-ə
Col·let	ko-le'	del Cas·ti·llo	del-käs-tē'-yō
Con·ca·to	kong-kä'-tō	De Mor·gan	di-môr'-gən
Con·do·rel·li	kon-do-rel'-lē	De·mours	də-moor'
Conn	kon	de Mus·set	də-mY-se'
Con·ra·di	kon-rä'-dē	Den·is Brown	den'-is broun'
Cooke	kUk	Den·ny-Brown	den'-ē-broun'
Coo·ley	koo'-lē	De·non·vil·liers	də-nôN-vē-lyā'
Coombs	koomz	de Quer·vain	də-ker-veN'
Coo·per	koo'-pər	De Sanc·tis	de-sängk'-tēs
Co·ri	kōr'-ē *or* kôr'-ē	Des·ce·met	des-(ə)-me'
Cor·ri·gan	kor'-i-gən	de To·ni	de-tô'-nē
Cor·ti	kōr'-tē	De·ver·gie	də-ver-zhē'
Cos·ten	kos'-tən	De·vic	də-vēk'
Co·tu·gno or Co·tun·ni·us	ko-too'-nyō kō-tUn'-ē-əs	Dia·mond	dī'-(ə)-mənd
		Diels	dēls
Coun·cil·man	koun'-səl-mən	Dietl	dē'-təl
Cour·voi·sier	koor-vwä-zyā'	Dieu·la·foy	dyœ-la-fwä'
Cou·ve·laire	koov-(ə)-ler'	Di·George	di-jôrj'
Cow·dry	kou'-drē	Di Gu·gliel·mo	di-gool-lyel'-mō
Cow·per	koo'-pər *or* kou'-pər	Di·vry	dē-vrē'
Cre·dé	krä-dā'	Do·giel	dô'-gyəlʸ

Word Guide 319

Döh·le	dœ'-lə	Eh·lers	ā'-lərs
Do·nath	dō'-nät	Ehr·lich	är'-lisʜ
Don·ders	don'-dərs	Ei·mer	ī'-mər
Don·nan	don'-ən	Eint·ho·ven	eynt'-hō-və(n)
Don·o·van	don'-ə-vən	Ei·sen·meng·er	ī'-zən-meng'-ər
Dopp·ler	dop'-lər	El·lis	el'-is
Doug·las	dug'-ləs	El·li·son	el'-i-sən
Down	doun	El·schnig	el'-shnik
Doyne	doin	Emb·den	emp'-dən
Dra·ger	drä'-gər	En·der	en'-dər
Dres·bach	dres'-bäk	En·do	en'-dō
Dress·ler	dres'-lər	Eng·el·mann	eng'-əl-män
Drink·er	dringk'-ər	Ep·stein	ep'-shtīn
Du·ane	doo-än'	pearl	
Du·bin	doo'-bin	Van Bogaert-	
Du·Bois	d(y)oo-bois'	Scherer-E. syn-	
formula, standard		drome	
Du·bois	dʏ-bwä'	Ep·stein	ep'-stīn
sign, abscess		E.-Barr virus	
Du·bois-Rey·	dʏ-bwä'-re-môN'	Erb	erp; *angl.* urb
mond		Er·len·mey·er	er'-lən-mī'-ər
Du·bo·vitz	doo'-bə-vits	Ernst	ernst
Du·chenne	dʏ-shen'	Esch·e·rich	esh'-ə-risʜ
Du·crey	doo-kre'	Es·march	es'-märsʜ; *angl.* es'-märk
Du·guet	dʏ-ge'		
Duke	d(y)ook	Est·lan·der	est'-län-dər
bleeding time test		Es·tren	es'-trən
Dukes	dyooks	Eu·sta·chi	eoo-stä'-kē
Filatov-D. dis-		Ev·ans	ev'-ənz
ease		Ew·ing	yoo'-ing
classification		Ex·ner	eks'-nər
Du·puy-Du·	dʏ-pwē'-dʏ-täN'	Fa·bri·ci·us	fa-brish'-ē-əs
temps		Fa·bry	fä'-brē
Du·puy·tren	dʏ-pwē-treN'	Fa·get	fä-zhe'
Du·rand	dʏ-räN'	Fahr	fär
Du·ran-Rey·nals	doo-rän'-rā-näls'	Fah·rae·us	
Du·ro·ziez	dʏ-rō-zyä'	or Fåh·rae·us	fō-rā'-us
Dyke	dīk	Faj·er·sztajn	fī'-ər-stīn
Eales	ēlz	Fal·lop·pio	fäl-lop'-pyō
Ea·ton	ē'-tən	or Fal·lo·pi·us	fə-lō'-pē-əs
Eberth	ā'-bert	Fal·lot	fa-lō'
Eb·ner	äb'-nər	Fan·co·ni	fäng-kō'-nē
Eb·stein	ep'-shtīn; *angl.* eb'-stīn	Far·ber	fär'-bər
		Fa·vre	fav'-r(ə)
Eck	ek	Fa·zio	fät'-tsyō
Eco·no·mo	ā'-kō-nō'-mō	Fech·ner	fesʜ'-nər
Eding·er	ā'-ding-ər	Fe·ge·ler	fā'-gə-lər
Ed·wards	ed'-wərdz	Feh·ling	fā'-ling

Medical Eponyms

Feil	fel	Fried·reich	frēd'-rīsн
Fe·lix	fā'-liks	Fröh·lich	frœ'-lisн
Fel·ty	fel'-tē	Froin	frweN
Fer·rein	fe-reN'	From·mel	from'-əl
Feul·gen	foil'-gən	Fro·riep	frō'-rēp
Fick	fik	Fuchs	fuks
Fi·la·tov	fē-lä'-təf	Furth	furt
Fin·kel·dey	fingk'-əl-dī	Gais·böck	gīs'-bœk
Fin·sen	fin'-sən	Ga·le·az·zi	gä-le-ät'-tsē
Fitz·Ger·ald	fits-jer'-əld	Ga·len	gā'-lən
Fitz-Hugh	fits-hyoo'	Gam·na	gäm'-nä
Flack	flak	Gams·torp	gäms'-torp
Flech·sig	flek'-sikh	Gan·dy	gäN-dē'
Flei·scher	flī'-shər	Gan·ong	gan'-ong
Flex·ner	fleks'-nər	Gan·ser	gän'-zər
Flow·er	flou'-ər	Ganz	ganz
Foer·ster	fœr'-stər	Gard·ner	gärd'-nər
Fo·gar·ty	fō'-gər-tē	Gar·ré	ga-rā'
Foix	fwä	Gart·ner	gärt'-nər
Fo·ley	fō'-lē	cyst, duct	
Fo·lin	fō'-lin	Gärt·ner	gert'-nər
Föl·ling	fœl'-ling	bacillus	
Fon·tan	fôN-täN'	phenomenon	
Fon·ta·na	fon-tä'-nä	Gas·ser	gäs'-ər
Forbes	fôrbz	Gas·taut	gas-to'
Forch·hei·mer	forsh'-hī-mər	Gau·cher	gō-shä'
For·dyce	fôr'-dīs	Gee	jē
Fo·rel	fo-rel'	Gei·ger	gī'-gər
Fos·ter Ken·ne·dy	fos'-tər ken'-ə-dē	Gé·li·neau	zhä-lē-nō'
		Gel·lé	zhə-lā'
Foth·er·gill	foтн'-ər-gil	Gen·gou	zhäN-goo'
Four·nier	foor-nyä'	Gén·na·ri	jen-nä'-rē
Fo·ville	fo-vēl'	Ger·hardt	gǎr'-härt
Fow·ler	fou'-lər	Ger·lach	ger'-läkh
Fox	foks	Ger·lier	zher-lyä'
Fran·ces·chet·ti	fräN-ses-ke-tē'	Gerst·mann	gerst'-män
Fran·çois	fräN-swä'	Ge·sell	gə-zel'
Frank	frängk	Ghon	gōn
Fre·det	frə-de'	Gia·co·mi·ni	jä-ko-mē'-nē
Frei	frī	Gian·nuz·zi	jän-nut'-tsē
Frei·berg	frī'-burg	Gia·not·ti	jä-not'-tē
Fren·kel	freng'-kəl	Giem·sa	gyem'-zä
Freud	froit; *angl.* froid	Gier·ke	gēr'-kə
Freund	froint	Gil·bert	zhēl-ber'
Frey	frī	Gil·christ	gil'-krist
Fri·de·rich·sen	frē'-тнə-rik-sən	Gilles de la Tou·rette	zhēl'-də-la-too-ret'
Fried·län·der	frēt'-len-dər		
Fried·man	frēd'-mən	Gil·lies	gil'-is

Word Guide 321

Gim·ber·nat	Spanish khēm-ber-nät'; Catalan zhēm'-	Guar·nie·ri	gwär-nye'-rē
Gi·ral·des		Gu·bler	gy-bler'
or ·dès	zhi-räl'-dəs	Gud·den	gud'-ən
Gjes·sing	yes'-sing	Gue·del	gyoo'-dəl
Glanz·mann	glänts'-män	Gué·rin	gā-reN'
Gla·ser	glä'-zər	Gui·di	gwē'-dē
Glau·ber	glou'-bər	(Latin Vidius)	
Glis·son	glē-soN'; angl. glis'-ən	Guil·lain	gē-leN'
Gold·blatt	gōld'-blat	Guth·rie	guth'-rē
Gol·den·har	gol-den-ar'	Gut·mann	goot'-män
Gold·flam	golt'-fläm	Haab	häp; angl. häb
Gold·stein	gōld'-stīn	Ha·ber	hä'-bər
hematemesis, hemoptysis		Hae·nel	he'-nəl or hä'-nəl
		Ha·ge·man	hä'-g(ə)-mən
Gold·stein	golt'-shtīn	Hah·ne·mann	hä'-nə-män
classification, G.-		Hai·ley	hä'-lē
Reichmann syndrome		Hal·ler	häl'-ər
		Hal·ler·vor·den	häl'-ər-for'-dən
		Hal·lo·peau	a-lo-pō'
Gol·gi	gol'-jē	Hal·sted	hôl'-sted
Goll	gol	Ham	ham
Gom·bault	gôN-bō'	Ham·man	ham'-ən
Good·pas·ture	gud'-pas(h)-chər	Hand	hand
Goor·magh·tigh	khōr'-mäkh-təkh	Ha·not	a-nō'
Go·pa·lan	gō'-pä-län	Han·sen	hän'-sən; angl. han'-
Gor·lin	gôr'-lin	Ha·ra·da	hä-rä'-dä
Gou·ge·rot	goozh-(ə)-rō'	Har·dy	här'-dē
Gow·ers	gou'-ərz	Har·ris	har'-is
Gra·de·ni·go	grä'-de-nē'-go	Har·ri·son	har'-i-sən
Grae·fe	gre'-fə or grä'-fə	Hart·mann	härt'-män
Gra·ham	grä'-əm	Hart·nup	härt'-nəp
Gram	gräm	Har·vey	här'-vē
Gras·set	gra-se'	Ha·shi·mo·to	hä-shi-mō'-tō
Gra·tio·let	gra-syo-le'	Has·ner	häs'-nər
Graves	grāvz	Has·sall	has'-əl
Gra·witz	grä'-vits	Has·sel·balch	häs'-əl-bälk
Gray	grā	Hau·dek	hou'-dek
Greig	greg	Ha·vers	hä'-vərz
Grei·ther	grī'-tər	Head	hed
Grep·pi	gräp'-pē; angl. grep'-ē	Heaf	hēf
Grey Tur·ner	grā tur'-nər	Heb·er·den	heb'-ər-dən
Gri·sel	grē-zel'	Heer·fordt	här'-fort
Grit·ti	grēt'-tē; angl. grit'-ē	He·gar	hā'-gär
Groe·nouw	groo'-nō	Hegg·lin	heg'-lin
Grön·blad	grœn'-bläd	Hei·den·hain	hī'-dən-hīn
Gru·ber	groo'-bər	Heim·lich	hīm'-lik
Grün·wald	gryn'-vält	Hei·ne·ke	hī'-nə-kə
Grütz	gryts	Heinz	hīnts

Heis·ter	hīs′-tər	How·ship	hou′-ship
Held	helt; *angl.* held	Hu·ët	hy-et′
Hel·ler	hel′-ər	Hu·guier	y-gyā′
Helm·holtz	helm′-holtz	Huh·ner	hyoo′-nər
Hel·weg	hel′-vey	Hü·ner·mann	hy′-nər-män
Hen·der·son	hen′-dər-sən	Hun·ner	hun′-ər
Hen·le	hen′-lə	Hun·ter	hun′-tər
He·noch	hā′-nokh	Hun·ting·ton	hun′-ting-tən
Hen·se·leit	hen′-zə-līt	Hur·ler	hur′-lər
Hen·sen	hen′-zən	Hürt·le	hyrt′-lə
He·ring	hā′-ring	Husch·ke	hush′-kə
Her·man·sky	her′-män-skē	Hutch·in·son	huch′-in-sən
He·roph·i·lus	hi-rof′-i-ləs	Hux·ley	huks′-lē
Hers	ers	Huy·gens	hœi′-gəns
Her·ter	hur′-tər	Hyrtl	hir′-təl
Hert·wig	hert′-vik *or* -vish	Imers·lund	im′-ərs-lynd
Herx·hei·mer	herks′-hī-mər	Im·lach	im′-ləkh
Heschl	hesh′-əl	In·gras·sia	ing-gräs-sē′-ä
Hes·sel·bach	hes′-əl-bäkh	Ir·vine	ur′-vin
Heub·ner	hoib′-nər	Ir·ving	ur′-ving
Hi·ga·shi	hē-gäsh′-ē	Isaacs	ī′-zəks
High·more	hī′-mōr	Ishi·ha·ra	i-shi-hä′-rä
Hill	hil	Ito	ē-tō′
Hip·poc·ra·tes	hi-pok′-rə-tēz	Ivy	ī′-vē
Hirsch·sprung	hir′-shprung	Iwa·noff	ē-vä-nof′ *or* ē-vä′-nəf
His	his	or Iva·nov	
Ho·bo·ken	hō′-bō-kən	Ja·bou·lay	zha-boo-le′
Hodg·kin	hoj′-kin	Jac·coud	zha-koo′
Hof·fa	hof′-ä	Ja·cob	jā′-kəb
Hoff·mann	hof′-män	membrane	
reflex, Werdnig-		Ja·co·bae·us	yä′-ko-bā′-us
H. disease		Ja·cob·son	yäk′-əp-sən; *angl.* jā′-
Hof·mann	hōf′-män		kəb-sən
bacillus		Ja·cod	zha-kō′
Hof·meis·ter	hōf′-mī-stər	Jac·quet	zha-ke′
Hol·lan·der	hol′-ən-dər	Ja·das·sohn	yä′-däs-zōn
Hol·len·horst	hol′-ən-horst	Jaf·fe	jaf′-ē
Holmes	hōmz	J.-Lichtenstein	
Holm·gren	holm′-grän	disease	
Holz·knecht	holts′-knekht	Jaf·fé	jä-fā′
Ho·mans	hō′-mənz	test, reaction	
Hor·ner	hor′-nər	Ja·kob	yä′-kop
Hor·te·ga	or-tā′-gä	J.-Creutzfeldt	
Hor·ton	hôr′-tən	disease	
Hous·say	oo-sī′	Ja·net	zha-ne′
Hous·ton	hoos′-tən	Jane·way	jān′-wā
Ho·vi·us	hō′-vē-us	Jan·sen	yän′-sən

Jan·sky	yän′-skē	Klein	klīn
Ja·risch	yä′-rish	muscle	
Je·ghers	jā′-gərz	Klei·ne	klī′-nə
Jen·dras·sik	yen′-dräsh-shik	K.-Levin syn-	
Jen·ner	jen′-ər	drome	
Jen·sen	yen′-sən	Kline	klīn
Jer·vell	yer′-vəl	test (for	
Jeune	zhœn	syphilis)	
Job	jōb	Kline·felter	klīn′-fel-tər
Jo·hans·son	yoo′-än′-son; *angl.* yō-han′-sən	Klip·pel	klē-pel′
		Klump·ke	klœmp′-kə
Joh·ne	yō′-nə	Klü·ver	klY′-vər
John·son	jon′-sən	Köb·ner	kœb′-nər
Jol·ly	zho-lē′	Koch	kokh
Jung	yʊng	Koch·er	kokh′-ər
Kall·mann	käl′-män	Ko·goj	kô′-goi
Kan·a·vel	kan′-ə-vel	Köh·ler	kœ′-lər
Kan·din·sky	kän-dʸin′-skē	Kö·nig	kœ′-nisH *or* -nik
Kan·do·ri	kän-do′-rē	Kop·lik	kop′-lik
Kan·ner	kän′-ər; *angl.* kan′-ər	Korff	korf
Ka·po·si	kä-pō′-zē; *angl.*-sē; *Hungarian* kop′-ō-shē	Korn·zweig	kôrn′-swīg
		Ko·rot·koff	
Kar·ta·ge·ner	kär′-tä-gä′-nər	or ·kov	kô′-rət-kəf
Kas·a·bach	kas′-ə-bäk	Kor·sa·koff	kor′-sə-kəf
Ka·ta·ya·ma	kä-tä-yä′-mä	Ko·ya·na·gi	ko-yä-nä′-gē
Ka·wa·sa·ki	kä-wä-sä′-kē	Ko·zhev·ni·kov	kä-zhev′-nē-kəf
Kay·ser	kī′-zər	Krab·be	kräb′-ə
Kea·ting-Hart	kē′-ting-härt′; *French* -art′	Krae·pe·lin	kre′-pə-lēn *or* krā′-art′
		Krau·se	krou′-zə
Keith	kēth	Krebs	krebz; *German* kräps
Ken·ny	ken′-ē	Kris·tel·ler	kris′-tel-ər
Ke·ran·del	kä-räN-del′; *angl.* ker′-ən-del′	Kro·mey·er	krō′-mī-ər
		Kro·neck·er	krō′-nek-ər
Kerck·ring	kerk′-ring	Kru·ken·berg	kroo′-kən-berk
Ker·ley	kur′-lē	Kufs	koofs
Ker·nig	ker′-nik	Ku·gel·berg	kY′-gəl-berʸ; *angl.* -burg
Ke·ty	kē′-tē		
Key	kā	Kuhnt	koont
Kien·böck	kēn′-bœk	Kul·chit·sky	
Kies·sel·bach	kē′-səl-bäkh	or Kul·tschitz·sky	kʊl-chit′-skē
Kil·lian	kil′-yän; *angl.* -yən		
Kim·mel·stiel	kim′-əl-shtēl	Küm·mel	kYm′-əl
Kin·nier Wil·son	ki-nēr′ wil′-sən	Kün·tscher	kYn′-chər
Kirsch·ner	kirsh′-nər; *angl.* kursh′-	Kupf·fer	kʊpf′-fər
		Kur·lov	kʊr′-ləf
Kjel·dahl	kel′-dal	Kuss·maul	kʊs′-moul
Klebs	kläps; *angl.* klebz	Küst·ner	kYst′-nər

Kveim	kveym	Legg	leg
La·bar·raque	la-ba-rak′	Leich·ten·stern	līsH′-tən-shtern
Lab·bé	la-bā′	Leish·man	lēsh′-mən
Ladd	lad	Lem·bert	läN-ber′
Laen·nec	le-nek′	Len·nox	len′-əks
La·fo·ra	lä-for′-ä	Lé·ri	lā-rē′
La·marck	la-mark′	Le·riche	lə-rēsh′
La·maze	la-maz′	Ler·moy·ez	ler-mwa-yä′
Lam·bert syndrome	lam′-burt	Lesch Let·te·rer	lesh let′-ə-rər
Lam·bert law	läm′-bert	Le·Veen Lev·en·thal	lə-vēn′ lev′-ən-thäl
La·my	la-mē′	Lé·vi	lā-vē′
Lance·field	lans′-fēld	dwarfism	
Lan·ci·si	län-chē′-zē	Le·vin	lə-vin′
Lan·dolt	läN-dolt′	Le·vine	lə-vēn′
Lan·dou·zy	läN-doo-zī′	Le·vret	lə-vre′
Lan·dry	läN-drē′	Lé·vy	lā-vē′
Land·stei·ner	länt′-shtī-nər	Roussy-L. syn-	
Lan·ge-Niel·sen	läng′-ə-nēl′-sən	drome	
Lang·er·hans	läng′-ər-häns	Le·wan·dow·sky	lā′-vän-dof′-skē
Lang·hans	läng′-häns	Lew·is	loo′-is
Lang·ley	lang′-lē	Le·wy	lā′-vē
Lan·ter·man	lan′-tər-mən; French läN-ter-man′	Ley·den Ley·dig	lī′-dən lī′-disH or -dik
La·ron	lä-ron′	Lher·mitte	ler-mēt′
Lar·sen	lär′sən	Lib·man	lib′-mən
L.-Johansson disease		Lich·ten·stein Licht·heim	lik′-tən-stīn lisHt′-hīm
Lars·son Sjögren-L. syn-	lär′-son	Lid·dle Lie·ber·kühn	lid′-əl lē′-bər-kyn
drome La·sègue	la-seg′	Lie·ber·mann Lin·dau	lē′-ber-män lin′-dou
Lau·rence	lô′-rəns	Lin·nae·us	li-nē′-əs
L.-Moon syn- drome		Swedish Lin·né Lip·pes	lin-nā′ lip′-əs or lip′-ēz
La·ve·ran	lav-(ə)-räN′	Lis·franc	lēs-fräN′
Law·rence	lô′-rəns	Lis·sau·er	lis′-ou-ər
L.-Seip syn- drome		Lis·ter Lit·tle	lis′-tər lit′-əl
Leão	lyouN	Lit·tre	lē′-tr(ə)
Le·ber	lā′-bər	Lo·bo	lō′-boo
Le·boy·er	lə-bwa-yä′	Locke	lok
Leede	lēd	Löf·fler	
Leeu·wen·hoek	lāoo′-vən-hook	or Loef·fler	lœf′-lər
Le·fè·vre	lə-fev′-r(ə)	Londe	lôNd
Le Fort	lə-fôr′	Loo·ser	lō′-zər
Le·gal	lā-gäl′	Lo·rain	lo-reN′

Word Guide

Lo·renz	lō′-rents	Ma·rey	ma-re′
Lou·is-Bar	lwē-bar′	Mar·fan	mar-fäN′; *angl.* mär′-fan
Løv·set	lœf′-sət		
Lö·wen·stein	lœ′-vən-shtīn	Ma·rie	ma-rē′
Low·er	lō′-ər	Ma·rín Amat	mä-rēn′-ä-mät′
Luc	lyk	Ma·ri·nes·co or ·cu	mä-rē-nes′-koo
Lu·cio	loo′-syō		
Lud·wig	loot′-vik; *angl.* lud′-wig	Ma·rion	ma-ryôN′
		Mar·jo·lin	mar-zho-leN′
Lu·er	loo′-ər	Ma·ro·teaux	ma-ro-tō′
Lukes	looks	Mar·shall	mär′-shəl
Lusch·ka	lʊsh′-kä	Mar·ti·not·ti	mär′-ti-not′-tē
Lu·tem·ba·cher	lY-teN-ba-ker′; *angl.* loo′-təm-bä′-kər	Mar·to·rell	Spanish mär-to-rel′; Catalan mur-too-rel[y]
Lutz (South American blastomycosis)	loots	Mas·son	ma-sôN′
		Mau·rer	mou′-rər
Lutz (epidermodysplasia verruciformis)	lʊts	Mau·ri·ceau	mo-rē-sō′
		Mauth·ner	mout′-nər
		May	mī
		May·er	mī-ər
		Ma·yo	mā′-ō
Ly·ell	lī′-əl	Maz·zo·ni	mät-tsō′-nē
Ly·on	lī′-ən	Mc·Ar·dle	mə-kär′-dəl
Mac·Con·key	mə-kong′-kē	Mc·Bur·ney	mək-bur′-nē
Mach·o·ver	mak′-ō-vər	Mc·Clin·tock	mə-klin′-tok
Mac·leod	mə-kloud′	Mc·Cune	mə-kyoon′
Mad·dox	mad′-əks	Mc·Kee	mə-kē′
Ma·de·lung	mä′-de-lʊng	Meck·el	mek′-əl
Maf·fuc·ci	mäf-fooch′-ē	Mei·bom	mī′-bōm
Ma·gen·die	ma-zheN-dē′	Meigs	megz
Mag·nus	mäg′-nʊs	Meiss·ner	mīs′-nər
Ma·joc·chi	mä-yok′-kē	Mel·e·ney	mel′-ə-nē
Ma·las·sez	ma-la-sā′	Mel·kers·son	mel′-kər-son
Mal·herbe	ma-lerb′	Men·del	men′-dəl
Mal·lo·ry	mal′-ə-rē	Men·del·son	men′-dəl-sən
Mal·pi·ghi	mäl-pē′-gē	Mé·né·tri·er	mā-nā-trē-ā′
Mann fistula	man	Mé·nière	mā-nyer′
		Men·kes	meng′-kəs
Mann stain test	män	Mer·cier	mer-syā′
		Mer·kel	mer′-kəl
		Merz·bach·er	merts′-bäkh-ər
Man·son	man′-sən	Mey·er	mī′-ər
Man·toux	mäN-too′	Mey·er·hof	mī′-ər-hôf
Ma·ra·ñón	mä-rä-nyon′	Mey·nert	mī′-nərt
Mar·burg	mär′-bʊrk	Mi·bel·li	mē-bel′-lē
Mar·che·sa·ni	mär′ke-zä′-nē	Mi·cha·e·lis	mɪsH-ä-ā′-lis
Mar·chia·fa·va	mär′-kya-fä′-vä	Mi·che·li	mē-ke′-lē
Mar·cus Gunn	mär′-kəs gun′	Mie·scher	mē′-shər

Mi·ku·licz	mē′-koo-lich	Na·both	nä′-bot
Milk·man	milk′-mən	Nae·ge·li	ne′-gə-lē
Mil·lard	mē-yar′	Naff·zi·ger	naf′′-zi-gər
Mil·li·kan	mil′-i-kən	Nä·ge·le	ne′-gə-lə
Mil·roy	mil′-roi	Na·geotte	na-zhot′
Min·kow·ski	min-kof′-ski	Naj·jar	na-jär′
Mi·ya·ga·wa	mē-yä-gä′-wä	Na·smyth	nä′-smith
M'nagh·ten	mək-nô′-tən	Neel·sen	näl′-zən
Mö·bius		Ne·gri	nä′-grē
or Moe·bius	mœ′-byus	Ne·gro	nä′-grō
Moel·ler	mœl′-ər	Ne·gus	nē′-gəs
Mohs	mōs	Neill	nēl
Mo·lisch	mō′-lish	Neis·ser	nī′-sər
Moll	mol	Né·la·ton	nä-la-tôN′
Mol·la·ret	mo-la-re′	Nel·son	nel′-sən
Mo·lo·ney	mə-lō′-nē	Nernst	nernst
Mo·na·kow	mä-nä′-kəf	Ness·ler	nes′-lər
Mönck·e·berg	mœng′-kə-berk	Neth·er·ton	neTH′-ər-tən
Mon·dor	môN-dôr′	Neu·feld	noi′-felt
Mon·ge	mong′-khe	Neu·mann	noi′-män
Mon·ro	mən-rō′	Neze·lof	nez-lof′
Mon·teg·gia	mon-täj′-jä	Niel·sen	nil′-sən
Mont·gom·ery	mənt-gum′-ə-rē	Nie·mann	nē′-män
Moon	moon	Ni·kol·sky	nē-kol′-skē
Moo·ren	mō′-rən	Nissl	nis′-əl
Moo·ser	mō′-sər	Ni·ta·buch	nē′-tä-bukh
Mo·rax	mo-raks′	No·card	no-kar′
Mo·rel	mo-rel′	Non·ne	non′-ə
Mor·ga·gni	mor-gä′-n^{y}ē	Noo·nan	noo′-nən
Mor·gan	môr′-gən	Noth·na·gel	nōt′-nä-gəl
Mo·ro	mō′-rō	Nuck	nœk
Mor·quio	mor′-kyō	Nu·el	ny-el′
Mor·ton	môr′-tən	Ny·han	nī′-ən
Mor·van	mor-väN′	Ober·stei·ner	ō′-bər-shtī′-nər
Mosch·ko·witz	mosh′-kə-witz	Od·di	od′-dē
Mount	mount	Ogu·chi	o′-gu-chē
Mu·cha	mukh′-ä	Ol·lier	o-lyä′
Muck·le	muk′-əl	Ol·szew·ski	ol-shef′-skē
Mül·ler		Op·pen·heim	op′-ən-hīm
or Muel·ler	myl′-ər	Oram	ô′-rəm
Münch·hau·sen	mynsh′-hou-zən	Or·be·li	är-b^{y}e′-lē
angl. Mun·chau·sen	munch′-ou-zən	Ort·ner	ort′-nər
		Or·to·la·ni	or′-to-lä′-nē
Münch·mey·er	mynsh′-mī-ər	Os·good	oz′-gud
Mun·ro Kerr	mun′-rō kär′	Os·ler	ōs′-lər
Mur·phy	mur′-fē	Ota	ô′-tä
Mus·set	my-se′	Ouch·ter·lo·ny	uk′-tər-lō′-nē
My·ers	mī′-ərz	Ow·ren	ôv′-rən

Word Guide

Pac·chio·ni	päk-kyō′-nē	Pi·ro·goff	pi-rä-gof′
Pa·ci·ni	pä-chē′-nē	Pir·quet	pir-ke′
Pag·et	paj′-ət	Pla·ci·do	plä′-sē-doo
Pa·jot	pa-zhō′	Plum·mer	plum′-ər
Pan·coast	pan′-kōst	Poi·seuille	pwa-zœi′
Pan·dy		Po·land	pō′-lənd
or Pán·dy	pän′-dē	Po·litz·er	pō′-lits-ər
Pa·neth	pä′-net	Pó·lya	pō′-lʸä or pō′-yä
Pa·pa·ni·co·laou	pä′-pä-nē′-ko-lou′	Pom·pe	pom′-pə
Pa·pil·lon	pa-pē-yôN′	Pos·ner	pōz′-nər
Pap·pen·heim	päp′-ən-hīm	Pott	pot
Par·a·cel·sus	par′-ə-sel′-səs	disease, abscess,	
Par·ham	par′-əm	paralysis	
Pa·ri·naud	pa-rē-nō′	Pot·ter	pot′-ər
Par·kin·son	pär′-kin-sən	Potts	pots
Par·rot	pa-rō′	operation, clamp	
Pa·si·ni	pä-zē′-nē	Pou·part	poo-par′
Pas·teur	pas-tœr′	Po·vey	pō′-vē
Pa·tau	pä′-tou	Pra·der	prä′-dər
Paul	pôl	Praus·nitz	prous′-nits
Pau·tri·er	pō-trē-ā′	Prei·ser	prī′-zər
Pav·lov	päv′-ləf	Pré·vost	prä-vō′
Paw·lik	päv′-lēk	Price-Jones	prīs-jōnz′
Pel	pel	Prinz·met·al	prints′-met-əl
Pel·ger	pel′-gər	Pros·kau·er	pros′-kou-ər
Pe·li·zae·us	pā′-li-tsā′-us	Prus·sak	pru-säk′
Pel·le·gri·ni	pel′-le-grē′-nē	Pur·ki·nje	pur′-ki-nʸe
Pel·liz·zi	pel-lēt′-tsē	Pur·tscher	pur′-chər
Pen·dred	pen′-drəd	Puus·sepp	poos′-sep
Per·lia	per′-lē-ä	Queck·en·stedt	kvek′-ən-shtet
Per·ron·ci·to	pe-rron-chē′-to	Quer·vain	ker-veN′
Per·thes	per′-tes	Quey·rat	ke-rä′
Pe·tit	pə-tē′	Quincke	kving′-kə
Pe·tri	pā′-trē	Ra·cou·chot	ra-koo-shō′
Pe·tze·ta·kis	pe-tse-tä′-kis	Rae·der	rā′-dər
Peutz	pœts	Rai·mist	rī′-mist
Pey·er	pī-ər	Ram·say Hunt	ram′-zē hunt′
Pey·ro·nie	pe-ro-nē′	Ram·stedt	räm′-shtet
Pfan·nen·stiel	pfän′-ən-shtēl	Ran·vier	räN-vyā′
Pfeif·fer	pfī′-fər	Rath·ke	rät′-kə
Phi·lippe	fē-lēp′	Ray·mond	re-môN′
Phys·ick	fiz′-ik	Ray·naud	re-nō′
Pia·get	pya-zhe′	Reck·ling·hau·sen	rek′-ling-hou′-zən
Pic	pēk		
Pick	pik	Red·lich	rät′-lisн
Pierre Ro·bin	pyer′ ro-beN′	Reed	rēd
Piltz	pilts	Ref·sum	ref′-sym
Pin·kus	ping′-kəs	Rei·chert	rī′-sнərt

Reid	rēd	vein	
Reil	rīl	spiral canal	
Reil·ly	rī'-lē	Ro·sen·thal	rō''-zən-thäl
bodies		syndrome (he-	
Reinsch	rīnsh	mophilia C)	
Reiss·ner	rīs'-nər	Ros·so·li·mo	rə-sä-lē'-mə
Rei·ter	rī'-tər	Roth	rōt
Re·mak	rā'-mäk	spots, vas aber-	
Re·naut	rə-nō'	rans	
Ren·du	räN-dY'	Roth or Rot	rot
Retz·i·us	ret'-sē-us	disease	
Re·ver·din	rə-ver-deN'	Roth·mund	rōt'-munt
Reye	rā	Ro·tor	rō-tor'
Rich·ard·son	rich'-ərd-sən	Rou·get	roo-zhe'
Rick·etts	rik'-əts	Rous	rous
Rid·doch	rid'-ok	Rous·sy	roo-sē'
Ri·de·al	ri-dē'-əl	Roux	roo
Rid·ley	rid'-lē	Rov·sing	row'-sing
Rie·del	rē'-dəl	Ru·bin	roo'-bən
Rie·ger	rē'-gər	Ru·bin·stein	roo'-bən-stīn
Riehl	rēl	Ruf·fi·ni	ruf-fē'-nē
Ri·ley	rī'-lē	Rum·pel	rum'-pəl
R.-Day syndrome		Rus·sell	rus'-əl
virus		Rust	rust
Ring·er	ring'-ər	Ruysch	rœis
Rin·ne	rin'-ə	Sa·bin	sā'-bin
Rio·lan	ryo-läN'	Sa·bou·raud	sa-boo-rō'
Rit·gen	rit'-gən	Sachs	saks
Rit·ter	rit'-ər	Tay-S. disease	
Ri·vi·nus	ri-vē'-nus; *angl.* ri-vī'-nəs	Sacks	saks
		Libman-S. endo-	
Ro·bin	ro-beN'	carditis	
Roe·de·rer	rœ'-də-rər	Salk	sô(l)k
Roent·gen		Sal·ter	sôl'-tər
or Rönt·gen	rœnt'-gən	Sa·lus	zä'-lus
Ro·ger	ro-zhā'	Sa·na·rel·li	sä-nä-rel'-lē
Rohr	rōr	San·fi·lip·po	san'-fi-lē'-pō
Ro·ki·tan·sky	rō'-ki-tän'-skē	Sang·er Brown	sang'-ər broun'
Ro·lan·do	ro-län'-do	San·to·ri·ni	sän'-to-rē'-nē
Rol·ler	rol'-ər	Sap·pey	sa-pe'
Ro·ma·ña	rro-mä'-nyä	Satt·ler	sät'-lər
Ro·ma·now·sky	rə-mä-nof'-skē	Sax·torph	säks'-torf
or ·nov·sky		Sayre	sār
Rom·berg	rom'-berk	Scan·zo·ni	skän-tsō'-nē
Ror·schach	rōr'-shäkh	Scar·pa	skär'-pä
Ro·sen·mül·ler	rō'-zən-mYl'-ər	Scha·fer	shä'-fər
Ro·sen·thal	rō'-zən-täl	syndrome	
Melkersson-R.		Schäf·fer	shef'-ər
syndrome		reflex	

Word Guide 329

Scham·berg	sham′-burg	Seme·laigne	sem-len^y′
Schatz	shäts	Se·near	sə-nēr′
Schatz·ki	shat′-skē	Sengs·ta·ken	sengz′-tä-kən
Schau·mann	shou′-män	Ser·to·li	ser′-to-lē
Schau·ta	shou′-tä	Se·ver	sē′-vər
Scheie	shī	Sé·za·ry	sā-za-rē′
Scheu·er·mann	shoi′-ər-män	Shar·pey	shär′-pē
Schick	shik	Shee·han	shē′-ən
Schiff	shif	Sher·ren	sher′-ən
Schil·der	shil′-dər	Sher·ring·ton	sher′-ing-tən
Schil·ling	shil′-ing	Shi·ga	shē′-gä
Schiötz	shœts	Shohl	shōl
Schir·mer	shir′-mər	Shone	shōn
Schlat·ter	shlät′-ər	Shope	shōp
Schlemm	shlem	Shrap·nell	shrap′-nəl
Schloss·man	shlos′-mən	Shwartz·man	shwôrts′-mən
Schmidt	shmit	Shy	shī
Schmorl	shmorl	Sia	s^yea; angl. sē′-ə
Schoe·ma·ker	skhō′-mä-kər	Sib·son	sib′-sən
Schön·lein	shœn′-līn	Si·card	sē-kar′
Schre·ger	shrā′-gər	Sid·bury	sid′-ber-ē
Schroe·der	shrā′-dər	Sie·mens	zē′-məns
Schroet·ter	shrœt′-ər	Sil·ber	sil′-bər
Schüff·ner	shyf′-nər	Sil·ver·skiöld	sil′-vər-shœld
Schül·ler	shyl′-ər	Sim·monds	zim′-onts
Schultz	shults	Si·mon	sī′-mən
disease, S.-Dale reaction		sign	
		Si·mon	zē′-mon
Schul·tze	shul′-tsə	position	
mechanism		Si·mon	sē-môN′
acroparesthesia		Binet-S. test	
bundle		Simp·son	simp′-sən
Schwal·be	shväl′-bə	Sip·ple	sip′-əl
Schwann	shvän	Sip·py	sip′-ē
Schwartz	shwôrts	Si·we	sē′-və
Watson-S. reaction		Sjö·gren	shœ′-grän
S.-Bartter syndrome		Sjö·qvist	shœ′-kvist
		Skene	skēn
Schwar·tze	shvär′-tsə	Skin·ner	skin′-ər
mastoidectomy		Skoog	skoog
Schweig·ger-Sei·del	shvī′-gər-zī′-dəl	Smith-Pe·ter·sen	smit′-pā′-tər-sən; angl. smith′-pē′tər-sən
Scott	skot	Sned·don	sned′-ən
Scrib·ner	skrib′-nər	Snel·len	snel′-ən
Se·bi·leau	sə-bē-lō′	Soem·mer·ing	zœm′-ər-ing
Seck·el	zek′-əl	So·mo·gyi	shō′-mō-d^yē; angl. sō′-mō-jē
Seip	seyp	So·tos	sō′-tōs
Sel·lick	sel′-ik	Sot·tas	so-täs′

Sou·lier	soo-lyä'	Suc·quet	sy-ke'
Spatz	shpäts	Su·deck	zoo'-dek
Speng·ler	shpeng'-lər	Su·gi·u·ra	su-gē-u'-rä
Spie·ghel	spē'-khəl	Sulz·ber·ger	sulz'-bur-gər
or Spi·ge·li·us	spi-jē'-lē-əs	Sut·ton	sut'-ən
Spie·gler	shpē'-glər	Sved·berg	svād'-bery; *angl.*
Spiel·mey·er	shpēl'-mī-ər		sved'-burg
Spi·nel·li	spē-nel'-lē	Swan	swän
Spreng·el	shpreng'-əl	Swen·son	swen'-sən
Ssa·ba·ne·jew	ssə-bä-nyä'-yəf	Swift	svift; *angl.* swift
Stacke	shtäk'-ə	Swy·er	swī'-ər
Sta·de·ri·ni	stä-de-rē'-nē	Syd·en·ham	sid'-ən-əm
Stäh·li	shte'-lē	Syl·vi·us	sil'-vē-əs
Stahr	shtär	Syme	sīm
Star·ling	stär'-ling	Sym·mers	sim'-mərz
Starr	stär	Szon·di	sōn'-dē
Star·ry	stär'-ē	Szy·ma·now·ski	shi-mä-nof'-skē
St. Clair Thom·son	sən-kler' tom'-sən	Ta·glia·coz·zi	täl-lyä-kot'-tsē
		Taille·fer	tī-y(ə)-fer'
Steele	stēl	Ta·ka·ha·ra	tä-kä-hä'-rä
S.-Richardson-Olszewski syndrome		Ta·ka·ya·su	tä-kä-yä'-su
		Tal·ma	täl'-mä
		Tan·ner	tan'-ər
Steell murmur	stēl	Tar·dieu	tar-dyœ'
		Ta·rin	ta-reN'
Stein	stīn	or Ta·ri·nus	tə-rī'-nəs
Stei·nert	shtī'-nərt	Tar·nier	tar-nyä'
Stein·mann	shtīn'-män	Ta·rui	tä-ru'-ē
Ste·no	stē'-nō	Taus·sig	tou'-sig
or Sten·sen	stän'-sən	Ta·wa·ra	tä-wä'-rä
Stent	stent	Tay	tä
Stern·berg	shtern'-berk	Tay·bi	tī'-bē; *angl.* tä'-bē
Ste·vens	stē'-vənz	Te·non	tə-nôN'
Stew·art	st(y)oo'-ərt	Ter·rier	te-ryä'
Stie·da	shtē'-dä	Tesch·en·dorf	tesh'-ən-dorf
Still	stil	Thay·sen	tī-sən
Stil·ling	shtil'-ing	The·be·sius	tā-bā'-zyus; *angl.* thē-bē'-zē-əs
Stokes	stōks		
Stook·ey	stuk'-ē	Thei·ler	tī'-lər
Strachan	strôn	Thi·bierge	tē-byerzh'
Strand·berg	stränd'-bery	Thiers	tyer
Strauss	shtrous; *angl.* strous	Thiersch	tērsh
Streiff	shtrīf	Tho·ma	tō'-mä
Strüm·pell	shtrym'-pəl	Tho·mas	to-mä'
Stu·art	st(y)oo'-ərt	Dejerine-T. atrophy	
Sturge	sturj		
Sturm	shturm	Thom·as	tom'-əs
Sturm·dorf	sturm'-dorf	heel, splint	
St. Vi·tus	sänt vī'-təs	pessary	

Word Guide 331

Thomp·son test (for urethritis)	tomp′-sən	Türk cell	tyrk
Thom·sen disease (myotonia congenita) antibody	tom′-sən	Tur·ner	tur′-ner
		Ty·rode	tī′-rōd
		Ty·son	tī′-sən
		Tzanck	tsänk
		Uhl	yool
		Uht·hoff	oot′-hof
Thom·son scattering	tom(p)′-sən	Ull·rich	ul′-risH
		Un·na	un′-ä
Thor·mäh·len	tor-mä′-lən	Un·ver·richt	un′-fer-risHt
Thorn syndrome (saltdepletion)	thôrn	Ur·bach	oor′-bäkh
		Ush·er	ush′-ər
		Va·len·tin	vä′-len-tēn
Thorn maneuver	torn	Val·sal·va	väl-säl′-vä
		van Bo·gaert	vän-bō′-khart
Thor·son	toor′-son	van Bu·chem	vän-bY′-khəm
Tie·tze	tē′-tsə	van Cre·veld	vän-krā′-vəlt
Ti·nel	tē-nel′	van den Bergh	vän-dən-berkh′; *angl.* van′-dən-burg′
Ti·se·li·us	tē-sā′-lē-us		
To·lo·sa	tō-lō′-sä	van der Hoe·ve	vän-dər-hoo′-və
Tomes	tōmz	van der Kolk	vän-dər-kolk′
Tooth	tooth	Van Slyke	van-slīk′
Tor·kild·sen	tur′-kil-sən	Va·quez	va-kez′
Torn·waldt or Thorn·waldt	tōrn′-vält	Va·ro·li·us or Va·ro·lio	va-rō′-lē-əs va-rō′-lē-o
Tou·raine	too-ren′	Va·ter	fä′-tər
Tou·rette	too-ret′	Vel·la	vel′-lä
Tou·ton	too-tōn′	Vel·peau	vel-pō′
Towne	toun	Ven·tu·ri	ven-too′-rē
Toyn·bee	toin′-bē	Ver·hoeff	vur′-hef
Trau·be	trou′-bə	Ver·ner	vur′-nər
Trea·cher Col·lins	trē′-chər kol′-inz	Ver·net	ver-ne′
		Ve·sa·li·us	ve-sä′-lē-əs
Treitz	trīts	Vicq d'Azyr	vēk-da-zēr′
Tren·de·len·burg	tren′-də-lən-burk	Vid·i·us (Italian **Guidi**)	vid′-ē-əs
Treves	trēvz		
Troi·sier	trwä-zyā′	Vieus·sens	vyœ-säNs′
Tro·lard	tro-lar′	Vil·la·ret	vē-la-re′
Tröltsch	trœlch	Vin·cent	veN-säN′; *angl.* vin′-sənt
Trous·seau	troo-sō′		
Tul·lio	tul′-lyō	Vine·berg	vīn′-burg
Türck tract, column	tyrk	Vin·son	vin′-sən
		Vir·chow	fir′-sHō *or* vir′-sHō
Tur·cot	tyr-kō′	Vo·ges	fō′-gəs
Turk Stilling-T.-Duane syndrome	turk	Vogt	fōkt
		Volk·mann	folk′-män
		von Gier·ke	fon-gēr′-kə
		von Grae·fe	fon-gre′-fə

Medical Eponyms

von Hip·pel	fon-hip′-əl	Weill sign (for pneumonia) W.-Reys-Adie syndrome	vey
von Kupf·fer	fon-kʊp′-fər		
von Lang·en· beck	fon-läng′-ən-bek		
von Mi·ku·licz	fon-mē′-koo-lich		
von Pir·quet	fon-pir-ke′	Wein·berg	vīn′-berk
von Reck·ling· hau·sen	fon-rek′-ling-hou′-zən	Weir Mitch·ell	wēr′ mich′-əl
		Weiss	vīs
von Sall·mann	fon-säl′-män; *angl.* von-sal′-mən	Weit·brecht	vīt′-brekht
		We·lan·der	vä′-län-dər
von Tröltsch	fon-trœlch′	Wenck·e·bach	vengk′-ə-bäkh
von Wil·le·brand	von-vil′-le-bränd	Werd·nig	vert′-nik
Waar·den·burg	vär′-dən-bœrkh	Werl·hof	verl′-hōf
Wag·ner	väg′-nər	Wer·nicke	ver′-ni-kə
Wal·den·ström	väl′-dən-strœm	Wert·heim	vert′-hīm
Wal·dey·er	väl′-dī-ər	Wes·ter·gren	ves′-tər-grän′
Walk·er	wô′-kər	West·phal	vest′-fäl
Wal·len·berg	väl′-lən-berk	We·ver	wē′-vər
Wal·ler	wol′-ər	Whar·ton	(h)wôr′-tən
Walt·hard	vält′-ärt	Whip·ple	(h)wip′-əl
War·burg	vär′-bʊrk	White	(h)wīt
War·ten·berg	vär′-tən-berk	Whit·field	(h)wit′-fēld
War·thin	wôr′-thin	Wick·ham	wik′-əm; *French* vē- kam′
Was·ser·mann	väs′-ər-män; *angl.* wäs′-ər-mən		
		Wi·dal	vē-dal′
Wa·ter·house	wô′-tər-hous	Wie·the	vē′-tə
Web·er	web′-ər	Wi·gand	vē′-gänt
Sturge-W. syn- drome, Osler- W.- Rendu dis- ease paralysis		Wil·der·vanck	vil′-dər-vängk
		Wil·kin·son	wil′-kin-sən
		Wil·lan	wil′-ən
		Wil·li	vil′-ē
		Wil·lis	wil′-əs
We·ber point, triangle test, W.-Fechner law glands, zone	vä′-bər	Wilms	vilms; *angl.* wilmz
		Wil·son	wil′-sən
		Wins·low	vins′-lō; *angl.* winz′-lō
		Win·ter·stei·ner	vin′-tər-shtī′-nər
		Win·trobe	win′-trōb
Wechs·berg	veks′-berk	Wir·sung	vir′-zʊng
Wechs·ler	weks′-lər	Wis·kott	vis′-kot
We·den·sky	vve-dʸen′-skē	Wiss·ler	vis′-lər
We·ge·ner	vä′-gə-nər	Wit·kop	wit′-kop
Wei·gert	vī′-gərt	Wohl·fart	vōl′-färt
Weigl	vī′-gəl	Wolfe graft	wʊlf
Weil stain W.-Felix test disease (icteric leptospirosis) basal layer	vīl		
		Wolff law (on bone development) body, duct	volf

Word Guide

Wolff	wulf	**Zei·gar·nik**	zī-gär′-nik
W.-Parkinson-White syndrome		**Zeis** gland, stye	tsīs
Wolff-Eis·ner	volf-īs′-nər	**Zeiss** counting chamber	tsīs
Wolf·ring	volf′-ringk		
Wol·man	wol′-mən		
Worm	vorm	**Zell·we·ger**	tsel′-vă-gər
Wright	rīt	**Zen·ker**	tseng′-kər
Wris·berg	vris′-berk; *angl.* ris′-burg	**Zie·hen**	tsē′-ən
		Ziehl	tsēl
Wu	woo	**Zieve**	zēv
Wu·che·rer	voo′-khə-rər	**Zinn**	tsin
Yer·sin	yer-seN′	**Zins·ser**	zin′-sər
Young	yung	**Zol·ling·er**	zol′-ing-ər
Zahn	tsän	**Zon·dek**	tson′-dek
Za·hor·sky	zä′-hor-skē	**Zoon**	zōn
Zap·pert	tsäp′-ərt	**Zuck·er·kandl**	tsuk′-ər-kän′-dəl